PROGRESS

in Bioceramics

Published by
The American Ceramic Society
735 Ceramic Place
Westerville, Ohio 43081 USA
www.ceramics.org

For information on ordering titles published by The American Ceramic Society, or to request a publications catalog, please contact our Customer Service Department at 614-794-5890 (phone), 614-794-5892 (fax),<info@ceramics.org> (e-mail), or write to Customer Service Department, P. O. Box 6136, Westerville, OH 43086-6136, USA.

Printed in the United States of America.

4 3 2 1–07 06 05 04

ISBN 1-57498-193-5

www.ceramics.org

www.ceramicbulletin.org

www.ceramicjournal.org

CONTENTS

Introduction ix

JOURNAL OF THE AMERICAN CERAMIC SOCIETY

Bioceramics 3
L. Hench
Vol. 81, No. 7, 1998

Novel Method to Manufacture Porous Hydroxyapatite by Dual-Phase Mixing 27
S.H. Li, J.R. de Wijn, P. Layrolle, and K. de Groot
Vol. 86, No. 1, 2003

Slow-Crack-Growth Behavior of Zirconia-Toughened Alumina Ceramics Processed by Different Method 35
A.H. De Aza, J. Chevalier, G. Fantozzi, M. Schehl, and R. Torrecillas
Vol. 86, No. 1, 2003

Composition and Crystallization of Hydroxyapatite Coating Layer Formed by Electron Beam Deposition 41
D.-H. Kim, Y.-M. Kong, S.-H. Lee, I.-S. Lee, H.-E. Kim, S.-J. Heo, and J.-Y. Koak
Vol. 86, No. 1, 2003

Synthesis of Nanosized and Microporous Precipitated Hydroxyapatite in Synthetic Polymers and Biopolymers 45
A. Sinha, S. Nayar, A. Agrawal, D. Bhattacharyya, and P. Ramachandrarao
Vol. 86, No. 2, 2003

Sintered Hydroxyapatite Latticework for Bone Substitute 49
F.C. Gomes de Sousa and J.R.G. Evans
Vol. 86, No. 3, 2003

Bioactivity and Mechanical Properties of Poly(Dimethylsiloxane)-Modified Calcia-Silica Hybrids with Added Titania 53
Q. Chen, N. Miyata, T. Kokubo, and T. Nakamura
Vol. 86, No. 5, 2003

Joining of Calcium Phosphate Invert Glass-Ceramics on a Beta-Type Titanium Alloy 59
T. Kasuga, M. Nogami, and M. Niinomi
Vol. 86, No. 6, 2003

Synthesis of Hydroxyapatite Nanopowders via Sucrose-Templated Sol-Gel Method 63
S. Bose and S.K. Saha
Vol. 86, No. 6, 2003

From CT Scan to Ceramic Bone Graft 67
J. Darsell, S. Bose, H.L. Hosick, and A. Bandyopadhyay
Vol. 86, No. 7, 2003

Preparation of Polymethylmethacrylate-Reinforced Functionally Graded Hydroxyapatite Composites 73
M. Ohgaki and K. Yamashita
Vol. 86, No. 8, 2003

Dispersing Behavior of Hydroxyapatite Powders Produced by Wet-Chemical Synthesis 77
M. Pretto, A.L. Costa, E. Landi, A. Tampieri, and C. Galassi
Vol. 86, No. 9, 2003

Improving the Durability of a Biomedical-Grade Zirconia Ceramic by the Addition of Silica 83
L. Gremillard, J. Chevalier, T. Epicier, and G. Fantozzi
Vol. 85, No. 2, 2002

Transparent Hydroxyapatite Ceramics Through Gelcasting and Low-Temperature Sintering 91
H. Varma, S.P. Vijayan, and S.S. Babu
Vol. 85, No. 2, 2002

Biomimetic Hydroxyapatite Coating on Metal Implants 95
P. Habibovic, F. Barrere, C.A. van Blitterswijk, K. de Groot, and P. Layrolle
Vol. 85, No. 3, 2002

Effects of Yttria-Stabilized Zirconia on Plasma-Sprayed Hydroxyapatite/Yttria-Stabilized Zirconia Composite Coatings 101
L. Fu, K.A. Khor, and J.P. Lim
Vol. 85, No. 4, 2002

Preparation of a Bioactive Poly(Methyl Methacrylate)/Silica Nanocomposite 109
S.-H. Rhee and J.-Y. Choi
Vol. 85, No. 5, 2002

Reaction Sintering and Mechanical Properties of Hydroxyapatite-Zirconia Composites with Calcium Fluoride Additions 113
H.-W. Kim, Y.-H. Koh, B.-H. Yoon, and H.-E. Kim
Vol. 85, No. 6, 2002

Formation and Properties of Hydroxyapatite-Calcium Poly (Vinyl Phosphonate) Composites 117
Y.E. Greish and P.W. Brown
Vol. 85, No. 7, 2002

Fabrication of Macrochannelled-Hydroxyapatite Bioceramic by a Coextrusion Process 125
Y.-H. Koh, H.-W. Kim, H.-E. Kim, and J.W. Halloran
Vol. 85, No. 10, 2002

Effect of Silicon Substitution on the Sintering and Microstructure of Hydroxyapatite 129
I.R. Gibson, S.M. Best, and W. Bonfield
Vol. 85, No. 11, 2002

Wear Simulation of Alumina-on-Alumina Prosthetic Hip Joint Using a Multidirectional Motion Pin-on-Disc Device .137
V. Saikko and J. Keranen
Vol. 85, No. 11, 2002

Calcium Phosphate Bioceramics with Various Porosities and Dissolution Rates 145
S.-H. Kwon, Y.-K. Jun, S.-H. Hong, I.-S. Lee, H.-E. Kim, and Y.Y. Won
Vol. 85, No. 12, 2002

Molten Salt Synthesis of Calcium Hydroxyapatite Whiskers 149
A.C. Tas
Vol. 84, No. 2, 2001

Gel-to-Ceramic Conversion During Hydroxyapatite Synthesis 155
M.-F. Hsieh, T.-S. Chin, L.-H. Perng, and H.-G. Perng
Vol. 84, No. 9, 2001

Hydroxyapatite Coating on Thermally Oxidized Titanium Substrates 159
M. Vatanatham and S. Kimura
Vol. 84, No. 9, 2001

American Ceramic Society Bulletin

Nanophase Ceramics as Improved Bone Tissue Engineering Materials 165
T.J. Webster
Vol. 82, No. 6, p. 23-28, 2003

3-D CT Images for Biomimetic Artificial Bone Design and Manufacture 171
J. Tian, X. Wang, C. Zhang, and Z. Guo
Vol. 81, No. 12, p. 39-41, 2002

No Bones About It—Rapid Prototyping—The Future for Bioceramic Implants 175
A. Emory
V. 80, No. 3, p. 23-26, 2001

Ceramic Transactions

The Role of Ceramics in an Age of Biology 181
L.L. Hench
Vol. 147, Bioceramics: Materials and Applications IV, p. 3-12, 2003

A Review of Bone Substitutes in Bone Remodeling: Influence of Materials Chemistry and Porosity 191
A. Cuneyt Tas
Vol. 147, Bioceramics: Materials and Applications IV, p. 15-24, 2003

Manufacturing of Thermally Sprayed Tricalcium Phosphate Coatings for Biomedical Applications 201
M. Baccalaro, R. Gadow, and K. von Niessen
Vol. 147, Bioceramics: Materials and Applications IV, p. 25-34, 2003

Electrochemical Deposition and Patterning of Calcium Phosphate Bioceramic Coating 211
K. Duan, Y. Fan, and R. Wang
Vol. 147, Bioceramics: Materials and Applications IV, p. 53-61, 2003

Two and Ten Year Retrievals of Zirconia Femoral Heads: XRD, SEM and Raman Spectroscopy Studies 221
D.D. Green, G. Pezzotti, S. Sakakura, M. Ries, and I.C. Clarke
Vol. 147, Bioceramics: Materials and Applications IV, p. 133-140, 2003

Ceramic Engineering and Science Proceedings (CESP)

3 Dimensional CT Analyses of Bone Formation in Porous Ceramic Biomaterials 231
M. Mizuno, M. Mukaida, Y. Ikeda, M. Yasutoshi, T. Nakamura, and M. Neo
Vol. 24, Issue 3, p. 185-190, 2003

Wear Characterization of Clinically used Hip Joint Prostheses by a HIP Simulator 237
Y. Takigawa, K. Jono, H. Takadama, M. Mizuno, and T. Nakamura
Vol. 24, Issue 3, p. 197-202, 2003

Fabrication of Biocompatible Calcium Phosphate Ceramics Using Eggshell 243
S.J. Lee and W.M. Kriven
Vol. 24, Issue 3, p. 203-208, 2003

Calcium Aluminate/Calcium Phosphate Composite Orthopedic Cement 249
M.L. Roemhildt, T.D. McGee, and S.D. Wagner
Vol. 24, Issue 3, p. 209-214, 2003

Fabrication of Composite for Bone Repairing from Alpha-tricalcium Phosphate and Hydroxypropylcellulose .255
T. Miyazaki, C. Ohtsuki, H. Iwasaki, S. Ogata, and M. Tanihara
Vol. 24, Issue 3, p. 215-220, 2003

Preparation of Bioactive Inorganic-Organic Hybrids by Hot Water Treatment 261
M. Kawashita, M. Kamitakahara, N. Miyata, T. Kokubo, and T. Nakamura
Vol. 24, Issue 3, p. 221-226, 2003

Apatite Formation on the PMMA Bone Cement Modified with Alkoxysilane and Calcium Salt in a Simulated Body Fluid 267
C. Ohtsuki, T. Miyazaki, A. Sugino, M. Tanihara, A. Mori, and K. Kuramoto
Vol. 24, Issue 3, p. 233-238, 2003

Formation of Hydroxyapatite Coatings on Alumina under Hydrothermal Conditions 273
J.-S. Ha and M.N. Rahaman
Vol. 24, Issue 3, p. 239-244, 2003

A Multi-Station Hip Joint Simulator Study and Wear Characterization of Commercial Hip Endoprostheses 279
K. Jono, Y. Takigawa, H. Takadama, M. Mizuno, and T. Nakamura
Vol. 24, Issue 3, p. 255-260, 2003

Processing of Bioactive Ceramics with Defined Porosity 285
C.M. Lofton, H. Huang, and W. Sigmund
Vol. 23, Issue 4, p. 729-734, 2002

Bioactive Surface Functionalization: Concept and Applications 291
H.-M. Kim
Vol. 23, Issue 4, p. 761-771, 2002

Affects of Alumina and Titania Nanoparticulates on Bone Cell Function 303
L.G. Gutwein and T.J. Webster
Vol. 23, Issue 4, p. 773-780, 2002

A Composite Approach to Tissue Engineering 311
A.R. Boccaccini, J.A. Roether, L.L. Hench, V. Maquet, and R. Jérôme
Vol. 23, Issue 4, p. 805-816, 2002

Increased Osteoblast Function on Nanofibered Alumina 323
T.J. Webster, L.G. Gutwein, and F. Tepper
Vol. 23, Issue 4, p. 817-824, 2002

Bioactive Glass-Ceramic Materials for Bone Substitutes 331
C.V. Brovarone, F. Smeacetto, and E. Verné
Vol. 23, Issue 4, p. 839-844, 2002

Fatigue Property of Zirconia for Hip Joint Prostheses 337
Y. Takigawa, Y. Yasutomi, M. Mizuno, and K. Shirakihara
Vol. 23, Issue 4, p. 845-850, 2002

Introduction

Bioceramics are generally defined as ceramic materials used for the repair, reconstruction and replacement of diseased or damaged parts of the musculo-skeletal system. Bioceramics fulfill a unique function as biomedical materials and have led to a remarkable advance in the quality of life for millions of people.

Bioceramics may be bioinert (alumina and zirconia), resorbable (tricalcium phosphate), bioactive (hydroxyapatite, bioactive glasses, and glass-ceramics), or porous for tissue ingrowth (hydroxyapatite-coated metals). Applications include replacements for hips, knees, teeth, tendons, and ligaments and repair for periodontal disease, maxillofacial reconstruction, augmentation and stabilization of the jawbone, spinal fusion, bone repair after tumor surgery, prosthetic heart valves, glass microspheres for cancer treatment, and more.

In the future, bioceramics will continue to be improved upon, new materials will be developed, new applications discovered, and they will continue to play an important role in improving and maintaining our quality of life.

This book contains a compilation of recent articles and papers published by The American Ceramic Society (ACerS). The articles originated from the *Journal of the American Ceramic Society*, the *American Ceramic Society Bulletin*, *Ceramic Engineering and Science Proceedings* (CESP), and *Ceramic Transactions* (CT).

The lead-off article by Larry L. Hench was published as a centennial feature article in the *Journal of the American Ceramic Society* and provides an excellent overview. Hench, a pioneer in bioceramics, developed Bioglass®, the first man-made material to bond to living bone. This article along with the additional 49 articles and papers on current research and development, provides a valuable reference resource for those involved in the field of bioceramics.

References to additional articles not included in this collection may be located by searching the following ACerS websites:

- *The Journal of the American Ceramic Society*: http://www.ceramicjournal.org/
- *Ceramic Transactions* and *CESP*: http://www.ceramics.org/ctindex.asp
- *American Ceramic Society Bulletin*: http://www.ceramicbulletin.org/

journal
of the American Ceramic Society

journal

J. Am. Ceram. Soc., 81 [7] 1705–28 (1998)

Bioceramics

Larry L. Hench*

Department of Materials, Imperial College of Science, Technology, and Medicine, University of London, London, United Kingdom

Ceramics used for the repair and reconstruction of diseased or damaged parts of the musculo-skeletal system, termed bioceramics, may be bioinert (e.g., alumina and zirconia), resorbable (e.g., tricalcium phosphate), bioactive (e.g., hydroxyapatite, bioactive glasses, and glass-ceramics), or porous for tissue ingrowth (e.g., hydroxyapatite-coated metals). Applications include replacements for hips, knees, teeth, tendons, and ligaments and repair for periodontal disease, maxillofacial reconstruction, augmentation and stabilization of the jaw bone, spinal fusion, and bone repair after tumor surgery. Pyrolytic carbon coatings are thromboresistant and are used for prosthetic heart valves. The mechanisms of tissue bonding to bioactive ceramics have resulted in the molecular design of bioceramics for interfacial bonding with hard and soft tissue. Bioactive composites are being developed with high toughness and elastic modulus that match with bone. Therapeutic treatment of cancer has been achieved by localized delivery of radioactive isotopes via glass beads. Clinical success of bioceramics has led to a remarkable advance in the quality of life for millions of people.

I. Introduction

Many millennia ago, the discovery that fire would irreversibly transform clay into ceramic pottery led to an agrarian society and an enormous improvement in the quality and length of life. Another revolution has occurred in the use of ceramics during the past four decades to improve the quality of life. This revolution is the innovative use of specially designed ceramics for the repair, reconstruction, and replacement of diseased or damaged parts of the body. Ceramics used for this purpose are termed "bioceramics." Bioceramics can be polycrystalline (alumina or hydroxyapatite), bioactive glass, bioactive glass-ceramic (A/W), or bioactive composite (polyethylene–hydroxyapatite).

Many specialty ceramics and glasses have been developed during this century for use in the health care industry, e.g., eyeglasses, diagnostic instruments, chemical ware, thermometers, tissue culture flasks, fiber optics for endoscopy, and carriers for enzymes and antibodies.[1] Ceramics also are used widely in dentistry as restorative materials, gold porcelain crowns, glass-filled ionomer cements, dentures, etc. The materials used in these applications are called dental ceramics.[2]

This review is devoted to the use of bioceramics as implants to repair parts of the body, usually the hard tissues of the musculo-skeletal system, such as bones, joints, or teeth, although use of carbon coatings for replacement of heart valves also is included. Many ceramic compositions have been tested for use in the body;[1,3] however, few have achieved human clinical application. Clinical success requires the simultaneous achievement of a stable interface with connective tissue and a match of the mechanical behavior of the implant with the tissue to be replaced. Only the few bioceramics that meet these severe requirements for clinical success are emphasized in this review. Historical developments of bioceramics have been presented by Hulbert *et al.*[3]

(1) Need for Bioceramics

Bioceramics are needed to alleviate pain and restore function to diseased or damaged parts of the body. A major contributor to the need for "spare parts" for the body is the progressive deterioration of tissue with age. Bone is especially vulnerable to fracture in older people because of a loss of bone density and strength with age.[4] Figure 1 summarizes the effect of time on bone strength and density from the age of 30 years onward. The effect is especially severe in women because of hormonal changes associated with menopause. Bone density decreases because bone-growing cells (osteoblasts) become progressively less productive in making new bone and repairing microfractures. The lower density greatly deteriorates the strength of the porous bone, called trabecular or cancellous bone (Fig. 2), in the ends of long bones and in vertebrae. An unfortunate consequence is that many old people fracture their hips or have collapsed vertebrae and spinal problems.

The great challenge facing the use of ceramics in the body is to replace old, deteriorating bone with a material that can func-

P. W. Brown—contributing editor

Manuscript No. 190448. Received December 30, 1997; approved May 15, 1998.
*Member, American Ceramic Society.

centennial feature

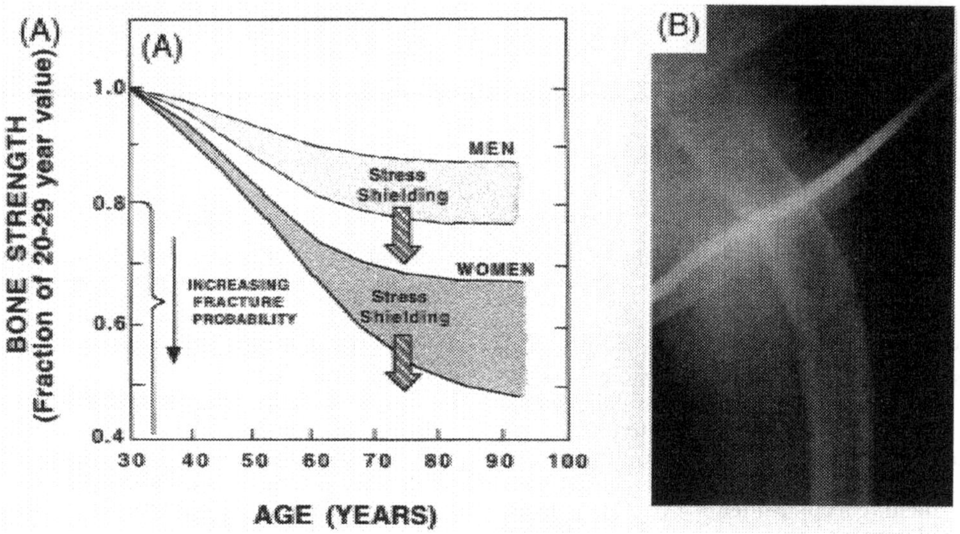

Fig. 1. (A) Effect of age on the strength of bone and probability of fracture. (B) Fractured femoral (thigh) bone caused by osteoporosis, which weakens bone. Stress shielding causes a further decrease in bone density and strength.

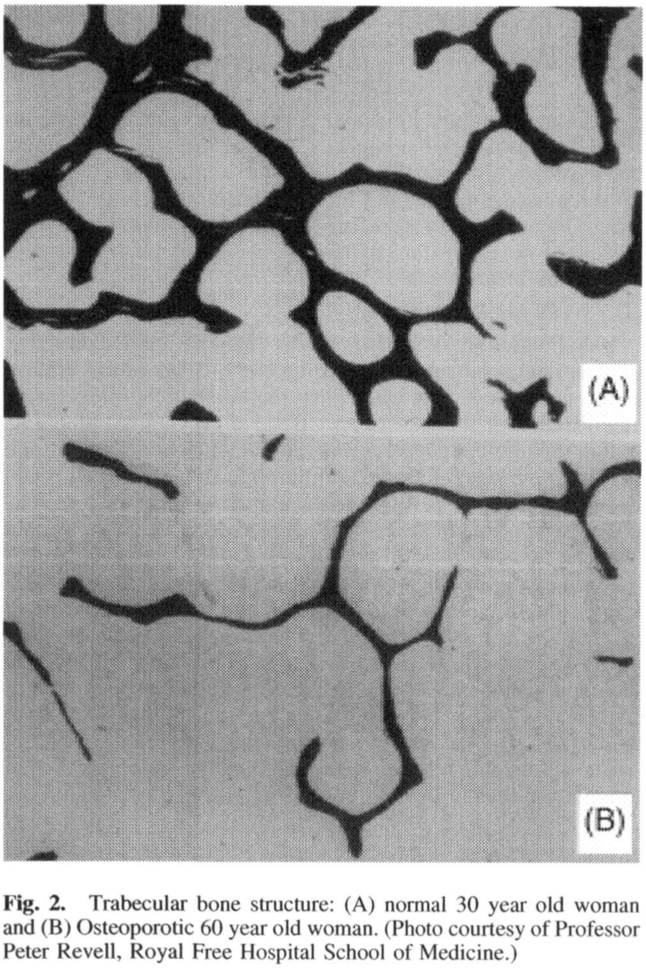

Fig. 2. Trabecular bone structure: (A) normal 30 year old woman and (B) Osteoporotic 60 year old woman. (Photo courtesy of Professor Peter Revell, Royal Free Hospital School of Medicine.)

tion the remaining years of the patient's life. Because the average life span of humans is now 80+ years and the need for spare parts begins at about 60 years of age, bioceramics need to last for 20+ years. This demanding requirement of survivability is under conditions of use that are especially harsh to ceramic materials: corrosive saline solutions at 37°C under variable, multiaxial, cyclical mechanical loads. The excellent performance of the specially designed bioceramics that have survived these clinical conditions represents one of the most remarkable accomplishments of ceramic research, development, production, and quality assurance during this century.

(2) Types of Bioceramic-Tissue Attachments

Survivability of a bioceramic requires formation of a stable interface with living host tissue. The mechanism of tissue attachment is directly related to the type of tissue response at the implant interface.[1,4,5] No material implanted in living tissues is inert; all materials elicit a response from living tissue. The four types of response (Table I) allow different means of achieving attachment of prostheses to the musculo-skeletal system. Table II summarizes the attachment mechanisms, with examples.

A comparison of the relative chemical activity of these different types of bioceramics is given in Fig. 3. The relative reactivity shown in Fig. 3(A) correlates very closely with the rate of formation of an interfacial bond of implants with bone (Fig. 3(B)).[4] Figure 3(B) is discussed in more detail in the section on bioactive ceramics.

The relative level of reactivity of an implant influences the *thickness* of the interfacial zone or layer between the material and tissue. Analysis of failure of implant materials during the past 20 years generally shows failure originating from the biomaterial–tissue interface.[4,5] When biomaterials are almost inert (type 1 in Table II and Fig. 3) and the interface is not chemically or biologically bonded, there is relative movement, and progressive development of a nonadherent fibrous capsule occurs in both soft and hard tissues. Movement at the biomaterial–tissue interface eventually leads to deterioration in function of the implant or of the tissue at the interface or of both. The thickness of the nonadherent capsule varies greatly, depending upon both the material (Fig. 4) and the extent of relative motion.

The fibrous tissue at the interface with dense, medical-grade Al_2O_3 implants can be very thin.[3,6] Consequently, if Al_2O_3 implants are implanted with a very tight mechanical fit and are loaded primarily in compression, they are successful clinically. In contrast, if an almost inert implant is loaded such that in-

Table I. Types of Implant–Tissue Response

If the material is toxic, the surrounding tissue dies.
If the material is nontoxic and biologically inactive (almost inert), a fibrous tissue of variable thickness forms.
If the material is nontoxic and biologically active (bioactive), an interfacial bond forms.
If the material is nontoxic and dissolves, the surrounding tissue replaces it.

Table II. Types of Bioceramic Tissue Attachment and Bioceramic Classification

Type of attachment	Type of bioceramic
Dense, nonporous, almost inert ceramics attach by bone growth into surface irregularities by cementing the device into the tissue, or by press-fitting into a defect (morphological fixation).	Al_2O_3 ZrO_2
For porous implants, bone ingrowth occurs, which mechanically attaches the bone to the material (biological fixation).	Porous hydroxyapatite Hydroxyapatite-coated porous metals
Surface-reactive ceramics, glasses, and glass-ceramics attach directly by chemical bonding with the bone (bioactive fixation).	Bioactive glasses Bioactve glass-ceramics Dense hydroxyapatite
Resorbable ceramics and glasses in bulk or powder form designed to be slowly replaced by bone.	Calcium sulfate (plaster of Paris) Tricalcium phosphate Calcium phosphate salts Bioactive glasses

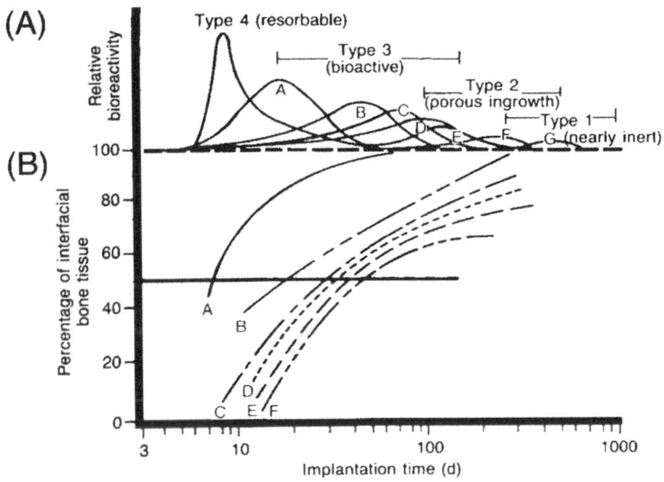

Fig. 3. Bioactivity spectrum for various bioceramic implants: (A) relative rate of bioreactivity and (B) time dependence of formation of bone bonding at an implant interface, where A is 45S5 bioactive glass, B is KGS glass-ceramic, C is S53P4, D is A/W glass-ceramic, E is dense synthetic HA, F is KGX glass-ceramic, and G is Al_2O_3.

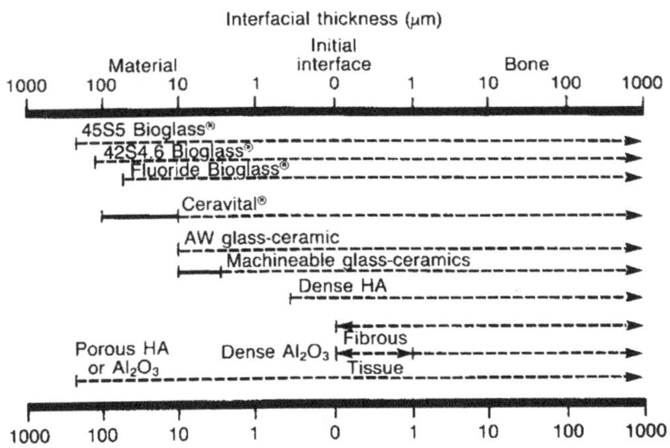

Fig. 4. Comparison of interfacial thickness of reaction layer of bioactive implants bonded to bone or thickness of nonadherant fibrous tissue in contact with inactive bioceramics in bone.

terfacial movement can occur, the fibrous capsule can become several hundred micrometers thick, and the implant loosens quickly. Loosening invariably leads to clinical failure, for a variety of reasons, including fracture of the implant or the bone adjacent to the implant. Bone at an interface with an almost inert implant is very often structurally weak because of disease, localized death of bone (especially if so-called bone cement, polymethylmethacrylate (PMMA), is used), or stress shielding that occurs because the higher elastic modulus of the implant prevents the bone from being loaded properly.

The concept behind microporous bioceramics (type 2 in Table II and Fig. 3) is the ingrowth of tissue into pores on the surface or throughout the implant, originated by Hulbert and co-workers[3] many years ago. The increased interfacial area between the implant and the tissues results in an increased resistance to movement of the device in the tissue. The interface is established by the living tissue in the pores. Figure 5 shows living bone that has grown into the pores of an Al_2O_3 bioceramic. This method of attachment often is termed "biological fixation." Biological fixation is capable of withstanding more-complex stress states than implants that achieve only "morphological fixation." However, the limitation associated with porous implants is that, for the tissue to remain viable and healthy, pores must be >100–150 μm in diameter. The large interfacial area required for the porosity is due to the need to provide a blood supply to the ingrown connective tissue. Vascular tissue does not appear in pores that measure <100 μm. If micromovement occurs at the interface of a porous implant, tissue is damaged, the blood supply may be cut off, the tissue dies, inflammation ensues, and the interfacial stability can be destroyed. When the material is a metal, the large increase in surface area can provide a focus for corrosion of the implant and loss of metal ions into the tissues, which can cause a variety of medical problems.[7,8] These potential problems can be diminished by using a bioactive ceramic material, such as hydroxyapatite (HA), as a coating on the porous metal.[9] The HA coating also speeds up the rate of bone formation in the pores.[9–13] However, the fraction of large porosity required for

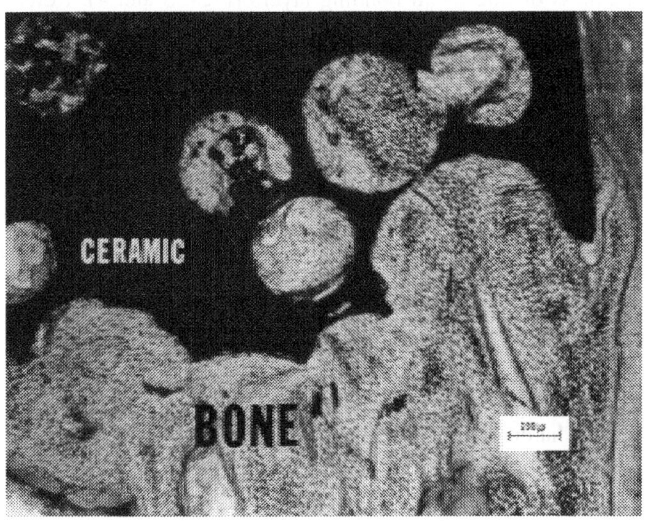

Fig. 5. Ingrowth of bone within >100 μm pores of Al_2O_3 bioceramic, after 8 weeks in rabbit. (Photo courtesy of Professor Sam Hulbert, Rose Hulman Institute of Technology.)

bone growth in any material degrades the strength of the material. Consequently, this approach to solving interfacial stability is best when the material is used as porous coatings on surgical metal alloys or as unloaded space fillers for bone ingrowth.

Resorbable biomaterials (type 4 in Table II and Fig. 3) are designed to degrade gradually over time and be replaced by the natural host tissue.[10–13] This leads to a very thin or nonexistent interfacial thickness (Fig. 4). This is the optimal solution to biomaterial problems if the requirements of strength and short-term performance can be met. Natural tissues can repair themselves and are gradually replaced throughout life by a continual turnover of cell populations. Thus, resorbable biomaterials are based on the same principles of repair that have evolved over millions of years. Complications in the development of resorbable bioceramics are

- Maintenance of strength and stability of the interface during the degradation period and replacement by the natural host tissue;
- Matching resorption rates to the repair rates of body tissues (Fig. 3(A)), which themselves vary enormously, depending upon type of tissue and its age and health.

Some resorbable materials dissolve too rapidly and some too slowly. Because large quantities of material can be replaced, it also is essential that a resorbable biomaterial consists only of metabolically acceptable substances. Otherwise, chronic inflammation and pain occur. This criterion imposes considerable limitations on the compositional design of resorbable biomaterials. Successful examples are resorbable polymers, such as polylactic–polyglycolic acid used for sutures, which are metabolized to CO_2 and H_2O and, therefore, are able to hold a wound together and then dissolve and disappear. Porous or particulate calcium phosphate ceramic materials, such as tricalcium phosphate (TCP), are successful materials for resorbable, hard tissue replacements when only low mechanical strength is required, such as in some repairs of the jaw or head.[10–13] Resorbable bioactive glasses are replaced rapidly with regenerated bone, as discussed below.

Another approach to the solution of the problems of interfacial attachment is the use of bioactive materials (type 3 in Table II and Fig. 3). The concept of bioactive materials is intermediate between resorbable and bioinert materials.[1,4,5] *A bioactive material is one that elicits a specific biological response at the interface of the material, which results in the formation of a bond between the tissues and the material,* shown first by the author and colleagues at the University of Florida in 1969.[14] This concept has been used to produce many bioactive materials with a wide range of bonding rates and thickness of interfacial bonding layers (Figs. 3 and 4). References 1, 3–5, and 15 discuss development of these interesting materials. The bioactive materials available commercially for clinical use are 45S5 bioactive glass, A/W bioactive glass-ceramic, dense synthetic HA, or bioactive composites, such as a polyethylene–HA mixture. All the above bioactive materials form an interfacial bond with adjacent tissue. However, the time dependence of bonding, the strength of the bond, the mechanism of bonding, and the thickness of the bonding zone differ for the various materials.

It is important to recognize that relatively small changes in the composition of a biomaterial can dramatically affect whether it is bioinert, resorbable, or bioactive. These compositional effects on surface reactions are discussed in the section on bioactive ceramics.

(3) *Almost-Inert Crystalline Bioceramics*

High-density, high-purity (>99.5%) Al_2O_3 (α-alumina) was the first bioceramic widely used clinically. It is used in total hip prostheses and dental implants because of its combination of excellent corrosion resistance, good biocompatibility, low friction, high wear resistance, and high strength.[1,3,6,16–18] Most Al_2O_3 devices are very-fine-grained, polycrystalline α-Al_2O_3. A very small amount of MgO (<0.5%) is used as a sintering aid and to limit grain growth during sintering.

Strength, fatigue resistance, and fracture toughness of polycrystalline α-Al_2O_3 are a function of grain size and concentration of sintering aid, i.e., purity. Al_2O_3 with an average grain size of <4 μm and a purity of >99.7% exhibits good flexural strength and excellent compressive strength. These and other physical properties are summarized in Table III with the International Standards Organization (ISO) requirements for medical-grade Al_2O_3 implants.[6] Extensive testing has shown that Al_2O_3 implants that meet or exceed ISO standards have excellent resistance to dynamic and impact fatigue and also resist subcritical crack growth.[19,20] An increase in average grain size to >7 μm can decrease mechanical properties by ~20%. High concentrations of sintering aids must be avoided, because they remain in the grain boundaries and degrade fatigue resistance, especially in the corrosive physiological environment.[1]

Methods exist for lifetime predictions and statistical design of proof tests for load-bearing ceramics. Applications of these techniques show that specific prosthesis load limits can be set for an Al_2O_3 device based upon the flexural strength of the material and its use environment.[19,21] Load-bearing lifetimes of 30 years at 12 kN loads, similar to those expected in total hip joints, have been predicted.[6] Results from aging and fatigue studies show that it is essential that Al_2O_3 implants be produced at the highest possible standards of quality assurance, especially if they are to be used as orthopedic prostheses in younger patients (<50 years old).

Al_2O_3 has been used in orthopedic surgery for more than 20 years as the articulating surface in total hip prostheses because of its exceptionally low coefficient of friction and minimal wear rates (Fig. 6).[3,6,19] The superb tribiologic properties (friction and wear) of Al_2O_3 occur only when the grains are very small (<4 μm) and have a very narrow size distribution. These conditions lead to very low surface roughness values (R_a = 0.02 μm, Table III). If large grains are present, they can pull out and lead to very rapid wear because of local dry friction and abrasion caused by the Al_2O_3 grains in the joint-bearing surfaces.[6]

Table III. Physical Characteristics of Alumina and Partially Stabilized Zirconia Bioceramics†

Physical characteristic	Alumina bioceramics	ISO alumina standard 6474	Partially stabilized zirconia	Cortical bone	Cancellous bone
Content (wt%)	Al_2O_3 > 99.8	Al_2O_3 > 99.50	ZrO_2 > 97		
Density (g/cm^3)	>3.93	>3.90	6.05	1.6–2.1	
Average grain size (μm)	3–6	<7	0.2–0.4		
Surface roughness, R_a (μm)	0.02		0.008		
Vickers hardness (HV)	2300	>2000	1300		
Compressive strength (MPa)	4500		2000	100–230	2–12
Bending strength (in Ringer's solution) (MPa)	595	>400	1000	50–150	
Young's modulus (GPa)	400		150	7–30	0.05–0.5
Fracture toughness, K_{IC} (MPa·m$^{-1/2}$)	5–6		15	2–12	
Slow crack growth (unitless)	30–52		65		

†Reference 4, Chs. 1 and 2.

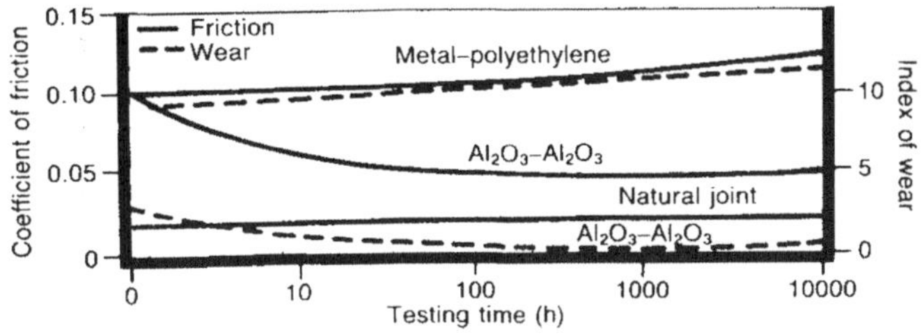

Fig. 6. Time dependence of coefficient of friction and wear of Al_2O_3–Al_2O_3 versus metal–polyethylene total hip joint (*in vitro* testing).

Al_2O_3–Al_2O_3 load-bearing wearing surfaces, such as in hip prostheses, must have a very high degree of sphericity produced by grinding and polishing the two mating surfaces. The Al_2O_3 ball and socket in a hip prosthesis are polished together and used as a pair. The long-term coefficient of friction of an Al_2O_3–Al_2O_3 joint is the closest of any synthetic material to the values of a normal joint. Wear of Al_2O_3–Al_2O_3 articulating surface is 2–10 times lower than metal–polyethylene surfaces (Fig. 6).

Low wear rates have led to use in Europe of Al_2O_3 noncemented cups press-fitted into the acetabulum (socket) of the hip. The cups are stabilized by bone growth into grooves or around pegs. The mating femoral ball surface also is Al_2O_3, which is press-fitted to a metallic stem (Fig. 7). Long-term results, in general, are excellent, especially for younger patients. However, stress shielding of the bone can occur.[6] This is due to the high Young's modulus of Al_2O_3 (Table III), which prevents the bone from being loaded—a requirement for bone to remain healthy and strong. The Young's modulus of cortical bone is 7–25 GPa, which is 10–50 times lower than Al_2O_3. Stress shielding may be responsible for cancellous bone atrophy and loosening of the acetabular cup in older patients with osteoporosis or rheumatoid arthritis.[6] Consequently, it is essential that the age of the patient, nature of the disease of the joint, and biomechanics of the repair be considered carefully before any prosthesis is used, including those made from Al_2O_3 ceramics. The primary use of Al_2O_3 in the United States is for the ball of the hip joint (Fig. 8) with the acetabular (socket) component being ultrahigh-molecular-weight polyethylene.

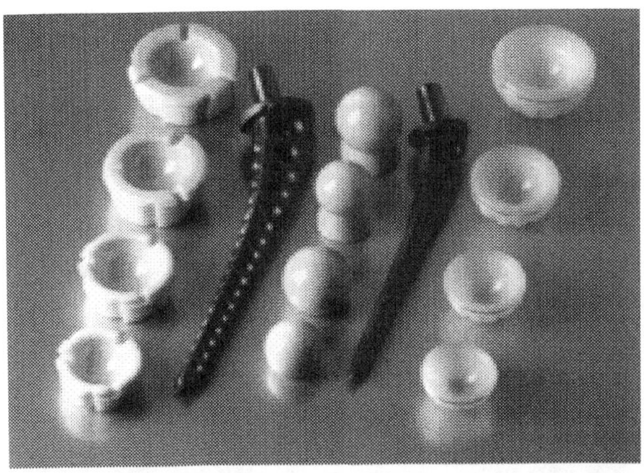

Fig. 7. Medical-grade Al_2O_3 used in total hip replacement: (left) Al_2O_3 acetabular cups mated with Al_2O_3 femoral balls; (center) Al_2O_3 balls also can be used with ultra-high-molecular-weight polyethylene cups; and (right) alternative metallic stem designs for morphological or cement fixation. (Photo courtesy of Dr. Gerd Willmann, CeramTec AG.)

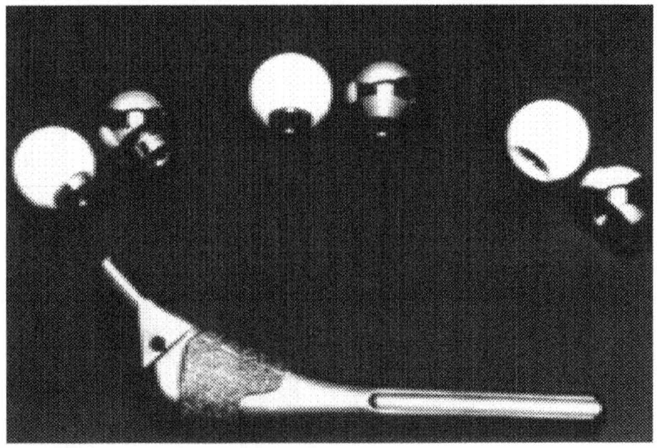

Fig. 8. Medical-grade Al_2O_3 used as femoral balls in total hip replacement. Note the porous coating on the metallic stem used for biological fixation. (Photo courtesy of Dr. Jack Parr.)

Other clinical applications of Al_2O_3 include knee prostheses, bone screws, alveolar ridge (jaw bone) and maxillofacial reconstructions, ossicular (middle ear) bone substitutes, keratoprostheses (corneal replacements), segmental bone replacements, and blade and screw and post-type dental implants.[1,3]

Zirconia (ZrO_2), in tetragonal form, stabilized by either magnesium or yttrium, also has been developed as a medical-grade bioceramic for use in total joint prostheses (Table III). The interest in ZrO_2 derives from its high fracture toughness and tensile strength. These improved properties make it possible to manufacture femoral heads for total hip prostheses that are smaller than the present generation of Al_2O_3 heads. ZrO_2 implants now are used clinically; only implant survivability data over 10 years will establish whether there is a clinical advantage.

II. Porous Ceramics

The potential advantage offered by a porous ceramic implant is the mechanical stability of the highly convoluted interface developed when bone grows into the pores of the ceramic.[22–24] The two primary clinical applications are

- Use of HA coatings on the porous surfaces of total joint prostheses as an alternative to cement fixation and as coatings on dental implants to achieve bioactive fixation;[4]
- Use of porous synthetic calcium phosphate ceramics to fill bone defects.[11–13,22–25]

The mechanical requirements of prostheses severely restrict the use of low-strength porous ceramics to low-load- or nonload-bearing applications.[3,22–25] A porous implant serves as a structural bridge and model or scaffold for bone formation. The microstructures of certain corals make an almost ideal material for forming structures with highly controlled pore sizes. White *et al.*[22,23] developed the replamineform process to duplicate the porous microstructure of corals that have a high degree of uniform pore size and interconnection. The first step is to machine the coral with proper microstructure into the desired shape. The coral genus, *Porites*, has pores with a size range of 140–160 μm pores, with all the pores interconnected.[22] Another coral genus, *Goniopora*, has a larger pore size, 200–1000 μm. The advantages of the replamineform process are that the pore size and microstructure are uniform, and there is complete interconnection of the pores. Clinical applications are reviewed by Schors and Holmes in Ref. 4.

Porous metal surfaces are produced on metallic orthopedic alloys by sintering balls or wires or meshes to the solid metal.[7] Synthetic HA ceramic coatings then are applied to the porous layers, usually by plasma-spray coating.[25,26] The bioactive coatings are applied to relatively small areas of a prosthesis, such as illustrated in Fig. 8. The rate of bone growth into the

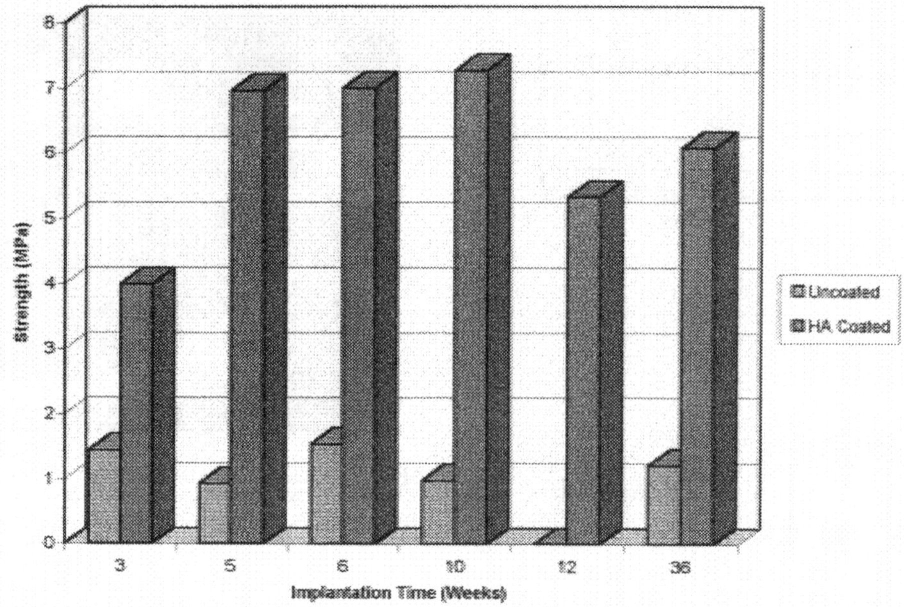

Fig. 9. Comparison of interfacial bond strength of porous titanium with and without plasma-sprayed HA coatings. (Data courtesy of Dr. Steve Cook.)

porous layer is accelerated by the bioactive HA ceramic, and the strength of the bone–implant interface also is enhanced (Fig. 9). Thus, bone bonding and biological fixation are restricted to specific areas, which reduces stress shielding in other areas of bone contact. This merger of the concepts of biological fixation, enhanced bone formation by a bioactive coating, and optimization of biomechanical stress transfer to the host bone is a major accomplishment of the past 20 years of research and development in orthopedic total joint replacement.

III. Bioactive Glasses and Glass-Ceramics

Certain compositions of glasses, ceramics, glass-ceramics, and composites have been shown to form a mechanically strong bond to bone.[4,5,14,27,30–40] These materials have become known as "bioactive ceramics."[4,5,25,40,41] Some even more specialized compositions of bioactive glasses bond to soft tissues as well as bone.[35,42] A common characteristic of bioactive glasses and bioactive ceramics is a time-dependent, kinetic modification of the surface that occurs upon implantation.[4,27,41] The surface forms a biologically active hydroxycarbonate apatite (HCA) layer that provides the bonding interface with the tissues. The HCA phase that forms on bioactive implants is equivalent chemically and structurally to the mineral phase in bone. It is that equivalence that is responsible for interfacial bonding.

Materials that are bioactive develop an adherent interface with tissue that resists substantial mechanical forces.[14,38,43,44] In many cases, the interfacial strength of adhesion is equivalent to or greater than the cohesive strength of the implant material or the tissue bonded to the bioactive implant. Figures 10 and 11 show bioactive implants bonded to bone with adherence at the interface sufficient to resist mechanical fracture. Failure occurs either in the implant (Fig. 10) or in the bone (Fig. 11) but not at the interface.

Bonding to bone was first demonstrated for a certain compositional range of bioactive glasses that contained SiO_2, Na_2O, CaO, and P_2O_5 in specific proportions[14] (Table IV). There were three important compositional features to these glasses that distinguished them from traditional soda–lime–

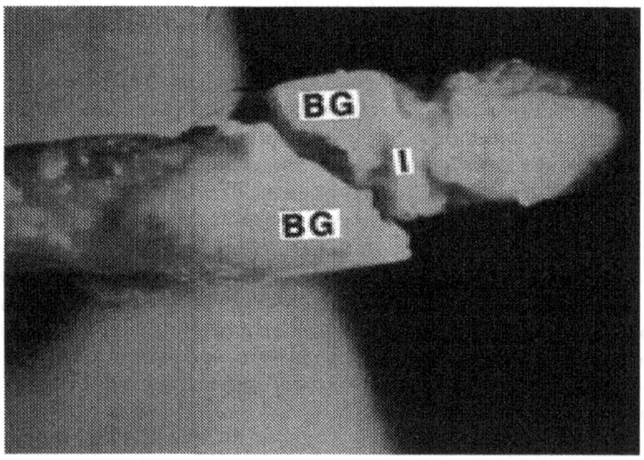

Fig. 10. Fracture of 45S5 bioactive glass [BG] segmental bone replacement in monkey due to torsional loading. Note the bonded interface [I] that survived the load to failure. (Photo courtesy of Professor George Piotrowski, University of Florida.)

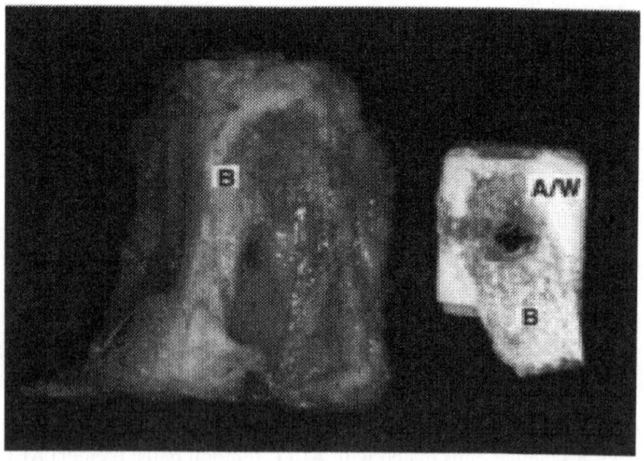

Fig. 11. Interfacial adherence of A/W bioactive glass-ceramic is stronger than either bone [B] or implant [A/W]. (Photo courtesy Professors T. Yamamura and T. Kokubo, Kyoto University.)

silica glasses: <60 mol% SiO_2, high Na_2O and CaO content, and high CaO:P_2O_5 ratio. These compositional features make the surface highly reactive when exposed to an aqueous medium, such as body fluids.

Many bioactive SiO_2 glasses are based upon the formula called "45S5," signifying 45 wt% SiO_2 (S means the network former). Glasses with substantially larger amounts of P_2O_5 do not bond to bone.[43] Substitutions in the 45S5 formula of 5–15 wt% B_2O_3 for SiO_2 or 12.5 wt% CaF_2 for CaO or crystallizing the glass compositions to form glass-ceramics has little effect on the ability of the material to form a bone bond.[43] However, addition of as little as 3 wt% Al_2O_3 to the 45S5 formula prevents bonding.[5,31,43–46]

The compositional dependence (in weight percent) of bone bonding and soft tissue bonding for the Na_2O–CaO–P_2O_5–SiO_2 glasses is illustrated in Fig. 12. All glasses in Fig. 12 contain a constant 6 wt% of P_2O_5. Compositions in the middle of the diagram (region A) form a bond with bone. Consequently, region A defines the bioactive bone-bonding boundary. Silicate glasses within region B, such as window or bottle glass or microscope slides, behave as almost inert materials and elicit formation of a fibrous capsule at the implant–tissue interface. Glasses within region C are resorbable and disappear within 10–30 d of implantation. Glasses within region D are not technically practical and, therefore, have not been tested as implants.

The collagenous constituent of soft tissues can adhere strongly to the bioactive silicate glasses that lie within the compositional range shown in Fig. 12 as region E. Figure 13(A) shows collagen from a 10 d *in vitro* test-tube experiment bonded to a 45S5 Bioglass surface by agglomerates of HCA crystallites growing on the surface. The collagen fibrils are woven into the interface by growth of the HCA layer. The dense HCA–collagen agglomerates mimic the nature of bonding between tendons and ligaments, composed entirely of collagen fibrils, and bone or teeth that are composites of HCA crystals and collagen.[47,48] There is similar attachment of a periodontal ligament (PL) to a tooth (Fig. 13(B)) as to the attachment of collagen fibers to a Bioglass sample (Fig. 13(A)).

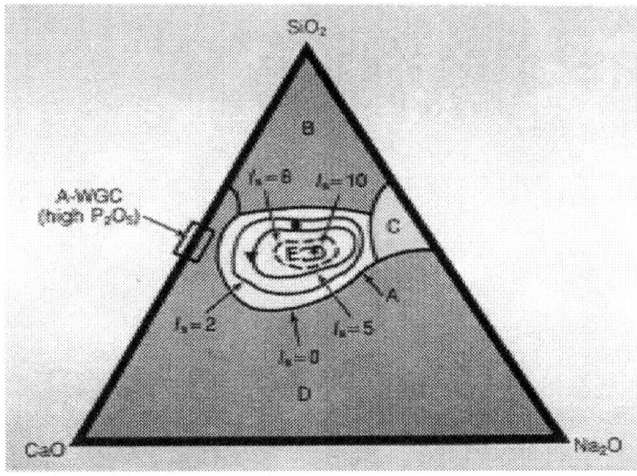

Fig. 12. Compositional dependence (in wt%) of bone bonding and soft tissue bonding of bioactive glasses and glass-ceramics. All compositions in region A are bioactive and bond to bone. They have a constant 6 wt% of P_2O_5. A/W glass-ceramic has higher P_2O_5 content (see Table IV for details). Compositions in region B are bioinert and lead to formation of a nonadherant fibrous capsule. Compositions in region C are resorbable. Region D is restricted by technical factors. Region E (soft tissue bonding) is inside the dashed line where the index of bioactivity, I_B, is >8.

The test tube collagen-bioactive glass experiment (Fig. 13(A)) produces a similar interfacial bond as that which occurs in living soft connective tissues, as first discovered by Wilson *et al.*[35,42] (Figs. 14 and 15). Figure 14 shows a disk of 45S5 bioactive glass immobilized in soft connective tissue by an adherant layer. There is no inflammation around the implant, because it does not move and abrade the cells or cause degradation products. The adherance of the collagen fibers to the bonding gel layer on the glass, illustrated in Fig. 15, is stronger than the coherance of the collagen fibers to themselves. This discovery is especially important, because many implants require a stable interface with both soft and hard connective tissues.

Table IV. Composition and Mechanical Properties of Bioactive Ceramics Used Clinically†

Property	Bioglass 45S5	S45PZ	Glass-ceramic Ceravital	Glass-ceramic Cerabone A/W	Glass-ceramic Ilmaplant L1	Glass-ceramic Bioverit	Sintered hydroxyapatite $Ca_{10}(PO_4)_6(OH)_2$ (>99.2%)	Sintered β-3CaO·P_2O_5 (>99.7%)
Composition (wt%)								
Na_2O	24.5	24	5–10	0	4.6	3–8		
K_2O	0		0.5–3.0	0	0.2	3–8		
MgO	0		2.5–5.0	4.6	2.8	2–21		
CaO	24.5	22	30–35	44.7	31.9	10–34		
Al_2O_3	0		0	0	0	8–15		
SiO_2	45.0	45	40–50	34.0	44.3	19–54		
P_2O_5	6.0	7	10–50	16.2	11.2	2–10		
CaF_2	0			0.5	5.0	3–23		
B_2O_3	0	2						
Phase‡	Glass	Glass	Apatite Glass	Apatite β-Wollastonite Glass	Apatite β-Wollastonite Glass	Apatite Phlogopite Glass	Apatite	Whitlockite
Density (g/cm³)	2.6572			3.07		2.8	3.16	3.07
Vickers hardness (HV)	458 ± 9.4			680		500	600	
Compressive strength (MPa)			500	1080		500	500–1000	460–687
Bending strength (MPa)	42§			215	160	100–160	115–200	140–154
Young's modulus (GPa)	35		100–150	218		70–88	80–110	33–90
Fracture toughness, K_{IC} (MPa·m$^{1/2}$)				2.0	2.5	0.5–1.0	1.0	
Slow crack growth, *n* (unitless)				33			12–27	

†Reference 15. ‡Apatite is $Ca_{10}(PO_4)_6(O,F)$, β-wollastonite is CaO·SiO_2, phlogopite is $(Na,K)Mg_3(AlSiO_{10})F_2$, and whitlockite is β-3CaO·P_2O_5. §Tensile.

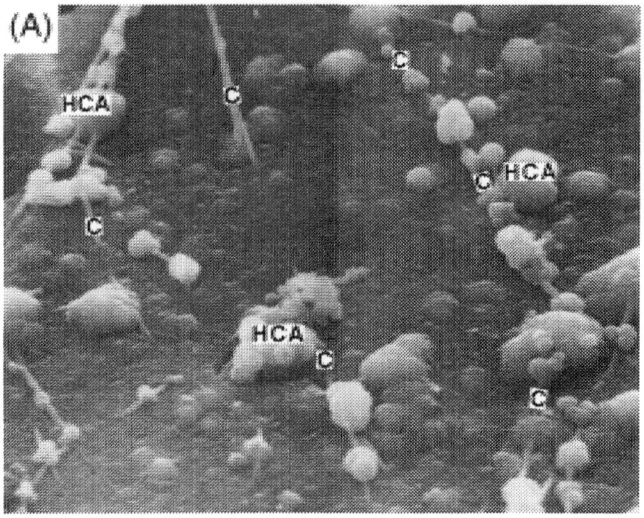

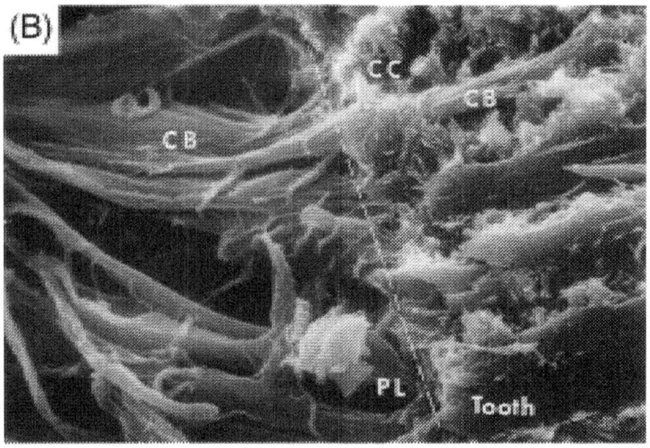

Fig. 13. (A) SEM micrograph of collagen fibrils [C] incorporated within the HCA layer [HCA] growing on a 45S5 bioactive glass substrate *in vitro*. (Photo courtesy of Professor Carlo Pantano, The Pennsylvania State University.) (B) SEM micrograph of tissue attachment to a tooth. Note the collagen bundles [CB] coming from the left in the periodontal ligament [PL] inserted deep into the calcified cementum [CC] on the surface of the tooth. (Photo courtesy of Dr. J. Brady.)

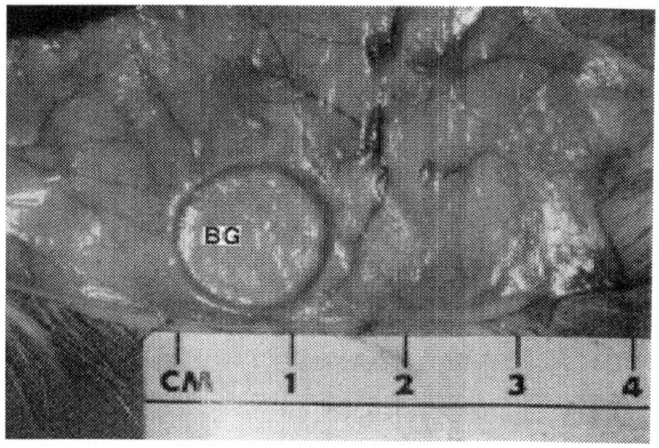

Fig. 14. Adherant soft connective tissue bonding immobilizes a 45S5 bioactive glass [BG] implant. (Photo courtesy of Dr. June Wilson.)

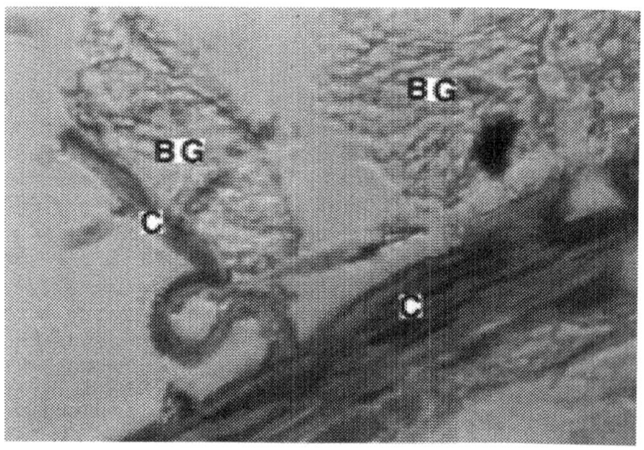

Fig. 15. Adhesion of collagen fibers [C] to bioactive glass bonding gel layer [BG] is stronger than cohesive bonding of collagen to itself. (Photo courtesy of Dr. June Wilson, University of Florida.)

The composite interface composed of HCA collagen on the bioactive glasses is ~30–60 μm of the 100–200 μm total interfacial thickness (Fig. 4). This junction thickness is equivalent to that at naturally occurring interfaces (Fig. 13(B)), where a transition occurs between materials with low Young's elastic moduli (tendons and ligaments) and those with moderately high Young's moduli (bones and teeth). The thicknesses of the hard tissue–bioactive ceramic interfaces are indicated in Fig. 4 for several clinically important bioactive materials. The interfacial thickness of the bonding zone decreases as the compositional boundary shown in Fig. 12 is approached.

Gross *et al.*[5,31,49–52] have shown that a range of low-alkali (0–5 wt%) bioactive SiO_2-based glass-ceramics also bond to bone. Small additions of Al_2O_3, Ta_2O_5, TiO_2, Sb_2O_3, or ZrO_2 inhibit bone bonding (Table IV).

The clinically most important bioactive glass-ceramic is the three-phase silica–phosphate material (Table IV) composed of apatite $[Ca_{10}(PO_4)_6(OH_1F_2)]$ and wollastonite ($CaO–SiO_2$) crystals and a residual $CaO–SiO_2$-rich glassy matrix, termed A/W glass-ceramic by Professors Yamamuro and Kokubo, its developers.[34,36–40] A/W glass-ceramic has excellent mechanical properties (Table IV) and forms a bond with bone that has a very high interfacial bond strength (Fig. 11).[37,38] Addition of Al_2O_3 or TiO_2 to the A/W glass-ceramic inhibits bone bonding, whereas incorporation of a second phosphate phase, β-whitlockite ($3CaO{\cdot}P_2O_5$) does not.

Another multiphase bioactive silica–phosphate, containing phlogopite mica $(Na,K)Mg_3(AlSi_3O_{10})F_2$ and apatite crystals, bonds to bone even though Al_2O_3 is present in the composition.[32] However, the Al^{3+} ions are incorporated within the crystal phase and do not alter the surface reaction kinetics of the material. An advantage of these mica-containing glass-ceramics, developed by Freidrich Schiller University, Jena, Germany, is their easy machinability.[53] Additional compositions of bioactive glasses have been developed at Abo Akademi and the University of Turku, Finland, for dental applications.[45,54,55] Compositions of these various bioactive glasses and glass-ceramics are compared in Table IV.

IV. Interfacial Reaction Kinetics

Bonding of bone to bioactive glasses involves 12 reaction stages summarized in Fig. 16(A). The first five stages occur very rapidly on the surface of most bioactive glasses because of fast ion exchange of alkali ions with hydrogen ions from body fluids (stage 1), network dissolution (stage 2), silica-gel polymerization (stage 3), and chemisorption and crystallization of the HCA layer (stages 4 and 5), as summarized in Table V. The surface reactions lead to the biochemical adsorption of growth factors (stage 6) and the synchronized sequence of cellular

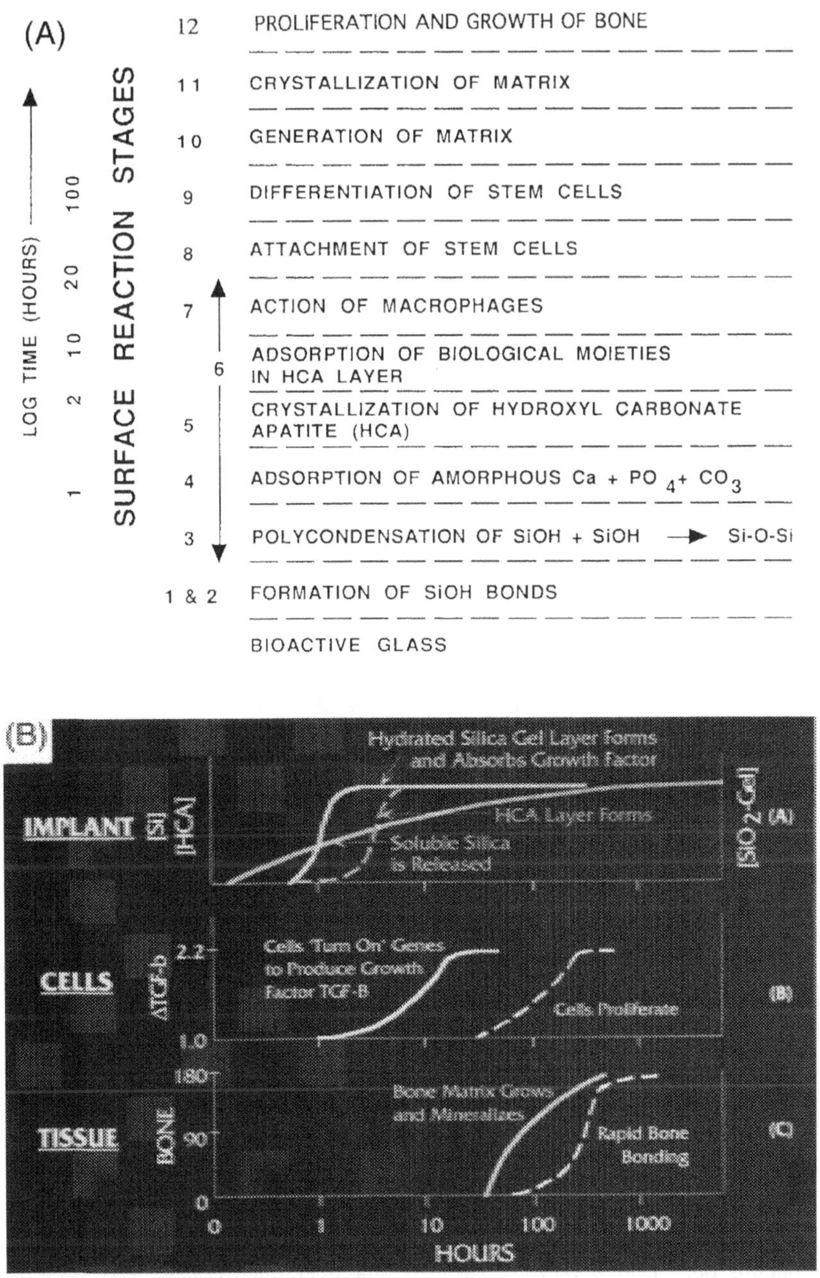

Fig. 16. (A) Sequence of interfacial reactions involved in forming a bond between bone and a bioactive glass. (B) Time dependence of reactions occurring on a bioactive implant surface and the effects on cells that lead to rapid bone bonding and bone proliferation.

events (stages 7–12) that result in rapid formation of new bone. The time dependence of the reaction stages is depicted in Fig. 16(B). Compositions in the center of the bioactive bonding field in Fig. 12 exhibit very rapid rates of stages 1–12. When the concentration of SiO_2 in the glass network exceeds ~55%, the rates of reaction slow greatly, as indicated by the iso-bioactivity contours in Fig. 12, and bonding to bone is very slow. At a concentration of 60% SiO_2, the rates of reaction are sufficiently slow that the material is biologically inert. Bioactive glass-ceramics, such as A/W glass-ceramic, are intermediate in reactions rates and bioactivity.

Surface compositional profiles resulting from stage 1 through stage 5 reactions have been measured for 45S5 bioactive glasses using Auger electron spectroscopy (AES) combined with argon-ion milling.[56–58] The results (Fig. 17) show that, after only 1 h *in vivo*, there has developed a calcium- and phosphorus-rich reaction layer heterogeneously nucleated and crystallized from the silica-gel layer formed on the glass surface. The calcium- and phosphorus-rich layer is identical in defect composition to biologically grown apatites, because it is grown *in situ*. With time, the interfacial bonding zone between living and nonliving material continues to grow by incorporating calcium and phosphorus ions from body fluids. The final result is a gradient in composition that extends over several hundred micrometers (Fig. 18), similar in dimension to the bonding zone that occurs naturally at bone interfaces. The compositional profiles correlate with electron microscopy of the bioactive glass implant bonding interface in bone[14,43,44,59] and provide the explanation for the high bonding strength of the interface.[60]

Kokubo[61,62] has shown that a calcium- and phosphorus-rich layer also is present at the bonding interface between the polycrystalline apatite- and wollastonite-based A/W glass-ceramic and bone. However, the SiO_2-rich layer was not present, even though a substantial concentration of soluble silicon was lost to solution. CaO–SiO_2-based glasses, without phosphate, form an

Table V. Reaction Stages of a Bioactive Implant†

Stage	Reaction
1	Rapid exchange of Na^+ or K^+ with H^+ or H_3O^+ from solution: $Si–O–Na^+ + H^+ + OH^- \rightarrow Si–OH^+ + Na^+(solution) + OH^-$ This stage is usually controlled by diffusion and exhibits a $t^{-1/2}$ dependence.
2	Loss of soluble SiO_2 in the form of $Si(OH)_4$ to the solution, resulting from breaking of Si–O–Si bonds and formation of Si–OH (silanols) at the glass solution interface: $Si–O–Si + H_2O \rightarrow Si–OH + OH–Si$ This stage usually is controlled by interfacial reaction and exhibits a $t^{1.0}$ dependence.
3	Condensation and repolymerization of a SiO_2-rich layer on the surface depleted in alkalis and alkaline-earth cations: O–Si(O)(O)–OH + HO–Si(O)(O)–O → O–Si(O)(O)–O–Si(O)(O)–O + H_2O
4	Migration of Ca^{2+} and PO_4^{3-} groups to the surface through the SiO_2-rich layer, forming a $CaO–P_2O_5$-rich film on top of the SiO_2-rich layer, followed by growth of the amorphous $CaO–P_2O_5$-rich film by incorporation of soluble calcium and phosphates from solution.
5	Crystallization of the amorphous $CaO–P_2O_5$ film by incorporation of OH^-, CO_3^{2-}, or F^- anions from solution to form a mixed hydroxyl, carbonate, fluorapatite layer.

†Reference 15.

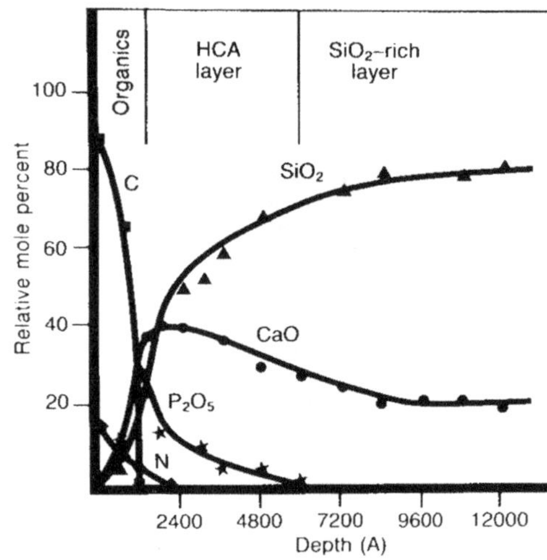

Fig. 17. Bilayer films formed on 45S5 bioactive glass after 1 h in rat bone, as measured by Auger electron spectroscopy and argon-ion beam milling.

apatite layer on their surfaces[62,63] when exposed for 2–30 d in simulated body fluid that contains only 1.0m*M* HPO_4^{2-}. The $CaO–SiO_2$-based glasses were confirmed to bond to living bone by the surface apatite layer.[62] Previously, Ogino *et al.*[57] showed that P_2O_5-free $Na_2O–SiO_2$ glasses form an apatite layer on their surfaces when exposed to an aqueous solution containing calcium and phosphate ions. Li, Clark, and Hench[64] demonstrated that highly porous sol–gel-derived glasses containing primarily SiO_2, with only 10 mol% of CaO and P_2O_5 and no Na_2O, form apatite layers in a *tris*-buffer solution. Earlier, Walker[65] demonstrated that even highly pure SiO_2 eventually forms a bone bond if the surface has a very high surface area, >400 m^2/g. Synthetic HA ceramic implants, which contain no SiO_2 or alkali ions, bond to bone by forming a new epitaxial apatite phase at the interface,[10,66,67] as discussed in a later section.

Consequently, it is concluded that bioactivity occurs only within certain compositional limits and very specific ratios of oxides in the $Na_2O–K_2O–CaO–MgO–P_2O_5–SiO_2$ systems. *A layer of biologically active HCA must form for a bond with tissues to occur. This is the common characteristic of all the known bioactive implant materials.* It is the rate of HCA formation (stage 4) and the time for onset of crystallization (stage 5) that varies greatly. When the rate becomes excessively slow, no bond forms, and the material is no longer bioactive.

The failure strength of a bioactively fixed bond appears to be a nonlinear function of the bonding rate of the implant. Interfacial strength appears to be *inversely* dependent on the *thickness* of the bonding zone. For example, 45S5 Bioglass with a very high bonding rate develops a gel-bonding layer of 100 μm (Fig. 18) that has a relatively low shear strength. In contrast, A/W glass-ceramic, with an intermediate rate of bonding, has an interface of 10–20 μm and a very high resistance to shear (note Fig. 7).[38,62] The interfacial area for bonding is time dependent, as shown in Fig. 3. Therefore, interfacial strength is time dependent and is a function of morphological factors, such as the change in interfacial area with time, progressive mineralization of the interfacial tissues, and resulting increase of elastic modulus of the interfacial bond, as well as a function of shear strength per unit of bonded area and the density and quality of bone bonded to the interface (Figs. 1 and 2). For example, a bioactive implant bonded to osteoporotic bone shears easily through the low-density trabecular bone.

V. Clinical Applications of Bioactive Glasses and Glass-Ceramics

Clinical applications of bioactive glasses and glass-ceramics have been reviewed by Gross *et al.*,[5] Yamamuro *et al.*,[40] and Wilson *et al.*[68,69] (see Table VI). Several of the most important clinical uses are described in this section. Bioactive glass and glass-ceramic implants have been used for more than 10 years to replace the small bones of the middle ear (ossicles) damaged by chronic infection, a clinical problem called "conductive hearing loss."[70–73] An example of a 45S5 bioactive glass middle ear implant, used as an ossicular prosthesis, is shown in Fig. 19. Survivability of the bioactive glass implants for middle-ear replacements is considerably longer than occurs when bioinert implants are used for the same purpose (Fig. 20). Bioinert implants do not bond to the eardrum and, therefore, gradually erode through the tissue and are extruded through the eardrum within 2–3 years.[73] In contrast, highly bioactive glasses form a bond with the collagen of the eardrum and also bond firmly to the remaining bone of the stapes footplate and, thereby, are anchored on both ends, which prevents extrusion. Sound conduction is excellent, and there is no fibrous tissue growth to impair sound transmission. Moreover, there is no micromotion at the implant–tissue interface; therefore, the implant remains stable and functions for the lifetime of the patient.[73]

Many patients are "profoundly deaf" because of loss of the auditory nerve fibers in the cochlea. Research has shown that such patients can sense electronic impulses applied to the cochlea, although at much lower frequency discrimination. These findings have led to the development of an extracochlear electrical implant that delivers electrical signals in real time en-

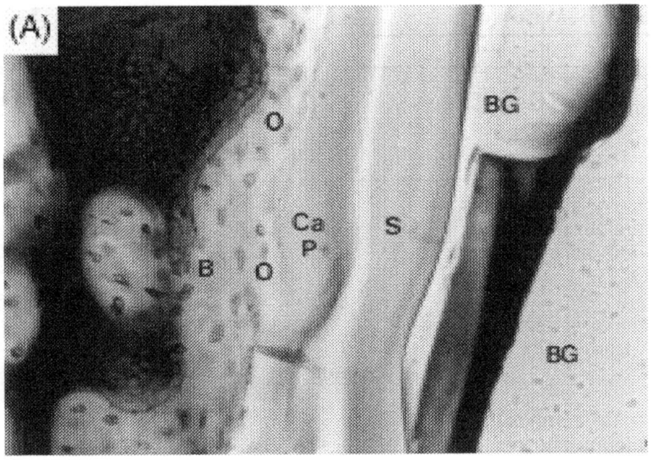

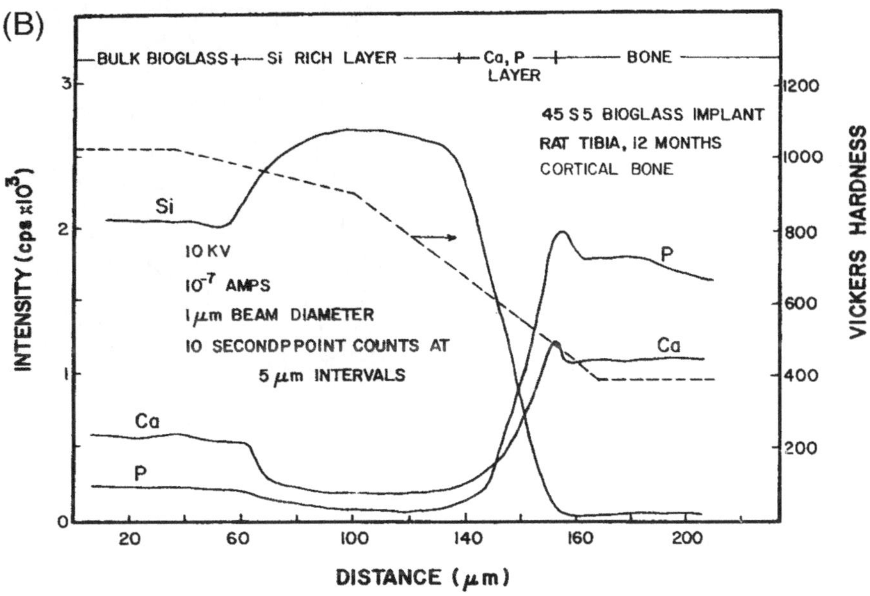

Fig. 18. (A) Optical micrograph of a 45S5 bioactive glass implant [BG] bonded to rat bone [B] after 1 year, showing osteocytes or bone cells [O] in conjunction with the HCA layer [Ca-P] formed on top of the silica gel [S]. (B) Electron microprobe analysis across the implant-bone interface shown in (A).

coded by a computer to match speech patterns.[74] A team led by Professor Fourcin and ENT Surgeon Douek in London reports successful clinical use of an array of four platinum electrodes insulated by medical-grade Al_2O_3 and anchored in the bone with a 45S5 bioactive glass sleeve. The Al_2O_3 provides mechanical and dielectric stability to the device, and the bioactive glass bonds both to the bone and the soft connective tissues as it protrudes through the skin. This hermetic, percutaneous living seal provides both mechanical stability and prevents infection from migrating down the electrodes, thereby protecting the patient who must unplug the electronics at night. Figure 21(A) shows the University of London extracochlear electrode array and its implantation site. Figure 21(B) shows the implant in place in a patient. Patients have used this type of auditory prosthesis for 5 years with success.

Another application of 45S5 Bioglass implants, based upon bonding to both soft tissues and bone, preserves the jawbone of patients who have had their teeth extracted prior to being fitted with dentures. This type of implant, called an Endosseous Ridge Maintenance Implant (ERMI), developed by Stanley *et al.*,[75] is injection molded in the shape of a cone with several sizes to match the size of roots of extracted teeth (Fig. 22). A mating drill bit of equal size is used to prepare the bone for the implant. X-rays (Fig. 23) show that the implants are stable after many years in bone and have prevented resorption (wearing away) of bone under the dentures. Survivability of bioactive glass ERMI implants after 10 years are dramatically greater than other bioactive implants that do not bond to soft tissue (Fig. 24).[75]

The clinical application of bioactive glasses that is most important is in the form of a particulate that is placed around teeth that have had periodontal (gum) disease, a clinical problem that affects tens of millions of people. The 45S5 bioactive glass material rapidly leads to new bone formation around the bioactive glass particles (Fig. 25).[68,69,76,77] The new bone forms by the reaction mechanisms summarized in Fig. 16. Because of the speed of formation of the new bone, the epithelial tissues are stopped from migrating down the tooth, a common problem if nothing is used to fill the space between the tooth and repairing bone. The junction between the tooth and the periodontal membrane is stabilized by use of bioactive glass particulate, and the tooth is saved. Clinical success is quite dramatic, as reported by periodontists[68,69] and oral surgeons.[68] The same particulate bioactive glass material has been used in a wide variety of clinical applications where bone grafting is needed to fill spaces or augment the natural repair process. An example is shown in Fig. 26, which are X-rays of a third molar site prior to surgical extraction (Fig. 26(A)) and 3 months after filling with 45S5 bioactive glass particulate (Fig. 26(B)).[68] An advantage of the rapid bone repair due to the bioactive material

Table VI. Clinical Uses of Bioceramics

Application	Materials[†]
Orthopedic	Al_2O_3 Stabilized ZrO_2 HA powders Bioactive glass powders
Coatings for bioactive bonding	HA Bioactive glass ceramics
Bone space fillers	Tricalcium phosphate Calcium phosphate salts
Dental implants	Al_2O_3 HA Bioactive glasses
Artificial tendon and ligament	PLA–carbon-fiber composite
Periodontal pocket obliteration	HA HA–PLA composite Tricalcium phosphate Calcium phosphate salts Bioactive glasses
Alveolar ridge augmentation	HA HA–autogenous bone composite Bioactive glasses
Maxillofacial reconstruction	Al_2O_3 HA PE–HA composite Bioactive glasses
Spinal surgery	Bioactive glass-ceramic HA
Therapeutic treatment of tumors	Rare-earth-doped aluminosilicate glasses
Artificial heart valves	Pyrolytic carbon coating
Otolaryngological	Al_2O_3 HA Bioactive glasses Bioactive glass ceramics PE–HA composite

[†]HA is hydroxyapatite, PE is polyethylene, and PLA is poly(lactic acid).

is that pain is minimized and the jawbone is rapidly stabilized. Similar procedures can be used to augment the jawbone when necessary to improve the stability of dental implants.[68,77]

Orthopedic applications, using 45S5 bioactive glass particulate, include bone grafting, repair of total hips and knees that have required revision surgery, and spinal fusion. The exciting finding is the hypothesis that bioactive glass is stimulating rapid proliferation of bone by activating a genetically controlled process that leads to production of growth factors.[41] The regenerated trabecular bone from this osteoconductive process is equivalent to normal bone, as shown by comparing the structure of the trabeculae in Fig. 27, created by filling the bone defect with 45S5 bioactive glass particulate with normal trabecular bone, shown in Fig. 2(A).

An especially important clinical application of bioactive implants is the use of A/W bioactive glass-ceramic in the repair of the spine. Professor T. Yamamuro recognized the clinical need of a bioactive ceramic with high strength and fracture toughness suitable for use as a replacement for vertebrae and, with Professor T. Kokubo and colleagues at Kyoto University, developed such a material in 1982.[36–40] The material is made by densifying 5-μm-sized glass powders into the desired shape, then precipitating oxyfluorapatite ($Ca_{10}(PO_4)_6(O,F_2)$) and wollastonite ($CaO–SiO_2$) phases to yield a crack- and pore-free, dense, homogenous glass-ceramic. The physical properties are summarized in Table IV. The high compressive and bend strengths, 1080 MPa and 215 MPa, respectively; high fracture toughness, 2.0 $MPa^{1/2}$; high interfacial bond strength to bone (Fig. 11); and excellent resistance to degradation of properties when exposed to physiological loading conditions (Fig. 28) provide confidence in the use of this material to replace surgically removed vertebrae.[63] In the past, when the vertebral column was extensively damaged by tumors or trauma, its reconstruction had been attempted by use of the patient's own

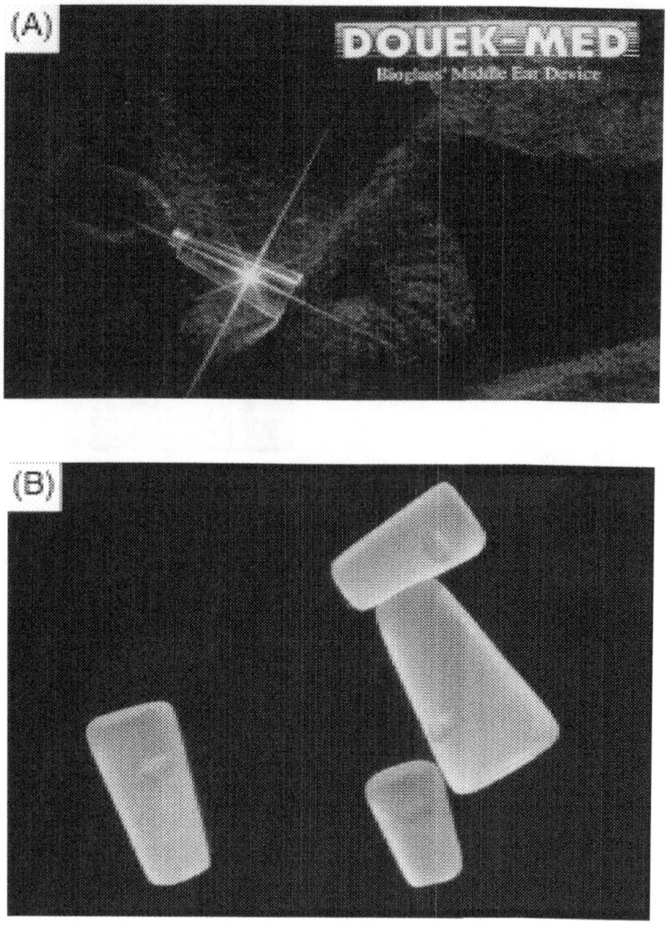

Fig. 19. (A) Schematic of bioactive glass (45S5) ossicular replacement prosthesis bonding to stapes footplate (left) and the eardrum (right). (B) Actual prostheses.

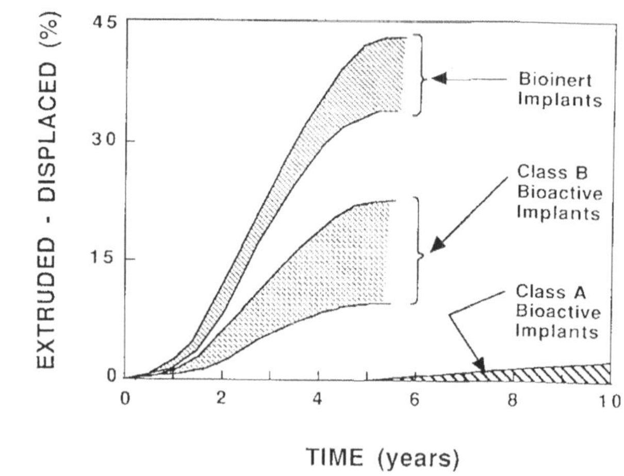

Fig. 20. Survivability comparison of bioinert implants. Class B bioactive implants (synthetic HA) and class A bioactive glass implants (45S5) used to replace middle-ear bones. (Analysis courtesy of Keith Lobel, University of Florida.)

(autogeneous) bone or cadaver (allograft) bone in combination with metals, PMMA bone cement, or Al_2O_3 ceramic. However, autogeneous allograft and bone have limited availability, and the long-term durability of non-bone-bonding implants was often unsatisfactory because of loosening and dislocation.[78,79] Since 1983, A/W glass-ceramic has been used successfully in vertebral replacement. Figure 29 shows four types of A/W prostheses. Use of bioactive glass-ceramic in repair of a burst

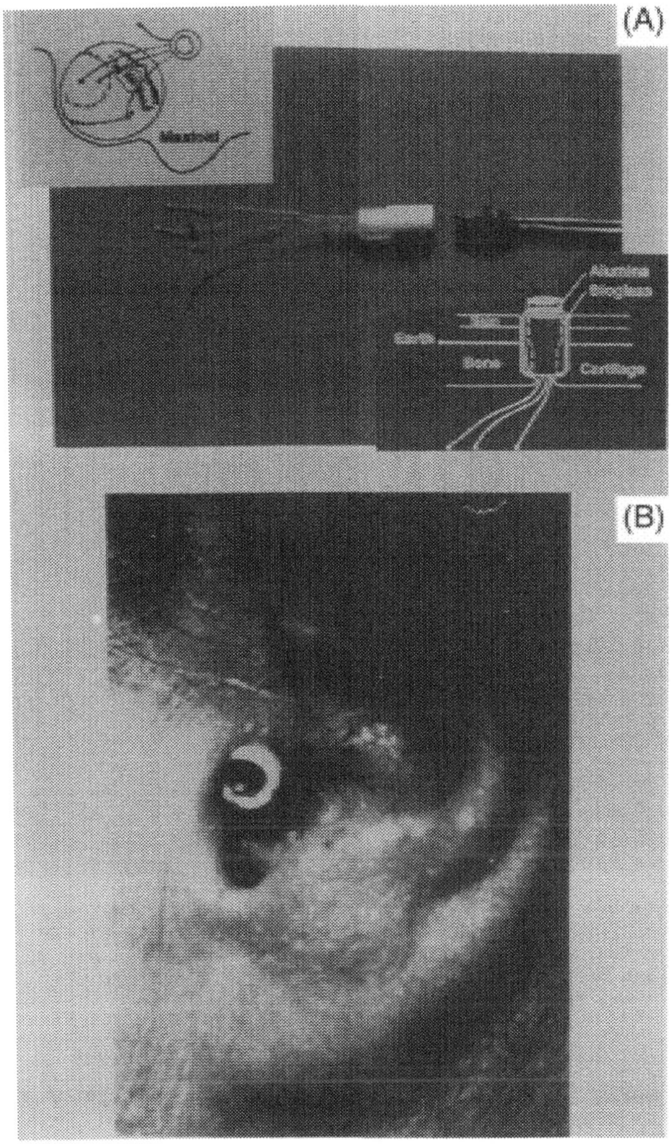

Fig. 21. (A) Extracochlear electric implant for the profound deaf showing electrode array (center), implantation site (upper left), and schematic of the components (lower right). (B) Implant in patient's ear, with electronics disconnected. (Photos courtesy Mr. Ellis Douek, Guy's Hospital, University of London.)

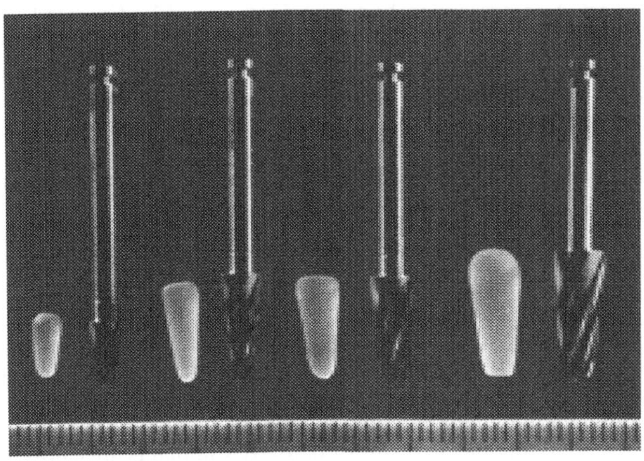

Fig. 22. Bioactive glass implants (45S5) and matching drill bits used to replace the roots of extracted teeth. (Photo courtesy of Dr. David Greenspan, U.S. Biomaterials Corp.)

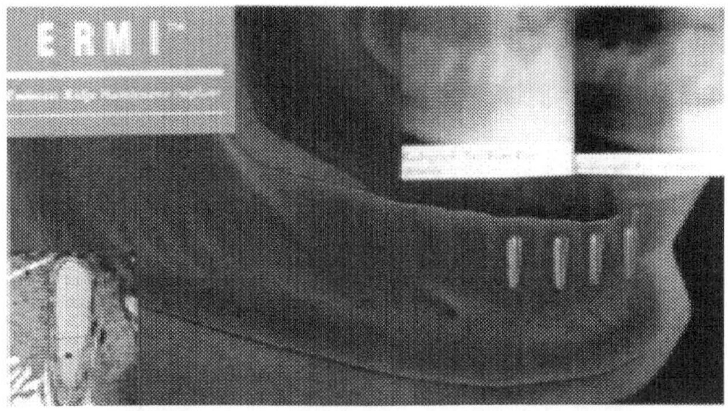

Fig. 23. Use of 45S5 bioactive glass endosseous ridge maintenance implants to maintain the thickness and width of the jawbone of denture wearers. Inserts show (lower left) bonding of alveolar bone to an implant and X-rays (far upper right) after implantation and (near right) after 2 years implantation.

fracture of the L_1 vertebra of a 48 year old man is shown in Fig. 30. Replacement of a L_2 vertebra that had malignant tumor metastasis with a A/W spacer is illustrated in Fig. 31. A case of spondyolisthesis with symptoms of lumbar canal stenosis repaired with bioactive glass-ceramic is shown in Fig. 32. The long-term (>10 years) successful use of A/W bioactive glass-ceramic is due to formation of trabecular bone bonded to all sides of the vertebral implant, as illustrated in Fig. 33, with a stable glass-ceramic–bone interface.

VI. Calcium Phosphate Ceramics

Calcium phosphate-based bioceramics have been in use in medicine and dentistry for 20 years.[3,10–13,25,33,66,67] Applications include coatings of orthopedic and dental implants, al-

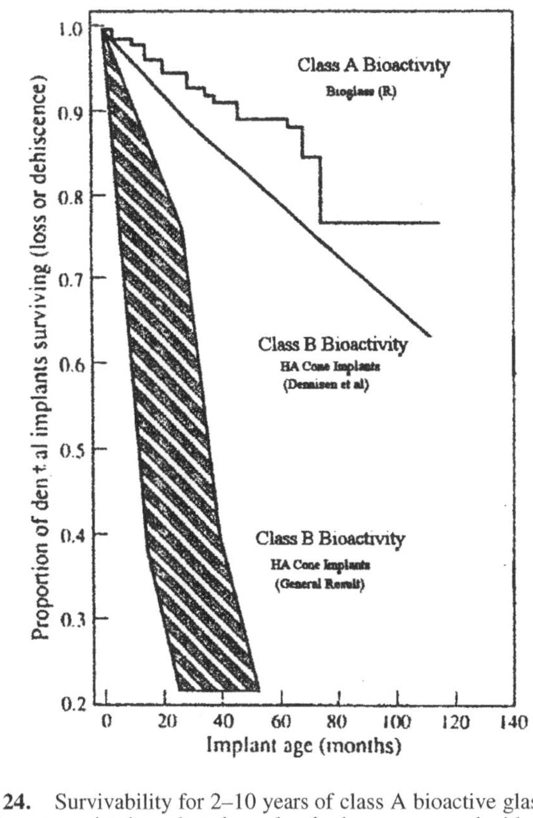

Fig. 24. Survivability for 2–10 years of class A bioactive glass cone implants to maintain endentulous alveolar bone compared with class B (synthetic HA) implants.

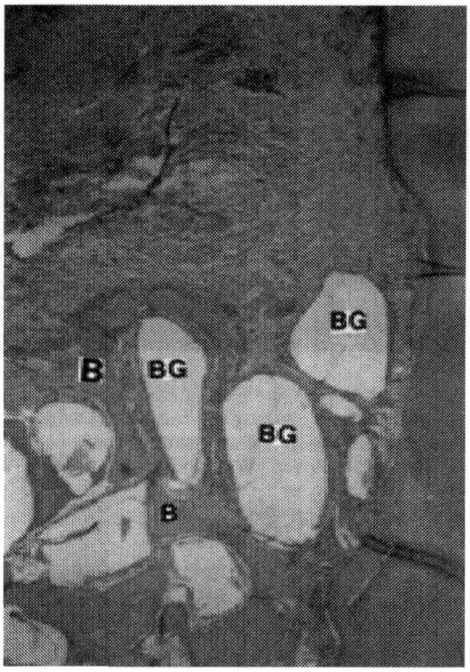

Fig. 25. Bioactive glass [BG] particulate used to enhance bone [B] formation around a tooth [T] and thereby restore its function following treatment of periodontal (gum) disease. (Photo courtesy of Dr. June Wilson.)

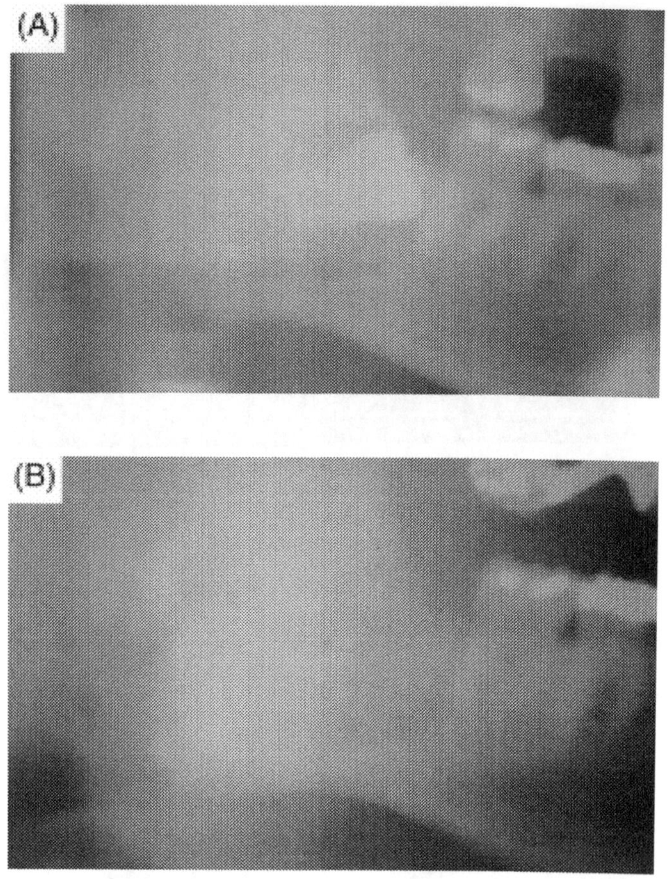

Fig. 26. Use of bioactive glass to fill bone defects: X-rays of (A) impacted third molar prior to extraction and (B) extraction site 3 months after filling with 45S5 bioactive glass particulate. Note that new bone has filled the space with an X-ray density equivalent to normal bone. (Photo courtesy of Dr. King Smith.)

veolar ridge augmentation, maxillofacial surgery, otolaryngology, and scaffolds for bone growth and as powders in total hip and knee surgery (Table VI). Different phases of calcium phosphate ceramics are used depending upon whether a resorbable or bioactive material is desired.

The stable phases of calcium phosphate ceramics depend considerably upon temperature and the presence of water, either during processing or in the use environment.[11] At body temperature, only two calcium phosphates are stable in contact with aqueous media, such as body fluids: at pH <4.2, the stable phase is $CaHPO_4{\cdot}2H_2O$ (dicalcium phosphate, brushite, C_2P), whereas, at pH >4.2, the stable phase is $Ca_{10}(PO_4)_6(OH)_2$ (HA). At higher temperatures, other phases, such as $Ca_3(PO_4)_2$ (β-tricalcium phosphate, C_3P, TCP) and $Ca_4P_2O_9$ (tetracalcium phosphate, C_4P) are present. The unhydrated, high-temperature calcium phosphate phases interact with water, or body fluids, at 37°C to form HA. Thus, the solubility of a TCP surface approaches the solubility of HA and decreases the pH of the solution, which further increases the solubility of TCP and enhances resorption. DeGroot,[10] Williams,[67] and LeGeros and LeGeros[81] have discussed the importance of the Ca:P ratio in determining solubility and tendency for resorbtion in the body. The presence of micropores in the sintered material can increase the solubility of these phases.[10–13,33]

Sintering of calcium phosphate ceramics usually occurs at 1000°–1500°C, following compaction of the powder into a desired shape.[10,33] The phases formed at high temperature depend on temperature and on the partial pressure of water (p_{H_2O}) in the sintering atmosphere. When water is present, HA can be formed and is a stable phase up to 1360°C, as shown in the phase equilibrium diagram for CaO and P_2O_5 with 500 mmHg (66 kPa) p_{H_2O} (Fig. 34). When there is no water, C_4P and C_3P are the stable phases.

The temperature range of HA stability increases with p_{H_2O}, as does the rate of phase transitions of C_3P or C_4P to HA. Because of kinetics barriers that affect the rates of formation of the stable calcium phosphate phases, it often is difficult to predict the volume fraction of high-temperature phases that are formed during sintering and their relative stability when cooled to room temperature.

Starting powders can be made by mixing, in an aqueous solution, the appropriate $CaNO_3:(NH_4)_3PO_4$ molar ratio that yields a precipitate of stoichiometric HA. The Ca^{2+}, PO_4^{3-}, and OH^- ions can be replaced by other ions during processing or in physiological surroundings; e.g., fluorapatite ($Ca_{10}(PO_4)_6(OH)_{2-x}F_x$, with $0 < x < 2$) and carbonate apatite ($Ca_{10}(PO_4)_6(OH)_{2-2x}(CO_3)_x$ or $Ca_{10-x+y}(PO_4)_{6-x}(OH)_{2-x-2y}$, where $0 < x < 2$ and $0 < y < x$) can be formed.[80] Fluorapatite is found in dental enamel and HCA is present in bone. Le Geros *et al.*[81] discussed the structure of these complex crystals. The mechanical behavior of calcium phosphate ceramics strongly influences their application as implants.[12] Tensile and compressive strength and fatigue resistance depend on the total volume of porosity. Porosity can be in the form of micropores (<1 μm diameter, due to incomplete sintering) or macropores (>100 μm diameter, created to permit bone growth).[82]

The Weibull modulus (m) of HA implants is low in physiological solutions (m = 12), which indicates low reliability under tensile loads. Consequently, in clinical practice, calcium phosphate bioceramics should be used as powders; small, unloaded implants; dental implants (with reinforcing metal posts); coatings on metal implants; low-loaded porous implants (where bone growth acts as a reinforcing phase); or bioactive phase in a polymer–bioactive ceramic composite.

The bonding mechanisms of dense HA implants appear to be very different from those described above for bioactive glasses.[33] A cellular bone matrix from differentiated osteoblasts appears at the surface, producing a narrow amorphous

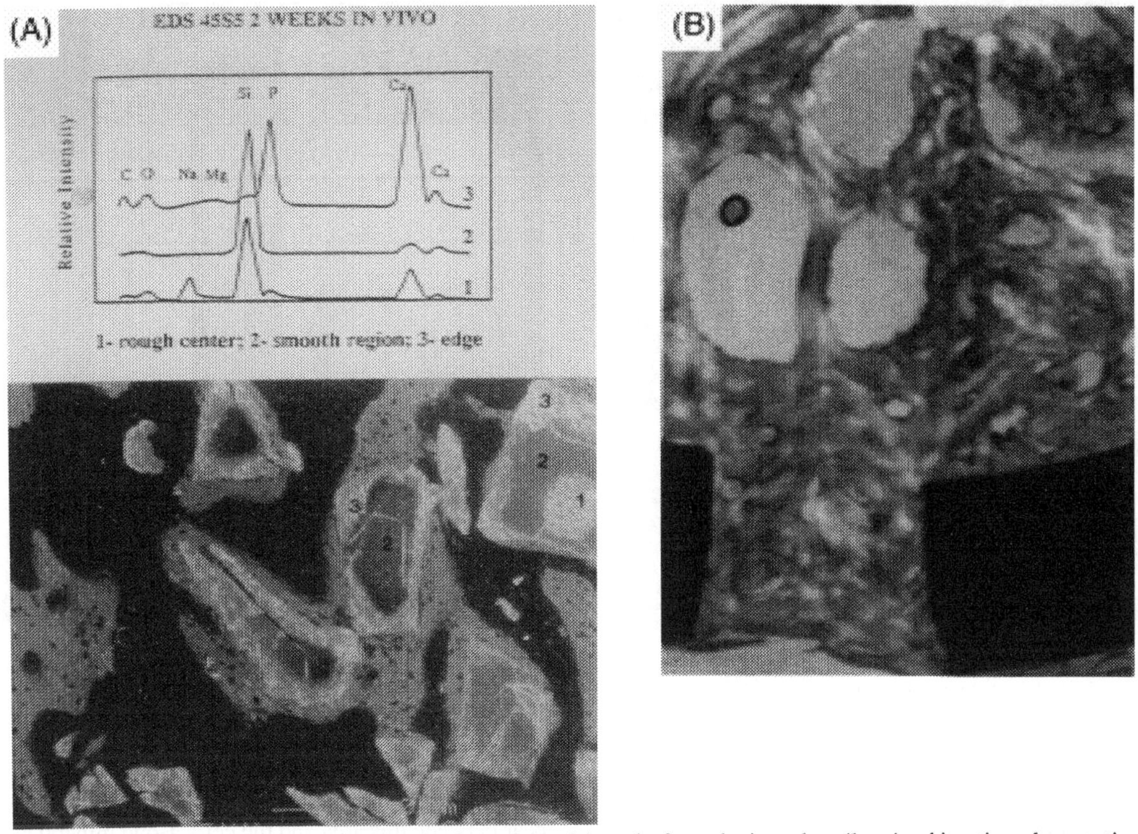

Fig. 27. (A) SEM micrograph of regenerated trabecular bone formed in only 2 weeks in a dog rib using bioactive glass particulate. Energy dispersive spectra of the compositional changes at the glass–bone interface is shown at the top of the figure. (Photo courtesy of Professor Marivalda Periera, Federal University of Minas Gerais, Brazil.) (B) Light microscopy micrograph of regenerated trabecular bone formed by use of bioactive glass (45S5) particulate inside a titanium cage fusing sheep vertebra. (Photo courtesy of Dr. Gary Lowery and Dr. June Wilson.)

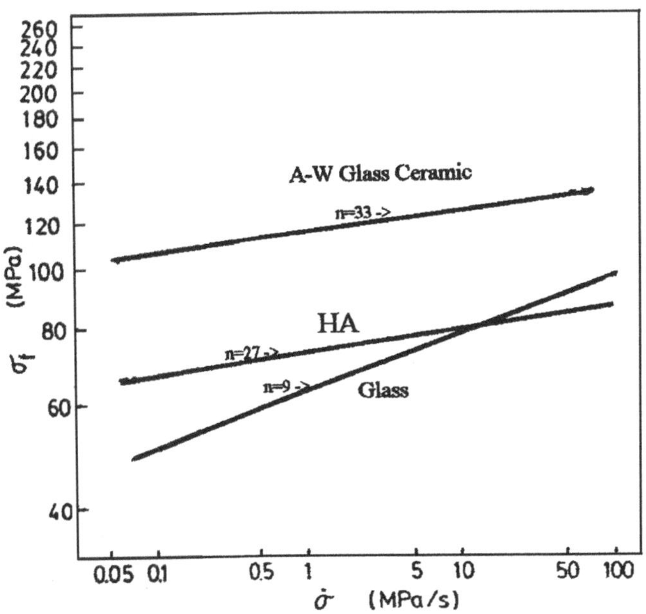

Fig. 28. Lifetime prediction diagrams for high-strength bioactive glass-ceramic A/W compared with dense HA ceramic and a bioactive glass. The A/W glass-ceramic withstands a flexural load of 65 MPa in the body for more than 10 years in contrast with HA, which is predicted to fail in <1 year. (Data courtesy of Professor T. Kokubo.)

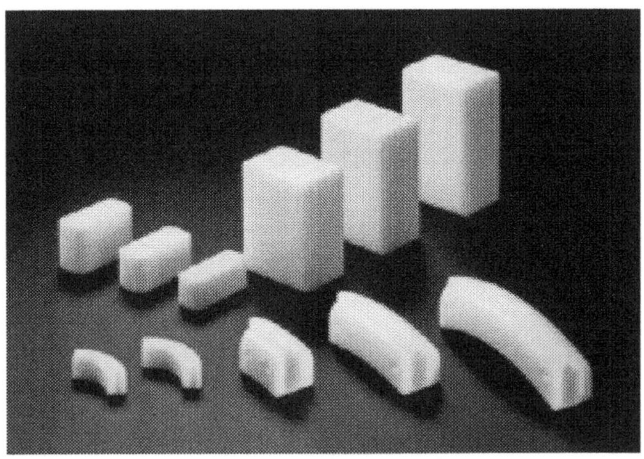

Fig. 29. Four types of bioactive glass-ceramic A/W prostheses for orthopedic applications: vertebral prostheses, iliac crest prostheses, intervertebral spacers, and laminoplasty spacers. (Photo courtesy of Nippon Electric Glass Co. and Professors T. Yamamuro and T. Kokubo, Kyoto University, Japan.)

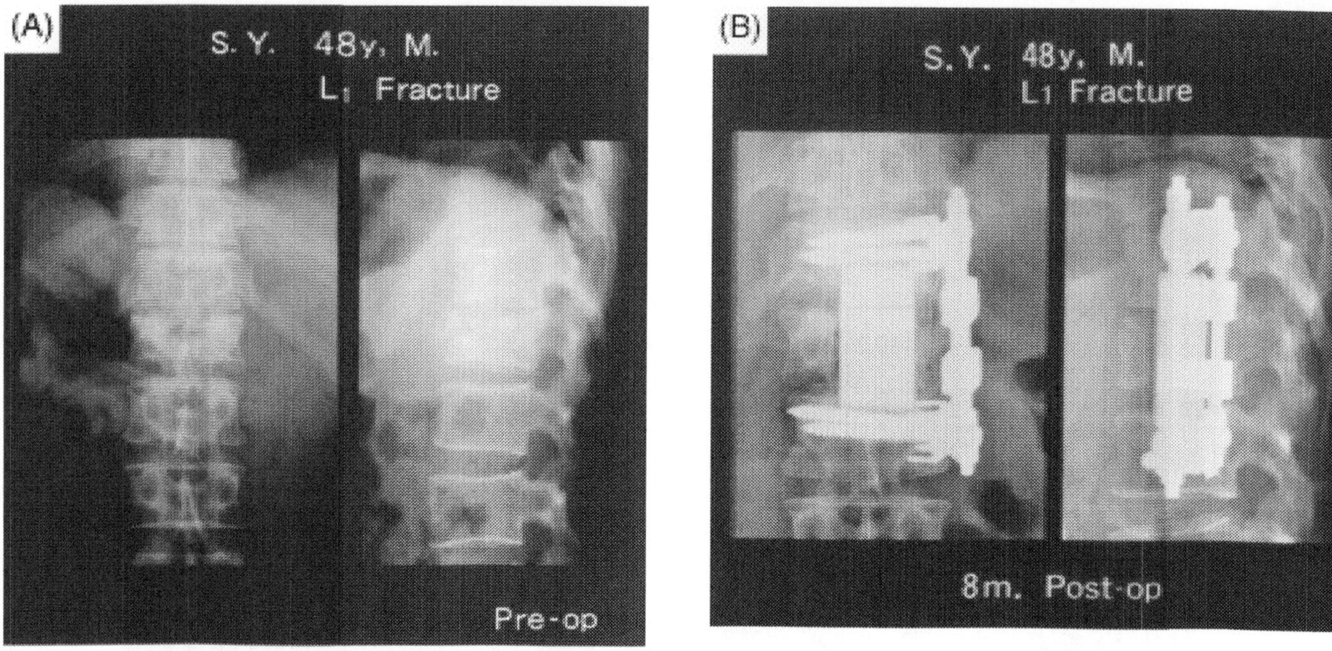

Fig. 30. X-rays of a case of burst fracture of the L_1 vertebra: (A) preoperative anterior–posterior and lateral views and (B) postoperative anterior–posterior and lateral views using bioactive glass-ceramic A/W prosthesis. (Photo courtesy of Professor T. Yamamuro.)

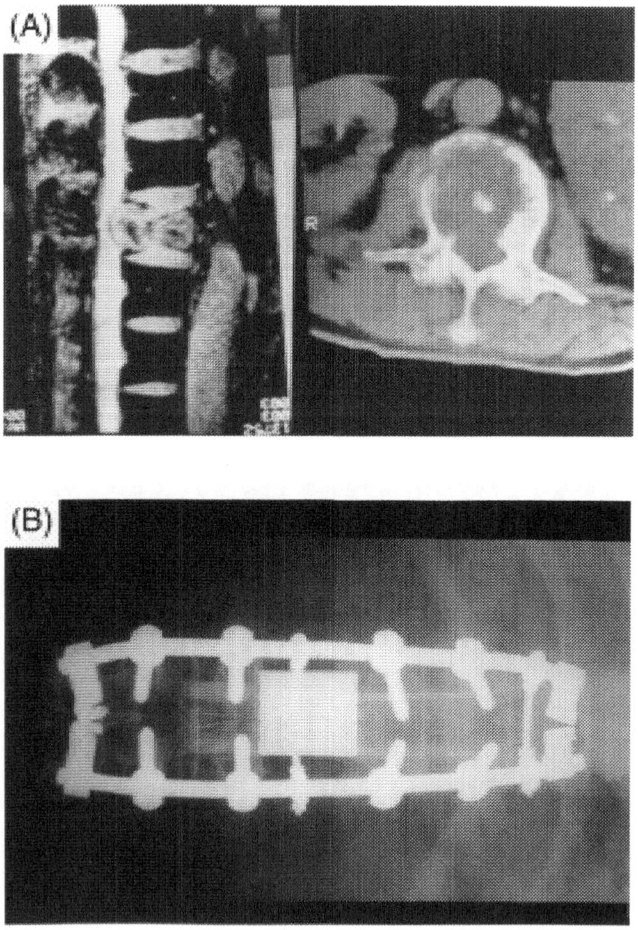

Fig. 31. Case of malignant tumor metastasis to L_2 vertebra: (A) preoperative MRI pictures and (B) postoperative anterior–posterior view using bioactive glass-ceramic A/W prosthesis to replace the vertebra. (Photo courtesy of Professor K. Tomita, Kamazawa University, Japan.)

electron dense band only 3–5 μm wide. Collagen bundles appear between this area and the cells. Bone mineral crystals have been identified in this otherwise amorphous area.[83] As the site matures, the bonding zone shrinks to a depth of only 0.05–0.2 μm. The result is normal bone attached through a thin epitaxial bonding layer to the bulk implant.[83] Ogiso *et al.*[84,85] have shown, through transmission electron microscopy (TEM) lattice image analysis of dense HA bone interfaces, an almost perfect epitaxial alignment of the growing bone crystallites with the apatite crystals in the implant (Fig. 35). A wide range of clinical applications of synthetic HA implants, both solid and porous, are described in Chs. 9–12 of Ref. 4 and in Refs. 3, 9–13, 22–26, 33, 66, 67, 73, 75, 77, 80, and 82.

VII. Composites

One of the primary restrictions on clinical use of bioceramics is the uncertain lifetime under the complex stress states, slow crack growth, and cyclic fatigue that result in many clinical applications. Two creative approaches to these mechanical limitations are use of bioactive ceramics as coatings, discussed above, and the biologically active phase in composites.[86–91] Bonfield argues[89] that analogous implant materials with similar mechanical properties should be the goal when bone is to be replaced. Because of the anisotropic deformation and fracture characteristics of cortical bone, which is itself a composite of compliant collagen fibrils and brittle HCA crystals, the Young's modulus varies ~7–25 GPa, the critical stress intensity ranges ~2–12 $MPa{\cdot}m^{1/2}$, and the critical strain intensity increases from as low as ~600 $J{\cdot}m^{-2}$ to as much as 5000 $J{\cdot}m^{-2}$, depending on orientation, age, and test condition.[103] In contrast, most bioceramics are much stiffer than bone and many exhibit poor fracture toughness (Table III). Figure 36 compares the strength and the elastic modulus of cortical and cancellous bone with various materials used for implants. The only materials that exhibit a range of properties equivalent to bone are composites. The approach used to achieve properties analogous to bone is to stiffen a compliant biocompatible synthetic polymer, such as polyethylene, with a higher-modulus ceramic second phase, such as HA powder.[102] The effect is to increase

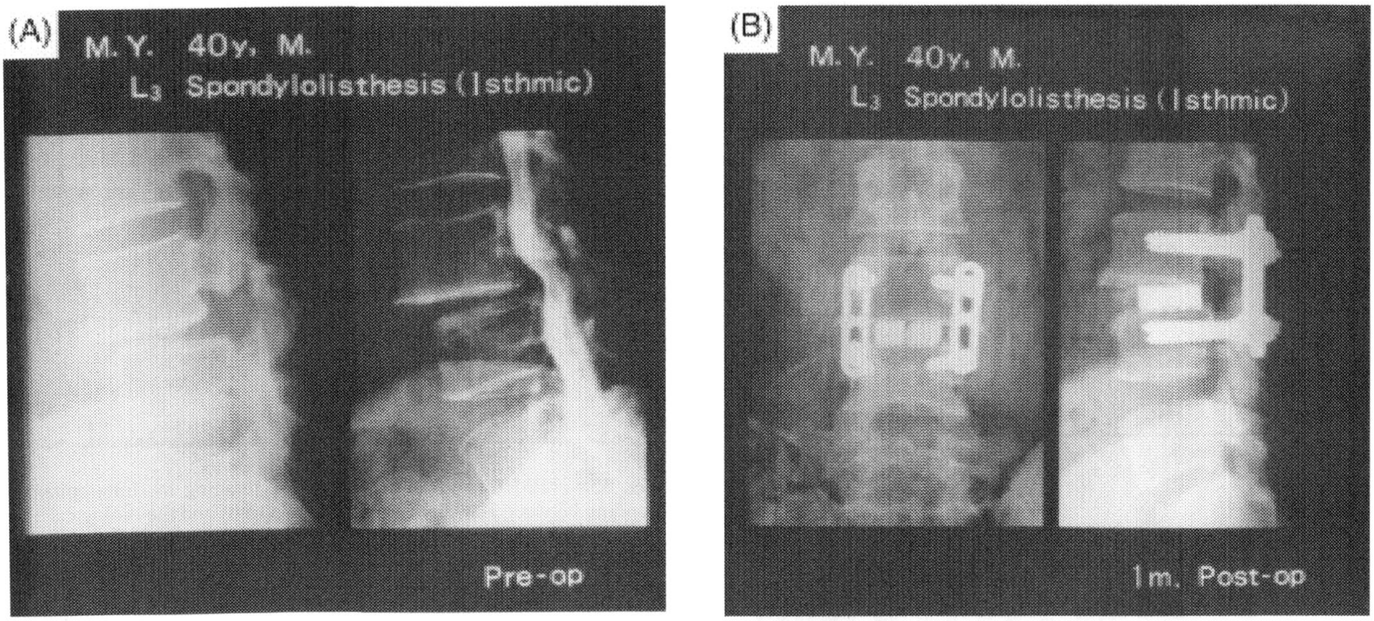

Fig. 32. Case of spondylolithesis with symptoms of lumbar canal stenosis: (A) preoperative lateral X-ray view (left) and lateral myelogram (right) and (B) postoperative anterior–posterior and lateral X-ray views using bioactive glass-ceramic A/W laminoplasty spacer. (Photo courtesy of Professor T. Yamamuro.)

Young's modulus from 1 to 8 GPa and to decrease the strain to failure from >90% to 3% (Fig. 37) as the volume fraction of HA increases to 0.5. The transition from ductile to brittle behavior occurs between 0.4 and 0.45 volume fraction HA. Bonfield reports[102] that the ultimate tensile strength of the composite remained within 22–26 MPa. At 0.45 volume fraction HA, the K_{IC} value was 2.9 ± 0.3 MPa·m$^{1/2}$, whereas, at <0.4 volume fraction HA, the fracture toughness was considerably greater because of the ductile deformation associated with crack propagation. Thus, the mechanical properties of the polyethylene–HA composite are similar to those of bone.

The bioactive phase is exposed by machining the surface of the composite. Bone-growing cells (osteoblasts) anchor onto the HA phase in the composite (Fig. 38) and proliferate.[91] Implant tests of the polyethylene–0.4 volume fraction HA composites demonstrated development of bone bonding between the natural hard tissue and the synthetic implant.[90]

Two clinical applications of the polyethylene–HA composite

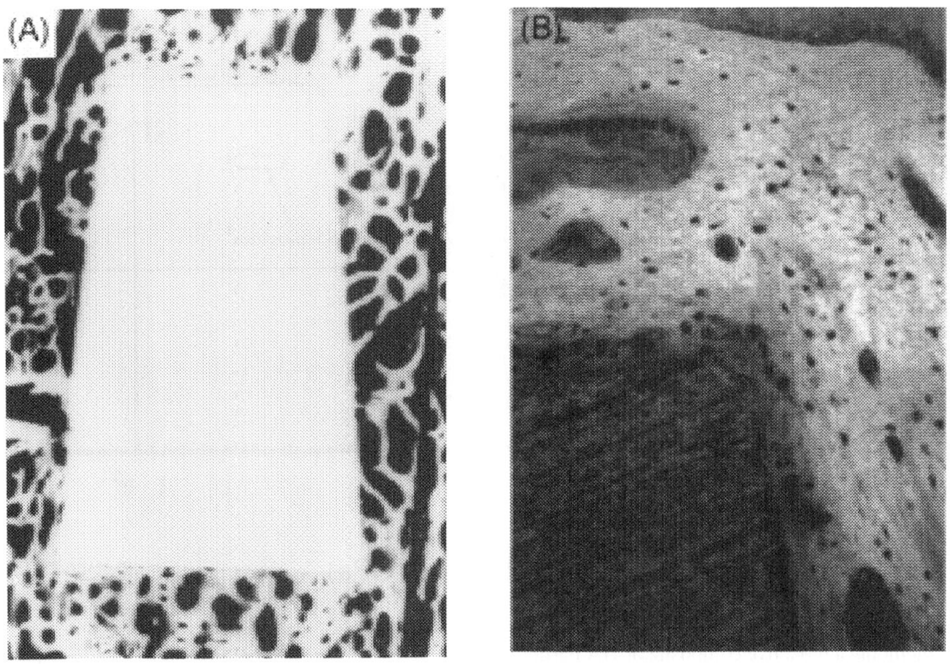

Fig. 33. Vertebral implant of bioactive glass-ceramic A/W in a sheep: (A) microradiograph showing trabecular bone bonding to all sides of the implant, 3 months following surgery and (B) histology of the bone bonding zone of the implant, 8 weeks after surgery. (Photo courtesy Professor T. Yamamuro.)

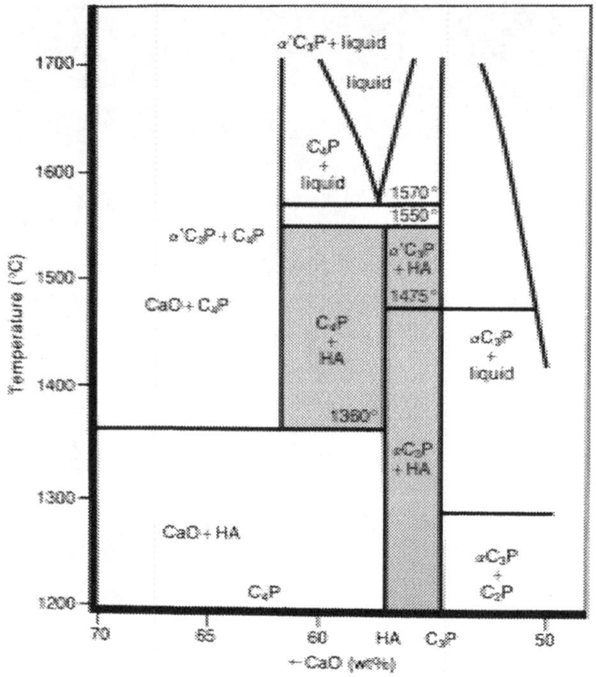

Fig. 34. Calcium phosphate phase equilibrium diagram with 500 mmHg p_{H_2O}. Shaded area is processing range to yield synthetic HA ceramic implants. (Diagram based upon the work[13] of Professor de Groot, University of Leiden.)

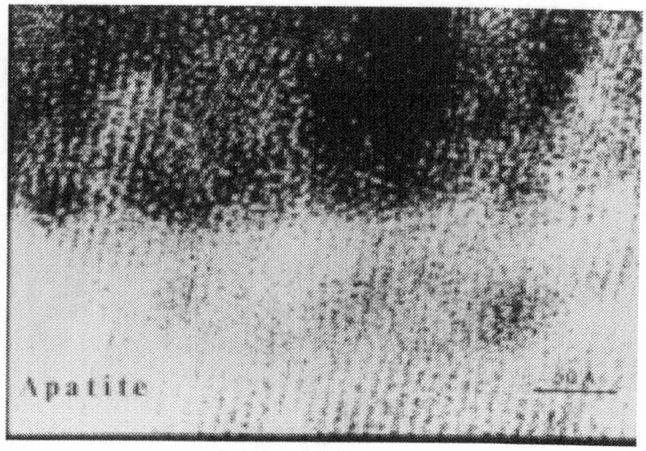

Fig. 35. TEM micrograph using lattice imaging to show epitaxial bonding between HA ceramic implant (bottom) and the biological HA phase of bone (top). (Photo courtesy of Dr. M. Ogiso.[84,85])

are shown in Figs. 39 and 40. It is used as ossicular prostheses (Fig. 39), where the stem of the device is made of the composite and the head is made of synthetic HA ceramic. The composite is very easily trimmed by the surgeon at the time of surgery to the size and configuration required for the patient. Figure 40(A) shows the use of the bioactive composite to repair a fractured orbital floor (eye socket) (Fig. 40(B)). The advantages offered by the composite are ease of shaping of the

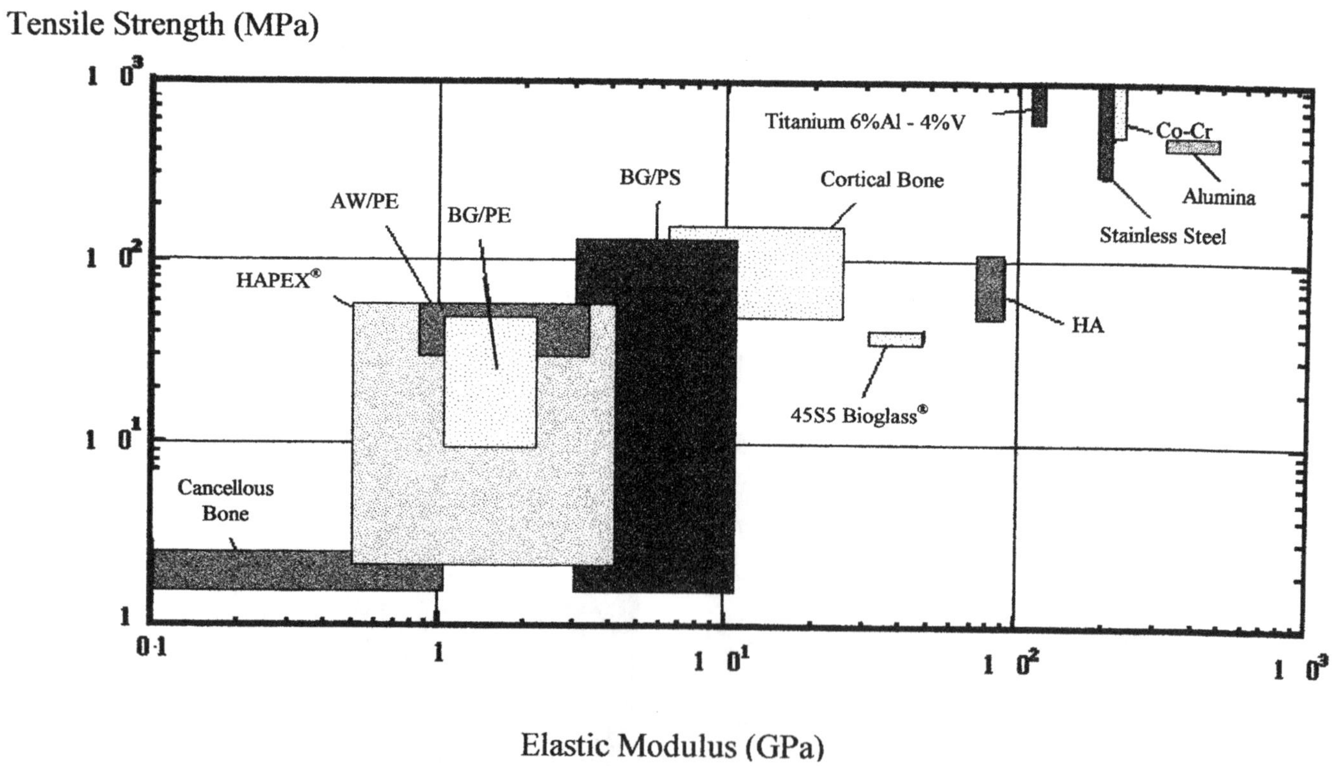

Fig. 36. Comparison of the range of mechanical properties, tensile strength, and elastic modulus of various biomaterials with cancellous, trabecular bone, and cortical bone, including a bioactive composite of HA particles in a polyethylene matrix: AW/PE is a bioactive composite of A/W particles in a polyethylene matrix; BG/PE is a bioactive composite of 45S5 bioactive glass particles in a polyethylene matrix; BG/PS is a bioactive composite of 45S5 bioactive glass or crystallized bioactive glass-ceramic particles in a polysulfone matrix; HA is dense, synthetic HA ceramic; Titanium–6%Al–4%V is an orthopedic alloy; Stainless Steel is 316L medical grade; Co-Cr is medical-grade orthopedic alloys; and Alumina is medical-grade Al_2O_3 (see Table III). (Graphic courtesy of I. Thompson and Y. Fujishiro.)

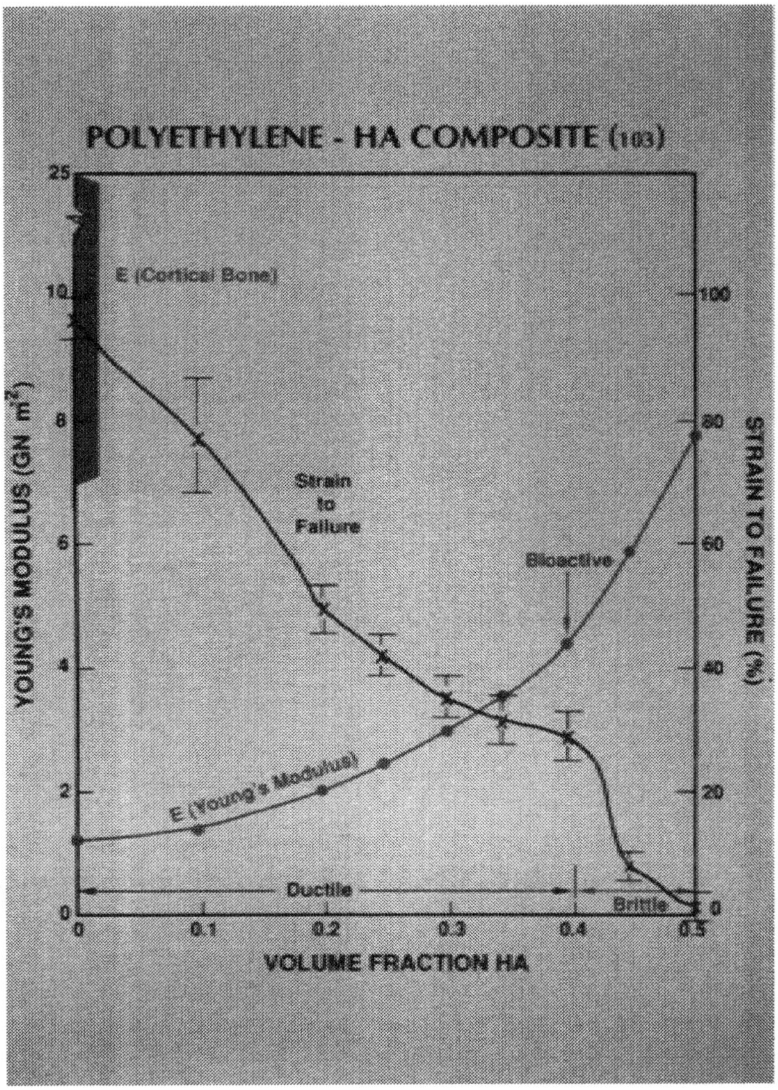

Fig. 37. Effect of HA on Young's Modulus and strain-to-failure of a polyethylene–HA composite. (Based upon data[89] of Professor Bill Bonfield, University of London IRC.)

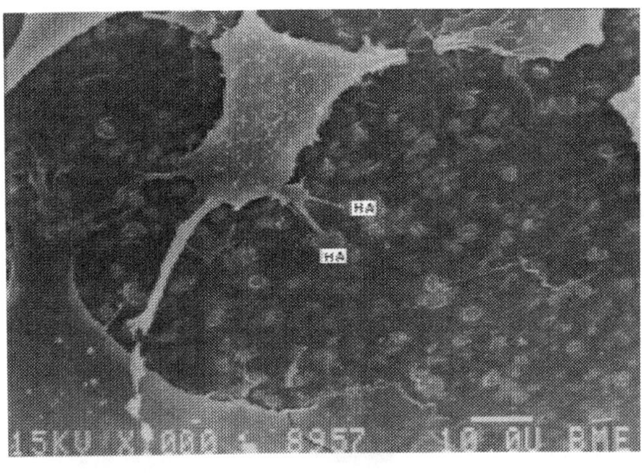

Fig. 38. SEM micrograph showing the anchoring of a bone-growing cell (osteoblast, OB) to HA particles in a bioactive composite of HA in a polyethylene matrix. (Photo courtesy of Professor Bill Bonfield and Dr. Elizabeth Tanner, University of London IRC.[91])

implant to meet the patient's needs at the time of surgery, formation of a bioactive bond to hold the implant in place, and mechanical properties that closely match those of the host tissues.

VIII. Coatings

(1) Carbon

For the ~40 000 patients per year in the United States that require heart valve replacement, the availability of high-performance carbon bioceramics can mean the difference between life and death. There are two classes of replacement heart valves: mechanical and tissue. Mechanical valves are made of synthetic, nonphysiological materials and represent about one-half of the valve replacements done at the present time. Tissue valves, also termed bioprosthetic valves, are usually fabricated from chemically preserved animal tissue, most often pig, mounted on a prosthetic frame, or can be a human aortic valve allograft. All types of replacement valves are a compromise over natural tissues and "within 10 years postoperatively valve-related complications occur in approximately 50% or more of patients having previously and currently used

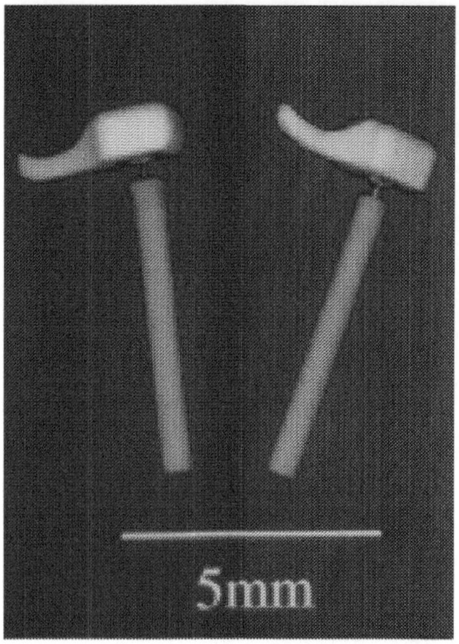

Fig. 39. Ossicular replacement prostheses. Head of the prosthesis is synthetic HA, and the stem is a bioactive composite of HA particles in a polyethylene matrix. (Photo courtesy of Professor Bill Bonfield and Dr. Elizabeth Tanner.)

substitute valves.''[92,93] The relative clinical merits of the two types of heart valves, mechanical versus tissue, are reviewed by Schoen *et al.*[93]

Because of their high mechanical reliability and resistance to blood clot formation, pyrolytic carbon-coated mechanical heart valves are often the valve replacement of choice. Bokros applied for a patent in 1967 describing the medical use of pyrolytic carbon coatings on metal substrates,[94] and the processing and applications in heart surgery were described soon thereafter.[95] The first time the low-temperature isotropic (LTI) carbon coatings were used in humans was as a prosthetic heart valve by DeBakey in 1969.[95] Many current prosthetic heart valves have LTI carbon coatings for the orifice and/or occluder (Fig. 41) because of the excellent resistance to blood clot formation and long fatigue life.[96] Almost a million lives have been prolonged through the use of this bioceramic in heart valves.[98]

Three types of carbon are used in biomedical devices: the LTI variety of pyrolytic carbon, glassy (vitreous) carbon, and the ultra-low-temperature isotropic (ULTI) form of vapor-deposited carbon.[97–99] These carbon materials are integral and monolithic materials (glassy carbon and LTI carbon) or impermeable thin coatings (ULTI carbon). These three forms do not suffer from the integrity problems typical of other available carbon materials. With the exception of the LTI carbons codeposited with silicon, all the carbon materials in clinical use are pure elemental carbon. Up to 20 wt% silicon has been added to LTI carbon without significantly affecting the biocompatibility of the material. The composition, structure, and fabrication of the three clinically relevant carbons are unique when compared with the more-common, naturally occurring form of carbon (i.e., graphite) and other industrial forms produced from pure elemental carbon.

The LTI, ULTI, and glassy carbons are subcrystalline forms and represent a lower degree of crystal perfection. There is no order between the layers such as there is in graphite; therefore, the crystal structure of these carbons is two-dimensional. Such a structure, called turbostratic, has densities of ~1400–2100 $kg\cdot m^{-3}$. High-density LTI carbons are the strongest bulk forms of carbon, and their strength can be increased further by adding

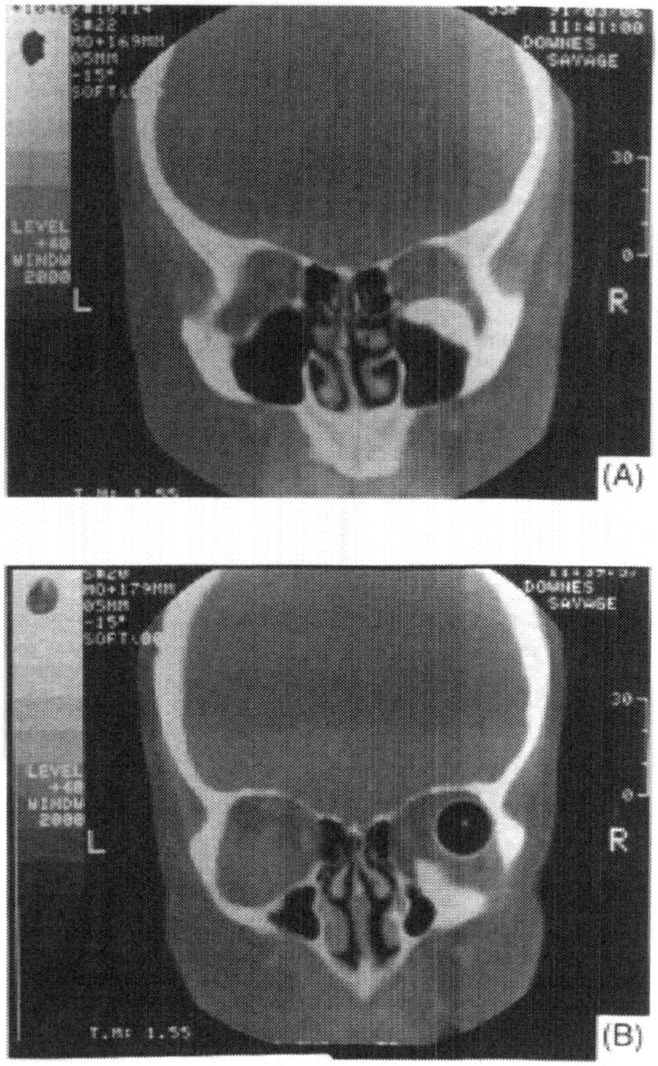

Fig. 40. X-ray of use of bioactive composite of HA particles in a polyethylene matrix in (A) repair of a fracture of the orbit of the eye shown in (B). (Photo courtesy of Professor Bill Bonfield and Dr. Elizabeth Tanner.)

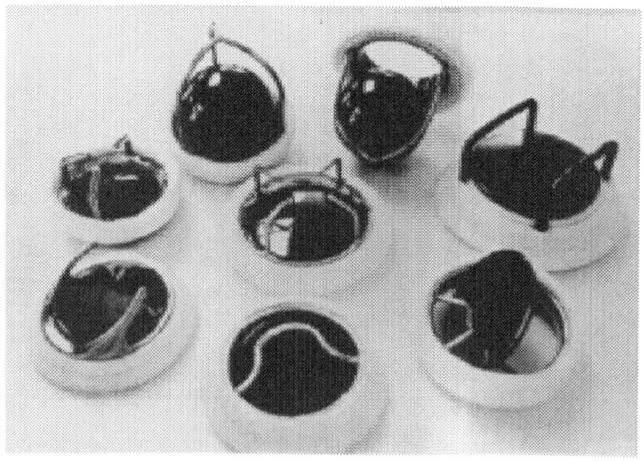

Fig. 41. Low-temperature isotropic (LIT) pyrolitic-carbon-coated heart valves. (Photo courtesy of Dr. Jack Bokros.)

silicon. ULTI carbon also can be produced with high densities and strengths, but it is available only as a thin coating (0.1–1.0 μm) of pure carbon. Glassy carbon is inherently a low-density material and, as such, is weak. Its strength cannot be increased through processing. Processing of all three types of medical carbons are discussed in Haubold *et al.*[98]

The mechanical properties of the various carbons are intimately related to their microstructures. It is possible to generate materials with low elastic moduli (20 GPa) and high flexural strength (275–620 MPa) in an isotropic carbon. There are many benefits as a result of this combination of properties, e.g., large strains (~2%) are possible without fracture. The turbostratic carbons are very tough when compared with ceramics, such as Al_2O_3. The energy to fracture for LTI carbon is ~5.5 $MJ \cdot m^{-3}$, compared with 0.18 $MJ \cdot m^{-3}$ for Al_2O_3; i.e., the carbon is ~25 times as tough.

The turbostratic carbon materials have extremely good wear resistance, part of which can be attributed to their toughness, i.e., their capacity to sustain large local elastic strains under concentrated or point loading without galling or incurring surface damage. The bond strength of the ULTI carbon to stainless steel and to Ti–6Al–4V exceeds 70 MPa, as measured with a thin-film adhesion tester. This excellent bond is achieved, in part, through the formation of interfacial carbides. The ULTI carbon coating generally has a lower bond strength with materials that do not form carbides.

Because of the extremely large number of loading cycles involved in a heart valve, 38 million beats/year,[99] an important characteristic of the turbostratic carbons is their fatigue resistance. In general, cyclic fatigue resistance of LTI carbon coatings on titanium or cobalt–chromium alloys is excellent. It is especially important to eliminate small cracks at the interface of the coating and the metallic substrate during processing and handling to assure long lifetimes under cyclic fatigue conditions, as discussed by Dauskardt and Ritchie.[99] Properties of the turbostratic carbons are listed in Ref. 98 with uses of glassy, LTI, and ULTI carbons in various medical areas.

(2) *Hydroxyapatite*

Another bioceramic coating that has reached a significant level of clinical application is the use of HA, as a coating on porous metal surfaces for fixation of orthopedic prostheses (Fig. 42). This approach combines types II and III methods of fixation (Table II) and originates from the observations of Ducheyne and colleagues[9] in 1980 that HA powder in the pores of a porous, coated-metal implant would significantly affect the rate and vitality of bone in growth into the pores. Many investigators have explored various means of applying the HA coating,[3,10,13,25,26] with plasma spray coating generally being preferred.[26,100] There is a substantial enhancement of the early stage interfacial bond strength of implants with a plasma-sprayed HA coating when compared with porous metals without the coating, as illustrated in Fig. 9.[101] Long-term animal studies and clinical trials of load-bearing dental and orthopedic prostheses suggest that some HA coatings may degrade or come off with time, depending upon the degree of crystallinity of the HA layer.[25,26] The clinical consequences continue to be debated and will not be conclusive until 10 year survivability statistics from multiple clinical centers have been reported.[102,103] However, early results are encouraging as an alternative to PMMA ''bone cement'' fixation of orthopedic devices.

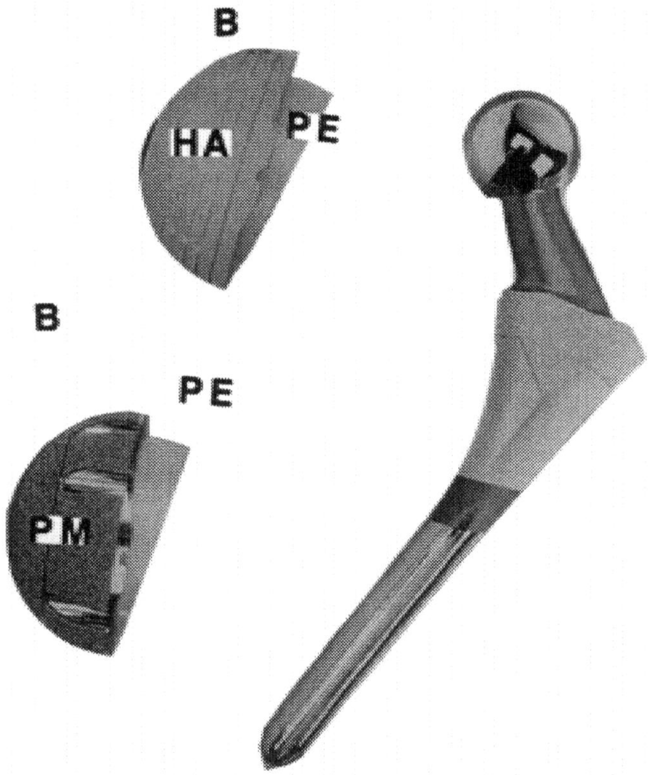

Fig. 42. Synthetic HA coatings on (A) femoral stem and (B) acetabular cup of a total hip prosthesis. Note the porous metal [PM] surface prior to coating and the ultra-high molecular-weight of polyethylene [PE] liner used in the cups to minimize friction. (Photo courtesy of Dr. Bernard Kapp, Stratec Medical.)

IX. Therapeutic Applications

A significant problem in the radiation treatment of cancer is the serious systemic side effects. Localization of the radiation at the site of the tumor decreases the radiation dosage required to kill the cancer cells and thereby minimizes side effect toxicities. An innovative approach to the localized delivery of radioactive yttrium-90 (Y^{90}) to treat liver cancer has been developed by Delbert Day at University of Missouri-Rolla using glass microspheres.[104] A yttria aluminosilicate (YAS) glass, containing Y^{89}, is made in the form of 25 μm microspheres. The microspheres, prior to use in hepatic arterial infusion therapy, are bombarded by neutrons that create Y^{90}, a radioactive isotope that is a short-half-life (64 h), short-range (2.5–3 mm in the liver) β-emitter. The microspheres are injected through a catheter placed in an artery, and the blood stream carries them to the liver, where a high proportion goes to the cancerous part because of the approximately 3 times increased blood supply. A localized dosage of up to 15×10^3 rads can be delivered in this manner, whereas a maximum of 3×10^3 rads of external radiation can be tolerated by the patient. The YAS glass microspheres have been safely used for more than 5 years to irradiate, up to 15×10^3 rads, malignant tumors in the liver in more than 100 patients. The rare-earth aluminosilicate glass system provides excellent chemical durability in the body, which is important, because it keeps the radioisotope concentrated in the target organ and prevents dissolution and migration via the circulation of blood. Application of this concept is being explored for treatment of tumors in the kidney and also for treatment of arthritic joints.[104]

X. Summary

Bioceramics has become an integral and vital segment of our modern health care delivery system. The full potential has only begun to be recognized as this century ends. Most of the developments to date have been based upon trial-and-error experiments. However, a theoretical foundation for the development of a new generation of bioceramics now exists. In the next century, the composition, microstructure, and molecular surface chemistry of various types of bioceramics will be tailored to match the specific biological and metabolic requirements of tissues or disease states. This "molecular-based pharmaceutical" approach to the design of bioceramics will be coupled with tissue and genetic engineering, sensor technology, and information processing to produce a range of products and applications not imagined presently. This new generation of bioceramics should enhance the quality of life of millions of people as they grow older.

Acknowledgments: The author acknowledges the long-term collaboration with June Wilson-Hench, wife and coresearcher, who helped establish the scientific understanding of bioactive glasses discussed herein; Dr. David Greenspan, who has led the effort to achieve clinical success; Alice Holt, who has provided the secretarial support throughout the 30 years of effort; the U.S. Army Medical Research and Development Command, that funded the first 10 years of studies; and the U.S. Air Force Office of Scientific Research, for financial support during the past 15 years.

References

[1]L. L. Hench and E. C. Ethridge, *Biomaterials: An Interfacial Approach.* Academic Press, New York, 1982.

[2]J. D. Preston, "Properties in Dental Ceramics"; in *Proceedings of the IV International Symposium on Dental Materials.* Quintessa, Chicago, IL, 1988.

[3]S. F. Hulbert, J. C. Bokros, L. L. Hench, J. Wilson, and G. Heimke, "Ceramics in Clinical Applications: Past, Present, and Future"; pp. 189–213 in *High Tech Ceramics.* Edited by P. Vincenzini. Elsevier, Amsterdam, The Netherlands, 1987.

[4]L. L. Hench and J. Wilson, *An Introduction to Bioceramics.* World Scientific, London, U.K., 1993.

[5]U. Gross, R. Kinne, H. J. Schmitz, and V. Strunz, "The Response of Bone to Surface Active Glass/Glass-Ceramics," *CRC Crit. Rev. Biocompat.*, **4**, 2 (1988).

[6]P. Christel, A. Meunier, J. M. Dorlot, J. M. Crolet, J. Witvolet, L. Sedel, and P. Boritin, "Biomechanical Compatibility and Design of Ceramic Implants for Orthopaedic Surgery'; p. 234 in *Bioceramics: Material Characteristics Versus In Vivo Behavior*, Vol. 523. Edited by P. Ducheyne and J. Lemons. Annals of New York Academy of Science, New York, 1988.

[7]L. L. Hench, "Cementless Fixation"; p. 23 in *Biomaterials and Clinical Applications.* Edited by A. Pizzoferrato, P. G. Marchetti, A. Ravaglioli, and A. J. C. Lee. Elsevier, Amsterdam, The Netherlands, 1987.

[8]J. Black, "Systemic Effects of Biomaterials," *Biomaterials*, **5**, 11 (1984).

[9]P. Ducheyne, L. L. Hench, A. Kagan, M. Martens, A. Burssens, and J. C. Mulier, "The Effect of Hydroxyapatite Impregnation of Skeletal Bonding of Porous Coated Implants," *J. Biomed. Mater. Res.*, **14**, 225 (1980).

[10]K. de Groot, *Bioceramics of Calcium-Phosphate.* CRC Press, Boca Raton, FL, 1983.

[11]K. de Groot, "Effect of Porosity and Physicochemical Properties on the Stability, Resorption, and Strength of Calcium Phosphate Ceramics"; see Ref. 6, pp. 227–34.

[12]K. de Groot and R. Le Geros; see Ref. 6, pp. 268, 272.

[13]K. de Groot, C. P. A. T. Klein, J. G. C. Wolke, and J. de Blieck-Hogervorst, "Chemistry of Calcium Phophate Bioceramics"; pp. 3–15 in *Handbook of Bioactive Ceramics*, Vol. II. Edited by T. Yamamuro, L. L. Hench, and J. Wilson. CRC Press, Boca Raton, FL, 1990.

[14]L. L. Hench, R. J. Splinter, W. C. Allen, and T. K. Greenlee Jr., "Bonding Mechanisms at the Interface of Ceramic Prosthetic Materials," *J. Biomed. Mater. Res.*, **2** [1] 117–41 (1971).

[15]L. L. Hench, "Bioceramics: From Concept to Clinic," *J. Am. Ceram. Soc.*, **74** [7] 1487–510 (1991).

[16]P. M. Boutin, "A View of 15 Year Results Obtained Using the Alumina–Alumina Hip Joint Replacement"; p. 297 in *Ceramics in Clinical Applications.* Edited by P. Vincenzini. Elsevier, New York, 1987.

[17]J. Black and G. Hastings, *Handbook of Biomaterial Properties.* Chapman and Hall, London, U.K., 1998.

[18]H. Plenk, "Biocompatibility of Ceramics in Joint Prostheses"; in *Biocompatibility of Orthopaedic Implants*, Vol. 1; pp. 269–85. CRC Press, Boca Raton, FL, 1982.

[19]G. Willmann, "Ceramic Components for Total Hip Arthroplasty," *Orthopaedics Int. Ed.*, **5** [4] 110–15 (1997).

[20]E. Dörre and W. Dawihl, "Ceramic Hip Endoprostheses"; pp. 113–27 in *Mechanical Properties of Biomaterials.* Edited by G. W. Hastings and D. F. Williams. Wiley, New York, 1980.

[21]J. E. Ritter, D. C. Greenspan, R. A. Palmer, and L. L. Hench, "Use of Fracture Mechanics Theory in Lifetime Predictions for Alumina and Bioglass-Coated Alumina," *J. Biomed Mater. Res.*, **13**, 251–63 (1979).

[22]R. T. Chiroff, E. W. White, J. N. Webber, and D. Roy, "Tissue Ingrowth of Replamineform Implants," *J. Biomed. Mater. Res. Symp.*, **6**, 29–45 (1975).

[23]E. W. White, J. N. Webber, D. M. Roy, E. L. Owen, R. T. Chiroff, and R. A. White, "Replamineform Porous Biomaterials for Hard Tissue Implant Applications," *J. Biomed. Mater. Res. Symp.*, **6**, 23–27 (1975).

[24]R. E. Holmes, R. W. Mooney, R. W. Bucholz, and A. F. Tencer, "A Coralline Hydroxyapatite Bone Graft Substitute," *Clin. Orthop. Relat. Res.*, **188**, 282–92 (1984).

[25]T. Yamamuro, L. L. Hench, and June Wilson (Eds.), Handbook of Bioactive Ceramics, Vol. II, *Calcium Phosphate and Hydroxylapatite Ceramics.* CRC Press, Boca Raton, FL, 1990.

[26]W. R. Lacefield, "Hydroxylapatite Coatings"; see Ref. 4, Ch. 12.

[27]L. L. Hench, "Bioactive Ceramics"; see Ref. 6, p. 54.

[28]C. A. Beckham, T. K. Greenlee Jr., and A. R. Crebo, "Bone Formation at a Ceramic Implant Interface," *Calcif. Tissue Res.*, **8**, 165–71 (1971).

[29]T. K. Greenlee Jr., C. A. Beckman, A. R. Crebo, and J. C. Malmborg, "Glass Ceramic Bone Implants," *J. Biomed. Mater. Res.*, **6**, 235–44 (1972).

[30]L. L. Hench and J. W. Wilson, "Surface-Active Biomaterials," *Science (Washington, D.C.)*, **226**, 630 (1984).

[31]U. Gross and V. Strunz, "The Interface of Various Glasses and Glass-Ceramics with a Bony Implantation Bed," *J. Biomed. Mater. Res.*, **19**, 251 (1985).

[32]W. Hohland, W. Vogel, K. Naurnann, and J. Gummel, "Interface Reactions between Machinable Bioactive Glass-Ceramics and Bone," *J. Biomed. Mater. Res.*, **19**, 303 (1985).

[33]M. Jarcho, "Calcium Phosphate Ceramics as Hard Tissue Prosthetics," *Clin. Orthop. Relat. Res.*, **157**, 259 (1981).

[34]T. Nakamura, T. Yamamuro, S. Higashi, T. Kokubo, and S. Itoo, "A New Glass-Ceramic for Bone Replacement: Evaluation of its Bonding to Bone Tissue," *J. Biomed. Mater. Res.*, **19**, 685 (1985).

[35]J. Wilson, G. H. Pigott, F. J. Schoen, and L. L. Hench, "Toxicology and Biocompatibility of Bioglass," *J. Biomed. Mater. Res.*, **15**, 805 (1981).

[36]T. Kokubo, S. Ito, S. Sakka, and T. Yamamuro, "Formation of a High-Strength Bioactive Glass-Ceramic in the System MgO–CaO–SiO_2–P_2O_5," *J. Mater. Sci.*, **21**, 536 (1986).

[37]T. Kitsugi, T. Yamamuro, and T. Kokubo, "Bonding Behavior of a Glass-Ceramic Containing Apatite and Wollastonite in Segmental Replacement of the Rabbit Tibia Under Load-Bearing Conditions," *J. Bone, Jt. Surg.*, **71A**, 264 (1989).

[38]S. Yoshii, Y. Kakutani, T. Yamamuro, T. Nakamura, T. Kitsugi, M. Oka, T. Kokubo, and M. Takagi, "Strength of Bonding between A-W Glass Ceramic and the Surface of Bone Cortex," *J. Biomed. Mater. Res.*, **22** [A] 327 (1988).

[39]T. Yamamuro, J. Shikata, Y. Kakutani, S. Yoshii, T. Kitsugi, and K. Ono, "Novel Methods for Clinical Applications of Bioactive Ceramics"; see Ref. 6, p. 107.

[40]T. Yamamuro, L. L. Hench, and J. Wilson (Eds.), *Handbook on Bioactive Ceramics: Bioactive Glasses and Glass-Ceramics*, Vol. I. CRC Press, Boca Raton, FL, 1990.

[41]L. L. Hench and J. K. West, "Biological Applications of Bioactive Glasses," *Life Chem. Rep.*, **13**, 187–241 (1996).

[42]J. Wilson and D. Nolletti, "Bonding of Soft Tissues to Bioglass®"; see Ref. 40, pp. 283–302.

[43]L. L. Hench and H. A. Paschall, "Direct Chemical Bonding between Bio-Active Glass-Ceramic Materials and Bone," *J. Biomed. Mater. Res. Symp.*, **4**, 25–42 (1973).

[44]L. L. Hench and A. E. Clark, "Adhesion to Bone"; Ch. 6 in *Biocompatibility of Orthopedic Implants*, Vol. 2. Edited by D. F. Williams. CRC Press, Boca Raton, FL, 1982.

[45]Ö. H. Andersson, G. Liu, K. H. Karlsson, L. Niemi, J. Miettinen, and J. Juhanoja, "*In Vivo* Behavior of Glasses in the SiO_2–Na_2O–CaO–P_2O_5–Al_2O_3–B_2O_3 System," *J. Mater. Sci., Mater. Med.*, **1**, 219–27 (1990).

[46]D. C. Greenspan and L. L. Hench, "Chemical and Mechanical Behavior of Bioglass-Coated Alumina," *J. Biomed. Mater. Res.*, **10** [4] 503–509 (1976).

[47]A. W. Ham, *Histology.* Lippincott, Philadelphia, PA, 1969.

[48]G. W. Hastings and P. Ducheyne (Eds.), *Natural and Living Materials.* CRC Press, Boca Raton, FL, 1984.

[49]U. M. Gross and V. Strunz, "The Anchoring of Glass Ceramics of Different Solubility in the Femur of the Rat," *J. Biomed. Mater. Res.*, **14**, 607 (1980).

[50]U. Gross, J. Brandes, V. Strunz, J. Bab, and J. Sela, "The Ultrastructure of the Interface Between a Glass Ceramic and Bone," *J. Biomed. Mater. Res.*, **15**, 291 (1981).

[51]U. M. Gross, C. Müller-Mai, and C. Voight, "Ceravital® Bioactive Glass-Ceramics"; see Ref. 4, pp. 105–23.

[52]U. Gross, W. Roggendorf, H. J. Schmitz, and V. Strunz, "Testing Procedures for Surface Reactive Biomaterials"; p. 367 in *Biological and Biomechanical Performance of Biomaterials.* Edited by P. Christel, A. Meunier, and A. J. C. Lee. Elsevier, Amsterdam, The Netherlands, 1986.

[53]W. Vogel, W. Hohland, K. Naumann, J. Vogel, G. Carl, W. Gotz, and P. Wange, "Glass-Ceramics for Medicine and Dentistry"; see Ref. 40, p. 353.

[54]Ö. H. Andersson, K. H. Karlsson, K. Kangasniemi, and A. Yli-Urop, "Models for Physical Properties and Bioactivity of Phosphate Opal Glasses," *Glastech. Ber.*, **61**, 300–305 (1988).

[55]K. Kangasniemi and A. Yti-Urpo, "Biological Response to Glasses in the SiO_2–Na_2O–CaO–P_2O_5–B_2O_3 System"; see Ref. 40, pp. 97–108.

[56]A. E. Clark, C. Y. Kim, J. K. West, J. Wilson, and L. L. Hench, "Reactions of Fluoride- and Nonfluoride-Containing Bioactive Glasses"; see Ref. 40, p. 73.

[57]M. Ogino, F. Ohuchi, and L. L. Hench, "Compositional Dependence of the Formation of Calcium Phosphate Films on Bioglass," *J. Biomed. Mater. Res.*, **14**, 55–64 (1980).

[58]A. E. Clark, C. G. Pantano, and L. L. Hench, "Auger Spectroscopic Analysis of Bioglass Corrosion Films," *J. Am. Ceram. Soc.*, **59** [1–2] 37–39 (1976).

[59]L. L. Hench, H. A. Paschall, W. C. Allen, and G. Piotrowski, "Interfacial Behavior of Ceramic Implants," *Natl. Bur. Stand. (U.S.) Spec. Publ.*, **415**, 19–35 (1975).

[60]L. L. Hench and H. A. Paschall, "Histo-Chemical Responses at a Biomaterials Interface," *J. Biomed. Mater. Res.*, **5** [1] 49–64 (1974).

[61]T. Kokubo, "Surface Chemistry of Bioactive Glass-Ceramics," *J. Non-Cryst. Solids*, **120**, 138–51 (1990).

[62]T. Kokubo, "Bonding Mechanism of Bioactive Glass-Ceramic A-W to Living Bone"; see Ref. 40, pp. 41–50.

[63]T. Kokubo, "A/W Glass-Ceramic: Processing and Properties"; see Ref. 4, Ch. 5, p. 75.

[64]R. Li, A. E. Clark, and L. L. Hench, "An Investigation of Bioactive Glass Powders by the Sol–Gel Process," *J. Appl. Biomater.*, **2**, 231–39 (1991).

[65]M. M. Walker, "An Investigation into the Bonding Mechanisms of Bioglass"; M.S. Thesis. University of Florida, Gainesville, FL, 1977.

[66]M. Jarcho, "Calcium Phosphate Ceramics as Hard Tissue Prosthetics," *Clin. Orthop. Relat. Res.*, **157**, 259 (1981).

[67]D. F. Williams, "The Biocompatibility and Clinical Uses of Calcium Phosphate Ceramics"; pp. 43–66 in *Biocompatibility of Tissue Analogs*, Vol. II. Edited by D. F. Williams. CRC Press, Boca Raton, FL, 1985.

[68]J. Wilson, A. E. Clark, E. Douek, J. Krieger, W. K. Smith, and J. S. Zamet, "Clinical Applications of Bioglass® Implants"; p. 415 in *Bioceramics 7.* Edited by D. H. Andersson, R. P. Happonen, and A. Y. Urpo. Butterworth-Heinemann, Oxford, U.K., 1994.

[69]C. A. Shapoff, D. C. Alexander, and A. E. Clark, "Clinical Use of a Bioactive Glass Particulate in the Treatment of Human Osseous Defects," *Compend. Contin. Educ. Dent.*, **18** [4] 352–63 (1997).

[70]R. Reck, S. Storkel, and A. Meyer, "Bioactive Glass-Ceramics in Middle Ear Surgery: An 8-Year Review"; see Ref. 6, p. 100.

[71]E. Merwin, "Review of Bioactive Materials for Otologic and Maxillofacial Applications"; see Ref. 40, pp. 323–28.

[72]J. Wilson, E. Douek, and K. Rust, "Bioglass® Middle Ear Devices: Ten Year Clinical Results"; pp. 239–46 in *Bioceramics*, Vol. 8. Edited by J. Wilson, L. L. Hench, and D. Greenspan. Pergamon/Elsevier, Oxford, U.K., 1995.

[73]K. Lobel, "Ossicular Replacement Prostheses"; pp. 214–36 in *Clinical Performance of Skeletal Prostheses.* Edited by L. L. Hench and J. Wilson. Chapman and Hall, London, U.K., 1996.

[74]J. Walliker, H. Carson, E. E. Douek, A. Fourcin, and S. Rosen, "An Extracochlear Auditory Prothesis"; p. 265 in *Proceedings of Cochlear Implant Symposium 90* (Diirer, Germany, Sept. 7–12, 1987). Edited by P. Bansai.

[75](a)H. R. Stanley, M. B. Hall, A. E. Clark, J. C. King, L. L. Hench, and J. J. Berte, "Using 45S5 Bioglass® Cones as Endosseous Ridge Maintenance Implants to Prevent Alveolar Ridge Resorptions—A 5 Year Evaluation," *Int. J. Oral Maxillofac. Implants.*, **12**, 95–105 (1997). (b)H. R. Stanley, A. E. Clark, and L. L. Hench, "Alveolar Ridge Maintenance Implants"; p. 255–70 in *Clinical Performance of Skeletal Prostheses.* Edited by L. L. Hench and J. Wilson. Chapman and Hall, London, U.K., 1996.

[76]J. Wilson and S. B. Low, "Bioactive Ceramics for Periodontal Treatment: Comparative Studies in the Patus Monkey," *J. Appl. Biomater.*, **3**, 123–69 (1992).

[77]A. E. Fetner, M. S. Hartigan, and S. B. Low, "Periodontal Repair Using Perioglas® in Nonhuman Primates: Clinical and Histologic Observations," *Compend. Contin. Educ. Dent.*, **15** [7] 932–39 (1994).

[78]T. Yamamuro, "Replacement of the Spine with Bioactive Glass-Ceramic Prosthesis"; see Ref. 40, pp. 343–52.

[79]T. Yamamuro, "A/W Glass-Ceramic: Clinical Applications"; see Ref. 4, Ch. 6, p. 89.

[80]R. Z. LeGeros and J. P. LeGeros, "Dense Hydroxyapatite"; see Ref. 4, Ch. 9, p. 139.

[81]R. F. LeGeros, G. Bone, and R. Z. LeGeros, "Type of H_2O in Human Enamel and in Precipitated Apatities," *Calcif. Tissue Res.*, **26**, 111 (1978).

[82]E. C. Shors and R. E. Holmes, "Porous Hydroxyapatite"; see Ref. 4, Ch. 10, p. 181.

[83]M. Jarcho, J. I. Kay, R. H. Gummaer, and H. P. Drobeck, "Tissue, Cellular, and Subcellular Events at a Bone-Ceramic Hydroxylapatite Interface," *J. Bioeng.*, **1**, 79 (1977).

[84]M. Ogiso, "TEM Analysis of Hydroxyapatite–Bone Interfacial Reactions," *J. Dent. Res.*, **60** [A] 419–24 (1981).

[85]M. Ogiso, H. Kaneda, J. Arasaki, K. Ishida, M. Shiota, T. Mitsuwa, T. Tabata, Y. Yamazaki, and T. Hidaka, *Trans. Soc. Biomat.*, **4**, 54 (1981).

[86]C. Doyle, "Bioactive Composites in Orthopedics"; see Ref. 40, pp. 195–208.

[87]P. Ducheyne and J. F. McGucken Jr., "Composite Bioactive Ceramic-Metal Materials"; pp. 185–86 in *Handbook of Bioactive Ceramics,* Vol. II. Edited by T. Yamamuro, L. L. Hench, and J. Wilson. CRC Press, Boca Raton, FL, 1990.

[88]U. Soltez, "Ceramics in Composites: Review and Current Status"; see Ref. 6, pp. 137–56.

[89]W. Bonfield, "Hydroxyapatite-Reinforced Polyethylene as an Analogous Material for Bone Replacement"; see Ref. 6, pp. 173–77.

[90]W. Bonfield, C. Doyle, and K. E. Tanner, "*In Vivo* Evaluation of Hydroxyapatite-Reinforced Polyethylene Composites"; p. 153 in *Biological and Biomechanical Performance of Materials.* Edited by P. Christel, A. Meunier, and A. J. C. Lee. Elsevier, New York, 1986.

[91]J. Huang, L. DiSilvo, M. Wang, K. E. Tanner, and W. Bonfield, "*In Vitro* Mechanical and Biological Assessment of Hydroxyapatite-Reinforced Polyethylene Composite," *J. Mater. Sci. Mater. Med.*, **8**, 775–79 (1997).

[92]P. Bloomfield, D. J. Wheatly, R. J. Prescott, and H. C. Miller, "Twelve-Year Comparison of a Bjork-Shiley Mechanical Heart Valve with a Porcine Bioprosthesis," *N. Engl. J. Med.*, **324**, 573–79 (1991).

[93]F. J. Schoen, R. J. Levy, and H. R. Piehler, "Pathological Considerations in Replacement Cardiac Valves," *J. Soc. Cardio. Path.*, **1** [1] 29–52 (1992).

[94]J. C. Bokros, U.S. Pat. No. 3 526 005, 1971.

[95]J. C. Bokros, L. D. LaGrange, and F. J. Schoen, "Control of Structure of Carbon for Use in Bioengineering"; pp. 103–71 in *Chemistry and Physics of Carbon*, Vol. 6. Edited by P. L. Walker Jr. Dekker, New York, 1972.

[96]A. Haubold, H. S. Shim, and J. C. Bokros, "Carbon in Medical Devices"; pp. 3–42 in *Biocompatibility of Clinical Implant Materials,* Vol. II. CRC Press, Boca Raton, FL, 1981.

[97]J. D. Bokros, "Carbon Biomedical Devices," *Carbon*, **18**, 355–71 (1977).

[98]A. D. Haubold, R. A. Yapp, and J. D. Bokros, "Carbons"; pp. 95–101 in *Concise Encyclopedia of Medical and Dental Materials.* Edited by D. Williams. Pergamon Press, New York, 1990.

[99]R. H. Dauskardt and R. O. Ritchie, "Pyrolytic Carbon Coatings"; see Ref. 4, Ch. 14, p. 261.

[100]C. P. A. T. Klein, J. G. C. Wolke, and K. de Groot, "Stability of Calcium Phosphate Ceramics and Plasma Sprayed Coating"; see Ref. 4, pp. 199–21.

[101]S. D. Cook, "*In Vivo* Evaluation of Hydroxylapatite Coatings for Orthopedic and Dental Applications"; pp. 71–86 in *Bioceramics*, Vol. 3. Edited by J. E. Hulbert and S. F. Hulbert. Rose Hulman Institute of Technology, Terre Haute, IN, 1992.

[102]J. E. Davies (Ed.), *The Bone-Biomaterial Interface.* University of Toronto Press, Toronto, Canada, 1991.

[103]S. Rao and A. Lecky, "Evaluation of the Success of Non-Cemented Porous and HA-Coated Metal-UHMWPE Total Hip Implant System"; pp. 33–41 in *Clinical Performance of Skeletal Prostheses.* Edited by L. L. Hench and J. Wilson. Chapman and Hall, London, U.K. 1996.

[104]D. E. Day and T. E. Day, "Radiotherapy Glasses"; see Ref. 4, Ch. 17, pp. 305–18. □

journal

J. Am. Ceram. Soc., 86 [1] 65–72 (2003)

Novel Method to Manufacture Porous Hydroxyapatite by Dual-Phase Mixing

Shi Hong Li, Joost R. de Wijn, Pierre Layrolle,* and Klaas de Groot

IsoTis NV, Bilthoven 3723 MB, The Netherlands

We have developed a novel method to construct porous hydroxyapatite (HA) by dual-phase mixing—in other words, generating a porous ceramic body and pore-forming template simultaneously. The technique is based on mixing two immiscible phases: HA slurry and polymethylmethacrylate (PMMA) resin. Naphthalene particles are necessary when greater porosity (>50%) is wanted. After shaping in a mold, the mixture is subjected to polymerization, drying, pyrolysis, and sintering. The porous HA has been thoroughly characterized with Fourier transformation infrared spectrometry, X-ray diffractometry, environmental scanning electron microscopy coupled with energy-dispersive X-ray analysis, and image analysis. The demanding specifications for bone ingrowth are met: (i) the size of pores and their fenestrations are adjustable, ~80% within 300–800 μm; (ii) uniform and isotropic porous structure is observed in three directions; (iii) pores are fully interconnected throughout; (iv) the porosity is adjustable up to 60%; and (v) sufficient mechanical strength is present for cell culture and implantation handling. The porous HA can be applied as either implant material or scaffold for bone-tissue engineering.

I. Introduction

THE following three phases can be identified when reviewing the development of biomaterials:

(1) Removal phase: in the past, diseased or damaged tissues were simply removed. This phase was before the use of biomaterials.

(2) Replacement phase: approximately three decades ago, transplantation and implantation became possible, and the latter practice provoked the rapid progress and wide application of biomaterials.

(3) Regeneration phase: with the rapid progression in material sciences and biology, we are now entering the third phase. Scientists are trying to form human bone by culturing bone-forming cells within a porous scaffold. Currently, tissue engineering, whether combined with gene therapy or not, has increasingly attracted attention in the area of biotechnology.

Orthopedic implants far exceed any other biomaterial applications, both in total weight currently implanted and current implantation rate.[1] One cannot summarize the history of orthopedic implants without mentioning the use of hydroxyapatite (HA), because of its excellent biocompatibility and osteoconductivity. HA has extensive application as a non-load-bearing implant material and as a coating on metal implants for load-bearing applications.[2] Therefore, it is logical to consider HA as a scaffold or carrier for hard-tissue engineering. In porous form, the surface area is greatly increased, which allows more cells or tissue to be carried, in comparison with dense HA. The interconnecting channels must guarantee the supply and circulation of the necessary nutrients, through the ingrowth of fibrous tissue, a vascular system, and bone tissue.

Porous ceramics can be grouped into two general categories: reticulate ceramics and foam ceramics. A reticulate ceramic is a porous material that is comprised of interconnected voids surrounded by a web of ceramic, whereas a foam ceramic has closed voids within a continuous ceramic matrix.[3] Because of the above-mentioned functional requirement, a tissue-engineering scaffold must take the reticulate form. Porous HA can be produced from natural sources or from completely synthetic routes, as summarized in Table I.

Of the techniques that have been mentioned, the H_2O_2 foaming method seems to be the most widely used in the last half-century. A thorough evaluation of all the materials made by the above-mentioned methods will focus on both material characterization and clinical results. The general requirements for the implant or tissue-engineering scaffold have been summarized in Table II, based on other publications.[22–24]

The merits and drawbacks of the materials from all the synthetic methods available will be discussed in the discussion section. In short, it is generally agreed that porous HA with a structure similar to human bone can be produced, but only with the help of Mother Nature, namely via the use of either natural bone or coral. Production of this porous structure entirely in the laboratory remains a challenging topic for material scientists worldwide. The critical point is control of the porous structure.

The porous HA ceramic generated by our recently developed method has a structure that is similar to natural bone. In principle, it is a negative replica method, with the unique feature that the negative template is prepared at the same time as the ceramic body. Basically, the process is a mixing procedure of two immiscible liquid phases in relative volumes, which guarantee the interpenetrating matrixes. Therefore, we have termed it a "dual-phase" mixing method.

II. Experimental Procedure

The current manufacturing procedure of porous HA is illustrated in a flowchart in Fig. 1. The process can also be figuratively described as follows: preparation a dough (mixture of naphthalene, PMMA resin and HA slurry) → demolding and drying → baking in an oven (pyrolysis into a porous form and final sintering).

(1) Preparation of Raw Materials

The raw HA powder (Merck, Darmstadt, Germany) was calcined at a temperature of 1000°C, using a heating and cooling rate of 100°C/h without a holding stage. HA powder (CAM, Leiden, The Netherlands) was calcined at 1000°C for 15 h and used as a reference material for X-ray diffractometry (XRD). Polymethylmethacrylate (PMMA) powder (Dentalbiolux International, Belgium) was mixed with 1% benzoyl peroxide (BPO, Merck Eurolab BV), which served as a radical polymerization initiator. Methylmethacrylate (MMA) monomer (Merck Eurolab BV) was mixed

D. Wilkinson—contributing editor

Manuscript No. 187548. Received July 30, 2001; approved May 7, 2002.
*Member, American Ceramic Society.

Table I. Methods Available to Make Porous Hydroxyapatite

Process	Description/comments
	Natural resources
Replamineform process	Replication of an echinoid skeletal macrostructure or coral (from White and co-workers[4,5])
Direct conversion of natural coral to HA	Occurs via hydrothermal reaction (from Roy and co-workers[6,7])
Changing natural cancellous bone to ceramic	As described by Hing *et al.*[8]
	Synthetic routes
Slurry foaming method	Foaming agents can be hydrogen peroxide (H_2O_2) (from Ryshkewitch[9] and Rejda *et al.*[10]), carbonate salt and acid (from Westerduin[11]), or kitchen baking powder (from Ribeiro *et al.*[12])
Solid-state reaction	Calcium carbonate and dicalcium phosphate forming HA, H_2O, and CO_2 (from Arita *et al.*[13])
Dry-state compression of HA powder with pore maker	Pore maker can be wax, polymer beads, or fugitive phase material. Process involves burning off these pore makers (from Yasuaki[14])
Starch consolidation	Starch suspension is mixed with dry HA powder under stirring; then, the material is dried and the starch is burned off (from Rodriguez-Lorenzo *et al.*[15])
Negative replica method	A polymer-bead network is used to create a negative replica of HA (from Richart *et al.*[16]), or cellulose sponge imbibition is used (from Martinetti *et al.*[17])
Positive replica method	A polymeric sponge method is used (slip casting), or a reticulate polymeric foam is used to create a positive replica of HA (from Woyansky *et al.*[3])
Negative–negative replica method	Cancellous bone is used to create a wax negative replica, then acid is used to remove the bone and a HA negative replica of the wax mold is formed (from Tancred *et al.*[18])
Combination of gelcasting and foaming	As described by Sepulveda *et al.*[19]
Rapid prototyping or solid freeform fabrication	As described by Brady and Halloran[20] and Wilson *et al.*[21]

with 2% N,N dimethyl-*p* toluidine (DMPT, Aldrich Chemical Co., Milwaukee, WI), which acted as an accelerator for the polymerization process. Particle sizes of the HA and PMMA powders were measured by Retsch Technology in Germany, using CRYSTAL-SIZER® equipment with the working principle of using incoherent light diffraction.

The HA slurry was prepared with the following chemical composition: 28.6 wt% demineralized water and 67.3 wt% calcined HA powder, 2.6 wt% ammonia solution (25%, Merck Eurolab BV), 1.5 wt% defloculant (Dolapix, Aschimmer and Schwarz GmbH, Germany) and 0.15 wt% binder (carboxymethyl cellulose (CMC), Pomosin BV, The Netherlands).

Naphthalene (Aldrich Chemical Co.) was used, both in crystal and flake form. The material was sieved, and particles in the size range of 600-1100 μm were selected.

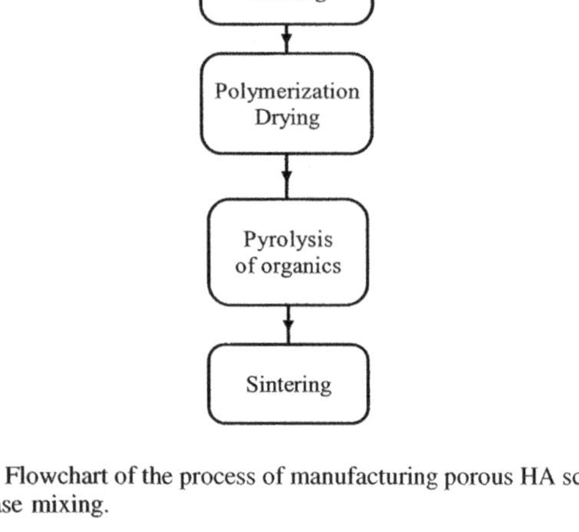

Fig. 1. Flowchart of the process of manufacturing porous HA scaffold by dual-phase mixing.

(2) Mixing of All the Ingredients

The HA slurry, naphthalene particles, MMA monomer, and PMMA powder were mixed homogeneously with a spatula in a Teflon™ (Dupont, Wilmington, DE) or polyethylene (PE) beaker. The volume ratio of HA slurry to the mixture of MMA/PMMA was 1:1. The addition of naphthalene was necessary only if greater porosity (>50%) was required. Subsequently, the mixture was transferred into PE or stainless-steel molds (40 mm in diameter, 50 mm in depth). After drying overnight, the mold was removed. Samples were further dried at room temperature or in an oven at a temperature of 50°C until they were completely dry and no further weight loss was observed.

(3) Pyrolysis of Organic Phases (PMMA, Naphthalene, and Binder)

Removal of naphthalene, PMMA, and other binders was performed in a furnace (Model 1100, Nabertherm, Germany) at a controlled heating rate to prevent blistering, cracking, or delamination that would be caused by (i) a mismatch of thermal expansion between the HA and organic phase or (ii) the expansion of exhaust gases. To optimize the heating profile, thermogravimetic analysis (TGA) (Perkin–Elmer, Norwalk, CT; software of Pyris windows) was performed on pure naphthalene, PMMA, and a mixture of HA, PMMA, and naphthalene. To understand the pyrolysis procedure *in situ*, photographs were taken in intervals of 10°C after a temperature of 150°C was attained. Based on the TGA studies and the photographs, a heating profile was selected:

$$\text{Room temperature (RT)} \xrightarrow{150\ \text{min}} 150°\text{C} \xrightarrow{600\ \text{min}}$$

$$350°\text{C} \xrightarrow{90\ \text{min}} 440°\text{C} \xrightarrow{210\ \text{min}} \text{RT}$$

(4) Sintering

After all the organic components had disappeared, at ~450°C, samples were finally sintered at 1250°C for 8 h in air or in a nitrogen atmosphere. A high-temperature furnace was used (Model HT-1600-GT-VAC, Linn High Therm, Germany).

(5) Characterization

The sintered porous HA was subjected to various characterization methods, including geometric, physical, chemical, and mechanical analyses. The analysis performed are summarized here (including all the instruments involved): stereo-optical microscopy (Model SMZ-10A, Nikon, Tokyo, Japan) coupled with a charge-coupled device (CCD) camera (Progressive 3CCD color video camera, Sony, Tokyo, Japan); Fourier transform infrared spectrometry (FT-IR) (Model Spectrum 1000, Perkin–Elmer); X-ray diffractometry (XRD) (Model Miniflex, Rigaku, Tokyo, Japan); environmental scanning electron microscopy (ESEM) (Model XL 30 ESEM-FEG, Philips, Eindhoven, The Netherlands) coupled with energy-dispersive micro-X-ray analysis (EDX); and a mechanical testing machine (Hounsfield, England).

(A) Porous Structural Parameters: As stated in Table II, the characterization of the porous structure includes pore size, uniformity of the porous structure, porosity, interconnectivity, size of the fenestration (or the "window between two adjacent pores"), and inner surface pattern of the pores.

To measure the pore size, a piece of porous HA was cut with a diamond saw and then the cross section was polished with a series of SiC sandpapers. After cleaning in an ultrasonic water bath and drying, the cross section was colored with stamp ink (Tianjin No. 4 stationery factory, PRC). This stained cross section was re-created digitally using a scanner. The image obtained was used for pore-size measurement, using image analysis.

Total porosity was determined by comparing the bulk density of a cylindrical sample with the theoretical density, namely 3.156 g/cm^3 for HA.

Pore interconnection is an important feature for porous materials, especially for tissue-engineering scaffolds. This parameter is not easy to determine, especially the quantification of the interconnectivity from a two-dimensional (2D) cross section. Therefore, a simple experiment was performed based on the principle that if all the pores are interconnected, one should be able to travel from one starting point to anywhere in the material through those pores in the vicinity. In practice, the porous HA was soaked in a black pigment suspension and subjected to centrifugation. After the nonattached black pigment was removed, the sample was sectioned, dried, and photographed. Pores that contained pigment indicated accessibility directly or via neighboring pores.

To examine the microstructure of the inner surface of the pores, the inner surfaces of porous HA with various porosities, prepared with or without adding naphthalene, were studied via ESEM. To clean and etch the porous HA, samples were soaked in a citric acid solution (2.1 wt%) for 1, 5, and 10 min with stirring. Then, they were cleaned thoroughly using demineralized water. Dried samples were sputtered with carbon, to make them electrically conductive, and analyzed via ESEM.

(B) Chemical Composition, Crystallinity, Purity, and Mechanical Properties: To characterize the chemical composition, FT-IR and XRD were used to study the functional groups and structural features. ESEM coupled with EDX was also used to provide some chemical information.

To examine the mechanical properties, ten cylinder samples (10 mm in diameter, 20 mm in depth) were prepared by grinding (Glass Technique BV, The Netherlands). Mechanical tests were performed with a computerized mechanical testing machine (Hounsfield) at a cross-head speed of 1 mm/min.

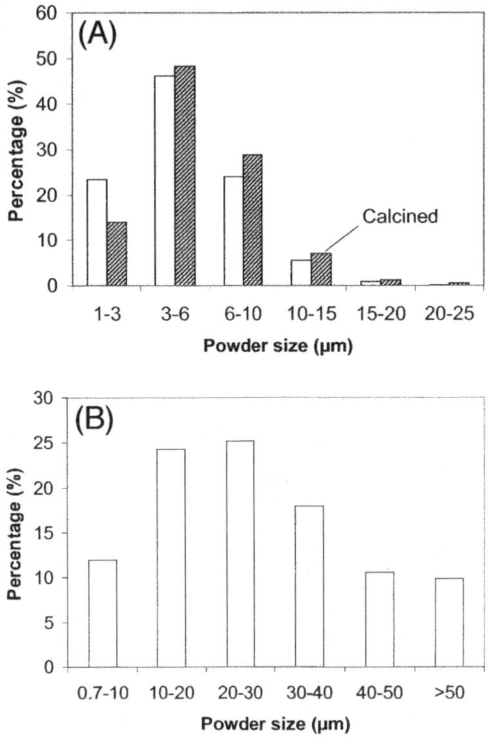

Fig. 2. Particle-size distribution of (A) HA powder (before and after calcination at 1000°C) and (B) PMMA resin powder.

III. Results

(1) Particle Size of HA and PMMA

Following calcination, the mean particle size of the HA powder increased slightly, as shown in Fig. 2(A). Another effect of calcination was the decrease of specific surface area (SSA) of the HA powder; this decrease in SSA was due to the fusion of some particles. The distribution of the particle size of PMMA powder is shown in Fig. 2(B); here, one can see that the majority (~50%) of particles were 10–30 μm in size.

(2) Pyrolysis: Removal of Naphthalene, PMMA, and Binder

Figure 3 shows the TGA curves of naphthalene and the HA/PMMA/naphthalene mixture sample. Naphthalene sublimated when it was held at a temperature of 50°C (a small amount of naphthalene changed to a gas). With additional heating, the gas disappeared completely at temperatures of <150°C. The TGA curve of the HA/PMMA/naphthalene mixture showed that most of the PMMA resin is pyrolyzed at 250°–350°C. To complete this pyrolysis process, the material was heated up to 440°C. To monitor

Table II. Requirements for Ceramic-Bone Tissue-Engineering Scaffold

Property	Factors
Material properties	Chemical composition (purity, crystallinity), raw-powder processing route (commercial or labmade), raw-powder particle size and its distribution, sintering parameters (temperature and time), mechanical properties
Porous structure properties	Pore size, fenestration size, and their distribution; pore shape (cylinder, sphere, etc.); porosity; interconnection; microporosity (bulk or surface); specific surface area; guidance of new bone formation in a certain direction
Material–cell/tissue interaction	Biocompatibility, fostering of uniform cell loading and retention, promotion of rapid vascular system ingrowth, resorption rate and degradation behavior
Geometric properties	Sample size, volume, and weight; sample shape (e.g., cylinder or block)

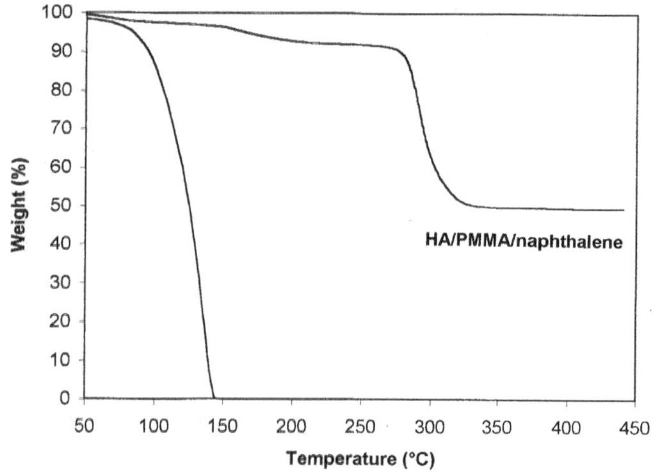

Fig. 3. TGA curves of naphthalene and mixture of HA/PMMA/naphthalene. Heating profile for HA/PMMA/naphthalene: room temperature (RT) → (150 min) 150°C → (600 min) 350°C → (90 min) 440°C → (210 min) RT. Heating profile for naphthalene: 50°C → (650 min) 700°C.

this process in the furnace, one photograph was taken at intervals of 10°C over a range of 150°–330°C. The photographs shown in Fig. 4 illustrate that the color of the PMMA turned darker as the temperature increased, up to 300°C. At temperatures ≥230°C, some of the PMMA resin started to flow out from the HA body; the maximum rate was observed at 280°–310°C. As the temperature increased, those portions of the PMMA resin that had flowed onto the crucible gradually disappeared. This observation was consistent with the TGA results. During the entire process, no combustion of PMMA in air was observed.

(3) Shrinkage of Porous Hydroxoyapatite

Assuming the diameter of a sample after demolding was D, then the diameter after pyrolysis would be 0.994D. After sintering, the diameter would be 0.768D; therefore, the linear shrinkage rate is 23%, corresponding to a volumetric decrease of ~50%.

(4) Characterization of the Final Porous Ceramic

An optical light micrograph was taken, as shown in Fig. 5(A). For comparison, the macroscopic picture of bovine bone is also shown in Fig. 5(B). Morphologic observation shows that, although both structures possess a well-interconnected porous structure, some differences still existed. Porous HA has a thicker cell wall than bovine bone, whereas the relative fenestration size in bovine bone was smaller.

(A) Pore-Size Distribution: Figure 6 shows a cross-sectional image of the porous HA, as used for image processing. The pore-size distribution is illustrated in Fig. 7. The majority of pores were 200–800 μm in size, which implies easy ingrowth of fibrous tissue, as well as the presence of a vascular system and, later, bone tissue. Less than 5% of the pores were <100 μm in size, as a result of the existence of small fugitive particles (PMMA powder, naphthalene, and binder particles) and inevitable air bubbles. The pore-size distribution (Fig. 7) is meaningful to show a general distribution trend; however, it is very difficult to be accurate for a real porous structure, such as that produced here. There are at least two reasons for this difficulty: (i) there is no clear, well-accepted definition of a "pore" and (ii) pore-size measurement for an individual pore based on a 2D image has a greater chance of giving a false value, even for regular spherical or cylindrical pores.

Evaluation of the sample filled with black pigment, under the help of a centrifuge, showed that all pores were black. This observation means that they were accessible to the stain and that the material was, therefore, thoroughly open.

(B) Bulk Density and Porosity: Cylindrical and cubic samples were used, and their weight and volume were measured. The bulk density was 1.215 g/cm^3. Using a value of 3.156 g/cm^3 to be the theoretical density of dense HA, the porosity of the porous HA was calculated to be 61.5%.

(C) Microstructure of Inner Surface of Pores: The porous HA with 50% porosity had a unique inner surface pattern (a microporous structure), as shown in Fig. 8. Hereafter, the expression "microporous structure" will be used in the sense that the pore diameters were mostly <5 μm in size. These structures were only observed on the pore surface. In the cross section of the solid portion of the ceramic, such texture was not observed. However, for those samples to which naphthalene was added in the HA slurry, the inner surfaces lost their microporous structure, more or less, as shown in Fig. 9(A). To regenerate the rough inner pore surface, samples were etched with a citric acid solution for 1, 5, and 10 min, as shown in Fig. 9(B)–(D), respectively. The inner surfaces of the pores were clean and exhibited a more-distinct microstructure, with increased soaking time.

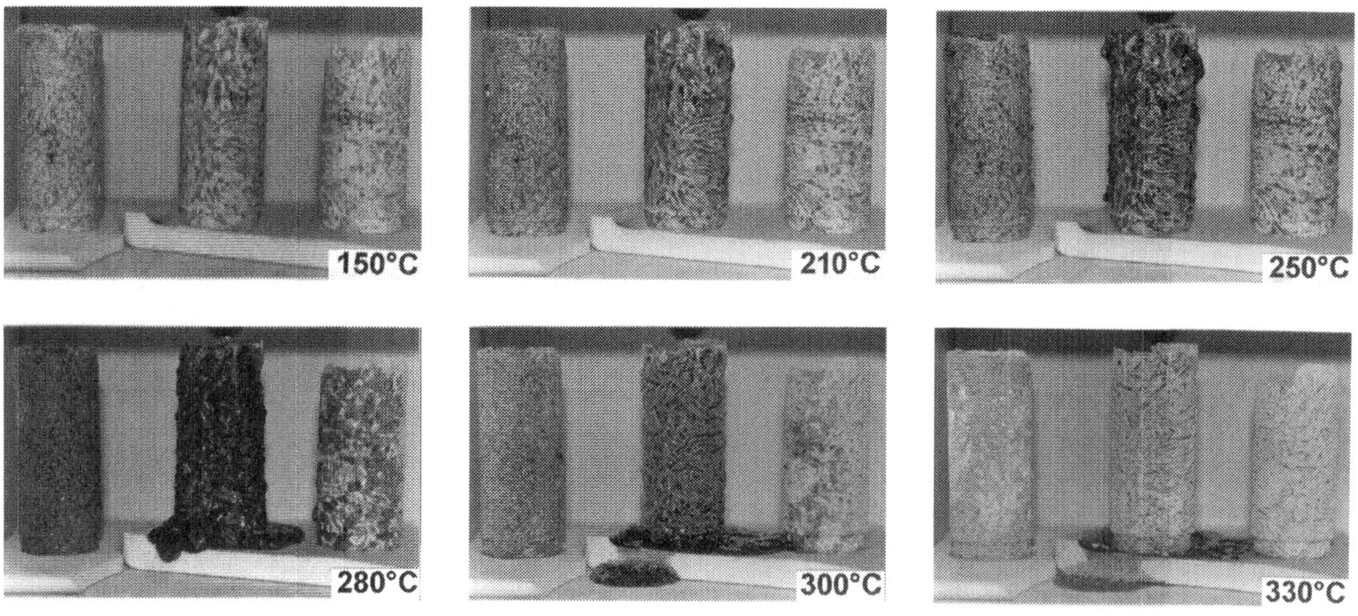

Fig. 4. Pyrolysis process of the mixture of HA/PMMA/naphthalene; the photographs show the morphology of samples at temperatures of 150°, 210°, 250°, 280°, 300°, and 330°C.

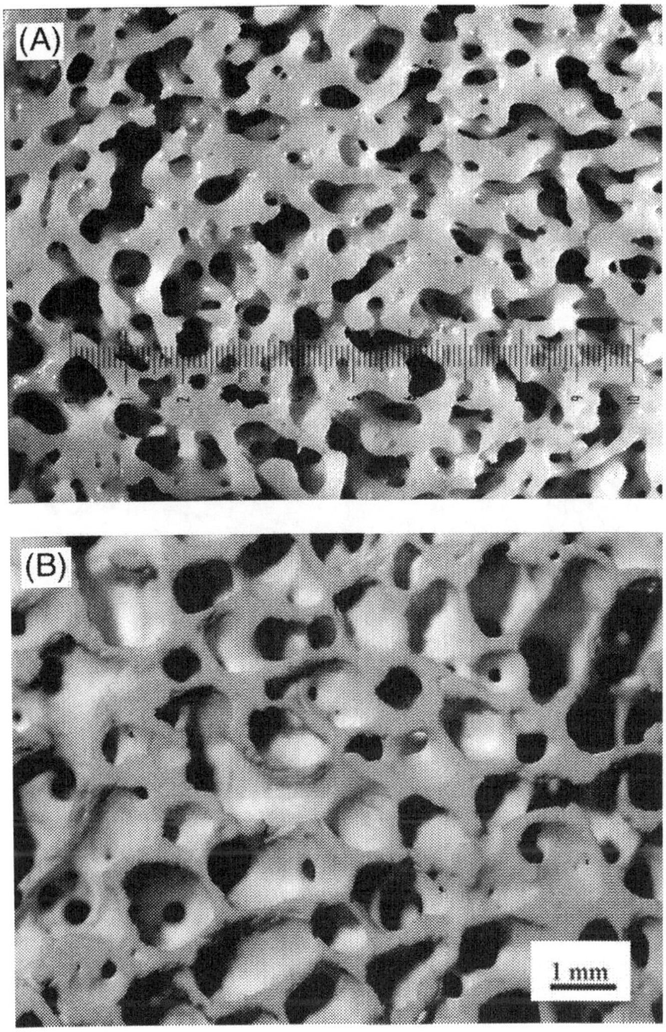

Fig. 5. Optical micrographs of (A) porous HA and (B) bovine bone.

(D) Chemical Composition and Crystal Structure: After sintering, the porous HA was characterized using FT-IR, as shown in Fig. 10. For comparison, the FT-IR spectra of PMMA and naphthalene are also shown. The results revealed that no organics (e.g., naphthalene and PMMA) remained after sintering at a temperature of 1250°C for 8 h. The peaks observed at 3580 and 630 cm^{-1} were assigned to the OH^- group, and the two peaks observed at 600 and 1030 cm^{-1} were assigned to PO_4^- groups.

Figure 11 shows the XRD pattern of porous HA and naphthalene. Clearly, no naphthalene remained; its highly crystalline peaks were completely absent. All the peaks of the ceramic were compared with JCPDS Powder Diffraction Data Card No. 9-432 and were assigned to HA. No other phase was observed.

(E) Mechanical Properties: The average compressive strength was 8.9 MPa for 50% porous HA and was only 4.8 MPa

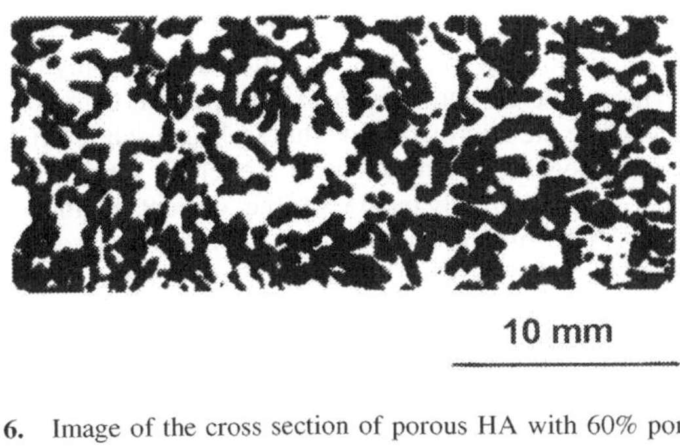

Fig. 6. Image of the cross section of porous HA with 60% porosity.

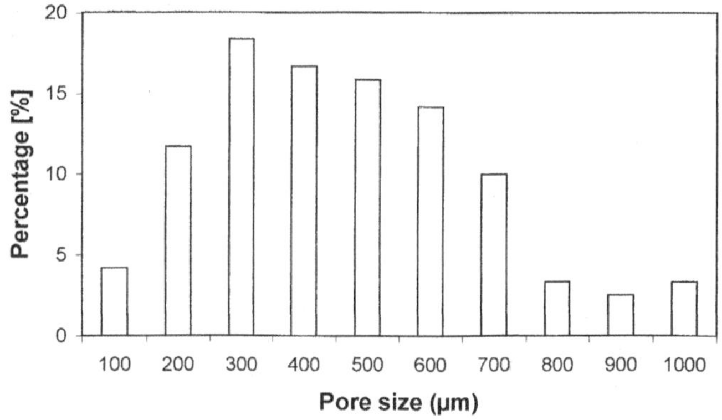

Fig. 7. Pore-size distribution of porous HA with 60% porosity.

for the HA with 60% porosity. These values correspond to studies that have been reported by Rejda and de Groot.[25]

IV. Discussion

A brief description and comparison of most of the synthetic routes of porous HA is summarized in Table III. The results of many clinical applications have been attributed to the merits and advantages of those methods. However, their remaining drawbacks sustain the driving forces for improved porous structure, especially where better control over interconnectivity and porosities is concerned.

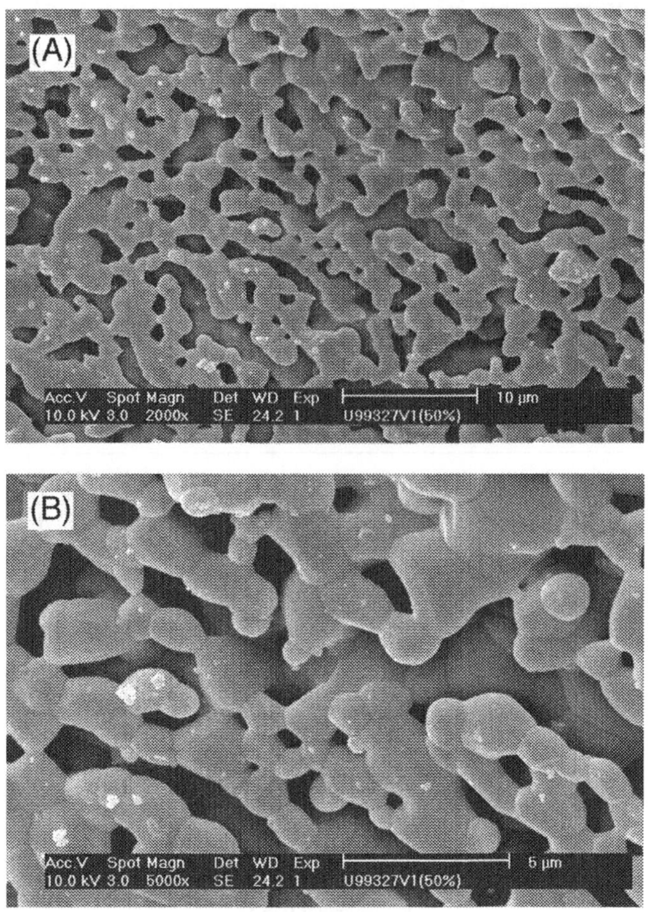

Fig. 8. ESEM images of the inner surface pattern of pores of porous HA with 50% porosity ((A) microporous structure and (B) higher magnification showing the detailed features).

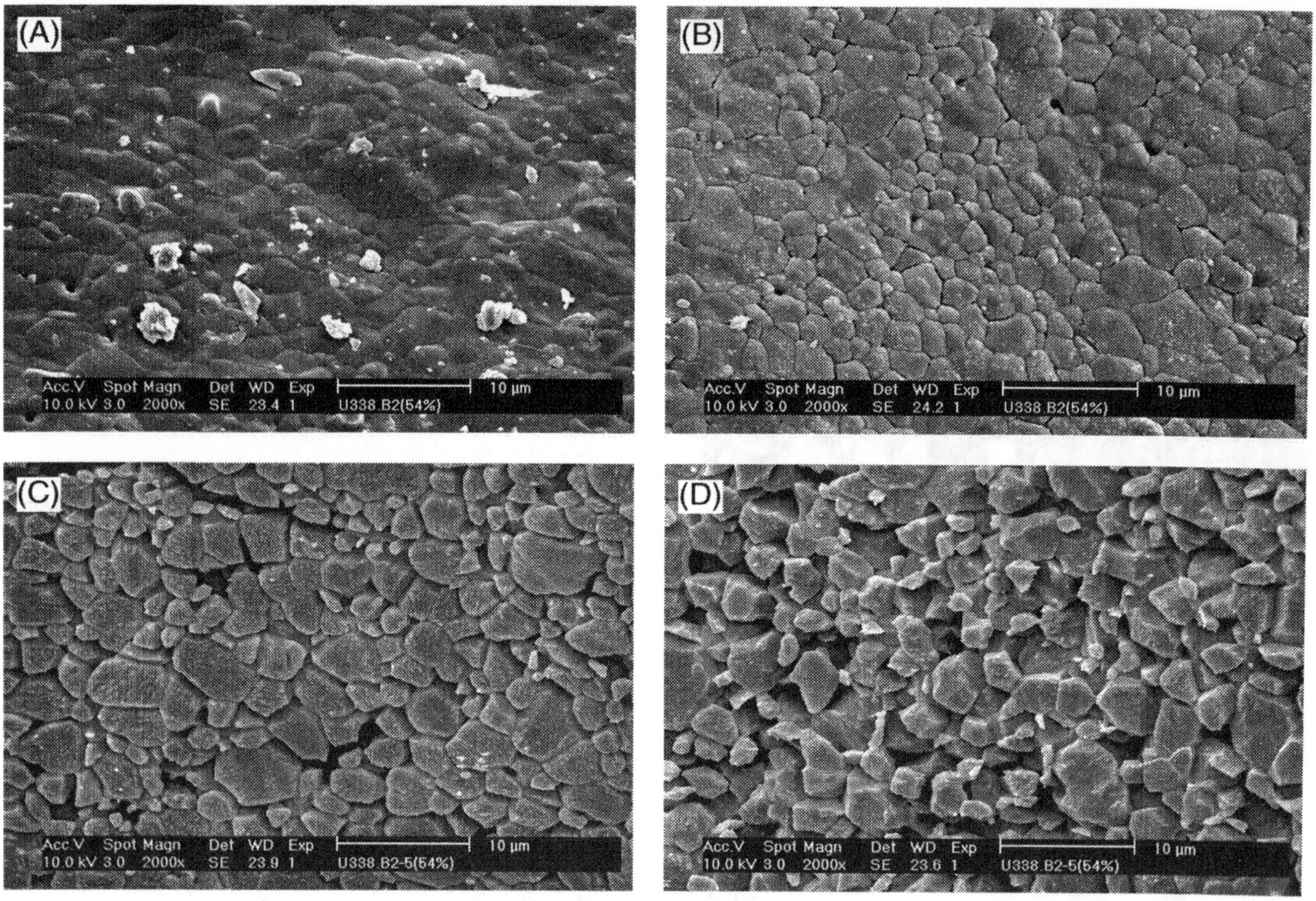

Fig. 9. Inner surface of the pores in porous HA with 60% porosity ((A) sample after sintering, without etching; (B) sample etched for 1 min; (C) sample etched for 5 min; and (D) sample etched for 10 min). In the etching tests, citric acid (2 wt%) was used.

Technically speaking, the current mixing technique is almost as simple as the H_2O_2 method, if the pyrolysis step is combined with the sintering. However, the porous structure is more controllable using the parameters of the mixing procedure—namely, the viscosity of the HA slurry, the components of the PMMA resin, the HA/PMMA ratio, the amount of naphthalene, the mixing speed and time, etc. In our experiment, for the same HA/PMMA ratio, a longer mixing time will generate thinner struts and a smaller pore size. For example, the majority of pores could be located within the range of 200–300 μm for HA with 50% porosity.

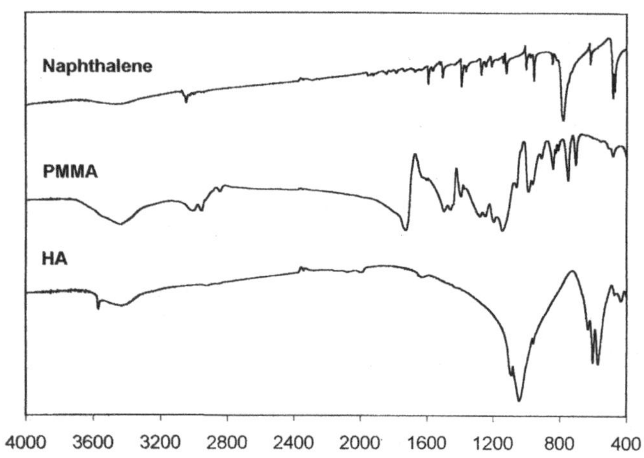

Fig. 10. FT-IR spectra of naphthalene, PMMA resin, and HA from the sintering of the mixture of HA/PMMA/naphthalene.

The novel feature of the current technique exists in the dual-phase mixing. At the very beginning, the two starting phases are separate—namely, a water-based HA slurry (containing naphthalene) and an organic PMMA resin. During the mixing process, they become dispersed and entangled phases, while retaining continuity. It is very important to understand that all the pores (the former acrylic phase) are, in principle, open. The interconnectivity is heavily dependent on the proportion of PMMA in the mixture, because this factor determines the probability of one portion of the PMMA meeting and coalescing with another portion.

The microtextures of the inner surfaces of pores are favorable for cell seeding and the ingrowth of tissue, even for later *in vivo* bone formation. Wilson[21] made porous HA with the same slurry as that used in the current study, using a so-called "rapid-prototyping method," which is a technique for manufacturing physical three-dimensional (3D) objects directly from computer-aided design (CAD) software. After seeding with goat bone-marrow cells for 4 h and statically culturing it for 7 d, the scaffold was implanted subcutaneously in a rat model. Bone formation was only observed at the surface, where microroughness was present. Citric acid was used to generate the microscale roughness, because it is a mild acid that does not degrade the mechanical properties significantly.

Another important advantage of the current method is the workability. After mixing the three ingredients, the viscosity of the mixture is still suitable for filling molds with complicated shapes. Therefore, if the shrinkage is taken into consideration beforehand, shaping of the products can be finished in one step. Recent experiments have shown that the shape of pores can be adjusted and oriented. Before completion of polymerization, the pores were

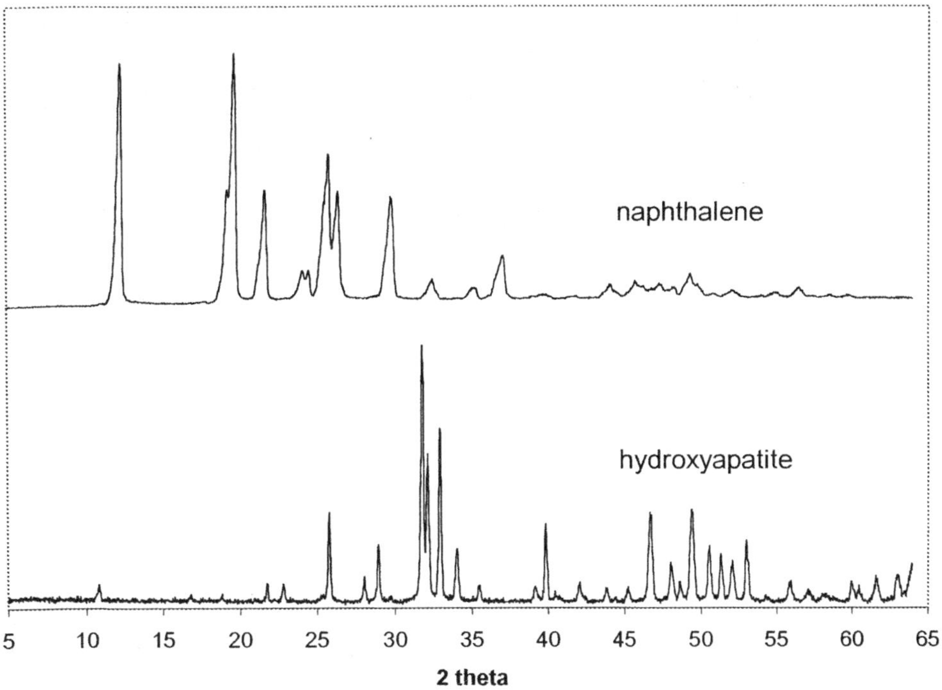

Fig. 11. XRD patterns of naphthalene and porous HA made by the dual-phase mixing method.

elongated and aligned in a certain direction, if shear force was applied,[26] which was difficult to achieve using the foaming method.

One would be curious about the effect of naphthalene in this process. In our experiments, if we used only HA and PMMA resin, then the upper limit of porosity was 50%. The addition of more resin to increase the porosity resulted in the collapse of the scaffold during sintering. After adding naphthalene, the porosity could be increased to 60 vol% without the occurrence of collapse. In our experiments, HA with 60% porosity is thoroughly open and

Table III. Comparison of the Merits and Drawbacks of Porous Hydroxyapatite Made Using Various Methods

Merits	Drawbacks
Conversion of natural coral to porous HA	
Commercially most successful Well-regulated pores Narrow pore-size distribution Excellent interconnection High porosity (55%–75%) High degree of isotropy Unique microtexture in the pore surface	Expensive Weak strength, so material is not suitable for load-bearing purposes
Changing natural bone to ceramic	
Good porous structure	Some health risks exist Cancellous bone properties vary greatly (e.g., porosity can vary from 60% to 80%); hence, there is no guarantee of consistency Sometimes, pore size may be <50 μm
H_2O_2 foaming	
Practically, it is easy to make	Less controllability in foaming Laminar pore structure with poor three-dimensional interconnection
Gelcasting and slip casting	
Easy method, in principle	Dilemma of sacrificing interconnection to gain strength, or vice versa
Negative replica of polymeric bead template	
Identical pores and fenestrations	Fenestration size is dependent on porosity (for example, if the pore size is 400–600 μm, then the interconnection would be 125 ± 25 μm and the porosity is 80%)
Rapid prototyping	
Easy to deign in various forms Meets most requirements, such as pore size and porosity	Low production rate Condition of being "open in all dimensions and directions" is questionable; at an angle of 45°, the pathway is completely blocked
Current dual-phase mixing	
Easy method and reproducible Good workability for different shapes Thoroughly open pores and complete interconnection Adjustable pore size and distribution	Mixing is a critical step; thus, an automatic mixer is preferred

interconnected throughout, whereas HA with 50% porosity is open but not fully interconnected. Naphthalene sublimates at temperatures <150°C, so during later stages, the melting PMMA was able to find space in which to flow or expand (depolymerizing into MMA monomers) without damaging the ceramic body, which is rather weak before sintering. The function of adding naphthalene can be summarized as follows:

(1) Increased porosity: After sublimation, the positions of naphthalene particles were left as pores.

(2) The overcoming of collapse during the pyrolysis process: This function is critical, because the volumetric percentage of organic phase was ≥50%, which is very high compared with the binders used in any other processing routes.

(3) Improvement of the interconnectivity: As mentioned earlier, HA with 50% porosity has pores that are open, but they are not always interconnected. After adding naphthalene, porosity was increased by 10%, which was enough to connect the pores.

(4) Removal of the surface dense layer: Without using naphthalene, the outer surface, which was in contact with either the PE or Teflon™ molds, lacked open pores. This lack of porosity was caused by the different interfacial affinity between the PMMA/mold and the HA/mold. Much more PMMA than HA accumulated on the outermost layer of the samples. As a result, more HA was observed in the next layer, which caused the formation of the dense layer after sintering. The addition of naphthalene changed this phenomenon significantly.

Previously, the porous structure of cancellous bone was considered the "gold standard" for implant materials. This ideal may not be true for tissue-engineering scaffolding, because the requirements for tissue-engineering scaffold are not the same as that for a piece of bone, especially when cells are seeded in the scaffold. If one examines the structure of bovine bone, as shown in Fig. 5, the fenestrations obviously are much smaller than the pores themselves. In the process of bone-tissue engineering, those osteoprogenitor cells must be cultured for a few days and then tissue must grow into the pores. If the fenestrations are too small, the growing cells (tissue) very likely may have blocked the "windows" between the adjacent pores. In this case, the cells located in the central portion of the scaffold will die, because of a lack of nutrients.

V. Conclusions

The dual-phase mixing described in this paper is very suitable for preparing porous hydroxyapatite (HA) for use as a tissue-engineering scaffold or an implant material. The novel feature is that both the porous ceramic body and pore-forming template are generated simultaneously. In this manner, thoroughly open pores are guaranteed. Fenestrations have the same size as the pores. By controlling the process parameters, such as the viscosity of the HA slurry, the hydroxyapatite/polymethylmethacrylate (HA/PMMA) ratio, or the mixing time and speed, it is possible to adjust porosity, pore size, and interconnectivity. This method renders the possibility of shaping complex porous product with molding before polymerization of PMMA resin. Porous HA ceramic with 50% porosity possesses a unique microtexture on the surface of the pores. The addition of naphthalene in the process could change this microtexture; however, regeneration is possible by mild etching in a citric acid solution.

After pyrolysis and final sintering, both the PMMA resin and the naphthalene vanished completely, as demonstrated by Fourier transform infrared spectroscopy and X-ray diffraction analysis; only pure HA remained. Finally, the material is strong enough for cell culture and implantation handling.

Acknowledgments

The authors thank the following colleagues: Fabienne Peters, for her enthusiastic help in the TGA experiments, and Yvonne Bovell, for her corrections of this manuscript. The discussions with Dr. Huipin Yuan and Mr. Jiaping Li were also very helpful during the preparation of this paper.

References

[1]H. R. Piehler, "The Future of Medicine: Biomaterials," *MRS Bull.*, **25** [8] 67–70 (2000).

[2]K. de Groot, "Bioceramics Consisting of Calcium Phosphate Salts," *Biomaterials*, **1**, 47–50 (1980).

[3]J. Saggio-Woyansky, C. E. Scott, and W. P. Minnear, "Processing of Porous Ceramics," *Am. Ceram. Soc. Bull.*, **71** [11] 1674–82 (1992).

[4]R. A. White, J. N. Weber, and E. W. White, "Replamineform: A New Process for Preparing Porous Ceramic, Metal and Polymer Prosthetic Materials," *Science*, **176**, 922–24 (1972).

[5]J. N. Weber, R. A. White, and J. Lebiedzik, "New Porous Biomaterials by Replication of Echinoderm Skeletal Microstructure," *Nature (London)*, **233**, 337 (1971).

[6]D. M. Roy, W. Eysel, and D. Dinger, "Hydrothermal Synthesis of Various Carbonate Containing Calcium Hydroxyapatite," *Mater. Res. Bull.*, **9**, 35 (1974).

[7]D. M. Roy and S. K. Linneham, "Hydroxyapatite Formed from Coral Skeletal Carbonate by Hydrothermal Exchange," *Nature (London)*, **247**, 220–22 (1974).

[8]K. A. Hing, S. M. Best, and W. Bonfield, "Characterization of Porous Hydroxyapatite," *J. Mater. Sci.: Mater. Med.*, **10**, 135–45 (1999).

[9]E. Ryshkewitch, "Compression Strength of Porous Sintered Alumina and Zirconia," *J. Am. Ceram. Soc.*, **36** [2] 65–68 (1953).

[10]B. V. Rejda, J. G. Peelen, and K. de Groot, "Tricalcium Phosphate as a Bone Substitute," *J. Bioeng.*, **1**, 93–97 (1977).

[11]W. Westerduin, M.S. Thesis. Technical University Delft, Delft, The Netherlands, 2000.

[12]A. S. Ribeiro, P. B. Malafaya, and R. L. Reis, "Two New Routes for Producing Porous Bioactive Ceramics: Polyurethane Precursors and Microwave Baking"; pp. 735–38 in *Bioceramics*, Vol. 11. Edited by R. Z. LeGeros and J. P. LeGeros. World Scientific Publishing Co. Pte., Ltd., New York, 1998.

[13]H. Arita, V. M. Castano, and D. S. Wilkinson, "Synthesis and Processing of Hydroxyapatite Ceramic Tapes with Controlled Porosity," *J. Mater. Sci.: Mater. Med.*, **6**, 19–23 (1995).

[14]S. Yasuaki, "Preparation of Adsorption Catalyst Material," Jpn. Pat. No. 09108567, 1995.

[15]L. M. Rodriguez-Lorenzo, J. M. F. Ferreira, and M. Vallet-Regi, "Processing of Porous Hydroxyapatite by Starch Consolidation"; see Ref. 12, pp. 89–92.

[16]O. Richart, M. Descamps, and A. Liebetrau, "Macroporous Calcium Phosphate Ceramics: Optimization of the Porous Structure and Its Effect on the Bone Ingrowth in a Sheep Model"; pp. 425–28 in *Proceedings of the 13th International Symposium on Ceramics in Medicine* (Bologna, Italy, Nov. 22–26, 2000). Edited by S. Giannini and A. Moroni. TransTech Publications, Aedermannsdorf, Switzerland, 2001.

[17]R. Martinetti, A. Belpassi, A. Nataloni, and C. Piconi, "Porous Hydroxyapatite Cell Carrier for Tissue Engineering"; *ibid*, pp. 507–10.

[18]D. C. Tancred, B. A. O. McCormack, and A. J. Carr, "A Synthetic Bone Implant Macroscopically Identical to Cancellous Bone," *Biomaterials*, **19**, 2303–11 (1998).

[19]P. Sepulveda, J. G. P. Binner, S. O. Rogero, O. Z. Higa, and J. C. Bressiani, "Production of Porous Hydroxyapatite by the Gel-casting of Foams and Cytotoxic Evaluation," *J. Biomed. Mater. Res.*, **50**, 27–34 (2000).

[20]G. A. Brady and J. W. Halloran, "Stereolithography of Ceramic Suspensions," *Rapid Prototyping J.*, **3**, 61–65 (1997).

[21]C. Wilson, J. de Bruijn, M. Kruijt, S. van Gaalen, W. Dhert, A. Verbout, and C. A. van Blitterswijk, "Design and Fabrication of Porous Hydroxyapatite Scaffolds for Bone Tissue Engineering Using Rapid Prototyping Techniques"; presented at the 47th Annual Meeting of the Orthopaedic Research Society (Feb. 25–28, 2001, San Francisco, CA).

[22]J. Bobyn, R. Pilliar, H. Cameron, and G. Weatherly, "The Optimum Pore Size for the Fixation of Porous-Surfaced Metal Implants by the Ingrowth of Bone," *Clin. Orthop.*, **150**, 263–70 (1980).

[23]J. J. Klawitter, J. G. Bagwell, A. M. Weinstein, and B. W. Sauer, "An Evaluation of Bone Growth into Porous High Density Polyethylene," *J. Biomed. Mater. Res.*, **10**, 311–23 (1976).

[24]K. Takaoka, H. Nakahara, H. Yoshikikawa, K. Masuhara, T. Tsuda, and K. Ono, "Ectopic Bone Induction on and in Porous Hydroxyapatite Combined with Collagen and Bone Morphogenetic Protein," *Clin. Orthop.*, **234**, 250–54 (1988).

[25]B. V. Rejda, Ph.D. Thesis; p. 65. Amsterdam Free University, Amsterdam, The Netherlands, 1977.

[26]S. H. Li, K. de Groot, and P. Layrolle, "Bioceramic Scaffold with Controlled Porous Structure for Bone Tissue Engineering," *Key Eng. Mater.*, **218–220**, 25–30 (2002). □

J. Am. Ceram. Soc., 86 [1] 115–20 (2003)

journal

Slow-Crack-Growth Behavior of Zirconia-Toughened Alumina Ceramics Processed by Different Methods

Antonio H. De Aza,† Jérôme Chevalier, and Gilbert Fantozzi

INSA—GEMPPM, UMR CNRS 5510, 69621 Villeurbanne, France

Martin Schehl and Ramón Torrecillas*

INCAR, Spanish Research Council (CSIC), 33080 Oviedo, Spain

A study of slow-crack propagation in zirconia-toughened alumina (ZTA) ceramics is presented. Different ZTA composites, using either unstabilized or yttria-stabilized zirconia, have been tested. The materials were prepared in the range 0–15 vol% ZrO_2, using two processing methods: powder mixing and a modified colloidal route. Crack propagation tests have been conducted for crack velocities from 10^{-12} to 10^{-2} m/s by means of a double-torsion method. The influence of the processing conditions and compositions on the microstructures and the effect of these microstructures on the slow-crack-growth behavior have been studied. The option that these composites may offer in terms of the lifetime of ceramic joint prostheses is discussed.

I. Introduction

With the publication of the article "Ceramic Steel?" by Garvie *et al.*,[1] it was shown that the fracture toughness of partially stabilized zirconia materials (PSZ) could be increased by stress-induced martensitic transformation of tetragonal zirconia particles (t-ZrO_2) to the monoclinic form (m-ZrO_2). The incorporation of zirconia (ZrO_2) inclusions into oxide ceramics, especially into alumina matrixes, to deliberately toughen them was undertaken shortly thereafter.[2] The mechanisms by which zirconia acts to toughen the composites are complementary:[3–7] they include transformation toughening, microcracking, and deflection. ZTA composites with high transformation toughening can be obtained if a high portion of tetragonal phase with the ability to transform under applied stress is retained at room temperature. To meet this requirement, the zirconia particles must have a size distribution ranging between the "critical" size for spontaneous transformation on cooling to room temperature after sintering, D_C, and the "critical" size for stress-induced transformation, D'_C. The practical implications in terms of particle size, size distribution, shape, composition, and temperature on the stability of the particles have been outlined by Claussen *et al.*[8] and Garvie.[9] The critical size of ZrO_2 particles for transformation to m-ZrO_2 has been the subject of a number of studies.[3–5,7–16] D_C size is reported to be in the range of 0.5–0.8 μm for unstabilized zirconia in an alumina ceramic matrix[14,15], and $D'_C \approx 0.1$ μm.[16] Processing is thus critical to obtain ZTA ceramics composites with maximum fracture toughness.[17] Today, there is a trend to develop more complex fabrication techniques[14–26] than traditional milling–mixing techniques. They include sol–gel[15,16,21] or colloidal processing,[22] which may allow the obtaining of a narrow size distribution of zirconia particles homogeneously dispersed in the alumina matrix. The addition of Y_2O_3 to ZrO_2 is another possibility to increase the stability of the t-ZrO_2 phase in ZTA systems.[3,4,18–20]

Although slow-crack-growth (SCG) resistance is a critical issue when considering the long-term behavior of ceramic materials, there is only a sparse collection of data in the literature concerning ZTA. It has been observed, in ZTA composites processed from a conventional route, that increasing the contribution of the ZrO_2 phase transformation not only increased the fracture toughness (K_{IC}) but also the required stress to induce crack propagation at a given rate.[19,27] However, little attention has been paid to the threshold (K_{I0}) in the stress-intensity factor under which no crack propagation occurs. This threshold determines a safety range of use for structural applications. The aim of this paper is to study SCG behavior as a function of the processing method and composition in ZTA. In the present investigation, ZTA composites were processed either by a classical route or a modified colloidal method to show the benefit of the latter method on SCG resistance. The overall SCG behavior, including the threshold, of the best ZTA composite processed in this research is measured. It is compared with that of other structural ceramics to keep in mind the option that these materials may offer to improve the lifetime of ceramic joint prostheses.[28]

II. Experimental Procedure

(1) Materials Processing

ZTA composites were prepared in the range of 0 vol% ZrO_2 (pure alumina) to 15 vol% ZrO_2. They were processed either by a conventional powder-mixing processing route or by a modified colloidal processing route.

Concerning the conventional powder-mixing technique, a high-purity alumina powder, α-Al_2O_3 > 99.9 wt% (HPA-0.5, Ceralox Division, Condea Vista Co., Tucson, AZ) with an average particle size of 0.49 μm and a specific surface area of 10 m^2/g (values given by the supplier), was used to process pure alumina samples. Stable suspensions, pH ≈ 4 in water media, of this alumina powder were homogeneously mixed with different amounts (10 and 15 vol%) of a (>99.9 wt% purity) monoclinic zirconia powder (TZ 0, Tosoh Corp., Tokyo, Japan) with a mean particle diameter of 0.47 μm and a specific surface area of 15.5 m^2/g (values given by the supplier). To homogenize, the batches were wet ground in a laboratory-scale annular gap mill[29] with high-purity alumina balls of 3 mm diameter, after which they were spray-dried. Quantitative X-ray diffraction (XRD) (Model D5000-Kristalloflex 710, Siemens, Karlsruhe, Germany) was performed to ensure that there was no preferential loss or segregation during the spray-drying process. The average particle size of the final batches,

N. Claussen—contributing editor

Manuscript No. 187654. Received June 7, 2001; approved September 5, 2002.
Supported by the Ministry of Education and Culture of Spain (PF9805271356) and MCYT MAT 2000-0941.

*Member, American Ceramic Society.
†Author to whom all correspondence should be addressed. Present address: ICV-CSIC, Campus de Cantoblanco 28049, Cantoblanco (Madrid) Spain, aaza@icv.csic.es

measured by laser diffraction (Model LS 130, Coulter Corp., Miami, FL), was between 0.33–0.4 μm. The specific surface area, measured by a 5-point BET method (Model ASAP 2010, Micromeritics Instrument Corp., Norcross, GA) was 10 ± 2 m^2/g for all batches processed from this classical route. The final particle size and BET-specific surface area are in fair agreement with the values given by the suppliers for the raw materials.

ZTA batches with the same zirconia proportion were also processed through a modified colloidal processing route developed by Schehl *et al.*[30] A composition with 7.5 vol% ZrO_2 was additionally processed. Stable suspensions of the above-mentioned alumina powder in absolute ethanol (99.97%) were doped by dropwise addition of a diluted (2/3 (vol%) zirconium alkoxide solution, 1/3 (vol%) ethanol absolute) zirconium alkoxide solution (zirconium(IV) propoxide 70 wt% solution in 1-propanol, Aldrich Chemical, Milwaukee, WI). The main difference with a standard solution method[15,26,31] using metal alkoxides is that the metal alkoxide is not hydrolized in the suspension. After drying under magnetic stirring at 70°C, the powders were thermally treated at 850°C for 2 h and were subsequently attrition milled, as a suspension in alcohol, with 3 mm alumina balls for 1 h. The powders were then dried and sieved to <45 μm. The specific surface area of the final powders ranged between 10 m^2/g for 7.5 vol% ZrO_2 and 14 m^2/g for 15 vol% ZrO_2 (they were all close to the initial specific surface area of alumina).

A composition with 7.5 vol% ZrO_2, stabilized by 2 mol% Y_2O_3, was additionally processed by the colloidal route described. For this purpose, the batch was also doped by dropwise addition of a diluted (2/3 (vol%) Y alkoxide, 1/3 (vol%) ethanol absolute) yttrium alkoxide (yttrium methoxyethoxide 15%–18% in methoxyethanol, Gelest ABCR GmbH & Co., Karlsruhe, Germany). The measured specific surface area was 10 m^2/g.

Next, all batches were uniaxially pressed at 20 MPa to a rectangular shape in a die (60 mm × 30 mm) to produce green compacts with just enough strength to be moved into an isostatic press, where they were cold isostatically pressed at 200 MPa. The temperature–time sintering conditions were studied by means of dilatometric analysis (Model DI-24, Adamel-Lhomargy Division d' Instruments S.A., Ivry-S/Seine, France). Final composites were sintered in air at 1550°C for 2 h, whereas the pure alumina samples were sintered at 1500°C for 2 h, with the aim of avoiding a high grain-growth rate. The bulk density of the obtained materials was measured by the Archimedes method.

(2) *XRD Analysis and Microscopy Observations*

The sintered samples were machined (2 mm × 20 mm × 40 mm) and polished with a series of diamond pastes up to 1 μm. XRD data, from unpolished, polished, and fractured surfaces, were obtained with a diffractometer using nickel-filtered Cu*K*α radiation. The tetragonal/monoclinic zirconia ratio was determined using the integrated intensity (measuring the area under the diffractometer peaks) of the tetragonal (101) and two monoclinic ($\bar{1}11$) and (111) peaks as described by Toroya *et al.*[32] For the purposes of comparison, the obtained volume fractions of tetragonal ZrO_2 ($V_t = 100 - V_m$; V_m denotes the volume fraction of monoclinic ZrO_2) were individually normalized to the volume fractions of ZrO_2 (V_{ZrO_2}) present in each composite as follows:

$$\frac{V_t \times V_{ZrO_2}}{100} = V_{t(composite)} \tag{1}$$

Additionally, the transformation of the tetragonal grains to monoclinic symmetry accompanying the propagating crack (ΔV_m) was investigated. This analysis was performed by XRD on the double-torsion sample crack plane after fracture from crack-propagation tests. Although the X-ray penetration is too deep to be considered as a real surface analysis, this test allowed a rough estimate of the stress-induced phase transformation in the materials to be obtained.

The average alumina and zirconia grain sizes were measured using micrographs via scanning electron microscopy (SEM; Model XL20, Philips, Eindhoven, The Netherlands) of polished and thermally etched surfaces using a linear intercept method (ASTM standard test method E112, American Society for Testing and Materials, West Conshohocken, PA) and using an image analyzer program (Scion Image, Scion Corp., Frederick, MD) where the diameter (*d*) was calculated from the projected particle area (*A*) using the well-known stereological expression:

$$d = 2\left(\frac{A}{\pi}\right)^{1/2} \tag{2}$$

(3) *Crack-Growth Measurements*

The double-torsion (DT) method was used to obtain the V–K_I (crack velocity versus stress-intensity factor) diagrams. The geometry of the DT specimen and the loading configuration can be found elsewhere.[33,34] No guiding groove was machined in the specimens to avoid any residual stress. Both sides of the specimens were polished, but the tensile surface was polished to a 1 μm finish to observe the crack with precision of ±2 μm using reflected-light microscopy (Model HP1, Karl Zeiss, Thornwood, NY). A notch of length $a_0 \approx 10$ mm was machined by a 0.3 mm diamond saw. A small natural crack was then induced in the specimen by slow precracking (loading rate 10 μm/min) up to ~12–13 mm ($\Delta a_0 \approx$ 2–3 mm). For a long time, the DT configuration has been considered to yield a stress-intensity factor independent of crack length. According to the specimen geometry, the conventional expression for K_I is given as:[34]

$$K_I = \frac{W_m}{T^2}\left[\frac{3(1+\nu)}{\psi \cdot W}\right]^{1/2} P = HP \tag{3}$$

with

$$\psi = 1 - 0.6302\left[2\left(\frac{T}{W}\right)\right] + 1.20\left[2\left(\frac{T}{W}\right)\right]\exp\left[\frac{-\pi}{2(T/W)}\right] \tag{4}$$

where P is the applied load, W_m the half-distance between the two points of flexion (moment arm), W the width, T the thickness of the specimen, and ν is the Poisson ratio.

However, it has been recently demonstrated that K_I was slightly dependent on the crack length,[35,36] and to obtain accurate V–K_I diagrams, a correction factor[35] should be introduced in the conventional expression of K_I (Eq. (3)). This correction is expressed with the following empirical equation:

$$K_{ICorr} = HP\left(\frac{a}{a_0}\right)^{6/32} \tag{5}$$

where a_0 is the notch length and a is the total crack length.

Subcritical-crack-growth laws were determined via two methods: relaxation tests and constant-loading tests. The load-relaxation method, which was first reported by Williams and Evans,[34] was used to obtain the SCG V–K_I diagrams in the velocity range 10^{-2}–10^{-7} m/s. This method does not allow measurements at very low velocity; however, it does present the advantage of being fast and, in principle, a full curve can be recorded in a single experiment. Precracked specimens were loaded at a constant rate of 0.2 mm/min, followed by subsequent stopping of the crosshead at constant displacement, when the crack started to propagate. The obtained load-relaxation versus time (P vs t) plot allows the determination of the V–K_I curve by a compliance calibration.[34,35] More details concerning the method for determination of V–K_I curves from P–t plots can be found elsewhere.[33–39]

Measurement of the crack velocities (V) under constant load presents the advantage of allowing the measurement of very low velocities. Thus, the specimens were subjected to different static loads under a prescribed duration, Δt. The crack length was

Table I. Designation and Main Characteristics of the Tested Materials

Ceramic material	Powder specific surface area (m^2/g)	Sintering conditions	% Theoretical density	Al_2O_3 grain size (μm)	ZrO_2 grain size (μm)	K_{IC} ($MPa{\cdot}m^{1/2}$) DT	Volume fraction (V_m) of monoclinic ZrO_2 after sintering	Stress-induced monoclinic content (ΔV_m %)	Designation
Alumina	10 ± 1.5	1500°C/2 h (air)	98.5	1.7		4.2 ± 0.2			Al_2O_3
Powder processing									
Al_2O_3–10 vol% ZrO_2		1500°C/2 h (air)	98	1.7	0.7	5.4 ± 0.2	45 ± 2	27	A10Z^{Pw}
Al_2O_3–15 vol% ZrO_2	11 ± 1.5	1550°C/2 h (air)	98	1.7	0.7	4.5 ± 0.2	81 ± 4	0	A15Z^{Pw}
Colloidal processing									
Al_2O_3–7.5 vol% ZrO_2	10 ± 1.5	1550°C/2 h (air)	98	1.2	0.4	5.5 ± 0.2	22 ± 1	21	A7.5Z
Al_2O_3–10 vol% ZrO_2	12 ± 1.5	1550°C/2 h (air)	98	1.2	0.4	5.9 ± 0.2	40 ± 2	29	A10Z
Al_2O_3–15 vol% ZrO_2	14 ± 1.5	1550°C/2 h (air)	98	1.2	0.4	5 ± 0.2	78 ± 4	0.5	A15Z
Al_2O_3–7.5 vol% ZrO_2 with 2 mol% Y_2O_3	10 ± 1.5	1550°C/2 h (air)	98	1.1	0.4	5.3 ± 0.2	19 ± 1	7	A7.5Z-2Y

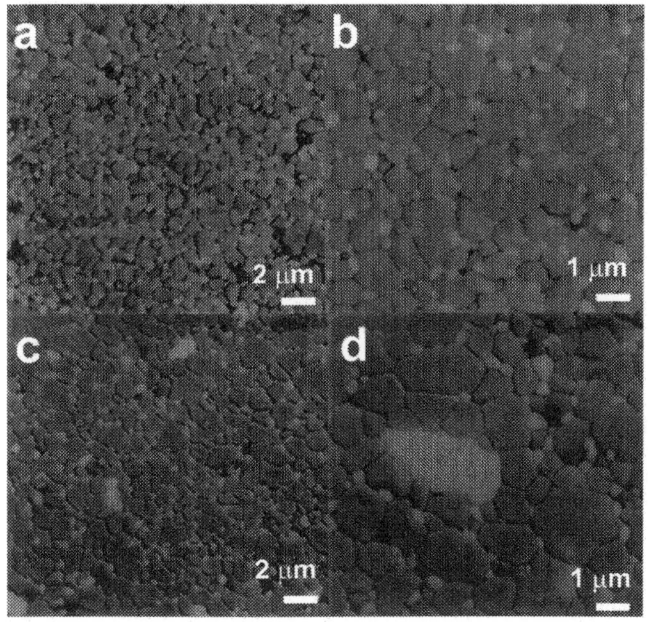

Fig. 1. Backscattered SEM images showing the microstructure of the Al_2O_3–10-vol%-ZrO_2 composites obtained. Samples show ZrO_2 grains (the brighter phase) distributed in a fine-grain Al_2O_3 matrix (the darker phase). (a) and (b): Nanocomposite processed by the colloidal processing route described (Al_2O_3 D_{50} = 1.2 ± 0.4 μm and ZrO_2 D_{50} = 0.4 ± 0.1 μm); (c) and (d): Composite processed by the conventional powder-mixing processing technique (Al_2O_3 D_{50} = 1.7 ± 0.6 μm and ZrO_2 D_{50} = 0.7 ± 0.4 μm).

measured via optical microscopy, with a precision of ±2 μm, and V is defined as the ratio of crack increment, Δa, to the duration, Δt:

$$V = \frac{\Delta a}{\Delta t} \tag{6}$$

From the obtained data, the threshold (K_{I0}) value was determined by extrapolation from the points on the V–K_I diagram, below which there is an abrupt drop of the crack velocity. On the other hand, the toughness (K_{IC}) was determined by extrapolation of the V–K_I curve to high-crack velocities (10^{-2} m/s).

III. Results and Discussion

The designation and main characteristics of each material are summarized in Table I.

Figures 1(a)–(d) show the final microstructures of the Al_2O_3–

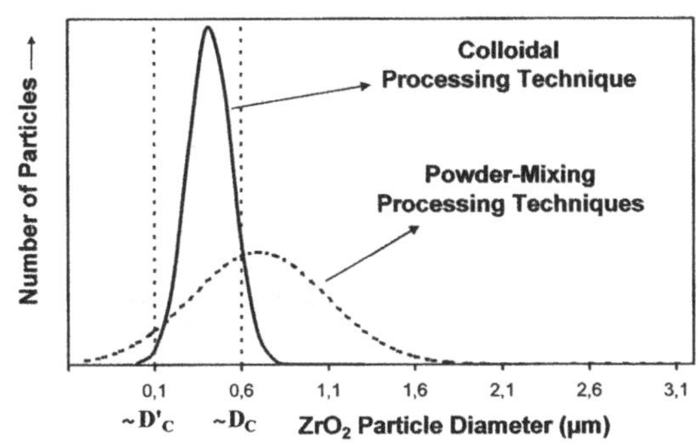

Fig. 2. ZrO_2 grain-size distribution in the alumina–10-vol%-zirconia composites obtained by conventional powder-mixing processing technique and a colloidal processing route (assuming a normal distribution of zirconia particle sizes). The values given for D_C and D'_C are reported values[14–16] for unstabilized zirconia in Al_2O_3–ZrO_2 composites.

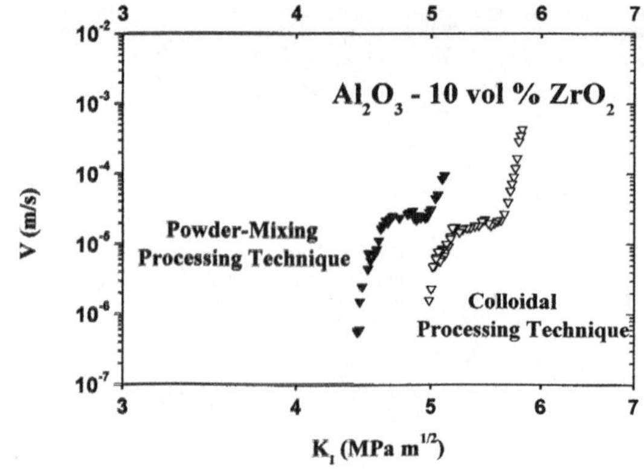

Fig. 3. Crack velocity (V) versus stress-intensity factor (K_I) for the alumina 10 vol% zirconia composites obtained by conventional powder-mixing processing technique and the colloidal processing route described; the finer microstructure obtained by colloidal processing leads to a displacement of the V–K_I diagram to higher K_I values.

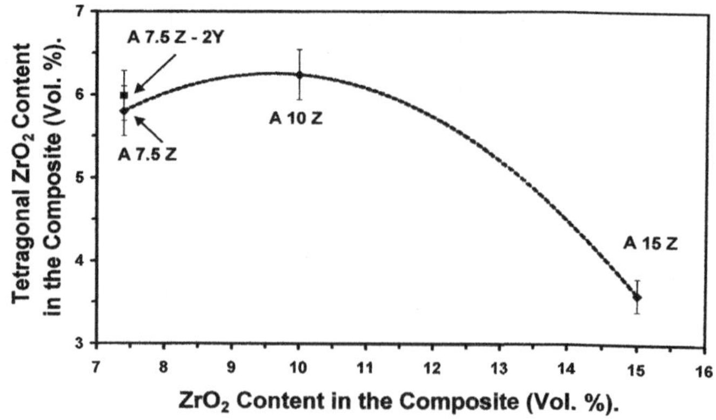

Fig. 5. Tetragonal zirconia retained after sintering in the ZTA composite ($V_{t(composite)} = (V_t V_{ZrO_2})/100$), as a function of zirconia content in the composite. Data from unpolished surfaces.

10-vol%-ZrO_2 composites obtained either by the powder-mixing processing technique or the colloidal processing route described. The figures show ZrO_2 grains (the brighter phase) distributed in an Al_2O_3 matrix (the darker phase). The composite obtained by the colloidal processing route (Figs. 1(a) and (b)) show nano-sized ZrO_2 particles ($D_{50} = 0.4 \pm 0{,}1$ μm) homogeneously distributed at Al_2O_3 grain boundaries ($D_{50} = 1.2 \pm 0.4$ μm), without agglomerates and a minimum number of microstructural flaws. The composite obtained by the conventional powder-mixing technique (Figs. 1(c) and (d)) show larger ZrO_2 particles ($D_{50} = 0.7 \pm 0.4$ μm) less homogeneously distributed in the Al_2O_3 matrix. Al_2O_3 also exhibits larger grains ($D_{50} = 1.7 \pm 0.6$ μm). Figure 2 compares the ZrO_2 grain-size distributions of the two A10Z composites, assuming a normal distribution of zirconia particle sizes. It is shown that the alumina zirconia composite processed by colloidal method has a narrow size distribution that is roughly between the critical size for spontaneous transformation on cooling to room temperature (D_C) and the critical size for stress-induced transformation (D'_C).[14–16] The above-mentioned fact leads to a more efficient transformation toughening in the material processed by the colloidal route. In this material, a transformation of the tetragonal grains toward monoclinic symmetry ahead of a propagating crack (ΔV_m) ~12% higher than for the composite processed by the conventional powder-mixing technique was found, highlighting higher transformability. As mentioned in the previous section, this analysis was performed by XRD on the DT crack plane after fracture from crack-propagation tests and gives a rough estimate of the stress-induced phase transformation in both materials. This more efficient transformation toughening leads to a shift of the obtained V–K_I diagrams toward higher K_I values for the composites processed by the colloidal route when compared with the same compositions processed by the powder-mixing technique. Figure 3 highlights this fact that is reflected in a higher crack growth resistance of the composite A10Z obtained by the colloidal processing route. This behavior was confirmed for all the compositions.

As the composites processed by the colloidal route exhibit better mechanical properties than those processed by the powder-mixing technique, from now on, the results and discussion will be focused on this type of composite.

The measured V–K_I diagrams of alumina and the composites, prepared with different volume fraction of unstabilized zirconia, are plotted in Fig. 4. The curves exhibit a trend to shift toward higher K_I values up to a maximum before dropping with increasing volume fraction. These results are in agreement with previously reported values on the toughness of Al_2O_3–ZrO_2 composites.[2,27] The increasing crack resistance of the composites can be explained by the transformation mechanism mentioned. The tetragonal ZrO_2 concentration in the ZTA composites ($V_{t(composite)}$) after sintering, plotted in Fig. 5, is calculated from Eq. (1) and from the values of monoclinic content measured by XRD that are shown in Table I. The A10Z composite is the one with the highest amount of tetragonal phase retained at room temperature in the whole composite. Additionally, Fig. 6 shows the stress-induced phase transformation of the metastable tetragonal grains toward monoclinic symmetry ahead of a propagating crack (ΔV_m%). The term ΔV_m% corresponds to the difference in percent between monoclinic content measured on fractured and sintered surface (Table I) and gives estimate of transformation toughening efficiency. Here,

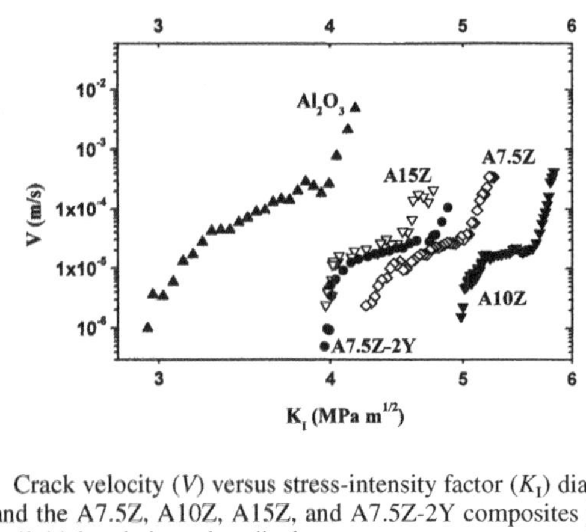

Fig. 4. Crack velocity (V) versus stress-intensity factor (K_I) diagrams for Al_2O_3 and the A7.5Z, A10Z, A15Z, and A7.5Z-2Y composites processed by the colloidal technique described.

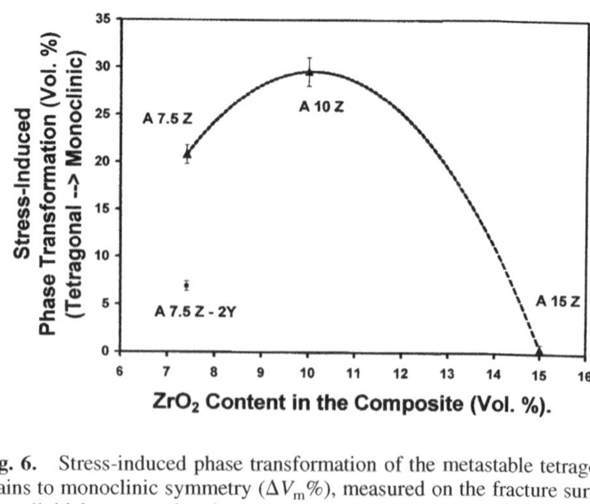

Fig. 6. Stress-induced phase transformation of the metastable tetragonal grains to monoclinic symmetry (ΔV_m%), measured on the fracture surface for colloidal processed series.

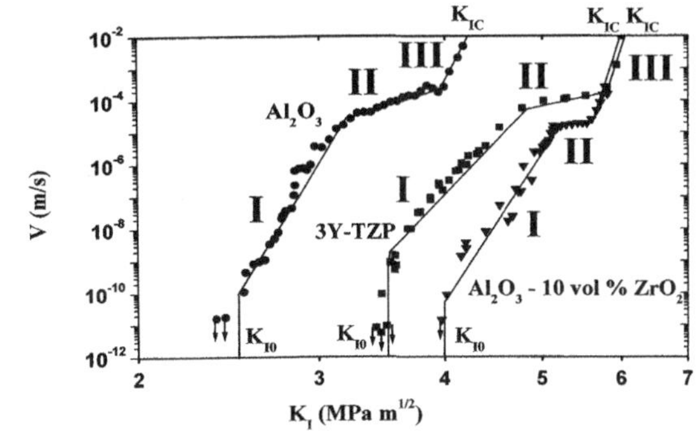

Fig. 7. Crack velocity (V) versus the stress-intensity factor (K_I) for Al_2O_3, Al_2O_3–10-vol%-ZrO_2 composite and 3Y-TZP;[40,41] the alumina–zirconia composite processed via the mentioned colloidal processing route exhibits the highest slow crack growth resistance. ((●) Al_2O_3, (▼) A10Z, and (■) 3Y-TZP.) Arrows indicate tests where no propagation could be observed, crack rate must be lower than the value plotted.

it can be seen that the A10Z composite has the highest effective transformation and the A15Z the lowest. As indicated by Claussen,[2] the amount of stress in the matrix increases with the amount of zirconia dispersed, and, beyond a maximum, the matrix is not able to retain the tetragonal ZrO_2 as a metastable phase. Additionally, it is worth noting that the critical ZrO_2 particle size for transformation is dependent on the volume fraction of ZrO_2 present in the matrix, as reported by Green.[5] For high-volume fractions of ZrO_2, the volume expansion (3%–5%) caused by the transformation leads to a high density of microcracks, which join up between the transformed particles. Consequently, the K_{IC} value decreases and the overall V--K_I curve is shifted toward lower K_I values.

Next, Fig. 4 also shows the measured V–K_I diagram of the A7.5Z composite processed with 2 mol% of Y_2O_3 (A7.5Z-2Y). The V–K_I curve of the composition with yttria is slightly shifted to lower K_I values compared with the batch A7.5Z. The V–K_I curve of this material lines up with the material A15Z. This lower crack resistance corresponds to a lower (if no) effective transformation toughening, as shown in Fig. 6 and Table I. The use of the 2 mol% of Y_2O_3 to stabilize the t-ZrO_2 limits the effectiveness of the transformation-toughening mechanism when an external stress is applied and processing modifications would be required to increase the size and/or the amount of the Y_2O_3-stabilized ZrO_2 particles. Figure 4 and Table I show that composites processed from the colloidal route always exhibit higher crack resistance than pure alumina, even for A15Z and A7.5Z-2Y where little or no transformation occurs. Note that transformation toughening is not the only mechanism acting to reinforce alumina in ZTA, and that complementary processes, i.e., crack deflection and microcracking, occur. These complementary toughening mechanisms already account for the crack resistance of ZTA, because they give an increase of ~1 MPa·$m^{1/2}$ of crack resistance compared with alumina. In any case, the material exhibiting the highest amount of phase transformation during crack extension (i.e., A10Z) presents the highest crack resistance.

Finally, the whole crack velocity diagrams of the A10Z composite obtained by the colloidal route and Al_2O_3 are compared in Fig. 7. Additionally, in the same figure, keeping in mind the option that these materials may offer to improve the lifetime of ceramic joint prostheses[28], both curves are compared with other results for a 3Y-TZP (3-mol%-yttria-stabilized zirconia) bioceramic.[40,41]

The overall curves obtained in air exhibits three distinct stages that have been fitted to a power law:[42]

$$V = AK_I^n \tag{7}$$

The different values of parameters A and n are reported in Table II. Thresholds below which no crack propagation occurs (K_{I0}) were observed at values indicated in the table. Figure 7 shows that the zirconia ceramic (3Y-TZP) exhibits a higher toughness than alumina but the thresholds of both materials are lower than that of the alumina–zirconia nanocomposite (also see Table II), meaning that the necessary stress to initiate crack growth is lower in alumina and 3Y-TZP. Additionally, the alumina-zirconia nanocomposite has a toughness close to that of zirconia but a higher threshold, a consequence of the steeper slope of its V–K_I diagram. SCG in ceramics is attributed to stress-assisted corrosion at the crack tip or any pre-existing defect in the ceramic. This is indeed the combined effect of high stresses at the crack tip and the presence of water or environmental species, temperature, and other extraneous variables (reducing surface energy at the crack tip) that induce crack propagation in a subcritical manner.[42] Alumina has lower susceptibility to water and thus to stress-assisted corrosion. As a consequence, the V–K_I curve of alumina presents a higher slope than the curve corresponding to zirconia. From an atomistic point of view, this means that the fracture energy of zirconia is lower in the presence of water, because the zirconia bonds are prone to chemisorption of the polar water molecules. The addition of a small amount of zirconia to alumina (in Fig. 7, 10 vol%) has two main advantages: first, alumina-zirconia composites exhibit crack propagation primarily through the alumina matrix. Thus, these composites possess a low susceptibility to stress-assisted corrosion from water. Second, these materials are reinforced by the presence of highly transformable zirconia particles, shifting the V–K_I diagram of alumina toward higher K_I values while preserving the slope of the curve, as it was theoretically shown previously.[43] Figure 7 and Table II show that the current results are in agreement with this previous work, primarily in the first stage of the curve, where the effect of the stress-assisted corrosion is higher.

In any case, the threshold K_{I0} represents the key parameter as far as durability is concerned[44] (as for orthopedic implants, which must survive *in vivo* for more than 10 years). From the well-known stress-intensity factor equation:

$$K_I = Y\sigma a^{1/2} \tag{8}$$

where Y is a shape factor related to the crack, σ the applied stress, and a the size of a pre-existing defect, it is expected that no failure occurs *in vivo* if the applied stress is lower than

$$\sigma_0 = \frac{K_{I0}}{Ya^{1/2}} \tag{9}$$

The K_{I0} value of the best ZTA composite processed in this research (10 vol% of ZrO_2) is twice that of pure alumina. This means that for the same pre-existing defects, this composite is expected to work at loads two times greater than monolithic alumina without any delayed failure.

Table II. Threshold (K_{I0}), Toughness (K_{IC}), and Slow-Crack-Growth Parameters (A and n) of Al_2O_3, A10Z, and 3Y-TZP Materials†

Material	Threshold (K_{I0}) MPa·$m^{1/2}$	Toughness (K_{IC}) MPa·$m^{1/2}$	1st stage		2nd stage		3rd stage	
			A	n	A	n	A	n
Al_2O_3	2.5 ± 0.2	4.2 ± 0.2	2×10^{-33}	56.8	3×10^{-11}	12	4×10^{-40}	59.7
A10Z	4.0 ± 0.2	5.9 ± 0.2	4×10^{-43}	53.5	5×10^{-9}	4.8	7×10^{-50}	59.6
3Y-TZP‡	3.5 ± 0.2	6.1 ± 0.2	1.8×10^{-26}	31.5	1.4×10^{-9}	6.6	9.3×10^{-53}	64

†Tested in air. ‡Data from Refs. 40 and 41.

IV. Conclusions

The following conclusions can be drawn:

(1) The microstructures of the alumina-zirconia composites obtained by the modified colloidal processing technique are very fine with a narrow distribution of zirconia particles homogeneously dispersed in the alumina matrix. This leads to a high portion of tetragonal phase retained after sintering with the ability to transform under applied stress. These composites show an increase of crack resistance compared with the composites processed with a classical powder-mixing route.

(2) The measured V–K_I diagrams of the composites are shifted toward higher K_I values with increasing transformable ZrO_2 volume fraction, up to ~10%. This trend is inverted at volume fractions beyond a maximum. The use of the 2 mol% of Y_2O_3 to stabilize the t-ZrO_2 could limit the effectiveness of the transformation toughening mechanism for the particle size obtained when an external stress is applied, and it would require processing modifications to increase crack resistance.

(3) The best alumina-zirconia composite developed in this study, A10Z, presents a threshold, K_{I0}, significantly higher than monolithic alumina and zirconia. This should offer the option of improving the safety range of use of orthopedic implants.

Acknowledgments

The authors wish to express their appreciation to L. A. Diaz and to J. L. Rodríguez for his kind help with sample preparations.

References

[1]R. C. Garvie, R. H. J. Hannink, and R. T. Pascoe, "Ceramic Steel?," *Nature (London)*, **258**, 703–704 (1975).

[2]N. Claussen, "Fracture Toughness of Al_2O_3 with an Unstabilized ZrO_2 Dispersed Phase," *J. Am. Ceram. Soc.*, **59** [1–2] 49–51 (1976).

[3]D. J. Green, R. H. J. Hannink, and M. V. Swain, *Transformation Toughening of Ceramics*; p. 232. CRC Press, Boca Raton, FL, 1989.

[4]R. H. J. Hannink, P. M. Kelly, and B. C. Muddle, "Transformation Toughening in Zirconia-Containing Ceramics," *J. Am. Ceram. Soc.*, **83** [3] 461–87 (2000).

[5]D. J. Green, "Critical Microstructures for Microcracking in Al_2O_3-ZrO_2 Composites," *J. Am. Ceram. Soc.*, **65** [12] 610–14 (1982).

[6]N. Claussen, J. Steeb, and R. F. Pabst, "Effect of Induced Microcracking on the Fracture Toughness of Ceramics," *Am. Ceram. Soc. Bull.*, **56** [6] 559–62 (1977).

[7]N. Claussen, "Stress-Induced Transformation of Tetragonal ZrO_2 Particles in Ceramic Matrices," *J. Am. Ceram. Soc.*, **61**, 85 (1978).

[8]N. Claussen and M. Rühle, "Design of Transformation-Toughened Ceramics"; pp. 137–63 in Advances in Ceramics, Vol. 3, *Science and Technology of Zirconia I*. Edited by A. H. Heuer and L. W. Hobbs. American Ceramic Society, Columbus, OH, 1981.

[9]R. C. Garvie, "Critical Size Effects in Alumina-Zirconia Alloys"; pp. 55–69 in Advanced in Ceramics, Vol. 24A, *Science and Technology of Zirconia III*. Edited by S. Sōmiya, N. Yamamoto, and H. Hanagida. American Ceramic Society, Westerville, OH, 1988.

[10]A. H. Heuer, N. Claussen, W. M. Kriven, and M. Rühle, "Stability of Tetragonal ZrO_2 Particles in Ceramic Matrices," *J. Am. Ceram. Soc.*, **65** [12] 642–50 (1982).

[11]F. F. Lange, "Transformation Toughening: Part I, Size Effects Associated with the Thermodynamics of Constrained Transformations," *J. Mater. Sci.*, **17** [1] 225–34 (1982).

[12]F. F. Lange and D. J. Green, "Effects of Inclusion Size on the Retention of Tetragonal ZrO_2: Theory and Experiments"; see Ref. 8, pp. 217–25.

[13]A. H. Heuer, "Stability of Tetragonal ZrO_2 Particles in Ceramic Matrices," *J. Am. Ceram. Soc.*, **65** [12] 642–50 (1982).

[14]G. L. Messing and M. Kumagai, "Low-Temperature Sintering of Seeded Sol–Gel-Derived, ZrO_2-Toughened Al_2O_3 Composites," *J. Am. Ceram. Soc.*, **72** [1] 40–44 (1989).

[15]V. V. Srdic and L. Radonjic, "Transformation Toughening in Sol–Gel-Derived Alumina-Zirconia Composites," *J. Am. Ceram. Soc.*, **80** [8] 2056–60 (1997).

[16]F. Thevenot and P. Homerin, "Composites Alumine-Zircone"; pp. 39–57 in *Ceramiques Composites a Particules, cas du Frittage-Reaction (FORCERAM)*. Edited by F. Thevenot. Septima, Paris, France, 1992.

[17]F. F. Lange, "Powder Processing Science and Technology for Increased Reability," *J. Am. Ceram. Soc.*, **72** [1] 3–15 (1989).

[18]F. F. Lange, "Transformation Toughening: Part 5, Effect of Temperature and Alloy on Fracture Toughness," *J. Mater. Sci.*, **17** [1] 225–62 (1982).

[19]P. F. Becher, "Slow Crack Behavior in Transformation-Toughened Al_2O_3-ZrO_2 (Y_2O_3) Ceramics," *J. Am. Ceram. Soc.*, **66** [7] 485–88 (1983).

[20]K. Tsukuma, K. Ueda, and M. Shimada, "Strength and Fracture Toughness of Hot Isostatic-Pressed Y_2O_3-Partially Stabilized ZrO_2/Al_2O_3 Composites," *J. Am. Ceram. Soc.* **68** [1] C-4 (1985).

[21]P. F. Becher, "Transient Thermal Stress Behavior in ZrO_2-Toughened Al_2O_3," *J. Am. Ceram. Soc.*, **64** [1] 37–39 (1981).

[22]I. A. Aksay, F. F. Lange, and B. I. Davis, "Uniformity of Al_2O_3-ZrO_2 Composites by Colloidal Filtration," *J. Am. Ceram. Soc.*, **66** [10] C-190–C-192 (1983).

[23]S. Hori, M. Yoshimura, and S. Sōmiya, "Al_2O_3–ZrO_2 Ceramics Prepared from CVD Powders"; pp. 794–805 in Advances in Ceramics, Vol. 12, *Science and Technology of Zirconia II*. Edited by N. Claussen, M. Rühle, and A. H. Heuer. American Ceramic Society, Columbus, OH, 1984.

[24]D. W. Sproson and G. L. Messing, "Preparation of Alumina-Zirconia Powders by Evaporative Decomposition Solutions," *J. Am. Ceram. Soc.*, **67** [7] C-92–C-93 (1984).

[25]S. Somiya, S. Kikugawa, and M. Yoshimura, "Fine Grained Al_2O_3-ZrO_2 Ceramics by Hydrothermal Reaction Sintering," *Am. Ceram. Soc. Bull.*, **63** [3] 459 (1984).

[26]B. Fegley Jr., P. White, and H. K. Bowen, "Preparation of Zirconia-Alumina Powders by Zirconium Alkoxide Hydrolysis," *J. Am. Ceram. Soc.*, **68** [2] C-60–C-62 (1985).

[27]G. Fantozzi and G. Orange, "Thermomechanical Properties of Zirconia Toughened Alumina Materials"; pp. 188–215 in *Processing of Advanced Ceramics*. Edited by J. S. Moya and S. De Aza. Societie de Espana Cerámica Vidro. Arganda del Rey, Madrid, Spain, 1986.

[28]J. Chevalier, A. H. De Aza, G. Fantozzi, M. Schehl, and R. Torrecillas, "Extending the Lifetime of Orthopaedic Implants," *Adv. Mater.*, **12** [21] 1619–21 (2000).

[29]W. Cremer, "Defined Grinding in a Grinding Chamber Formed as an Annular Gap," *Interceram*, [5] 59–61 (1989).

[30]M. Schehl, L. A. Díaz, and R. Torrecillas, "Alumina Nanocomposites from Powder-Alkoxide Mixtures," *Acta Mater.*, **50**, 1125–39 (2002).

[31]S. Hirano, T. Yogo, and K. Kikuta, "Processing of Functional Ceramics by Metallorganic Route," *J. Ceram. Soc. Jpn.*, **99** [10] 1026–35 (1991).

[32]H. Toroya, M. Yoshimura, and S. Sōmiya, "Calibrated Curve for Quantitative Analysis of the Monoclinic-Tetragonal ZrO_2 System by X-Ray Diffraction," *J. Am. Ceram. Soc.*, **67** [6] C-119–C-121 (1984).

[33]A. G. Evans, "A Method for Evaluating the Time-Dependent Failure Characteristics of Brittle Materials and Its Application to Polycrystalline Alumina," *J. Mater. Sci.*, **7**, 1137–46 (1972).

[34]D. P. Williams and A. G. Evans, "A Simple Method to Study Slow Crack Growth," *J. Test. Eval.*, **1** [4] 264–70 (1973).

[35]J. Chevalier, M. Saadaoui, C. Olagnon, and G. Fantozzi, "Double-Torsion Testing a 3Y-TZP Ceramic," *Ceram. Int.*, **22**, 171–77 (1996).

[36]M. Ciccotti, "Realistic Finite-Element Model for Double-Torsion Loading Configuration," *J. Am. Ceram. Soc.*, **83** [11] 2737–44 (2000).

[37]E. R. Fuller Jr., "An Evaluation of Double Torsion Testing– Analysis"; pp. 3–19 in Proceedings of the 11th Symposium of Fracture Mechanics: Part II, ASTM STP 678, *Fracture Mechanics Applied to Brittle Materials*. Edited by S. W. Freiman. American Society for Testing and Materials, Philadelphia, PA, 1979.

[38]B. J. Plekta, E. R. Fuller, and B. G. Koepke, "An Evaluation of Double Torsion Testing–Experimental"; *ibid*, pp. 19–38.

[39]M. E. Ebrahimi, J. Chevalier, and G. Fantozzi, "Slow Crack Growth of Alumina Ceramics," *J. Mater. Res.*, **15**, 142–47 (2000).

[40]J. Chevalier, "Slow Crack Growth Behavior of 3Y-TZP Biomedical Ceramics" (in Fr.); Ph.D. Thesis. National Institute of Applied Sciences of Lyon, Lyon, France, 1996.

[41]J. Chevalier, C. Olagnon, and G. Fantozzi, "Subcritical Crack Propagation in 3Y-TZP Ceramics: Static and Cyclic Fatigue," *J. Am. Ceram. Soc.*, **82** [11] 3129–38 (1999).

[42]B. Lawn, *Fracture of Brittle Solids*, 2nd Ed., Cambridge Solid State Science Series; p. 378. Cambridge University Press, Oxford, U.K., 1993.

[43]J. Chevalier, C. Olagnon, and G. Fantozzi, "Crack Propagation and Fatigue in Zirconia-Based Composites," *Composites (Guildford UK)*, Part A, 30, 525–30 (1999).

[44]G. Willmann, "Ceramic Femoral Heads for Total Hip Arthroplasty," *Adv. Eng. Mater.*, **2** [3] 114–22 (2000). □

journal

J. Am. Ceram. Soc., 86 [1] 186–88 (2003)

Composition and Crystallization of Hydroxyapatite Coating Layer Formed by Electron Beam Deposition

Dong-Hwan Kim, Young-Min Kong, Su-Hee Lee, In-Seop Lee, and Hyoun-Ee Kim*

School of Materials Science and Engineering, Seoul National University, Seoul, 151-742, Korea

Seong-Joo Heo and Jai-Young Koak

Department of Prosthodontics and Intellectual Biointerface Engineering Center, College of Dentistry, Seoul National University, Seoul, Korea

To improve the biocompatibility of Ti-based metal implants, a hydroxyapatite (HA) coating layer was formed on the surface by electron-beam deposition. The dissolution rate of the coating layer was strongly dependent on the layer's calcium/phosphorus (Ca/P) ratio. Layers with a Ca/P ratio close to that of crystalline HA (Ca/P = 1.67) showed good stability in a physiologic saline solution. When the layer was crystallized by heat treatment in air at temperatures between 400° and 500°C, the stability was enhanced further while maintaining good interfacial bonding strength with the substrate. Preliminary *in vivo* tests on rabbits indicated that heat treatment and the resultant enhancement in stability are beneficial for bone attachment to the implants.

I. Introduction

To improve the bioactivity of various metal implants, hydroxyapatite (HA; $Ca_{10}(PO_4)_6(OH)_2$) or other calcium phosphates are often used as coatings.[1] Because of their chemical and crystallographic similarities to the inorganic components of human bones, HA or calcium phosphate layers promote the direct bonding or the earlier stabilization of implants with the surrounding bones or tissues.[2] For actual applications, in addition to bioactivity, the coating layer should possess a high bonding strength with the metal substrate and a low dissolution rate in a body fluid environment.[1–3]

Various techniques have been used to deposit HA or other calcium phosphate layers on metal implants.[3–7] Regardless of the coating methodology used, amorphous layers with unacceptably high dissolution rates are generally formed on metal substrates. Therefore, the coatings are thermally crystallized at elevated temperatures. During these thermal treatments, many cracks are formed due to a thermal expansion mismatch between the coating and the metal substrate, which severely reduces the bonding strength of the coating layer with the substrate.[8–11]

In this study, thin calcium phosphate surface coatings were deposited on Ti-based alloys by electron-beam deposition. The Ca/P ratio of the layer was controlled by adding extra CaO to the HA targets.[6] Effects of the Ca/P ratio on the coating layer's dissolution rate and crystallization behavior on heat treatment were monitored. The relationship between the heat treatment conditions and the bonding strength of the layer was also investigated and related to the crystallization behavior. Screw-shaped Ti alloy implants were coated and heat-treated for preliminary *in vivo* tests. The implants were placed in the proximal tibial metaphysis of rabbits for 6 weeks, and the bioactivity of the coating layer was evaluated by measuring the removal torque of the implants.

II. Experimental Procedure

Thin HA coating layers were electron-beam deposited on a commercial-purity Ti substrate (Supra Alloys, Inc., Camarillo, CA). Two types of specimens were prepared: flat disks for physical and *in vitro* analyses and screws for *in vivo* tests. Disks with a diameter of 25 mm and a thickness of 2 mm were ground and polished with diamond pastes down to 1 μm. Screws with a length of 4.0 mm, an outer diameter of 3.75 mm, and a pitch height of 0.5 mm were prepared.

After the chamber was evacuated down to 10^{-7} torr, an electron beam (Telemark, Fremont, CA) of 8.5 kV and ~0.1 A was directed onto the source target. Targets were made using a commercially available HA powder (Alfa Aesar Co., Ward Hill, MA). Up to 30 wt% of CaO powder (Cerac Co., Milwaukee, WI) was added to the HA, and the mixtures were sintered in air at 1200°C for 2 h. Composition, thickness, and bond strength of the deposited layers were analyzed using techniques reported previously.[6]

The deposited coating layer was heat-treated in air at temperatures between 300° and 600°C for 1 h. Two different procedures were used to measure the dissolution rate of the layer in a physiologic saline solution. Before the heat treatments, the dissolution rate was measured using a surface profiler.[6] After the heat treatments, the dissolution rate was measured by monitoring the concentrations of the solution in which the specimen was immersed.

Eleven female New Zealand white rabbits were used for the *in vivo* tests. All animals were between 9 and 10 months old. After general anesthesia, four implants were placed in each rabbit, two in each proximal tibial metaphysis. The holes for the implantation were drilled with a low-speed rotary instrument with profuse saline irrigation. The diameters of the drills were successively increased, and the insertion sites were finalized with a 3.75 mm tap without countersinking. After a healing period of 6 weeks, the rabbits were sacrificed and the bond strength between the bone and the implant was measured with a torque measurement device (Shinsung Co., Seoul, Korea).

III. Results and Discussion

All of the coating layers formed on the surface of the Ti substrate were in an amorphous state. The composition of layers

T. Kokubo—contributing editor

Manuscript No. 187618. Received June 27, 2001; approved October 23, 2002.
This work was sponsored by the National Research Laboratory (NRL) Program of the Ministry of Science and Technology of Korea.
*Member, American Ceramic Society.

estimated by EDS was different from that of targets. The EDS was calibrated using standard specimens of known composition. When pure HA was used as a target, the Ca/P ratio of the layer was much lower than the stoichiometric HA (Ca/P = 1.67). The Ca/P ratio of the deposited layer was increased by adding extra CaO to the HA.[6] When 17.5% of CaO was added to the HA, the target had a Ca/P ratio of 2.4 and the resultant coating layer had 1.62, which is very close to that of stoichiometric HA. The Ca/P ratio of the coating layer is known to vary widely depending on the deposition procedures.[5,12–14]

The dissolution rate of the coating layer in the physiologic saline solution decreased with increasing Ca/P ratio until it reached the value for stoichiometric HA. However, when the Ca/P ratio exceeded 1.67, the dissolution rate increased again.[6] It still remains unclear which level is the optimum dissolution rate for such coatings in a biological environment.[15] Therefore, in the present experiment, coating layers with very low dissolution rate were prepared by heat treatment in air and tested *in vivo*. The dissolution rate of the coating layer was further reduced by heat treatment in air. XRD patterns of the layers (Ca/P = 1.62) after treatments at various temperatures are shown in Fig. 1. Up to 300°C, the coating layer remained amorphous, as shown in Fig. 1(A), but at 400°C, the layer was partially crystallized into HA. This crystallization occurred more extensively as the temperature was increased to 500°C and finally to 600°C. Layers with different Ca/P ratios were also crystallized into HA; however, the crystallization temperature required was much higher than that required for the stoichiometric HA composition. Figure 2 shows the crystallization temperature of the layers with different Ca/P ratios to achieve similar degree of crystallization as the stoichiometric HA layer at 500°C.

The crystallization of the coating layers by heat treatment has been known for a long time.[4] At the same time, it is also well known that the interfacial bonding strength between the coating layer and the substrate decreases by such treatment.[8–11] When the treatment temperature was too high, thermal stress developed on the layer because of the difference in the thermal expansion coefficients (CTE; $\alpha_{HA} = 16 \times 10^{-6}$/°C, $\alpha_{Ti} = 10 \times 10^{-6}$/°C) causing a cracking and/or delamination of the layers. However, in this experiment, up to 500°C, the bonding strength remained almost unchanged, as shown in Fig. 3.

The dissolution rate of the coating layers after heat treatment was estimated by monitoring the concentration changes of the saline solution in which the specimens were immersed. The

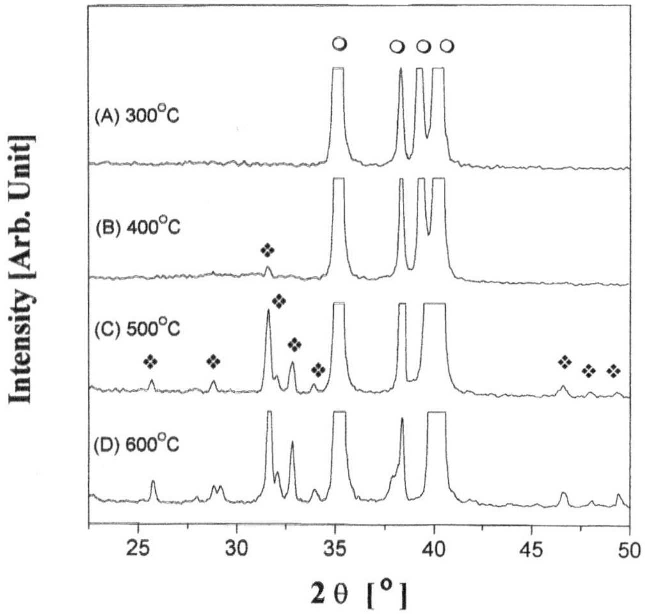

Fig. 1. X-ray diffraction patterns of the coating layers (Ca/P = 1.62) heat-treated at various temperatures in air: (○) Ti, (❖) HA.

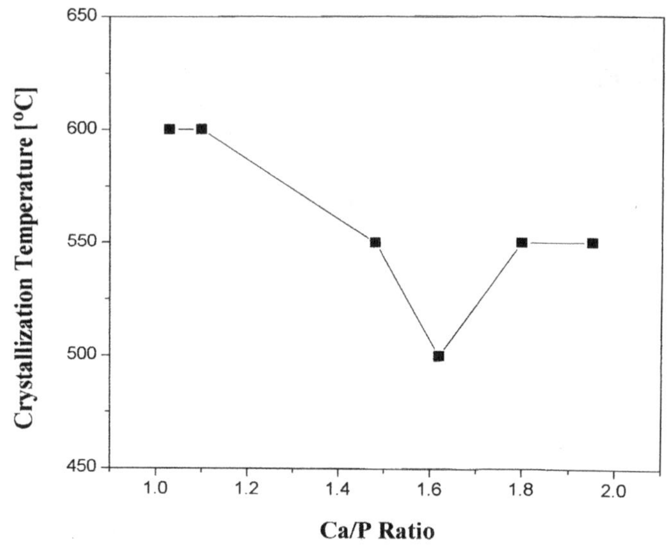

Fig. 2. Effect of Ca/P ratio on the crystallization temperature of the coating layers.

surface profiler could not be used because of the increased surface roughness. Figure 4 shows the dissolution rates of the crystallized layers compared with that of as-deposited specimens. When the layer was crystallized by heat treatment at 450°C, the dissolution rate was reduced, as shown in Fig. 4, and was further reduced by increasing the heat treatment temperature to 500°C. Therefore, heat treatment at temperatures between 400° and 500°C is suitable to crystallize the coating layers without decreasing the bonding strength.

The effect of crystallization and the resultant improvement in the dissolution behavior on biological performance was estimated by *in vivo* tests on rabbits. Screw-shaped Ti implants were blasted with 75 μm Al_2O_3 particles at a pressure of 5 kgf/cm^2. The implants were subsequently coated with HA (Ca/P = 1.62) and heat-treated for 1 h at 500°C in air for the crystallization. Four implants were placed in each of seven rabbits: two heat-treated ones on the right proximal tibial metaphysis and two implants without heat treatment on the left. Out of 28 implants, except for two heat-treated specimens and one without heat treatment, all were successfully osseointegrated.

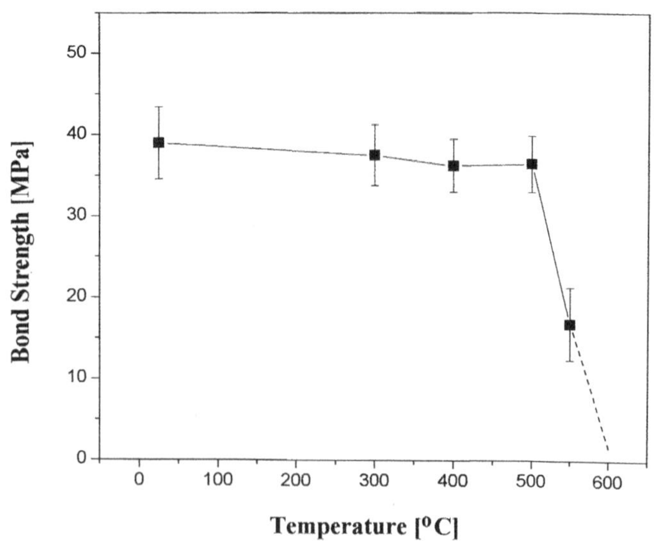

Fig. 3. Bond strength of the coating layers to the metal substrate after heat treatment.

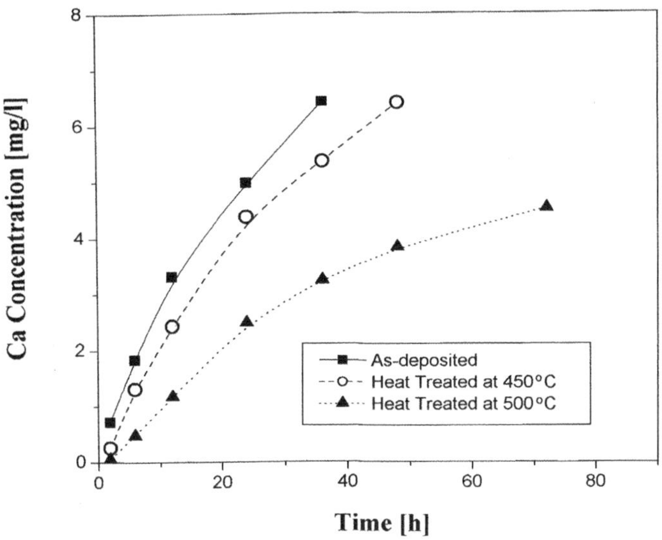

Fig. 4. Dissolution behavior of the coating layers in the physiologic solution after heat treatment in air.

The removal torques of the implants after 6 weeks of healing are itemized in Table I. The average removal torque of the heat-treated implants was significantly higher than that of the untreated controls. Greater removal force is generally interpreted as an increase in the bone healing around the implants and an improved osseointegration. The heat-treated coating layers permitted the bone tissue to grow onto implant surfaces, while the layers without the treatment were apparently dissolved too quickly for the new bone tissue to extend onto the substrate surface. For the purpose of comparison, the removal torque of the implants without the HA coating were similarly tested in four rabbits. The removal torque required for implants without a coating lay between that of the heat-treated and untreated specimens with the HA coating. These results suggest that the biocompatibility of the metal implants is controllable and may be enhanced further by adjusting the dissolution rate of the coating layers.

IV. Summary

The bioactivity of metal implants was enhanced by coating with HA. The dissolution rate of the HA coating layer in physiologic saline solution is an important factor for biological performance. The dissolution rate of the layer was controlled by changing the Ca/P ratio and by crystallization through heat treatment in air. When the Ca/P ratio of the coating layer was much different from the stoichiometric HA value (Ca/P = 1.67), high crystallization temperatures were necessary (≥550°C), and that led to cracking and delamination of the layers. When the Ca/P ratio of the layer was 1.62, complete crystallization commenced at 450°C without any cracking or delamination. Preliminary *in vivo* tests indicate that heat treatment and the resultant reduction in dissolution rate are beneficial to bone attachment to implants.

Table I. Removal Torque of Implants after 6 Weeks

Removal torque (N·cm)		
Coated		
Without heat treatment	Heated-treated at 450°C	Without coating (sand blasted)
24	34	34
10	32	34
12	24	34
10	32	36
34	28	20
24	38	20
14	20	20
14	24	10
16	36	20
20	24	22
10	24	34
20	36	36
	26	20
		22
Average (±1 standard deviation)		
17.3 (7.3)	29.1 (5.8)	25.8 (8.4)

References

[1]K. Soballe and S. Overgaard, "The Current Status of Hydroxyapatite Coating of Protheses," *J. Bone Jt. Surg.*, **78-B**, 689–91 (1996).

[2]L. Willam, M. D. Jaffe, F. David, and M. D. Scott, "Total Hip Arthroplasty with Hydroxyapatite-Coated Prostheses," *J. Bone Jt. Surg.*, **78-A** [12] 1918–34 (1996).

[3]C. Y. Yang, B. C. Wang, E. Chang and B. C. Wu, "Bond Degradation at the Plasma-Sprayed HA Coating/Ti-6Al-4V Alloy Interface: An *In Vitro* Study," *J. Mater. Sci. Mater. Med.*, **6**, 258–65 (1995).

[4]T. S. Chen and W. R. Lacefield, "Crystallization of Ion Beam Deposited Calcium Phosphate Coatings," *J. Mater. Res.*, **9** [5] 1284–90 (1994).

[5]Z. S. Luo, F. Z. Cui, and W. Z. Li, "Low-Temperature Crystallization of Calcium Phosphate Coatings Synthesized by Ion-Beam-Assisted Deposition," *J. Biomed. Mater. Res.*, **42**, 80–86 (1998).

[6]J. M. Choi, Y. M. Kong, S. Kim, H.-E. Kim, C. S. Hwang, and I. S. Lee, "Formation and Characterization of Hydroxyapatite Coating Layer on Ti-Based Metal Implant by Electron-Beam Deposition," *J. Mater. Res.*, **14**, 2980–85 (1999).

[7]F. Z. Cui, Z. S. Luo, and Q. L. Feng, "Highly Adhesive Hydroxyapatite Coatings on Titanium Alloy Formed by Ion Beam Assisted Deposition," *J. Mater. Sci.: Mater. Med.*, **8**, 403–405 (1997).

[8]B. Locardi, U. Pazzaglia, C. Gabbi, and B. Profilo, "Thermal Behaviour of Hydroxyapatite Intended for Medical Applications," *Biomaterials*, **14**, 437–41 (1993).

[9]P. Ducheyne, W. V. Raemodonck, J. C. Heughebaert, and M. Heughebaert, "Structural Analysis of Hydroxyapatite Coatings on Titanium," *Biomaterials*, **7**, 97–103 (1986).

[10]K. A. Gross, V. Gross, and C. C. Berndt, "Thermal Analysis of Amorphous Phase in Hydroxyapatite Coatings," *J. Am. Ceram. Soc.*, **81** [1] 106–12 (1998).

[11]W. Tong, J. Chen, Y. Cao, L. Lu, J. Feng, and X. Zhang, "Effect of Water Vapor Pressure and Temperature on the Amorphous-to-Crystalline HA Conversion during Heat Treatment of HA Coatings," *J. Biomed. Mater. Res.*, **36**, 242–45 (1997).

[12]F. Z. Cui and Z. S. Luo, "Biomaterials Modification by Ion-Beam Processing," *Surf. Coat. Technol.*, **112**, 278–85 (1999).

[13]X. Li, J. Weng, W. Tong, C. Zuo, X. Zhang, P. Wang, and Z. Liu, "Characterization of Hydroxyapatite Film with Mixed Interface by Ar^+ Ion Beam Enhanced Deposition," *Biomaterials*, **18**, 1487–93 (1997).

[14]K. van Dijk, C. H. M. Maree, J. Verhoeven, F. H. P. M. Havraken, and J. A. Jansen, "A Complete Characterization of $Ca_5(PO_4)_3OH$ Sputter-Deposited Films by Ion Beam Analysis: RBS and ERD," *J. Biomed. Mater. Res.*, **42**, 366–71 (1998).

[15]H. Zeng, K. K. Chittur, and W. R. Lacefield, "Dissolution/Reprecipitation of Calcium Phosphate Thin Films Produced by Ion Beam Sputter Deposition Technique," *Biomaterials*, **20**, 443–51 (1999). □

J. Am. Ceram. Soc., **86** [2] 357–59 (2003)

journal

Synthesis of Nanosized and Microporous Precipitated Hydroxyapatite in Synthetic Polymers and Biopolymers

Arvind Sinha, Suprabha Nayar, and Archana Agrawal

National Metallurgical Laboratory, Jamshedpur 831007, India

Debasish Bhattacharyya

Indian Institute of Chemical Biology, Kolkata 700 032, India

Patcha Ramachandrarao

Banaras Hindu University, Varanasi 221005, India

In situ **precipitation of microporous and nanosized hydroxyapatite particles (5–40 nm) has been conducted in poly(vinyl alcohol) and bovine serum albumin gels. The process, which is similar to biomineralization, is highly controlled with respect to microstructural features, such as size and shape, and to precipitation of hydroxyapatite phase having a calcium:phosphorus stoichiometric ratio of 1.67. Nanosized precipitated hydroxyapatite particles show remarkable thermal stability and do not decompose to other calcium phosphate phases, even at higher temperatures.**

I. Introduction

Out of the six principal calcium salts of orthophosphoric acid, precipitated hydroxyapatite (PHA) is most similar to the apatite present in bone, and it is known for its excellent biocompatibility and nontoxicity.[1] PHA is the as-precipitated phase of hydroxyapatite (HA) in aqueous solution, and it normally exists in a poorly crystalline state.[2] Several techniques based on wet, dry, hydrothermal, and alkoxide methods have been developed for the synthesis of PHA and HA.[3–6] However, the chemistry of PHA is very complex, and, when attempts have been made to precipitate it in solution, uncontrolled agglomerates of apatite products that have a calcium:phosphorus ratio ranging from 1.5 to 1.66 have been produced.[7] Apatite structures are normally characterized by the presence of channels along their hexagonal axes, and ions in these channels are less rigorously bound in comparison with those in the bulk.[8] This results in many specific structural, thermal, and chemical properties associated with PHA that makes the material suitable for bone implantation and for chromatographic separation as catalysts, ion exchangers, and drug-delivery systems.[9]

Nature produces a variety of minerals in nano and bulk sizes with an optimum degree of crystallinity and porosity through the process of biomineralization. Recent experiments have revealed biomimetics (polymer matrix mediated *in situ* synthesis of inorganic materials) as a powerful tool for the synthesis of monodispersed nanoparticles and hierarchical structures produced by the self-assembly, self-construction, and self-organization of basic building components.[10,11] In the present manuscript, we discuss a biomimetic approach for the synthesis of monodispersed nanosized PHA particles and microporous polymer–HA composites with a calcium:phosphorus molar ratio of 1.67. The supramolecular matrices used are bovine serum albumin (BSA) and poly(vinyl alcohol) (PVA). This simple process provides nanosized and porous PHA–bio/synthetic polymer composites that can be directly used for various orthopedic applications.

II. Experimental Procedure

In situ synthesis of nanosized and microporous HA particles was conducted using gels of PVA and BSA, respectively. Two 54 mL sets of freshly prepared 0.4 *M* calcium nitrate tetrahydrate solution were made alkaline using 11 mL of 1:2 ammonia:water solution. A 70 mL aqueous solution of 0.1g of BSA (i.e., 0.1% Fraction V powder, SRL, India) in 100 mL of double-distilled water was added to one of the above sets, and 70 mL aqueous solution of 4% PVA was added to the other set. The calcium nitrate–BSA system was gently stirred to avoid denaturation of the protein, but the calcium nitrate–PVA system was vigorously stirred for 10 min, and both solutions were poured into Petri dishes and allowed to form transparent gels by incubating at 75°C in a hot-air oven for 24 h. A 77 mL amount of 0.156 *M* diammonium hydrogen phosphate was made alkaline using 7 mL of 1:1 ammonia:water, and this was added to the above gels. Milky white coloration was observed almost instantaneously, and the gels were allowed to stand for 48 h, after which they were decanted, and the mineralized gels washed thoroughly with deionized water. The HA formed was structurally characterized using scanning electron microscopy (SEM; Model JSM-840 A, JEOL, Tokyo, Japan), transmission electron microscopy (TEM; Model CM 200, Philips, Eindhoven, The Netherlands), X-ray diffractometry (XRD; Model PTS 3003, Seifert), Fourier-transform infrared spectroscopy (FTIR), and differential thermal analysis (DTA, Model A-320, Seiko) techniques.

III. Results and Discussion

The applications of synthetic polymers and biopolymers as preorganized matrices for controlled nucleation and growth of minerals is of paramount importance in biomimetic studies.[12] Gelation of PVA solution under optimum conditions leads to the formation of a noncovalent spatial network. The major types of intermolecular links in the junction knot are hydrogen bonding between –OH groups of neighboring polymer chains. Syndiotactic sites in the chains are responsible for the formation of hydrogen

R. Condrate—contributing editor

Manuscript No. 186907. Received June 17, 2002; approved September 4, 2002.

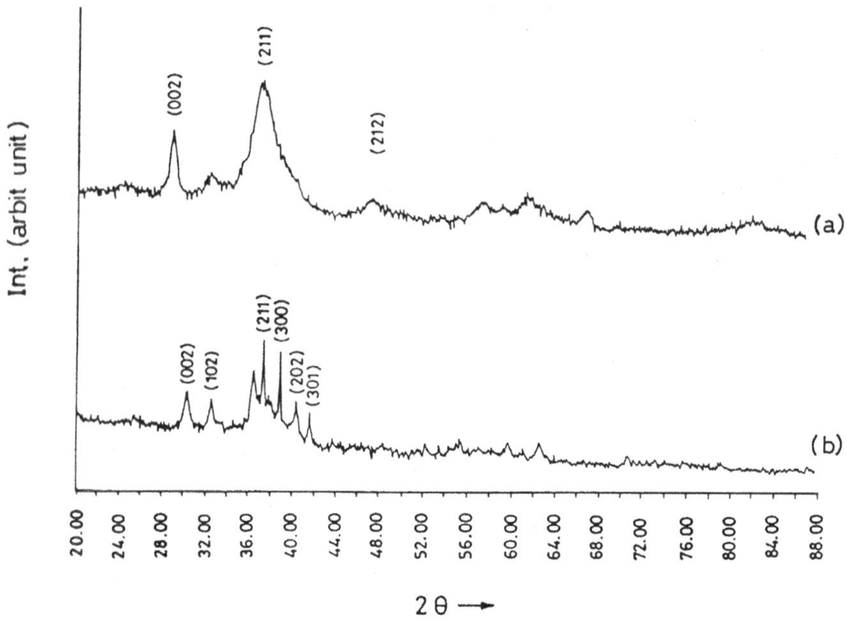

Fig. 1. XRD pattern of nanosized HA particles in (a) PVA gel and (b) BSA gel.

bonds, while the isotactic sites participate in intermolecular interactions to sterically entrap cations.[13] Similarly, BSA is a globular protein that has nanosized cavities in its native folded form. The specific spatial chemistry of nanosized cavities present in the quaternary structure of BSA attracts cations through interfacial molecular recognition.[14] Based on their conformation, the above organic systems dictate size, morphology, and orientation of inorganic particles and kinetically control the nucleation and growth process.

The formation of PHA phases in PVA and BSA has been confirmed using XRD. Characteristic (002), (112), (211), and (212) reflections in the diffraction pattern of the calcium phosphate *in situ* synthesized in PVA confirms the formation of the HA phase (Fig. 1(a)). An underlying broadening of peaks reflects the nanometer range of the particle size. Peak analysis of the (211) reflection (scanned at $0.5° \text{min}^{-1}$) using the Scherer formula ($L = 0.9\lambda/B \cos\theta$, where λ is the wavelength of the X-ray, B the full width at half maximum, and θ the Bragg angle) predicts an average particle size of 5 nm embedded in the PVA matrix. The analysis, however, does not take into account the instrumental and strain-induced components of the peak broadening. Similarly, the XRD pattern of PHA precipitated in BSA exhibits characteristic reflections from (002), (102), (211), (300), (202), and (301) planes of the pure HA phase (Fig. 1(b)). The Bragg peaks obtained in this sample are relatively sharper with respect to the particles produced in the PVA matrix. Peak width analysis of a slow-scanned (211) reflection of the diffraction pattern indicates an average size of 25 nm, as compared with 35 nm obtained by plotting the size distribution curve based on TEM micrographs. No decrease in the peak broadening can be observed, even after storing the sample for >30 d. This indicates the absence of aggregation-based growth of nanosized particles in the organic matrix.

SEM studies of PHA–PVA composite film manifest the presence of regularly arranged and interconnected uniform-sized pores of the order of 1–2 μm (Fig. 2(a)), a requirement of the osteoblast process attributed to the preorganized porous PVA matrix. The limited solubility of PVA in water makes it possible to form a micellelike structure that leads to the huddling of hydrophilic groups to form tubular conformations that minimize the surface energy. As a result of solvent loss, the tubules assemble themselves into a long-range-ordered structure under mild conditions of gelation.[15,16] During gelation, the present calcium ions sterically entrap on the diffused surface of the PVA, transform the texture of the gel from regularly arranged tubular array to a fibrillike interconnected porous structure. These cations then react with phosphate ions at alkaline pH to precipitate the apatite phase, which keeps the porous network intact. A high nucleation rate of apatite particles followed by a very slow growth rate in highly viscous PVA matrix leads to the formation of poorly crystalline PHA particles in the nanosized range. Stability of 4–5 nm PHA particles can be explained as surface-energy minimization as a result of interaction of supercritical nuclei with PVA. In the absence of the matching of interatomic distances in PVA and HA, this process resembles the biologically induced precipitation of

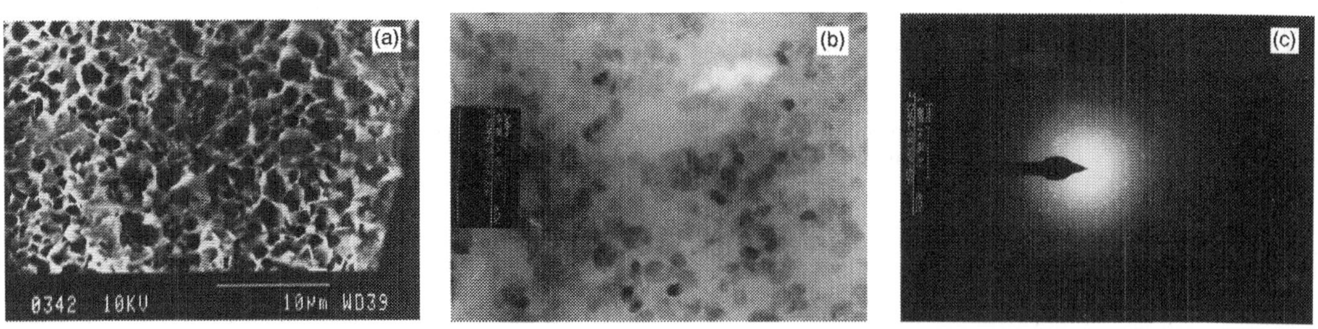

Fig. 2. (a) SEM micrograph of *in situ*-synthesized microporous PVA–PHA composite. (b) TEM micrograph exhibiting monodispersed and nanosized HA particles (30–40 nm) in a BSA matrix. (c) SAD pattern from PHA particles in BSA gel, revealing a polycrystalline ring from (100) reflection of HA.

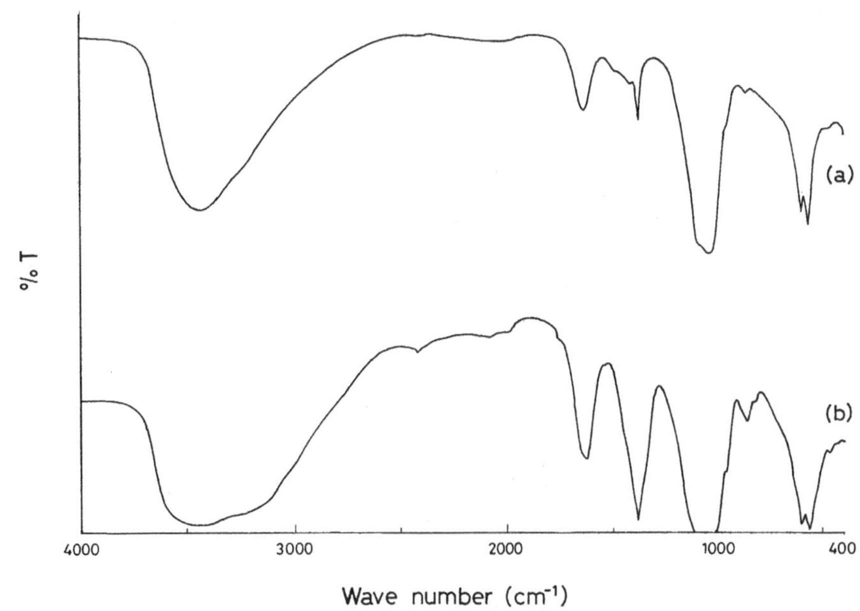

Fig. 3. FTIR spectra of (a) PHA–PVA composite and (b) PHA–BSA composite.

biominerals, where the organic matrix provides a functional surface for heterogeneous nucleation and constrained space for precipitation.

TEM microstructures of PHA precipitated in a BSA matrix reveal monodispersion of nanosized particles of uniform size (30–40 nm) and elliptical morphology (Fig. 2(b)). This is attributed to the nucleation and growth of HA particles limited to self-organized nanosized cages present in the quaternary structure of BSA. Similar to Ferritin, BSA facilitates the matrix-mediated precipitation process into these cages as a result of electrostatic, structural, and stereochemical interactions at the organic–inorganic interface.[13] The only ring present in the selected-area diffraction (SAD) pattern of these particles can be indexed as (100) (Fig. 2(c)). The energy-dispersive X-ray (EDX) analysis of the PVA/BSA–PHA film and atomic absorption spectroscopy (AAS) confirm a calcium:phosphorous ratio of 1.67, which confirms the formation of stochiometric HA phase.

FTIR studies also confirm the *in situ* precipitation of nanosized HA particles in organic matrices. Although the usual hydroxyl-stretching vibration of apatite occurs at 3573 cm^{-1},[17] there are evidences, e.g., FTIR of chicken bone, that interference of organic matrices brings about changes in the FTIR spectra. In contrast, when the crystals are isolated free of organic constituents, the apatite nature is readily identifiable.[18] Hence, in the PHA–PVA composite, the bands at 3435 and 635 cm^{-1} may correspond to hydroxyl-ion stretching and deformation bands, respectively, and bands at 1740 and 1384 cm^{-1} may be attributed to –C=O and $-CH_2$ asymmetric bending, a signature of PVA formed by the hydrolysis of poly(vinyl acetate). The double bands centered at $\sim$603 cm^{-1} are due to bending modes of P–O bonds in phosphate groups, while the band at 1079 cm^{-1} is due to stretching modes of P–O bonds. (Fig. 3(a)). Along with the characteristic bands corresponding to hydroxyl and phosphate groups of HA, two well-defined peaks of BSA are obtained at 1638 and 1384 cm^{-1} in BSA–PHA composites (Fig. 3(b)). PHA particles synthesized in PVA and BSA matrices exhibit a rare thermal stability, because no transformation or their decomposition to other calcium phosphate phases can be observed, even by heating the samples to 1200°C in air as, confirmed by DTA studies.

IV. Conclusions

This communication reports a biomimetic synthesis route to produce porous PVA–PHA composites and monodispersed and nanosized PHA particles in BSA. A case similar to biologically induced precipitation in PVA matrix replicates the porous network of the matrix, whereas, because of the specific electrostatic interactions at the protein cages, the nucleation of HA nanoparticles takes place as a result of matrix-mediated mineralization.

References

[1]A. Makishima and H. Aohi, *Bioceramics* (in Jpn.); p. 267. Edited by T. Yamaguchi and H. Yanagida. Hihodo, Tokyo, Japan, 1984.

[2]M. Bohner, "Calcium Orthophosphates in Medicine: From Ceramics to Calcium Phosphate Cements," *Injury, Int. J. Care Injured*, **31**, S-D-37–47 (2000).

[3]A. L. Boskey and A. S. Posner, "Conversion of Amorphous Calcium Phosphate to Microcrystalline Hydroxyapatite. A pH-Dependent, Solution-Mediated, Solid–Solid Conversion," *J. Phys. Chem.*, **77**, 2313 (1973).

[4]T. Okuyama, T. Ogawa, and M. Ebihara, *Gypsum Lime*, **210**, 323 (1987).

[5]T. Nagaya and H. Kuwahara, "Calcium Phosphate Type Hydroxyapatite for Chromatographic Separation and Process for Producing Same," U.S. Pat. No. 4 781 904, Nov. 1988.

[6]M. Kikuchi, Y. Suetsugu, J. Tanaka, S. Ito, S. Ichinose, K. Shiniyama, Y. Hiraoka, Y. Mandal, and S. Nakatani, "The Biomimetic Synthesis and Biocompatibility of Self-Organized Hydroxyapatite/Collagen Composites," *Bioceramics*, **12**, 393 (1999).

[7]P. Brown and R. J. Martin, "An Analysis of Hydroxyapatite Surface Layer Formation," *Phys. Chem. B*, **103**, 1671–75 (1999).

[8]J. C. Heughebaert and G. Bonel, "Composition, Structure, and Properties of Calcium Phosphate of Biological Interest"; p. 9 in *Biological and Biochemical Performance of Biomaterials*. Edited by P. Christel, A. Meunier, and A. J. C. Lee. Elsevier Science, Amsterdam, The Netherlands, 1986.

[9]A. Uchida, Y. Shinto, N. Araki, and O. Ono, "Slow Release of Anticancer Drugs from Porous Calcium Hydroxyapatite Ceramics," *J. Orthop. Res.*, **10**, 440–45 (1992).

[10]S. Mann, B. R. Heywood, S. Rajam, and J. D. Brichall, "Controlled Crystallization of $CaCO_3$ Under Steric Acid Monolayers," *Nature (London)*, **334**, 692 (1988).

[11]L. Addadi and S. Weiner, "Interaction of Acidic Proteins and Crystals: Stereochemical Requirements in Biomineralization," *Proc. Natl. Acad. Sci. U.S.A.*, **82**, 4110 (1985).

[12]S. Mann, "Molecular Tectonic in Biomineralization and Biomimetic Materials Chemistry: Review Article," *Nature (London)*, **365**, 499 (1993).

[13]A Sinha, A. Agrawal, S. K. Das, B. Ravi Kumar, V. Rao, and P. Ramachandrarao, "On the Growth of Monoclinic Calcium Carbonate in Poly(vinyl alcohol)," *J. Mater. Sci. Lett.*, **20**, 1569–72 (2001).

[14]S. Nayar, A. Sinha, S. Das, S. K. Das, and P. Ramachandrarao, "*In Situ* Synthesis of Nanosized Cadmium Sulfide Using Bovine Serum Albumin," *J. Mater. Sci. Lett.*, **20**, 2099–100 (2001).

[15]H. Y. Yasuda, S. Mahara, T. Nishiyama, and Y. Umakoshi, "Preparation of Hydroxyapatite/Tricalcium Phosphate Composites by Colloidal Process," *Sci. Technol. Adv. Mater.*, **3**, 29–33 (2002).

[16]A. Sinha, J. Chakraborty, S. K. Das, S. Das, V. Rao, and P. Ramachandra Rao, "Oriented Arrays of Nanocrystalline Magnetite in Polymer Matrix Produced by Biomimetic Synthesis," *Mater. Trans. JIM*, **42** [8] 1672–75 (2001).

[17]K. C. Blakeslee and A. Condrate, "Vibrational Spectra of Hydrothermally Prepared Hydroxyapatites," *J. Am. Ceram Soc.*, **54** [11] 559–63 (1971).

[18]L. K. Spearing, C. Rey, H. M. Kim, and M. J. Glimcher, *Synthesis and Processing of Nanocrystalline Powder*; pp. 57–68. Edited by D. Bourell. The Minerals, Metals, and Materials Society, Warrendale, PA, 1996. □

J. Am. Ceram. Soc., **86** [3] 517–19 (2003)

Sintered Hydroxyapatite Latticework for Bone Substitute

F. Cristina Gomes de Sousa and Julian R. G. Evans

Department of Materials, Queen Mary, University of London, London, E1 4NS, United Kingdom

Hydroxyapatite suspensions were extruded through a range of nozzles from 100 to 330 μm diameter from a stepper-driven syringe. Regular latticework scaffolds were built by fused deposition modeling (FDM), a solid freeforming method, on a three-axis table using 330 μm diameter filament. The scaffolds were sintered at 1250°C to 97% density retaining the hydroxyapatite crystal structure. The scaffolds were introduced to cultured human osteoblast cells and, after 48 h, the surfaces were thoroughly covered with active cells.

I. Introduction

An intriguing miscellany of porous materials has been proposed for insertion into human beings in the quest for a support to encourage and enhance bone growth following orthopaedic surgery. They include ostrich eggshell,[1] hen's eggshell,[2] marine coral,[3] deproteinized bovine bone,[4] plaster of Paris,[5] calcium carbonate,[6] and various forms of calcium phosphate[7,8] and hydroxyapatite.[9] Mammalian studies suggest that calcium phosphate is resorbed and bone regenerated after 4–12 weeks.[10]

Natural materials present the body with a porous calcium-containing mineral that provides a scaffold for biomineralization. However, there is little control over the pore size, distribution, or diameter of connecting channels that are essential for the development of blood vessels to conduct nutrient to growing bone and to remove waste products. Ceramic foaming methods have therefore emerged as a way of providing a more controlled material. Many techniques are available for creating ceramic foams.[11] Hydroxyapatite foams have been made by water-based[12,13] and polymer-based[14] methods but there remains incomplete control of the architecture in such foaming processes.

It is against this background that solid freeforming methods need to be assessed. Selective laser sintering has been used to make porous hydroxyapatite material[15] as has indirect stereolithography, in which a pyrolyzable mold is generated from computed tomographic data.[16] Hutmacher[17] has used extrusion freeforming to make polycaprolactone filled with 7 vol% hydroxyapatite to provide a bioconsumable latticework scaffold for bone substitute. Extrusion freeforming, otherwise known as fused deposition modeling (FDM) or fused deposition of ceramics (FDC), has been widely used for functional ceramics[18] and is particularly suited to scaffold construction because the characteristic problem of stepped surfaces does not occur in latticework. What is more, the method opens up the prospect of multinozzle or variable nozzle work[19] in which a scaffold could have large (150 μm) pores for blood vessels intersecting a very fine porous (10–20 μm) structure providing strength and accommodation for active osteoblast cells. Extrusion freeforming can produce fine (60 μm) diameter zirconia threads by extrusion using a modified sapphire ink-jet printing nozzle.[20] We aim to apply this method to the preparation of sintered hydroxyapatite latticework and thereby to encourage its wider use in solid freeforming of bioscaffolds.

II. Experimental Details

Table I gives details of materials, their sources, and formulation. Organic components were dissolved in solvent, powder was added, and the mixture subjected to ultrasonic mixing under a probe (type IKA U200S, Carl Stuart, Ltd., Staffs, U.K.). Partial drying left a paste which was loaded into a syringe (Type: HGB 81320 1 mL, Hamilton GB, Ltd., Carnforth, U.K.) driven by a linear actuator (four-phase, 88 N linear force, type N, RS components Northants, U.K.) over a three axis table (Parker Hannifin Automation, Dorset, U.K.). The table (Fig. 1) was driven by Easitools™ software to form latticework patterns ("log-pile" structures). The extrusion dies were (a) 100 μm i.d. sapphire nozzle (INZA0402054K, Lee Products, Ltd., Gerrards Cross, U.K., (b) 190 μm i.d. sapphire nozzle (INZA0705014K supplied *ibidem*), and (c) luer lock syringe needle (23 g: 330 μm i.d.) with 6 mm land length and polished end. The extrusion speed was independently controlled. The lattices were heated at 5°C/min to 350°C in flowing air and then sintered at 1225° or 1250°C for 5 h. X-ray diffraction was done on a Siemens D5000 diffractometer and scanning electron microscopy on a Jeol 6300.

Cell culture was conducted under the supervision of Dr. Lucy Di Silvio at the Institute of Orthopaedics, Stanmore, U.K., following a well-established[21] procedure for assessment of biomaterials with human osteoblast sarcoma (HOS) cells cultured in Dulbecco's modified Eagle's medium supplemented *inter alia* with 10% fetal calf serum. Cells were seeded at a density of 2×10^6 cells mL^{-1} and incubated for 48 h at 37°C in a humidified atmosphere with 5% CO_2. The cells were viewed in a Jeol JSM 5500LV scanning electron microscope after dehydration with alcohols, staining, further dehydration, and coating with palladium.

III. Results and Discussion

X-ray diffraction of the powder and the sintered material showed that it was single-phase hydroxyapatite corresponding to JCPDS Card 9-432. The powder was fine and agglomerated. The sintered density after 5 h measured on compacted disks was 91% at 1225°C and 97% at 1250°C. At 1225°C the grain size was ~4 μm and most pores were 1–5 μm. The selection of PVB as a binder was based on adhesion properties,[22] dispersant action for ceramics,[23] and its widespread use in tape casting.[24]

Figure 2 shows sintered filaments made by extrusion through 100 and 190 μm sapphire nozzles and through a 330 μm stainless steel tube. This indicates the possibility of making very fine latticework structures. In previous work[20] with thermoplastic filament extrusion, it was not possible to build with filaments below about 190 μm diameter because solidification occurred before deformation and welding. Similarly, with the solvent method used here, it was not possible to build regular lattices with

J. W. Halloran—contributing editor

Manuscript No. 186819. Received September 12, 2002; approved November 15, 2002.

Table I. Details of Materials, Sources, and Compositions

Material	Grade	Source	Density (kg·m^{-3})	Concn (wt%)
Hydroxyapatite	GPR	Merck KgaA, Darmstadt, Germany	3160	77.0
Poly(vinyl butyral)	BN18	Wacker Chemicals, U.K.	1100	11.5
Poly(ethylene glycol)	20000 mol wt	BDH Merck, Poole, U.K.	1210	11.5
Propan-2-ol†	GPR	BDH Merck, Poole, U.K.	789	—

†Diluted to form a paste; loss on drying 50 wt%.

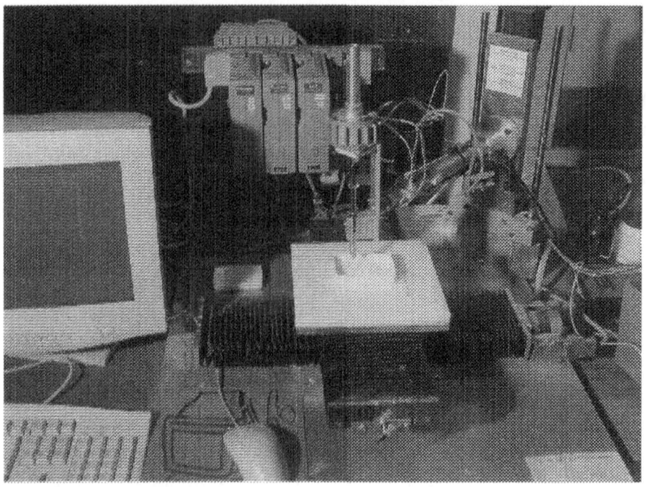

Fig. 1. Arrangement of the extruder over the three-axis table.

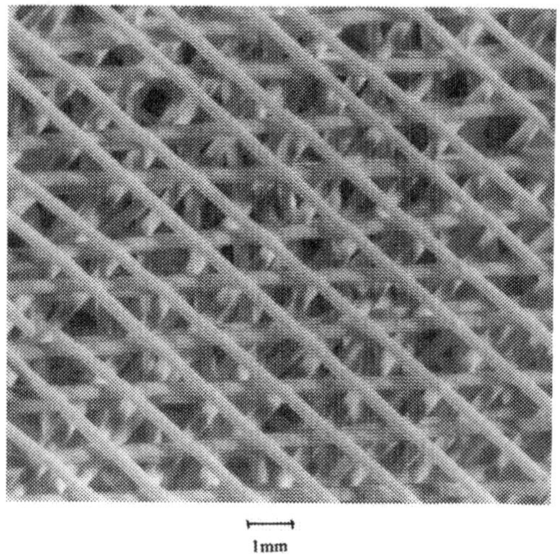

Fig. 3. Hydroxyapatite latticework with a 0°–45°–90° lay-up ($V_c \sim 0.25$).

190 μm filament with propan-2-ol solvent because rapid evaporation had a similar effect. A higher molecular weight solvent may ameliorate this restriction. However, 300 μm filament was easily processed.

The nozzle was positioned 3 mm above the building plane. The syringe plunger velocity V_R, was controlled to give an extrusion velocity V_r, of 20 ms^{-1} based on the dependence on radius of the syringe (R) and die (r), namely

$$V_R = V_r\left(\frac{r}{R}\right)^2 \quad (1)$$

The filament spacing was chosen to give a ceramic volume fraction of about 0.25. For a "log-pile" structure with cylindrical filaments of radius r, and intercenter spacing a, the ceramic volume fraction is

$$V_c = \frac{\pi r}{2a} \quad (2)$$

Thus for a given filament, $V_c \propto 1/a$. When the filaments touch and $a = 2r$ the maximum packing efficiency of 78.5% is reached. Clearly higher volume fractions can be obtained with noncylindrical filaments.

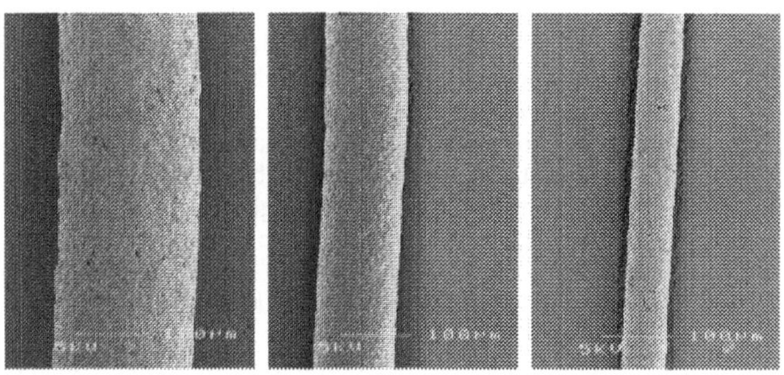

Fig. 2. Sintered filaments deposited from nozzles of diameter (a) 330, (b) 190, and (c) 100 μm.

Figure 3 shows a ceramic scaffold with a 0°–45°–90° lay-up. A few filaments have fractured during drying because each layer dries while attached to its predecessor that has already undergone shrinkage. Slight shrinkage deformation causing a concave curvature was also attributed to drying effects.

The welding mechanism at the junction is similar to the solvent welding-before-firing technique that can be used in general for ceramics made by injection molding, extrusion, or tape casting.[25] The sintered and fractured weld seen in Fig. 4 indicates that fluidity is retained for much longer than in welds made by thermoplastic extrusion freeforming of fine filament ceramics.[20] The disk-shaped weld occupies a larger area than the thermoplastic welds where the limitation is rapid cooling. The selection of solvent for volatility thus becomes the main factor controlling filament diameter and hence the ability to form multipore size arrays, which is clearly the next step in the evolution of this approach.

Figure 5 shows the dense array of HOS cell relics on the sintered surface of the hydroxyapatite scaffold as revealed by scanning electron microscopy. This *in vitro* testing protocol has

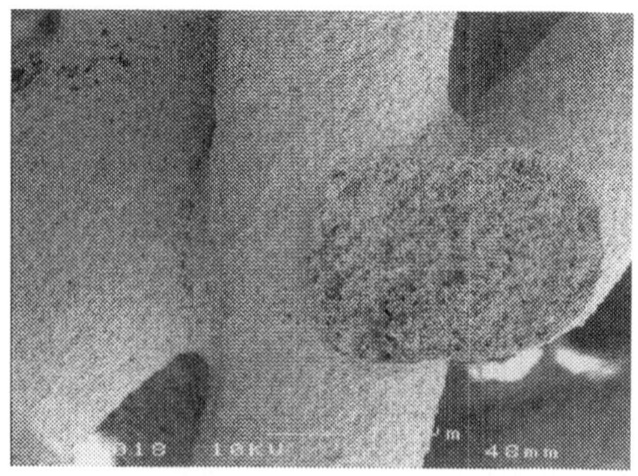

Fig. 4. Detail of the welds formed between successive layers in a lattice sintered at 1225°C (scale bar represents 100 μm).

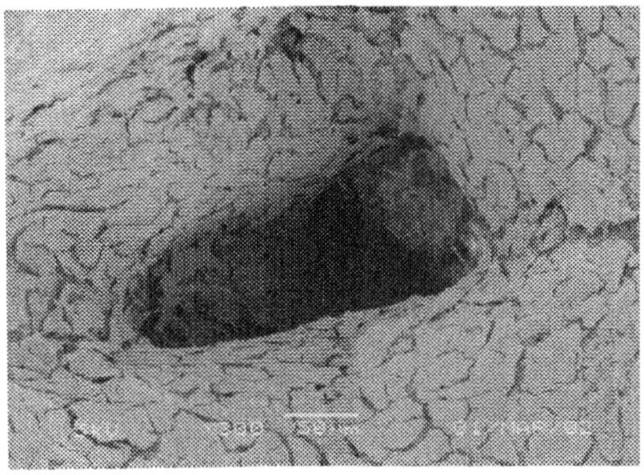

Fig. 5. Attachment of human osteoblast-like cells to the sintered scaffold showing dense coverage after 48 h incubation.

become an established stage in the assessment of biomaterials. The attachment of cells occurs by placing of filopodia on the ceramic surface and it presages biomineralization. In this micrograph the surface density of attachment after 48 h incubation indicates the viability of this material for further biological study.

IV. Conclusions

Extrusion freeforming of crowded ceramic suspensions offers a route for preparing sintered ceramic scaffolds in the form of regular or multichannel lattices. The welds produced by solvent extrusion of 330 μm diameter filament extended over a wide contact area. Solvent volatility restricted finer filament work (<200 μm), as does rapid cooling in thermoplastic extrusion freeforming. Human osteoblast sarcoma cells were cultured on the sintered hydroxyapatite scaffold and formed a dense covering after 48 h, indicating the biocompatibility of the scaffold.

Acknowledgments

We are grateful to Ms. Thushari Herath and Dr. Lucy Di Silvio for conducting the cell culture work at the Institute of Orthopaedics, Stanmore Orthopaedic Hospital, London, U.K.

References

[1]L. Dupoirieux, "Ostrich Eggshell as a Bone Substitute: A Preliminary Report of Its Biological Behaviour in Animals—A Possibility in Facial Reconstructive Surgery," *Br. J. Oral Maxillofacial Surg.*, **37**, 467–71 (1999).

[2]L. Dupoirieux, D. Pourquier, and F. Souyris, "Powdered Eggshell—A Pilot-Study on a New Bone Substitute for Use in Maxillofacial Surgery," *J. Cranio-Maxillo-Facial Surg.*, **23**, 187–94 (1995).

[3]B. Loty, F. X. Roux, B. George, J. P. Courpied, and M. Postel, "The Use of Coral as a Bone Substitute," *Int. Orthopaedics.*, **14**, 255–59 (1990).

[4]J. Catanese, J. D. B. Featherstone, and T. M. Keaveny, "Characterisation of the Mechanical and Ultrastructural Properties of Heat-Treated Cortical Bone for Use as a Bone Substitute," *J. Biomed. Mater. Res.*, **45**, 327–36 (1999).

[5]N. G. Georgiade, J. Hanker, G. Ruff, and S. Levin, "The Use of Particulate Hydroxyapatite and Plaster of Paris in Aesthetic and Reconstructive Surgery," *Aesthetic Plast. Surg.*, **17**, 85–92 (1993).

[6]A. Lucas, J. Gaude, C. Carel, J. F. Michel, and G. Cathelineau, "A Synthetic Aragonite-Based Ceramic as a Bone Graft Substitute and Substrate for Antibiotics," *Int. J. Inorg. Mater.*, **3**, 87–94 (2001).

[7]I. R. Zerbo, A. L. J. J. Bronckers, G. L. de Lange, G. J. van Beek, and E. H. Burger, "Histology of Human Alveolar Bone Regeneration with a Porous Tricalcium Phosphate—A Report of Two Cases," *Clinical Oral Implants Res.*, **12**, 379–84 (2001).

[8]K. Shimazaki and V. Mooney, "Comparative Study of Porous Hydroxyapatite and Tricalcium Phosphate as Bone Substitute," *J. Orthopaedic Res.*, **3**, 301–10 (1985).

[9]J. F. Kay, "Current Uses of Hydroxyapatite as a Bone Substitute," *Am. Am. Ceram. Soc. Bull.*, **62**, 871–71 (1983).

[10]I. Manjubala, M. Sivakumar, R. V. Sureshkumar, and T. P. Sastry, "Bioactivity and Osseointegration Study of Calcium Phosphate Ceramic of Different Chemical Composition," *J. Biomed. Mater. Res.*, **63**, 200–208 (2002).

[11]J. Saggio-Woyanski, C. E. Scott, and W. P. Minnear, "Processing of Porous Ceramics," *Am. Ceram. Soc. Bull.*, **71**, 1674–82 (1992).

[12]P. Sepulveda and J. G. P. Binner, "Processing of Cellular Ceramics by Foaming and *In Situ* Polymerisation of Organic Monomers," *J. Eur. Ceram. Soc.*, **19**, 2059–66 (1999).

[13]P. Sepulveda, J. G. P. Binner, S. O. Rogero, O. Z. Higa, and J. C. Bressiani, "Production of Porous Hydroxyapatite by the Gel-Casting of Foams and Cytotoxic Evaluation," *J. Biomed. Mater. Res.*, **50**, 27–34 (2000).

[14]E. Ebaretonbofa and J. R. G. Evans, "Low Density Hydroxyapatite Foam Scaffolds for Bone Substitute," *J. Porous Mater.*, in press.

[15]N. K. Vail, L. D. Swain, W. C. Fox, T. B. Aufdlemorte, G. Lee, and J. W. Barlow, "Materials for Biomedical Applications," *Mater. Design.*, **20**, 123–32 (1999).

[16]T. M. G. Chu, J. W. Halloran, S. J. Hollister, and S. E. Feinberg, "Hydroxyapatite Implants with Designed Internal Architecture," *J. Mater. Sci.—Mater. Med.*, **12**, 471–78 (2001).

[17]D. W. Hutmacher, T. Schantz, I. Zein, K. W. Ng, S. H. Teoh, and K. C. Tan, "Mechanical Properties and Cell Cultural Response of Polycaprolactone Scaffolds Designed and Fabricated via Fused Deposition Modelling," *J. Biomed. Mater. Res.*, **55**, 203–16 (2001).

[18]A. Safari and S. C. Danforth, "Solid Freeform Fabrication of Novel Piezoelectric Ceramics and Composites for Transducer Applications," *Ferroelectrics*, **231**, 731–45 (1999).

[19]A. A. Tseng and M. Tanaka, "Advanced Deposition Techniques for Freeform Fabrication of Metal and Ceramic Parts," *Rapid Prototyping J.*, **7**, 6–17 (2001).

[20]I. Grida and J. R. G. Evans, "Extrusion Freeforming of Ceramics through Fine Nozzles," *J. Eur. Ceram.*, in press.

[21]M. J. Dalby, L. di Silvio, E. J. Harper, and W. Bonfield, "*In Vitro* Adhesion and Biocompatibility of Osteoblast-like Cells to Poly(methyl methacrylate) and Poly-(ethyl methacrylate) Bone Cements," *J. Mater. Sci.—Mater. Med.*, **13**, 311–14 (2002).

[22]D. A. Schupp and W. W. Gerberich, "Effects of Film Thickness on the Work of Fracture between Adhesive and Glass," *J. Adhes.*, **35**, 269–83 (1991).

[23]S. Bhattacharjee, M. K. Paria, and H. S. Maiti, "Poly(vinyl butyral) as a Dispersant for Barium Titanate in a Nonaqueous Suspension," *J. Mater. Sci.*, **28**, 6490–45 (1993).

[24]H. Hellebrand, "Tape Casting"; pp. 189–265 in *Materials Science and Technology*, Vol. 17A. Edited by R. W. Cahn, P. Haasen, and E. J. Kramer. VCH, Weinheim, Germany.

[25]H. Rashid, K. Lindsey, and J. R. G. Evans, "Joining Ceramics before Firing by Solvent Welding," *J. Eur. Ceram. Soc.*, **7**, 165–75 (1991). □

J. Am. Ceram. Soc., **86** [5] 806–10 (2003)

Bioactivity and Mechanical Properties of Poly(dimethylsiloxane)-Modified Calcia–Silica Hybrids with Added Titania

Qi Chen, Noboru Miyata,* and Tadashi Kokubo*

Department of Material Chemistry, Faculty of Engineering, Kyoto University, Kyoto 606-8501, Japan

Takashi Nakamura

Department of Orthopedic Surgery, Faculty of Medicine, Kyoto University, Kyoto 606-8507, Japan

Hydrolysis and polycondensation of poly(dimethylsiloxane) (PDMS), tetraethoxysilane (TEOS), and calcium nitrate, added with tetraisopropyltitanate (TiPT) at a TiPT/(TiPT + TEOS) molar ratio of 0.15, gave a pore- and crack-free transparent monolithic organic-inorganic hybrid material. It was speculated to be composed of a Si–O–Ti–O$^-$ network modified with methyl groups, and a Ca^{2+} ion ionically bonded to the network. The hybrid obtained showed a high apatite-forming ability on its surface in a simulated body fluid that is indicative of high bioactivity, as well as mechanical properties such as bending strength, Young's modulus, and strain at failure, analogous to those of the human cancellous bone. This hybrid material is expected to be useful as a new type of bioactive bone-repairing material.

I. Introduction

SINCE the discovery of Bioglass® by Hench *et al.* in 1971,[1] various types of glasses, glass-ceramics, and sintered ceramics have also been found to bond to living bone, and are already used clinically as important bone-repairing materials.[2–4] Recently, it was revealed that some metals, such as titanium and its alloys, can bond to living bone when they are previously subjected to alkali and heat treatments.[5,6] Elastic moduli of these materials, however, are higher than those of natural bone. In contrast, organic polymers generally show lower elastic moduli, but they do not show bioactivity. A copolymer of poly(ethylene oxide) and poly(butylene terephthalate) called Polyactive® shows bioactivity,[7] but it is biodegradable. The essential requirement for an artificial material to bond to living bone is the formation of a bonelike apatite layer on its surface in the living body. Mechanical properties of the material should also be taken into account. Materials having higher elastic modulus than that of natural bone are liable to induce resorption of the surrounding bone because of stress shielding. Therefore, development of a new type of bioactive materials with mechanical properties analogous to those of natural bone is strongly required.

Organically modified sol–gel-derived ceramics are currently attracting much attention because of their unique properties. These hybrid materials are synthesized by chemically incorporating organic polymer into the inorganic network at the molecular level to improve the extensibility of pure oxide ceramics. Some of these materials are known as "ormosils" (*or*ganically *mo*dified *sil*icates)[8] and "ceramers."[9] The properties of the synthesized materials are anticipated to be highly dependent on the composition, molecular weight, and chemistry of the polymer as well as the process history. Tetraethoxysilane (TEOS) has been used as a main inorganic component of many systems, and poly(dimethylsiloxane) (PDMS) is an important organic component for the synthesis of the hybrids, because the terminal Si–OH groups of the latter can react with the Si–OH groups of hydrolyzed TEOS to form cross-linking of Si–O–Si. Although the structures and properties of the ormosils have been studied extensively during the last decade,[10–20] they have mainly been in the field of optical applications. Tsuru *et al.*[21] reported for an *in vitro* experiment that some ormosils containing Ca(II) can show bioactivity. Their mechanical properties, however, have not been reported. Young's moduli, hitherto reported for the ormosils, are 10–80 MPa.[10,11,15,16,19] These values are lower than those of human cancellous bone, ~50–500 MPa.[22] Titanium alkoxide can also be used to form the hybrids with PDMS.[23–26] Incorporation of titanium gives a high cross-linking density and an increased elastic modulus of the PDMS-modified materials.

In the present work, effects of incorporation of TiO_2 into PDMS-modified $CaO–SiO_2$ hybrids on their bioactivity and mechanical properties were investigated. A synthesis route different from Mackenzie's method[16] was used in the present study to incorporate highly reactive titanium alkoxide into the ormosils. Bioactivities of the products were evaluated by examining apatite formation on their surfaces in a simulated body fluid (SBF) with ion concentrations nearly equal to those of the human blood plasma.[27] It is already confirmed for various types of materials that the material that forms the apatite on its surface in SBF also forms the apatite in the living body and bonds to living bone.[28,29]

II. Experimental Procedure

(1) *Preparation of Hybrids*

Tetraethoxysilane (TEOS, $Si(OC_2H_5)_4$), tetraisopropyltitanate (TiPT, $Ti(OCH(CH_3)_2)_4$), calcium nitrate ($Ca(NO_3)_2{\cdot}4H_2O$), and hydrochloric acid (HCl 35%) (Nacalai tesque, Inc., Kyoto, Japan) were used as starting inorganic constituents. Poly(dimethylsiloxane) (PDMS, HO-$[Si(CH_3)_2\text{-O-}]_nH$, Aldrich Chemical Co., Milwaukee, WI) with average molecular weight of 1100 was used as the organic component. The starting materials with the compositions given in Table I were subjected to hydrolysis and polycondensation by the following procedure. TEOS was first prehydrolyzed in aqueous solution containing isopropyl alcohol (IPA) and tetrahydrofuran (THF), and the catalyst 35% HCl. Two hours later, PDMS was added to the solution. Fifteen hours later, TiPT and a mixture of calcium nitrate, H_2O, and IPA were mixed with the solution. The solutions were aged in a covered plastic container at ambient condition for 1 d. After partial evaporation, the solvents were kept at 40°C for gelation for 7 d. The formed gels were dried

P. W. Brown—contributing editor

Manuscript No. 188835. Received January 3, 2000; approved December 30, 2002.
Supported by The Special Coordination Fund of the Science and Technology Agency of Japan, Research on Creation of Biointegrated Materials to Improve Physically Handicapped People's Quality of Life.

*Member, American Ceramic Society.

Table I. Compositions and Properties of Examined Samples

Sample	Composition in molar ratio[†] TiPT / (TiPT + TEOS)	PDMS / (TiPT + TEOS)	$Ca(NO_3)_2$ / (TiPT + TEOS)	H_2O / (TiPT + TEOS)	Pore volume (cm^3/g)	Average diameter of pores (μm)	Induction period for apatite formation (d)
Ti0	0	0.109	0.15	2.0	0.039	0.0257	7
Ti5	0.05	0.109	0.15	2.0	0.091	0.0143	14
Ti10	0.10	0.109	0.15	2.0	0.087	0.0142	3
Ti15	0.15	0.109	0.15	2.0	0.079	0.0144	3
Ti30	0.30	0.109	0.15	2.0	0.155	0.227	1

[†] PDMS: poly(dimethylsiloxane), $[-Si(CH_3)_2-O-]_n$; TiPT: tetraisopropyltitanate, $Ti(OCH(CH_3)_2)_4$); TEOS: tetraethoxysilane, $Si(OC_2H_5)_4$).

at 60°C for 3 d and then heated at 150°C for 1 d. Monolithic disks ~70 mm in diameter and 6 mm thick were obtained.

(2) *Measurement of Density and Pore Structure*

Densities of the obtained samples were measured by the Archimedes method using water at 23°C. Pore-size distributions were measured by the mercury intrusion method (Poresizer 9320, Micromeritics Instrument Corp., Norcross, GA).

(3) *Soaking in Simulated Body Fluid*

The specimens 10 mm × 10 mm × 2 mm were cut, polished with No. 400 abrasive disk (one-step polishing), washed with distilled water and dried at 40°C. Acellular SBF with inorganic ion concentrations (Na^+ 142, K^+ 5.0, Mg^{2+} 1.5, Ca^{2+} 2.5, Cl^- 147.8, HCO^{3-} 4.2, HPO_4^{2-} 1.0, SO_4^{2-} 0.5 m*M*) nearly equal to those of human blood plasma was prepared by dissolving reagents NaCl, $NaHCO_3$, KCl, $K_2HPO_3{\cdot}3H_2O$, $MgCl_2{\cdot}6H_2O$, $CaCl_2$, and Na_2SO_4 (Nacalai tesque, Inc.) into distilled water and buffered to pH 7.4 at 36.5°C with $(CH_2OH)_3CNH_2$ and 1*M* HCl (Nacalai tesque, Inc.).[27] The specimens were soaked in 30 mL of SBF at 36.5°C. After soaking for various periods, the specimens were removed from the fluids, washed moderately with ion-exchanged distilled water, and dried at 40°C for 1 d.

(4) *Analysis of Sample Surface and Measurement of Element Concentrations of SBF*

The surfaces of the specimens were analyzed by thin-film X-ray diffraction (TF-XRD; Model 2651A, Rigaku Co., Tokyo, Japan) and Fourier transform infrared reflection spectroscopy (FT-IRRS; Model System 2000, Perkin-Elmer, Norwalk, CT). In the TF-XRD, the surface of the specimens was fixed at an angle of 1° against the direction of the incident beam. This technique enables the detection of a surface layer ~1 μm thick. The surfaces of the specimens were also observed under scanning electron microscopy (SEM; Model S2500CX, Hitachi, Tokyo, Japan) after coating a thin Au-Pd film.

Changes in element concentrations of SBF with the soaking of the specimens were measured by inductively coupled plasma (ICP) atomic emission spectroscopy (Model SPS1500, Seiko Instruments, Makuhari, Japan).

(5) *Measurement of Mechanical Properties*

Rectangular bar specimens of 3 mm × 4 mm × 30 mm were cut from the disks and polished using diamond pastes down to No. 2000 finish. Bending test of the specimens was conducted with a testing machine (Model AGS-10kNG, Shimadzu Co., Kyoto, Japan) using a three-point loading over a 20 mm span at a crosshead speed of 0.5 mm/min. Eight specimens were tested for each composition. The Young's modulus was determined from the slope of the initial linear elastic portion of the load–deflection curve, loading geometry, and specimen dimensions based on the simple linear elastic beam analysis. For materials having linear or approximately linear behavior up to the point of fracture, the maximum tensile edge stress and strain were calculated from the load and deflection data using simple elastic beam theory. For materials that exhibited a large nonlinear portion in the load–deflection curve, corrections were made based on the assumption that, beyond the initial linear portion, stress was approximated to be proportional to strain raised to a power. The exponent was estimated from a logarithmic plot of the experimental load-deflection data. The strain at failure and ultimate strength of the specimens were thus evaluated. It is possible that the neutral axis may shift somewhat from the centroid of the cross-sectional area of the beam as deformation largely progresses, but this was not taken into account in the present calculations.

III. Results

(1) *Structure of the Hybrids*

The homogeneous and transparent samples were obtained without cracking for all the examined compositions by the method described above. Figure 1 shows the bulk densities of the obtained samples. They increased with increasing TiPT content in the starting compositions. The pore volume and the average diameter of pores of the samples are shown in Table I. The pore volumes were <0.1 cm^3/g for all samples except sample Ti30. The average diameter of the pore was <0.03 μm for all samples except sample Ti30. Sample Ti30 contained pores of larger size (0.227 μm). These results indicate that except for Ti30 the samples are essentially pore-free and homogeneous.

Figures 2 and 3 show TF-XRD patterns and FT-IR reflection spectra of the surfaces of some samples as-prepared and soaked in SBF for various time periods. Assignments of main peaks on XRD patterns and IR spectra were made by referring to the previous literatures.[29–32] It can be seen from X-ray patterns of the as-prepared samples in Fig. 2 that all samples have an amorphous structure. IR spectra of the as-prepared samples in Fig. 3 show that all the samples are essentially composed of a Si–O network modified with methyl groups.

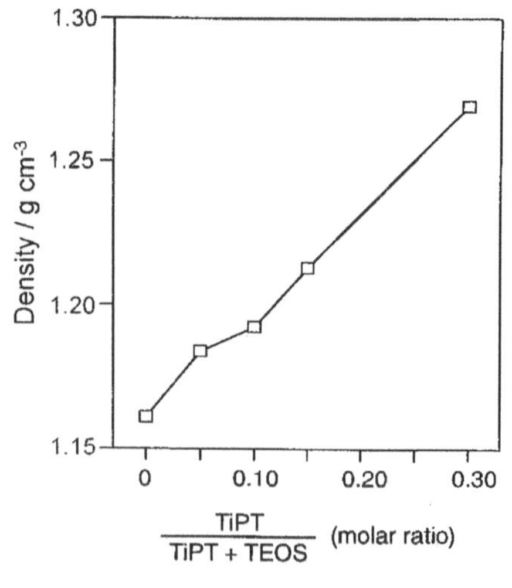

Fig. 1. Bulk densities of the samples.

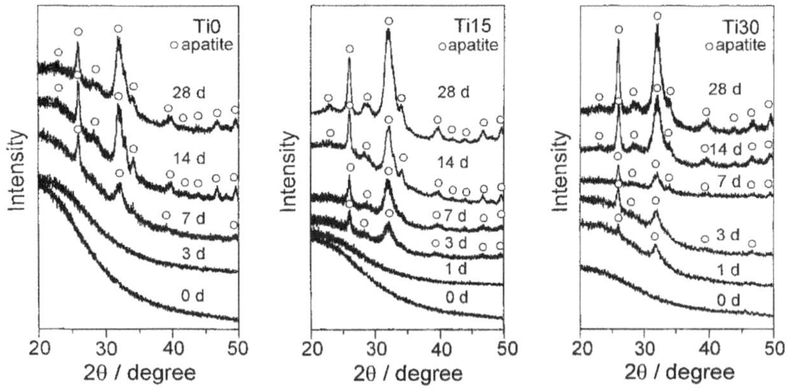

Fig. 2. TF-XRD patterns from the surfaces of samples Ti0, Ti15, and Ti30 as-prepared and soaked in SBF for various periods.

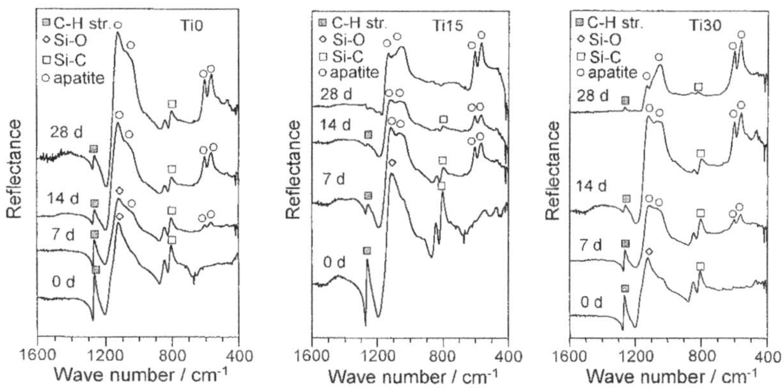

Fig. 3. FT-IR reflection spectra from the surfaces of samples Ti0, Ti15. and Ti30 as-prepared and soaked in SBF for various periods.

(2) Apatite-Forming Ability of Hybrids

Figure 4 shows SEM photographs of the surfaces of sample Ti15 soaked in SBF for 0, 3, and 14 d. It can be seen from Figs. 2–4 that all samples form an apatite on their surfaces in SBF sooner or later. The induction periods for apatite formation, which was determined by TF-XRD, are shown in Table I. It can be seen from Figs. 2–4 and Table I that apatite-forming ability of the samples in SBF increases with increasing TiPT content except for sample Ti5.

(3) Element Concentration Changes in SBF

Figure 5 shows changes in element concentrations in SBF with soaking of the samples. Titanium was not detected by ICP in SBF for all samples within 28 d. Figure 5 shows the increase in the calcium concentration and the decrease in the phosphorus concentration in SBF with increasing TiPT content in the starting compositions, except for Ti5. The increase in the silicon concentration in SBF increased with increasing TiPT content.

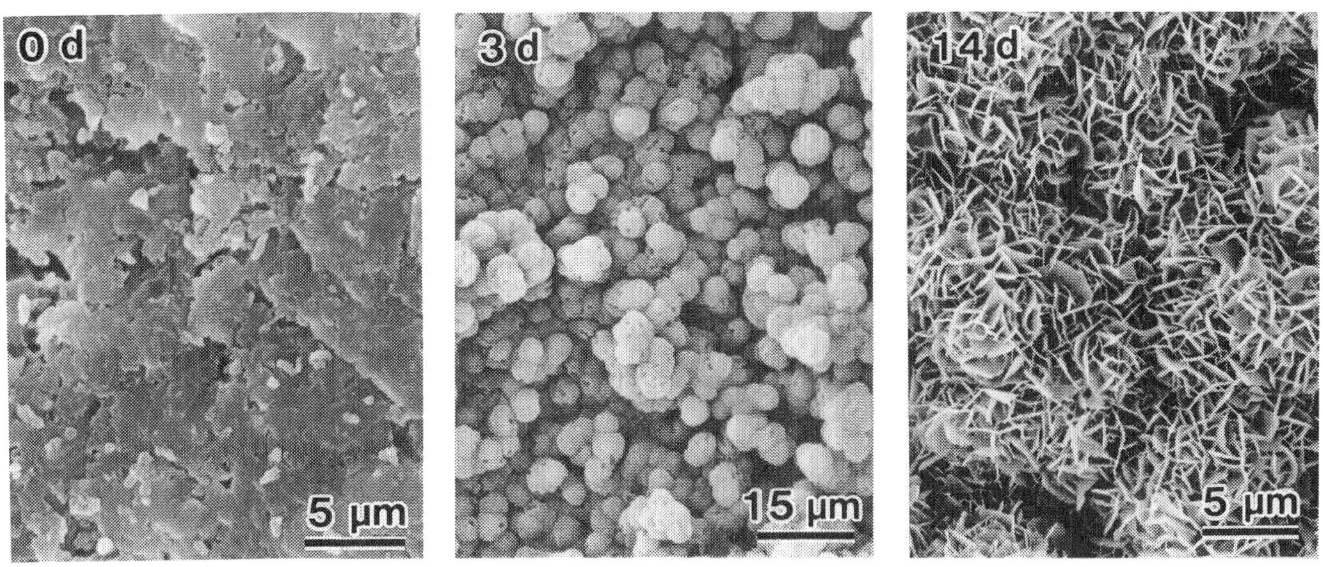

Fig. 4. SEM photographs of the surfaces of sample Ti15 soaked in SBF for various periods.

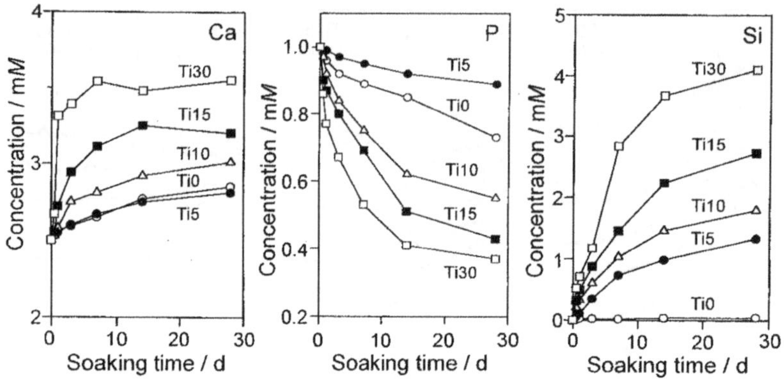

Fig. 5. Changes in element concentrations of SBF owing to soaking of the samples.

(4) Mechanical Properties of Samples

In Fig. 6, representative stress–strain curve established by a three-point bending test is shown for each composition. Strain at failure, bending strength, and Young's modulus obtained from these curves for each sample are shown in Figs. 7 and 8, in comparison with those of the human cancellous bone.[22] The magnitude of the strain at failure decreased with increasing TiPT content. The bending strengths were 10–15 MPa for all samples. The Young's modulus of the samples increased from 150 to 300 MPa with increasing TiPT contents.

IV. Discussion

It is apparent from the results described above that essentially pore- and crack-free, homogeneous, and transparent monolithic disks are obtained by the present sol–gel method, except for sample Ti30. Their bulk densities are >1.15 g/cm^3. These results are in contrast with the conventional ormosil, porosities, and bulk densities of which were $>50\%$ and 0.3–0.9 g/cm^3.[17] The bulk density of the samples increased with increasing TiPT content in the starting compositions (see Fig. 1). This indicates that the titanium oxide is incorporated into the Si–O network to give a compact structure, as suggested by Morsi and El-Shennawi.[33] TF-XRD patterns in Fig. 2 and FT-IR reflection spectra in Fig. 3 for the surface of the as-prepared samples showed that the samples have an amorphous structure essentially composed of a Si–O network modified with methyl groups. The titanium is speculated to be incorporated into this network structure. The lack of release of the titanium from the samples into SBF also supports this speculation. The calcium ion might be ionically bonded to the Si–O$^-$ and Ti–O$^-$ of the network, as in the conventional calcium silicate glasses.

All the hybrid materials formed an apatite on their surfaces in SBF. The induction period for the apatite formation increased a little by the addition of a small amount of titanium oxide, but decreased with increasing content of titanium oxide. This indicates that hybrids such as Ti10, Ti15, and Ti30 show a high bioactivity. The apatite-forming ability of the present hybrids is closely related to the rate of the release of the calcium ion in SBF (see Fig. 5). This is interpreted as follows: Hybrids that release the calcium ion at a high rate form a larger number of Si–OH and Ti–OH groups by exchanging with H_3O^+ ion in SBF and rapidly increase the ionic activity product of the apatite in the surrounding SBF,

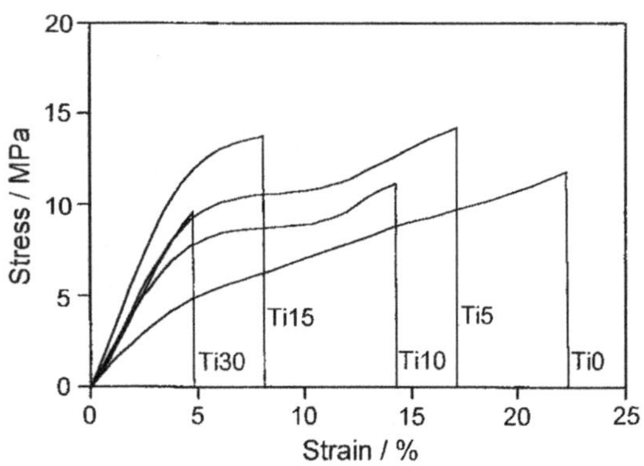

Fig. 6. Representative stress–strain curves of the samples measured by three-point bending test.

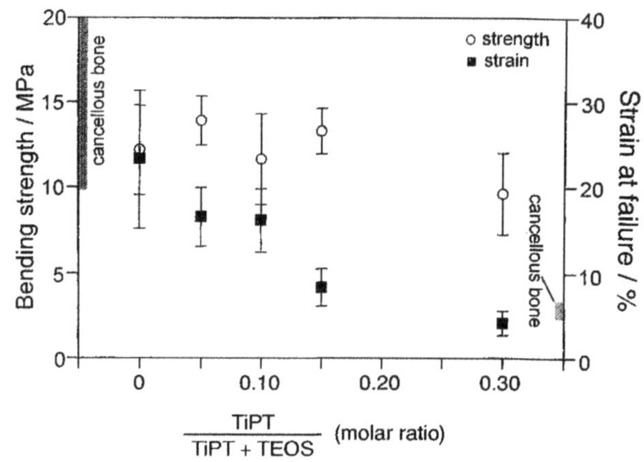

Fig. 7. Bending strength and strain at failure of the samples, compared with those of the human cancellous bone.[22]

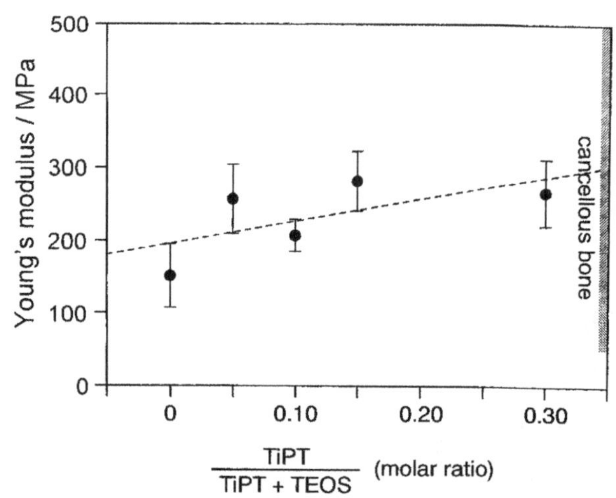

Fig. 8. Young's modulus of the samples. The vertical shaded band in the right side represents the range of Young's modulus values exhibited by the human cancellous bone.[22]

because the calcium is a component of the apatite. Si–OH and Ti–OH groups thus formed induce the apatite nucleation,[34] and the increased ionic activity product accelerates the apatite nucleation. Once the apatite nuclei are formed, they grow spontaneously by consuming the calcium and phosphate ions in SBF, as shown by the decrease in the phosphorous concentration in SBF in Fig. 5, because SBF is already supersaturated with respect to the apatite even under normal conditions. The reason hybrids Ti10 and Ti15 showed higher rates of calcium release than hybrids Ti0 and Ti5 is not known. The high rate of the calcium release for Ti30 might be attributed to the presence of pores, because the release rate of silicon is also high for Ti30.

The magnitude of the strain at failure is too large for Ti0. It decreased with increasing TiO_2 content, and its values went down to those exhibited by the human cancellous bone for Ti15 and Ti30 (see Fig. 7). The bending strengths were in the range of those of the human cancellous bone for all the compositions except for Ti30, which contains a small amount of pore (see Fig. 7 and Table I). Young's modulus of the hybrids increased with increasing TiO_2 content (see Fig. 8). This might be attributed to the formation of compact structure by the incorporation of Ti–O into the Si–O network structure. Young's moduli of the hybrids all fall into the range of those exhibited by the human cancellous bone. Thus, dense and homogeneous organic–inorganic hybrids with high bioactivity as well as limited mechanical properties analogous to those of human cancellous bone can be obtained by the present method. The composition with a TiPT/(TiPT + TEOS) molar ratio of 0.15 is found to be most favorable for obtaining such hybrid.

V. Summary

Hydrolysis and polycondensation of PDMS, TEOS, and calcium nitrate, with added TiPT at a TiPT/(TiPT + TEOS) molar ratio of 0.15 give a pore- and crack-free transparent monolithic hybrid. It shows a high apatite-forming ability in SBF, as well as limited mechanical properties such as bending strength, Young's modulus, and strain at failure, analogous to those of the human cancellous bone. This hybrid material is expected to be useful as a new kind of bioactive bone-repairing materials.

Acknowledgment

The experiment guidance of pore volume measurements of Dr. K. Nakanishi is greatly appreciated.

References

[1]L. L. Hench, R. J. Splinter, W. C. Allen, and T. K. Greenlee Jr., "Bonding Mechanism at Interface of Ceramic Prosthetic Materials," *J. Biomed. Mater. Res.*, **2**, 117–41 (1971).

[2]M. Jarcho, J. L. Kay, R. H. Gumaer, and H. P. Drobeck, "Tissue, Cellular and Subcellular Events at Bone–Ceramic Hydroxyapatite Interface," *J. Bioeng.*, **1**, 79–92 (1977).

[3]T. Kokubo, M. Shigematsu, Y. Nagashima, M. Tashiro, T. Nakamura, T. Yamamuro, and S. Higashi, "Apatite- and Wollastonite-Contaning Glass-Ceramics for Prosthetic Application," *Bull. Inst. Chem. Res., Kyoto Univ.*, **60**, 260–68 (1982).

[4]L. L. Hench, "Bioceramics," *J. Am. Ceram. Soc.*, **81**, 1705–28 (1998).

[5]H.-M. Kim, F. Miyaji, T. Kokubo, and T. Nakamura, "Preparation of Bioactive Ti and Its Alloys Via Simple Chemical Surface Treatment," *J. Biomed. Mater. Res.*, **32**, 409–17 (1996).

[6]W.-Q. Yan, T. Nakamura, M. Kobayashi, H.-M. Kim, F. Miyaji, and T. Kokubo, "Bonding of Chemically Treated Titanium Implants to Bone," *J. Biomed. Mater. Res.*, **37**, 267–75 (1997).

[7]C. A. Van Blitterswijk, D. Bakker, and H. Leenders, "Interfacial Reactions Leading to Bone-Bonding with PEO/PBT Copolymer (Polyactive™)"; pp. 153–71 in *Bone-Bonding Biomaterials*. Edited by P. Ducheyne, T. Kokubo, and C. A. Van Blitterswijk. Reed Healthcare Communications, Leiderdorp, The Netherlands, 1992.

[8]H. Schmidt, "New Type of Non-Crystalline Solids between Inorganic and Organic Materials," *J. Non-Cryst. Solids.*, **73**, 681–91 (1985).

[9]G. L. Wilkes, B. Orler, and H. Huang, "'Ceramers': Hybrid Materials Incorporating Polymeric/Oligomeric Species into Inorganic Glasses Utilizing a Sol–Gel Approach," *Polym. Prepr.*, **26**, 300–302 (1985).

[10]Y. P. Ning, M. X. Zhao, and J. E. Mark, "Siloxane–Silica Composites Prepared by Sol–Gel Technique with Hydrolysis Water Generated in situ"; pp. 745–51 in *Chemical Processing of Advanced Materials*. Edited by L. L. Hench and J. K. West. Wiley, New York, 1992.

[11]H.-H. Huang, B. Orler, and G. L. Wilkes, "Ceramers: Hybrid Materials Incorporating Polymeric/Oligomeric Species with Inorganic Glasses by a Sol–Gel Process, 2: Effect of Acid Content on the Final Properties," *Polym. Bull.*, **14**, 557–64 (1985).

[12]H.-H. Huang, B. Orler, and G. L. Wilkes, "Structure–Property Behavior of New Hybrid Materials Incorporating Oligomeric Species into Sol–Gel Glasses, 3: Effect of Acid Content, Tetraethoxysilane Content, and Molecular Weight of Poly(dimethylsiloxane)," *Macromolecules*, **20**, 1322–30 (1987).

[13]H. Schmidt and G. Philipp, "Inorganic/Organic Polymers for Contact Lenses by the Sol–Gel Process"; pp. 580–91 in *Glass. . . Current Issues*. Edited by A. F. Wright and G. Dupuy. Martinus Nijhoff, Dordrecht, The Netherlands, 1988.

[14]H. Schmidt, "Processing and Optical Properties of Inorganic–Organic Composites"; pp. 727–35 in *Chemical Processing of Advanced Materials*. Edited by L. L. Hench and J. K. West. Wiley, New York, 1992.

[15]S. Motakef, T. Suratwala, R. L. Roncone, J. M. Boulton, G. Teowe, and D. R. Uhlmann, "Processing and Optical Properties of Inorganic–Organic Hybrids (Polycerams), II: PDMS-Based Waveguides," *J. Non-Cryst. Solids*, **178**, 37–43 (1994).

[16]J. D. Mackenzie, Y. J. Chung, and Y. Hu, "Rubbery Ormosils and Their Applications," *J. Non-Cryst. Solids*, **147–148**, 271–79 (1992).

[17]Y. J. Chung, S. Ting, and J. D. Mackenzie, "Rubbery Ormosils," *Mater. Res. Soc. Symp. Proc.*, **180**, 981–86 (1990).

[18]Y. Hu and J. D. Mackenzie, "Rubber-like Elasticity of Organically Modified Silicates," *J. Mater. Sci.*, **27**, 4415–20 (1992).

[19]J. D. Mackenzie, "Structures and Properties of Ormosils," *J. Sol–Gel Sci. Technol.*, **2**, 81–86 (1994).

[20]Y. Hoshino and J. D. Mackenzie, "Viscosity and Structure of Ormosil Solution," *J. Sol-Gel Sci. Technol.*, **5**, 83–92 (1995).

[21]K. Tsuru, C. Ohtsuki, A. Osaka, T. Iwamoto, and J. D. Mackenzie, "Bioactivity of Sol–Gel Derived Organically Modified Silicates, Part I: In vitro Examination," *J. Mater. Sci.: Mater. Med.*, **8**, 157–61 (1997).

[22]L. L. Hench and J. Wilson, "Introduction"; pp.12–14 in: *An Introduction to Bioceramics*. Edited by L. L. Hench and J. Wilson. World Scientific, Singapore, 1993.

[23]R. H. Glaser and G. L. Wilkes, "Structure Property Behavior of Polydimethylsiloxane and Poly(tetramethylene oxide) Modified TEOS Based Sol–Gel Materials, V: Effect of Titaniumisopropoxide Incorporation," *Polym. Bull.*, **19**, 51–57 (1988).

[24]S. B. Wang and J. E. Mark, "*In-situ* Precipitation of Reinforcing Titania Fillers," *Polym. Bull.*, **17**, 271–77 (1987).

[25]J. Wen and J. E. Mark, "Synthesis, Structure, and Properties of Poly(dimethylsiloxane) Networks Reinforced by *in situ*-precipitated Silica-Titania, Silica-Zirconia, and Silica–Alumina Mixed Oxides," *J. Appl. Polym. Sci.*, **58**, 1135–45 (1995).

[26]C. S. Parkhurst, W. F. Doyle, L. A. Silverman, S. Singh, M. P. Andersen, D. McClurg, G. E. Wnek, and D. R. Uhlmann, "Siloxane Modified SiO_2–TiO_2 Glasses Via Sol–Gel," *Mater. Res. Soc. Symp. Proc.*, **73**, 769–73 (1986).

[27]T. Kokubo, H. Kushitani, S. Sakka, T. Kitsugi, and T. Yamamuro, "Solution Able to Reproduce *in vivo* Surface-Structure Changes in Bioactive Glass-Ceramics A-W," *J. Biomed. Mater. Res.*, **24**, 721–34 (1990).

[28]T. Kokubo, "Bioactive Glass Ceramics: Properties and Applications," *Biomaterials.*, **12**, 155–63 (1991).

[29]L. L. Hench, "Bioceramics: from Concept to Clinic," *J. Am. Ceram. Soc.*, **74**, 1487–510 (1991).

[30]S. Diré and F. Babonneau, "Structural Evolution during Pyrolysis of Sol–Gel Derived Hybrid Materials," *J. Sol–Gel Sci. Technol.*, **2**, 139–42 (1994).

[31]X. Li and T. A. King, "Spectroscopic Studies of Sol-Gel-derived Organically Modified Silicates," *J. Non-Cryst. Solids.*, **204**, 235–42 (1996).

[32]I. Rehman and W. Bonfield, "Characterization of Hydroxyapatite and Carbonated Apatite by Photo Acoustic FTIR Spectroscopy," *J. Mater. Sci.: Mater. Med.*, **8**, 1–4 (1997).

[33]M. M. Morsi and A. W. A. El-Shennawi, "Some Physical Properties of Silicate Glasses Containing TiO_2 in Relation to Their Structure," *Phys. Chem. Glasses.*, **25**, 64–68 (1984).

[34]P. Li, C. Ohtsuki, T. Kokubo, K. Nakanishi, N. Soga, and K de Groot, "The Role of Hydrated Silica, Titania, and Alumina in Inducing Apatite on Implants," *J. Biomed. Mater. Res.*, **28**, 7–15 (1994). □

J. Am. Ceram. Soc., 86 [6] 1031–33 (2003)

Joining of Calcium Phosphate Invert Glass-Ceramics on a β-Type Titanium Alloy

Toshihiro Kasuga* and Masayuki Nogami*

Graduate School of Materials Science and Engineering, Nagoya Institute of Technology, Nagoya 466-8555, Japan

Mitsuo Niinomi

Department of Production Systems Engineering, Toyohashi University of Technology, Toyohashi 411-8580, Japan

A bioactive calcium phosphate invert glass-ceramic containing β-$Ca_3(PO_4)_2$ crystals could be joined strongly with a Ti–29Nb–13Ta–4.6Zr alloy consisting of a β-titanium phase by heating the metal on which the mother glass powders with a composition $60CaO{\cdot}30P_2O_5{\cdot}7Na_2O{\cdot}3TiO_2$ (mol%) were placed, at 800°C for 1 h in air; the tensile joining strength was estimated to be ~26 MPa on average. A compositionally gradient layer was developed on the metallic substrate during the heating. When the metal with glass powders on it was heated at 850°C in air, the phosphate glassy phase flowed viscously, permeating the oxide layer formed around the surface of the metal, which was thicker than that formed by heating at 800°C; a compositionally gradient layer was not developed, and a strong joining was not realized. The joining between the glass-ceramic and the metal is suggested to be controlled by viscous flow of the glassy phase in the glass-ceramic and by reaction of the glassy phase with the oxide phase formed around the surface layer of the metal.

I. Introduction

β-TYPE titanium alloys are currently attractive metals for biomedical applications, because they have high mechanical strength and low modulus of elasticity.[1,2] Niinomi and co-workers[3–5] have developed a new β-type titanium alloy, Ti–29Nb–13Ta–4.6Zr (denoted TNTZ, hereafter), composed of elements sufficiently tolerated by living tissues. The alloy shows a high tensile strength of ~1 GPa and low Young's modulus of 60–80 GPa.

Some portions in artificial substitutes for hard tissues may require bioactivity, which is the ability to form a chemical bond with living bone. Bioactive hydroxyapatite or β-$Ca_3(PO_4)_2$ (β-TCP) coatings on titanium or titanium alloys prepared using various coating processes, such as a plasma spraying[6] or sputtering,[7] have been investigated. Recently, the authors have reported that the calcium phosphate invert glass-ceramic $60CaO{\cdot}30P_2O_5{\cdot}7Na_2O{\cdot}3TiO_2$ (mol%) can be joined easily by heating TNTZ, on which the mother glass powders are placed, at 800°C in air.[8,9] The glass-ceramic layer containing β-TCP crystal is strongly joined. In simulated body fluid, a bonelike apatite phase forms on the coating.[8] This preparation process is easy and simple and, hence, is advantageous in terms of the fabrication performance.

In the present work, we found a unique behavior of the reaction between the glassy phase in the glass-ceramic and the oxide layer around the surface of the TNTZ substrate during heating at 800° or 850°C, and we determined the optimum heating condition for realization of the fine joining.

II. Experimental Procedure

Calcium phosphate invert glass was prepared using a composition of $60CaO{\cdot}30P_2O_5{\cdot}7Na_2O{\cdot}3TiO_2$ (mol%).[10] The mixture of the starting materials, which were reagent-grade $CaCO_3$, H_3PO_4 (85% liquid), Na_2CO_3, and TiO_2, was placed with water in a Teflon beaker and stirred to form a slurry. The slurry was dried at ~200°C. The resulting product was melted in a platinum crucible at 1350°C for 0.5 h. The melt was poured onto a stainless-steel plate and quickly pressed with an iron plate, which resulted in the formation of glasses with thicknesses of 0.3–1.0 mm. Forty grams of the glasses were pulverized to <10 μm in diameter (the average size was 1.0–1.5 μm) using a zirconia ball mill with zirconia balls in 50 mL of methanol. After the pulverization, the slurry was poured into a polyethylene vessel and dried at ~100°C. Twenty grams of the dried glass powders were mixed with 20 mL of methanol to form a slurry for subsequent dip-coating.

TNTZ alloy obtained was cut into a disk shape of 20 mm diameter with 1 mm thickness, and the surfaces were sandblasted to a roughness of ~2 μm (examined using scanning electron microscopy (SEM)). The disk was washed using acetone in an ultrasonic bath, and it was subsequently dried at 100°C. After the disk-shaped metal was dipped into the glass-powder slurry described above, it was drawn up at a speed of 1.4 mm/s and then dried at 100°C. The substrate with the glass powder layer was placed in an electric furnace and was heated in air at 5°C/min to 800° or 850°C and held at the temperature for 0.5–1 h. Finally the power of the furnace was shut off to cool the sample to room temperature in the furnace.

Crystalline phases in the coating layer were examined using X-ray diffractometry (XRD), and the microstructure was observed using SEM, incorporating X-ray microanalysis using energy dispersive spectrometry (EDS). The bonding strength of the glass-ceramic layer to the substrate was measured using a tensile method that modified ASTM C-633 ("Standard Test Method for Adhesion or Cohesion Strength of Thermal Spray Coatings," ASTM Designation C633-01, Annual Book of Standards, Vol. 02.05, ASTM International, West Conshohocken, PA).[8] At least five specimens were used, and the average tensile bonding strength was estimated. Oxidation behavior of the substrate metals was determined using thermogravimetric analysis (TGA) of the metals heated in air. TNTZ alloy shaped into a plate (5 mm × 5 mm × 1 mm) was

J. W. Burdon—contributing editor

Manuscript No. 186667. Received September 26, 2002; approved January 13, 2003.

Supported in part by a Grant-in-Aid for Scientific Research (No. 13555173) from Japan Society for the Promotion of Science.

*Member, American Ceramic Society.

Table I. Tensile Bonding Strength of the Glass-Ceramic Layer to the Substrate

	Tensile bonding strength (MPa)		
Heating condition	Average value†	Maximum value	Minimum value
800°C, 1 h	26 ± 5	31	18
850°C, 0.5 h	15 ± 4	22	11
850°C, 1 h	7 ± 2	12	5

†± means the standard deviation.

heated from room temperature at a rate of 5°C/min to 800° or 850°C and held at that temperature for 1 h.

III. Results and Discussion

Table I shows the tensile bonding strengths between the glass-ceramic and the substrate of the samples prepared under some heating conditions. When the sample is heated for 1 h at 800°C, the strength is estimated to be ~26 MPa on average and is the highest value in the present work. The value is significantly higher than that of plasma-splayed hydroxyapatite coatings on titanium (<7 MPa).[11] On the other hand, when the sample is heated at 850°C for 0.5 or 1 h, the strength is estimated to be ~15 or ~7 MPa on average, respectively.

No significant differences in XRD patterns of the coating layers among all the samples prepared by heating at 800° and 850°C can be seen; β-TCP crystal is identified with small amounts of β-$Ca_2P_2O_7$ and TiO_2 (rutile) crystals, as reported in our earlier works.[8,9] Figure 1 shows TGA curves of TNTZ. The weight of TNTZ increases gradually with increasing temperature because of the occurrence of oxidization around the surface. The weight increase after 1 h of holding at 850°C is ~1.4 times as large as that at 800°C. Figure 1 implies that the oxide layer at the surface of the TNTZ substrate after the heating at 850°C is relatively thicker than that after the heating at 800°C. However, because the oxygen concentration decreases gradually with increasing distance from the surface, it is difficult to estimate the thickness of the oxide layers concretely.

Figure 2 shows the cross-sectional SEM images around the joining interface between the glass-ceramic and TNTZ of the samples prepared by heating at 800° or 850°C for 1 h and the results of elemental concentration analysis by EDS along the indicated line in the SEM images. The images in Fig. 2 show that the thicknesses of the coating layers are estimated to be ~15 μm. The image of the sample obtained by heating at 800°C shows a compositionally gradient layer around the interface. Figure 2 also shows a phase containing a small amount of calcium element on the substrate; the thickness of the phase is estimated to be ~1 μm, and the composition of the phase is semiquantitatively estimated from an EDS spectrum method to be Ca:P:Na:Ti:Nb:Ta:Zr = 4:42:12:34:3:1:4 in cationic percentage. The phase is based on sodium titanium phosphate. It seems that the phosphorus element permeates slightly (<1 μm) into the substrate. On the other hand, no compositionally gradient layer can be seen around the interface in the sample obtained by heating at 850°C. Concentrations of calcium and phosphorus show minimums around the interface between the glass-ceramic and the substrate. The phosphorus element permeates to a 2–3 μm depth from the surface of the substrate and gives a peak of the concentration.

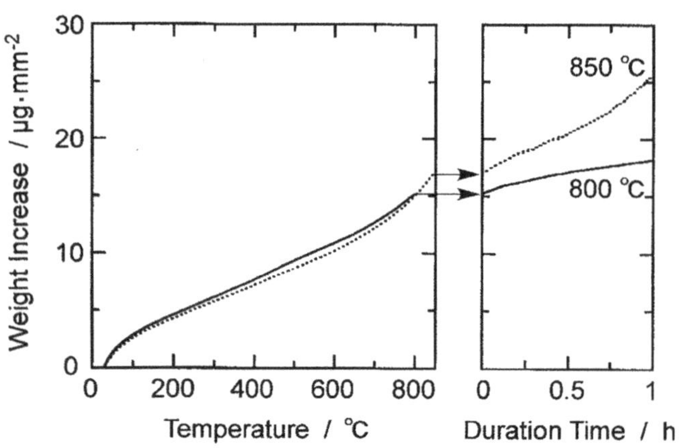

Fig. 1. TGA curves of TNTZ alloy. TNTZ plate (5 mm × 5 mm × 1 mm) was heated from room temperature at a rate of 5°C/min to 800° or 850°C, and, subsequently, it was held at that temperature for 1 h (heating at (—) 800° and (· · ·) 850°C).

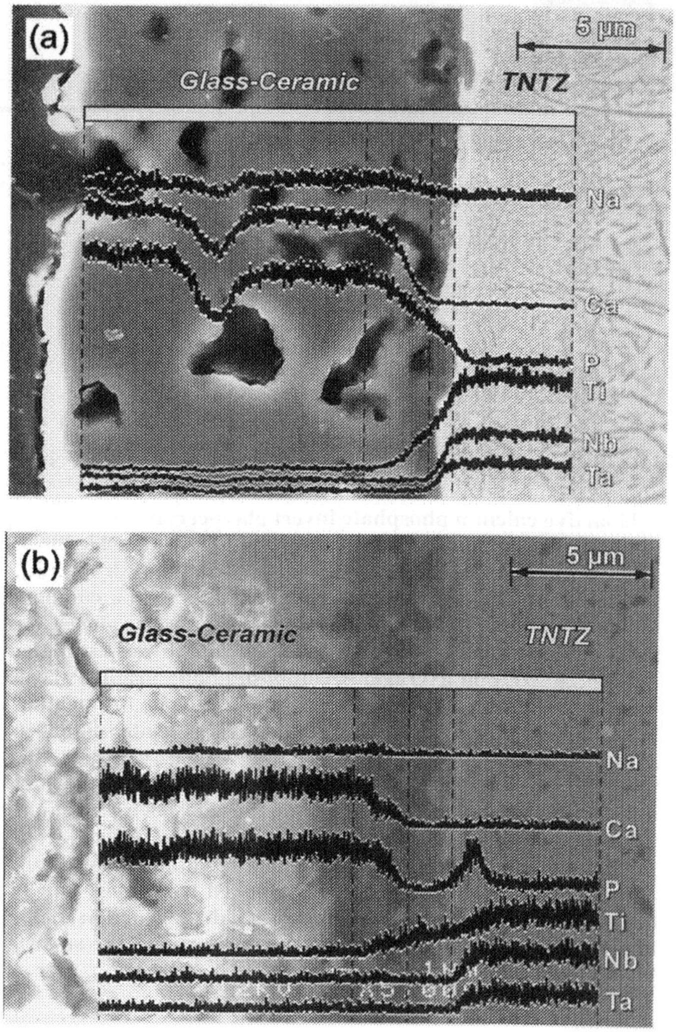

Fig. 2. Elemental concentrations of the cross section around the interface between the glass-ceramic and the substrate measured using EDS analysis along the indicated line in the SEM images: (a) sample obtained by heating at 800°C for 1 h and (b) sample obtained by heating at 850°C for 1 h. Zirconium concentration profiles were not measured, because the EDS peak position of the *L*-line from zirconium overlaps with that of the *K*-line from phosphorous. Zirconium content in the substrate is small.

Figure 3 shows the cross-sectional SEM images around the joining interface between the glass-ceramic and TNTZ of the samples prepared at 800° or 850°C for 1 h after the tensile bonding strength test and the results of elemental concentration analysis along the indicated line in the images. In the case of the sample prepared at 800°C, fracture occurs in the glass-ceramic layer having porosity; the bonding strength at the interface layer is higher than the tensile strength of the glass-ceramic. On the other hand, in the case of the sample prepared at 850°C, no residual glass-ceramic layer appears on the substrate after the test. In the concentration profiles, a characteristic peak in the substrate of the

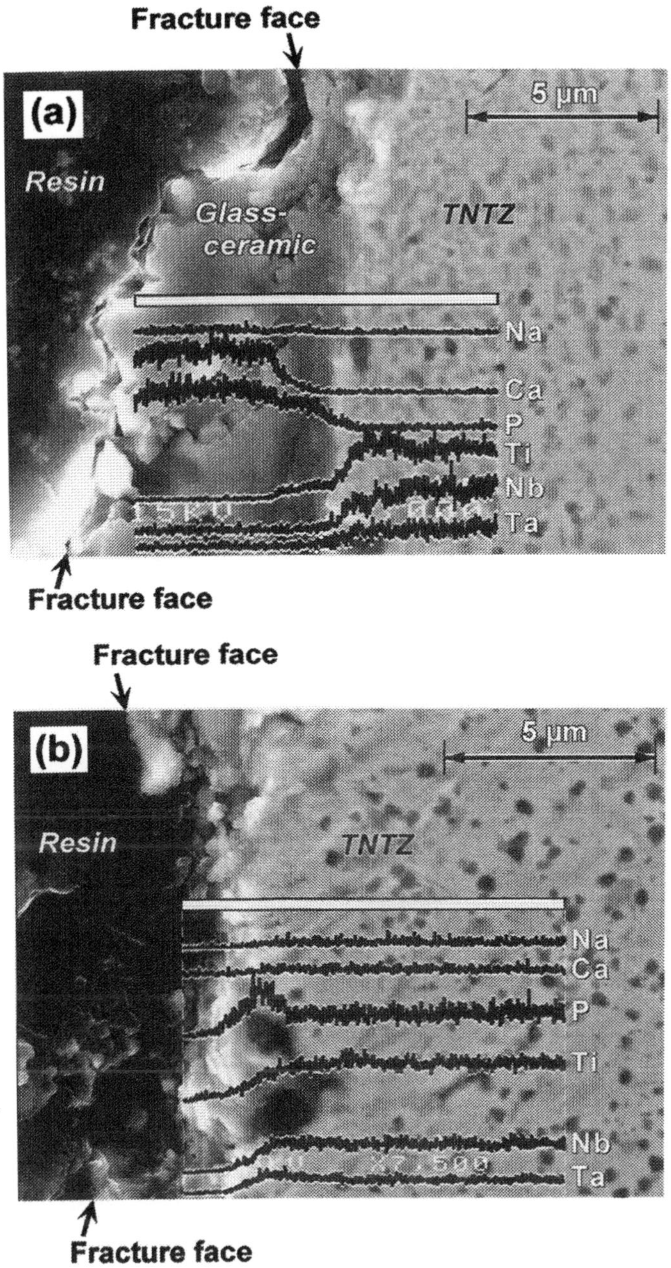

Fig. 3. Cross-sectional SEM images around the surface of the substrate after the tensile bonding test of the samples and elemental concentrations measured by EDS analysis along the indicated line in the images: (a) the sample obtained by heating at 800°C for 1 h and (b) the sample obtained by heating at 850°C for 1 h.

phosphorus concentration is shown in Fig. 2(b); the fracture occurs at the interface between the glass-ceramic and the substrate.

During heating at 800°C for 1 h in air, β-TCP and β-$Ca_2P_2O_7$ crystals are precipitated in the glass and, subsequently, the β-$Ca_2P_2O_7$ crystal is partially melted by reaction with the residual glassy phase.[8,10,12] The phosphate melt flows viscously, which results in densification of the crystallized glass powders. The surface of the TNTZ alloy is oxidized during heating, which results in the formation of a thin layer consisting of titania-based oxides. A part of the phosphate melt permeates into the oxide layer around the alloy to react strongly. Because the oxide layer is relatively thin, the residual melt after reaction with the layer can stand on the substrate. The glass-ceramic layer containing β-TCP crystal thus can be strongly joined through the melt with the substrate. When the sample is cooled, the melt can be vitrified. On the other hand, when the sample is heated at 850°C, the oxide layer formed around the surface of the TNTZ alloy is thicker. The phosphate melt in the crystallized glass powders flows and actively reacts with the thick oxide layer. A large amount of the phosphate melt around the surface of the substrate permeates into the titania-based oxide layer and reacts with the oxides. Because there exists almost no interface layer based on the sodium titanium phosphate for joining the glass-ceramic with the substrate, the sample shows poor tensile bonding strength, which may have originated from thermal stresses generated by the difference of thermal expansions between the glass-ceramic and the reacted surface layer of the substrate. The joining between the glass-ceramic and the metal is suggested to be controlled by viscous flow of the melt formed by the partial melting in the glass-ceramic and by reaction of the glassy phase with the oxide layer formed around the surface of the metal.

IV. Summary

A fine, strong coating consisting of a $60CaO{\cdot}30P_2O_5{\cdot}7Na_2O{\cdot}3TiO_2$ glass-ceramic containing β-$Ca_3(PO_4)_2$ crystal can be prepared easily by reaction of the glassy phase with an oxide layer formed on a Ti–29Nb–13Ta–4.6Zr alloy during heating at 800°C for 1 h in air. During the heating, the phosphate melt that forms in the crystallized glass powders flows viscously, which results in densification of the crystallized glass powders, while the surface of the TNTZ alloy is oxidized to form a titania-based oxide layer. The phosphate melt densifies the crystallized glass powders and permeates into the oxide layer to react strongly. The residual melt after the reaction stands on the substrate. As a result, a compositionally gradient layer is developed on the alloy and the glass-ceramic layer is strongly joined through the melt with the substrate.

References

[1]M. Long and H. J. Rack, "Review: Titanium Alloys in Total Joint Replacement—A Materials Science Perspective," *Biomaterials*, **19**, 1621–39 (1998).

[2]M. Morinaga, M. Kato, T. Kamimura, M. Fukutomi, I. Harada, and K. Kudo, "Theoretical Design of β-Type Titanium Alloys"; pp. 276–83 in *Titanium '92 Science and Technology*. Edited by F. H. Froes and I. L. Caplan. Minerals, Metals, and Materials Society, Warrendale, PA, 1993.

[3]M. Niinomi, "Mechanical Properties of Biomedical Titanium Alloys," *Mater. Sci. Eng.*, **A243**, 231–36 (1998).

[4]D. Kuroda, M. Niinomi, M. Morinaga, Y. Kato, and T. Yashiro, "Design and Mechanical Properties of New β-Type Titanium Alloys for Implant Materials," *Mater. Sci. Eng.*, **A243**, 244–49 (1998).

[5]M. Niinomi, D. Kuroda, K. Fukunaga, M. Morinaga, Y. Kato, T. Yashiro, and A. Suzuki, "Corrosion Wear Fracture of New β-Type Biomedical Titanium Alloys," *Mater. Sci. Eng.*, **A263**, 193–99 (1999).

[6]C. P. A. T. Klein, J. G. C. Wolke, and K. de Groot, "Stability of Calcium Phosphate Ceramics and Plasma-Sprayed Coating"; pp. 199–221 in *An Introduction to Bioceramics*. Edited by L. L. Hench and J. Wilson. World Scientific, Singapore, 1993.

[7]W. R. Lacefield, "Hydroxylapatite Coatings"; pp. 223–38 in *An Introduction to Bioceramics*. Edited by L. L. Hench and J. Wilson. World Scientific, Singapore, 1993.

[8]T. Kasuga, T. Mizuno, M. Watanabe, M. Nogami, and M. Niinomi, "Calcium Phosphate Invert Glass-Ceramic Coatings Joined by Self-Development of Compositionally Gradient Layers on a Titanium Alloy," *Biomaterials*, **22**, 577–82 (2001).

[9]T. Kasuga, M. Nogami, M. Niinomi, and T. Hattori, "Bioactive Calcium Phosphate Invert Glass-Ceramic Coating on β-Type Ti–29Nb–13Ta–4.6Zr Alloy," *Biomaterials*, **24**, 283–90 (2003).

[10]T. Kasuga and Y. Abe, "Novel Calcium Phosphate Ceramics Prepared by Powder Sintering and Crystallization of Glasses in the Pyrophosphate Region," *J. Mater. Res.*, **13**, 3357–60 (1998).

[11]Y. C. Tsui, C. Doyle, and T. M. Clyne, "Plasma-Sprayed Hydroxyapatite Coatings on Titanium Substrates, Part 1: Mechanical Properties and Residual Stress Levels," *Biomaterials*, **19**, 2015–26 (1998).

[12]T. Kasuga, M. Sawada, M. Nogami, and Y. Abe, "Bioactive Ceramics Prepared by Sintering and Crystallization of Calcium Phosphate Invert Glasses," *Biomaterials*, **20**, 1415–20 (1999). □

J. Am. Ceram. Soc., 86 [6] 1055–57 (2003)

Synthesis of Hydroxyapatite Nanopowders via Sucrose-Templated Sol–Gel Method

Susmita Bose* and Susanta Kumar Saha

School of Mechanical and Materials Engineering, Washington State University, Pullman, Washington 99164–2920

The present research describes synthesis of hydroxyapatite (HAp) nanopowders using a sol–gel route with calcium nitrate and ammonium hydrogen phosphate as calcium and phosphorous precursors, respectively. Sucrose is used as template material, and alumina is added as a dopant to study its effects on particle size and surface area. Synthesized powders are characterized using X-ray diffractometry, BET surface-area analysis, and transmission electron microscopy. Results show that alumina stabilizes the HAp crystalline phase. Average particle size of mesoporous HAp samples is between 30 and 50 nm with surface area of 51–60 m^2/g.

I. Introduction

Calcium phosphate-based materials are used in various orthopedic and dental applications because of their chemical and morphologic similarities to natural bone.[1] The major phase found in bone is hydroxyapatite (HAp, $Ca_{10}(PO_4)_6(OH)_2$) with a Ca:P ratio of 1.67:1. There are other important calcium phosphate phases as well, including α- and β-tricalcium phosphate (TCP) with a Ca:P ratio of 1.5:1. For successful applications of calcium phosphate-based ceramics in load-bearing bone grafts, higher strength and toughness are necessary. Unfortunately, because of poor sinterability, HAp ceramics show low strength and poor reliability, especially in a wet environment,[2] which makes them unsuitable for even low-load-bearing applications.[3] Synthesis of ultrafine HAp powder can be an important step in processing parts with high sintered density. It is believed that nanostructured calcium phosphate ceramics can improve the sintering kinetics because of higher surface area and subsequently improve mechanical properties. Thus, our effort is focused toward the development of synthetic routes to produce calcium phosphate-based nanopowders.

Synthesis of HAp has been performed several ways, which include the conventional methods, such as solid-state reaction[4] and modern chemical routes (coprecipitation,[5,6] sol–gel,[7–11] hydrothermal,[12] and emulsion[13] techniques). Layrolle *et al.*[7] have synthesized HAp powders with average surface area of 26 m^2/g and average particle size of 200 nm with a strongly agglomerated morphology with an average agglomerate size of 45 μm. Lim *et al.*[13] have reported synthesis of HAp powders with specific surface area between 42 and 80 m^2/g and average particle size between 0.53 and 1.15 μm with agglomerated morphology. Among the various synthesis methods, the sol–gel method is quite common for processing of nanostructured materials. The sol–gel method offers a molecular-level mixing of the precursors, which is capable of improving chemical homogeneity of the resulting powders to a significant extent.

The objective of the current work is to develop a synthetic chemical route to make mesoporous nanocrystalline HAp powder using an aqueous solution of calcium nitrate, ammonium hydrogen phosphate, and sucrose. Alumina, which is known as a bioinert ceramic, was used as a dopant to improve mesoporosity as well as surface area. Magnesium nitrate (0.5 mol% with respect to alumina content) is also added to alumina-containing samples to form magnesium oxide as a sintering aid.

II. Experimental Procedures

Starting materials used in this work included high-purity calcium nitrate ($Ca(NO_3)_2{\cdot}4H_2O$), ammonium hydrogen phosphate ($(NH_4)_2HPO_4$), aluminum nitrate ($Al(NO_3)_3{\cdot}9H_2O$), magnesium nitrate ($Mg(NO_3)_2{\cdot}6H_2O$), and sucrose (all from Alfa Aesar, Ward Hill, MA). Aqueous solutions of all the starting materials were made dissolving them in deionized water. Initial strengths of all metal and phosphate salt solutions were maintained to 2*M*. Initial concentration of the sucrose solution was 5*M*. The Ca:P ratio in the precursor was maintained at 1.67:1 in all the cases. The metal-ion:sucrose ratio was varied from 1:5 to 1:35. In some samples, a selected amount of aluminum and magnesium salts were added. 10 mL of 2.0*M* calcium nitrate solution was mixed with 20 mL of 5.0*M* sucrose solution. 6 mL of 2.0*M* ammonium hydrogen phosphate was added to this solution with constant magnetic stirring. Concentrated nitric acid was added to dissolve the precipitate, and the pH of the solution was adjusted to 1. The solution was aged at 80°C for 2 h and then evaporated on a hot plate at 200°C to obtain a transparent gel. The gel was dried in an oven at 150°C for a couple of hours. After it was dried, the gel converted to a black fluffy mass, which was crushed in an agate mortar and dried further on the hotplate at 400°C. This heat treatment converted the black powder to a gray-colored powder, which was then considered as the precursor powder. For the alumina-doped samples, 1 mol% of magnesium oxide with respect to alumina was added to the starting solution mixture. Required amounts of aluminum and magnesium nitrates were added to the calcium salt solution before it was mixed with the ammonium hydrogen phosphate solution. The precursor powders then were heat-treated in air at various temperatures between 650° and 850°C for 1 h in a muffle furnace.

Powder X-ray diffractometry (XRD) of the heat-treated samples was obtained using a fully automated diffractometer with CoK_a radiation and a Ni filter (Philips, Eindhoven, The Netherlands). The XRD data were collected at room temperature over the 2θ range of 20°–70° at a step size of 0.02° 2θ and a count time of 0.5 s/step. Samples were investigated for their microstructural and morphologic features using transmission electron microscopy (TEM; Model JEM-120, JEOL, Tokyo, Japan). Powder surface area was measured using five-point BET surface-area analysis

T. Troczynski—contributing editor

Manuscript No. 186842. Received July 12, 2002; approved February 7, 2003.
Supported by the National Science Foundation under Grant Nos. CTS-0103105 and CTS-0134476.

*Member, American Ceramic Society.

(Model Tristar, Micromeritics, Norcross, GA). Powders were dried in a sample holder at 350°C in nitrogen atmosphere for 12 h before BET surface-area analysis.

III. Results and Discussion

Addition of sucrose to the metal-ion solution makes the solution viscous with no precipitation or segregation of ions from the homogeneous solution. Sucrose is used as a polymeric matrix for calcium and phosphorus ions. When the volume of the solution is decreased via evaporation, the solution forms a transparent gel. At this stage, sucrose also helps to prevent the separation of calcium and phosphorus ions. With further heating, the transparent gel foams because of the presence of organic sucrose in solution. Complete evaporation of the solution occurs along with liberation of heat and gases because of the decomposition of organic matrix, which helps to form a fluffy dried mass. The fluffy dried mass, when calcined, results in the formation of mesoporous nanocrystalline HAp powders.

Precursor powders are calcined at elevated temperatures to examine the formation of the HAp phase. Room-temperature XRD patterns for 850°C for 1 h calcined powders of some selected samples are shown in Fig. 1. Samples with a Ca:P ratio of 1.67:1, pure, and with 2.5% alumina-doped HAp show the formation of HAp and β-TCP crystalline phases, along with some calcium oxide (CaO) phase. As alumina concentration is increased to 5%, both TCP and calcium oxide phases disappear and phase-pure HAp is formed. The formation of calcium oxide is directly linked with the TCP phase formation. In TCP, the Ca:P ratio is 1.5:1. In all our experiments, starting materials were taken in a Ca:P ratio of 1.67:1. Because of the formation of TCP, which has lower Ca:P ratio compared with the starting material, excess calcium is released as calcium oxide in the final product. Figure 2 shows the relative amounts of HAp phase present in the calcined powders as a function of Ca:sucrose ratio. As the Ca:sucrose mole ratios are varied in the precursor, the HAp phase content in calcined powders is also changing. The HAp phase content decreases with the increase in sucrose content in the precursor. This is because of the increasing amount of carbonaceous material due to a higher amount of sucrose in the precursor. During calcination, the heat formation due to the oxidation reaction of carbonaceous materials present in the precursor causes dehydration of HAp. The dehydration results in an increasing amount of β-TCP formation. Thus, higher sucrose content in the precursor favors the formation of the β-TCP phase over the HAp phase.

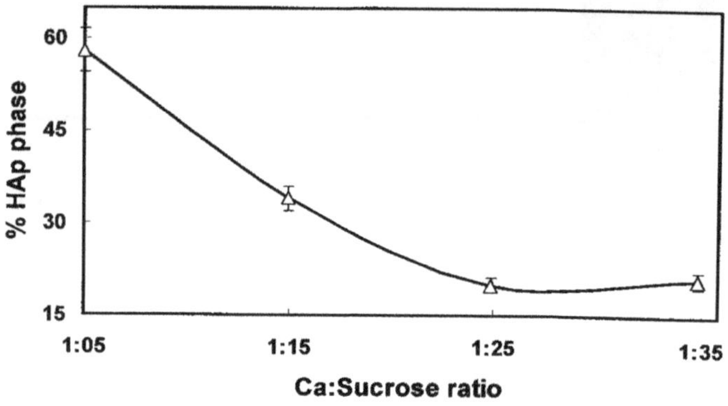

Fig. 2. Influence of Ca:sucrose ratio on the amount of HAp phase formation after calcinations at 850°C for 1 h.

Addition of alumina in the calcium phosphate system is found to retain the HAp crystalline phase. Alumina acts as a Lewis acid, which can make chemical interaction with the hydroxyl (OH) group of HAp and stabilize the HAp phase during drying and calcination steps.[14] Lone-pair electrons of the hydroxyl group make a coordinate bond with the vacant orbital of the aluminum and stabilizes the hydroxyl groups in HAp. Calcined powders doped with 5 mol% of alumina exhibit a 100% phase-pure HAp. The experimental results show that alumina stabilizes the HAp phase during the heat-treatment process.

BET surface-area analysis results are shown in Fig. 3. There is a significant increase in the surface area with an increase in the Ca:sucrose mole ratio for powders calcined at 650°C for 1 h. This increase is caused by the presence of a large amount of carbonaceous material present in the precursor powder. However, for a Ca:sucrose ratio greater than 1:25, a saturation in increasing surface area because of higher sucrose in the precursor is observed. One mole of sucrose liberates 23 mol of gases. At higher calcination temperatures, the variation of surface area with various Ca:sucrose ratios is less significant because of potentially significant particle–particle agglomeration. Addition of alumina increases the surface area of the calcined powders. In our previous work,[15] we have shown that mesoporous alumina powder with high surface area can be prepared using sucrose as a template material. With the increase in the amount of alumina in the calcium phosphate system, surface area also increases, which infers that

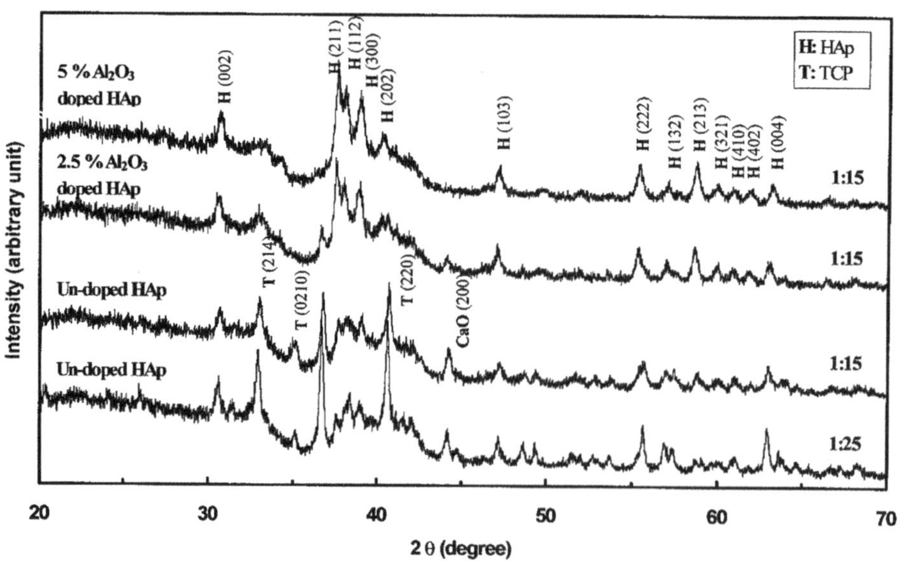

Fig. 1. XRD patterns for the samples obtained using a Ca:sucrose ratio of 1:15 after calcination at 850°C for 1 h.

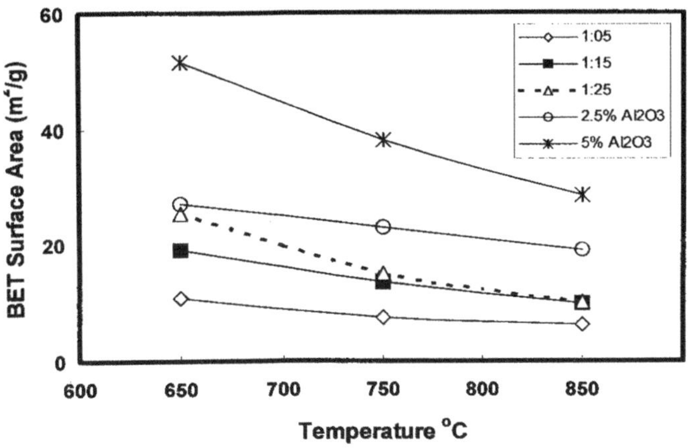

Fig. 3. Influence of calcination temperatures on BET surface area. Ca:sucrose ratio is varied from 1:5 to 1:25 for undoped samples. 2.5%- and 5%-alumina-doped samples with a Ca:sucrose ratio of 1:15 are also shown here.

sucrose has a more significant effect in increasing surface area in the case of oxide-based ceramic powders.

Figure 4 shows a TEM micrograph of calcined powders outlining the particle size and morphology of HAp powders obtained by calcination at 650°C for 1 h from the precursor with 5 mol% of alumina doped with a Ca:sucrose ratio of 1:15. The average particle size shown here is 30 nm with a mesoporous morphology. By increasing the calcination temperature to 850°C, the particle size increases to 60 nm although the morphology remains the same. The undoped calcium phosphate system, calcined at 650°C for 1 h and obtained from the precursor with a Ca:sucrose ratio of 1:15, shows an average size of 50 nm with a spherical morphology. The powders obtained from the precursor with a Ca:sucrose ratio of 1:5 are agglomerated with an average particle size of 100 nm. The amount of sucrose and the addition of alumina have significant effects on surface area and phase purity of HAp nanopowders.

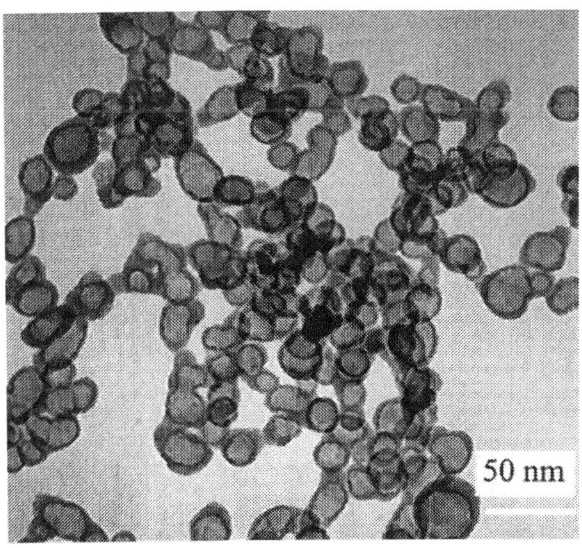

Fig. 4. Bright-field TEM micrograph of 5%-alumina-doped HAp powders calcined at 650°C for 1 h with a Ca:sucrose ratio of 1:15.

IV. Conclusion

Nanocrystalline HAp powders have been synthesized using a sol–gel method from aqueous solutions of calcium and phosphorus ions containing sucrose as a gelling agent. Some samples were doped with alumina. Presence of alumina in the HAp system helps stabilize the HAp crystalline phase during heating. Sucrose keeps the metal ions in solution through complex formation. Dehydration and thermal decomposition of metal-ion–sucrose mass produce a large amount of gases, which helps to create porosity and high surface area in the final product. The HAp powders obtained by this process have a uniform morphology with an average particle size between 30 and 50 nm. Results show that the presence of alumina also increases the surface area of the powders.

Acknowledgment

The authors would like to acknowledge Professor Amit Bandyopadhyay for experimental assistance and helpful discussions.

References

[1]L. L. Hench, "Bioceramics: From Concept to Clinic," *J. Am. Ceram. Soc.*, **74**, 1487–510 (1991).

[2]G. de With, H. J. A. van Dijk, N. Hattu, and K. Prijs, "Preparation, Microstructure, and Mechanical Properties of Dense Polycrystalline Hydroxyapatite," *J. Mater. Sci.*, **16**, 1592–98 (1981).

[3]W. Suchanec and M. Yoshimura, "Processing and Properties of Hydroxyapatite-Based Biomaterials for Use as Hard Tissue Replacements," *J. Mater. Res.*, **13**, 94–117 (1998).

[4]R. R. Rao, H. N. Roopa, and T. S. Kannan, "Solid-State Synthesis and Thermal Stability of HAP and HAP-β-TCP Composite Ceramic Powders," *J. Mater. Sci.: Mater. Med.*, **8**, 511–18 (1997).

[5]A. C. Tas, F. Korkusuz, M. Timicin, and N. Akkas, "An Investigation of the Chemical Synthesis and High-Temperature Sintering Behavior of Calcium Hydroxyapatite (HA) and Tricalcium Phosphate (TCP) Bioceramics," *J. Mater. Sci.: Mater. Med.*, **8**, 91–96 (1997).

[6]S. H. Rhee and J. Tanaka, "Hydroxyapatite Coating on a Collagen Membrane by a Miomimetic Method," *J. Am. Ceram. Soc.*, **81**, 3029–31 (1998).

[7]P. Layrolle, A. Ito, and T. Tateishi, "Sol–Gel Synthesis of Amorphous Calcium Phosphate and Sintering into Microporous Hydroxyapatite Bioceramics," *J. Am. Ceram. Soc.*, **81**, 1421–28 (1998).

[8]A. Jillavenkatesa and R. A. Condrate Sr., "Sol–Gel Processing of Hydroxyapatite," *J. Mater. Sci.*, **33**, 4111–19 (1998).

[9]C. M. Lopatin, V. Pizziconi, T. L. Alford, and T. Laursen, "Hydroxyapatite Powders and Thin Films Prepared by a Sol–Gel Technique," *Thin Solid Films*., **326**, 227–32 (1998).

[10]H. K. Verma, S. N. Kalkura, and R. Sivakumar, "Polymeric Precursor Route for the Preparation of Calcium Phosphate Compounds," *Ceram. Int.*, **24**, 467–70 (1998).

[11]G. Kordas and C. C. Trapalis, "Fourier-Transform and Multi-Dimensional EPR Spectroscopy for the Characterization of Sol–Gel-Derived Hydroxyapatite," *J. Sol-Gel Sci. Technol.*, **9**, 17–24 (1997).

[12]H. S. Liu, T. S. Chin, L. S. Lai, S. Y. Chiu, K. H. Chung, C. S. Chang, and M. T. Lui, "Hydroxyapatite Synthesized by a Simplified Hydrothermal Method," *Ceram. Int.*, **23**, 19–25 (1997).

[13]G. K. Lim, J. Wang, S. C. Ng, C. H. Chew, and L. M. Gan, "Processing of Hydroxyapatite via Microemulsion and Emulsion Routes," *Biomaterials*, **18**, 1433–39 (1997).

[14]D. J. Shanefield, *Organic Additives and Ceramic Processing*, 2nd ed.; p. 13. Kluwer, Boston, MA, 1996.

[15]R. N. Das, A. Bandyopadhyay, and S. Bose, "Nanocrystalline α-Alumina Using Sucrose," *J. Am. Ceram. Soc.*, **84**, 2421–23 (2001). □

journal

J. Am. Ceram. Soc., 86 [7] 1076–80 (2003)

From CT Scan to Ceramic Bone Graft

Jens Darsell,† Susmita Bose,*,† Howard L. Hosick,‡ and Amit Bandyopadhyay*,†

School of Mechanical and Materials Engineering and School of Biological Sciences and Molecular Biosciences, Washington State University, Pullman, Washington 99164

An indirect fused deposition process was used to fabricate controlled-porosity alumina bone grafts using a computer-aided-design file created from computed tomography (CT) scans of a horse's short pastern bone. Structures with both uniform and gradient porosity were fabricated to show the effectiveness of this process for the fabrication of custom orthopedic implants. Cytotoxicity and cell proliferation studies were conducted with different cell lines to show that these bone grafts are biocompatible. Uniaxial compression tests were also conducted to understand the influence of porosity on the mechanical properties of these structures.

I. Introduction

During the past four decades, the use of ceramics has revolutionized the quality of human life. Many specialty ceramics and glasses have been developed for the use of the health care industry, e.g., eyeglasses, diagnostic instruments, thermometers, tissue culture flasks, carriers for enzymes and antibodies, and ceramics in dentistry as restorative material.[1–5] Novel ceramic materials that are used for the repair and reconstruction of diseased or damaged parts of the musculoskeletal system are called bioceramics. Bioceramic materials are preferred as bone grafts over other materials such as metals, because of their low density, chemical inertness, and compositional similarities with human bones and tissues. Numerous ceramic and glass compositions have been developed and tested for their use in the human body; however, only a few have achieved successful human clinical applications.

Bone is a naturally occurring porous ceramic material. The porosities in human bone are predominantly in the range of 1–100 μm. The canaliculi and vasculature channels are 1–5 μm in diameter. Osteocyte lacunae and Volksmann's canals are typically 5–15 μm in diameter, and the larger Haversian canals are between 50 and 100 μm in diameter. Significant research has already been done for the development of dense and porous bone implants using inert, bioactive, and bioresorbable materials. It was reported that microporous implants with controlled pore size in the range of 100–600 μm are osteoconductive.[6] A minimum pore size of 100 μm is necessary for tissue in-growth into the bone grafts to maintain blood supply in the connective tissues. As the bone cells grow within the interconnected pore channels, the implant serves as a structural bridge or scaffold for bone formation. Although porous bone implants improve the bonding between the scaffolds and body tissue through biological fixation, the higher-porosity content lowers the mechanical strength and reliability of implants. This is particularly important for ceramic scaffolds because higher porosity reduces their ability to act as a load-bearing component.

Various bone substitutes that are currently being used include *autograft* (tissue from another location of the body of the same individual), *allograft* (tissue from different individuals of the same species), *xenograft* (tissue implanted from a different species), and *bone graft* (artificial bone). Though autograft is the most suitable for orthopedic applications, it requires at least two operations and may result in patient morbidity (hemorrhage, infection, and pain). Both allograft and xenograft may be rejected by the patient's body and may also pose a serious threat for transmittal of fatal diseases. Because of these reasons, development and applications of bone grafts are becoming popular.

In this work, controlled-porosity alumina ceramic bone grafts were processed from computed tomography (CT) data of a short pastern bone of a horse's knuckle. Initially, the CT scan information was converted to a computer-aided-design (CAD) file of the bone. The CAD file was then used to create polymeric prototypes of the knuckle. The indirect fused deposition process was then used to create the ceramic prototypes having controlled uniform or gradient porosity by infiltrating desired ceramic slurry into the polymeric prototype or mold. Cytotoxicity and cell-proliferation studies were conducted using modified human osteoblast cells to understand the influence of various structural parameters on the cell-growth behavior using these porous ceramic scaffolds. The processing science described here can be used to fabricate custom-made bone grafts having tailored structural parameters.

II. Solid Freeform Fabrication in Biomedical Applications

Solid freeform fabrication (SFF) or rapid prototyping (RP) is a layered manufacturing approach to fabricate three-dimensional objects on a fixtureless platform directly from a CAD file. Some of the commercial SFF processes include stereolithography (SLA), selective laser sintering (SLS), fused deposition modeling (FDM), and sanders prototype (SP).[7] The utilization of SFF processes to fabricate models derived from medical imaging data sources has received some attention in recent years. The SFF-fabricated patient-specific anatomic models have emerged as worthwhile tools for surgical planning as well as mechanisms of information dissemination to patients. Griffith *et al.*[8] and Garg *et al.*[9] have independently examined the use of SLA to produce bioceramic implants. Both groups have demonstrated fabrication of small hydroxyapatite objects. In these cases, solids loading in ceramic slurry is typically limited to about 50% by volume. Because of the large volume of resin, there is a concern about complete removal of resin decomposition products as well as maintaining dimensional tolerance and structural integrity particularly for large parts. Griffin *et al.*[10] have used laminated object manufacturing (LOM) to fabricate high-density anatomic models using alumina, zirconia, and hydroxyapatite. In another approach, the fused deposition of ceramics (FDC) process was used to directly fabricate green ceramic parts of tricalcium phosphate (TCP) from their CAD file.[11] Like direct SLA parts, high volume fraction of thermoplastic binders is of serious concern for the FDC processed parts as well. Complete removal of thermoplastic binders, as well as maintaining dimensional tolerance and structural integrity during

J. W. Halloran—contributing editor

Manuscript No. 187879. Received March 7, 2001; approved February 24, 2003.
This work received financial support from the National Science Foundation through CAREER Grant No. DMI 9874971.

*Member, American Ceramic Society.
†School of Mechanical and Materials Engineering.
‡School of Biological Sciences and Molecular Biosciences.

densification, requires significant process optimization. In recent years, Chu *et al.* have used the indirect SLA to produce controlled-porosity hydroxyapatite (HAp) parts using a 40 vol% flowable suspension.[12]

In the present work, the indirect FDM process is used to fabricate porous bone grafts. In the indirect process, a polymeric mold or negative of the desired structure can be fabricated using any SFF machine with commercially available feed stock material. The molds can then be infiltrated with desired materials. For fabrication of ceramic structures, the infiltrated mold structure will then be subjected to a binder removal and sintering cycle to remove the mold polymer and the densification of the ceramic structure. For the fabrication of porous ceramic structures, the FDM process has the ability to control pore structure in all three dimensions. Moreover, simple changes to FDM tool-path can also be used to create structures with different porosities.

III. From CT Scan to Polymer Model

Computed tomography (CT or CAT scan) is a diagnostic procedure in which a cross-sectional X-ray picture of a "slice" of the body is made. In this process, the patient lies on a table and the X-ray machine rotates around the patient, as the table is moved horizontally. Images from these X-rays are then processed via a computer. The main advantage for CT is that it produces excellent contrast for bony structures while allowing good picture quality for soft tissues as well. For our work, a CT scan was first created of a short pastern bone or knuckle of a horse that was placed in a bag of water to simulate the density of surrounding tissues. The short pastern bone is located in the hoof of the horse, as shown in Fig. 1. This bone was used because of the desired size and availability. The bone was scanned using a Philips Tomoscan M CT scanner at the Washington State University Veterinary Teaching Hospital. The bone was scanned with 45 slices at a slice interval of 1 mm. A gantry tilt was not used during the scan. The two-dimensional images were saved in a DICOM (digital imaging and communication in medicine) standard format on the Philips system. An evaluation copy of Materialises Interactive Medical Image Control System (MIMICS) version 6.0[13] was used to convert these images into a CAD file. The MIMICS software did not automatically recognize the images or the patient information. As a result, the 45 CT scan images were opened manually using the software. A CT scan distinguishes between two different materials of different densities by light intensity. Less dense materials like air have lower light intensity values and appear dark. Higher density materials such as bone have a higher light intensity and appear lighter or whiter in color. A mask of the desired density of the bone was created, which allowed for the cleanest selection of the bone while separating the bone from the water and any air pockets. Figure 2 shows a few selected two-dimensional images of the CT scan for the short pastern bone of the horse's knuckle. The selected mask region was then grown into a three-dimensional representation and converted into and saved as a stereolithography (*.stl*) file.

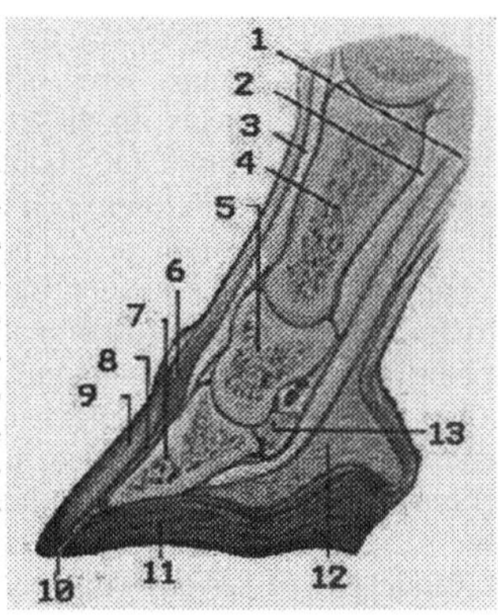

Fig. 1. Anatomy of a horse's hoof.

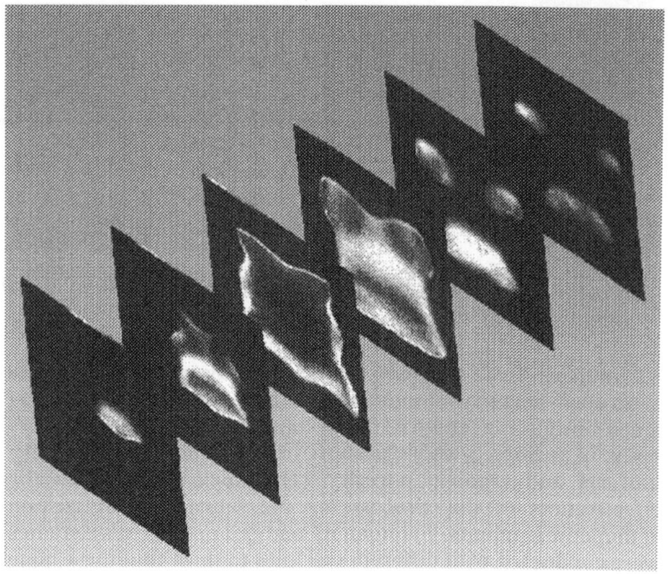

Fig. 2. Six of the 45 two-dimensional CT scan images of the horse knuckle.

An *.stl* file is a tessellated representation of a surface model. The *.stl* file was used as an input file for the Stratasys™ Quickslice™ software to develop a tool-path for the commercial FDM 1650 (Stratasys™, Eden Prairie, MN).

IV. Processing of Ceramic Bone Graft

Processing of ceramic bone grafts consists of three stages of optimization work mold design, slurry composition development, and binder burnout and sintering cycle development. Molds were designed and fabricated by FDM 1650 using commercially available ICW-06 thermoplastic wax filament material. Molds were designed and fabricated with different raster width and raster gap from 0.62 to 1.5 mm. The top 5 mm of the mold had only perimeter but no raster filling, which is also called the lip, to hold excess ceramic slurry during infiltration. The bottom four layers of the mold had no raster gap to avoid leaking of slurry during infiltration. Raster width varied from 0.38 to 0.64 mm. By changing the polymer raster width and the raster gap of the molds, internal pore structures can be tailored.[14] After binder removal of slurry-infiltrated ceramic structures, pores can be formed mimicking the polymeric mold architecture. The shape or the macrostructure is controlled via the *.stl* file generated from the CT scan. The *.stl* file and tool-path modification in the FDM allows for the simultaneous control of the micro- as well as the macrostructure of the parts.

Ceramic slurry development work started with commercially available high-purity alumina powders from Baikowski International Corp., with different surface areas, 10D (8.6 m^2/g) and 30D (26.6 m^2/g), and Sedigraph d_{50} for 10D = 0.45 μm and for 30D = 0.41 μm (supplied by the vendor). A Brookfield viscometer was used to determine the optimum weight percent of dispersant needed for the preparation of water-based ceramic slurry by measuring the viscosity at different shear rates and solids loading for each solution. The ideal slurry should have the highest solids loading with the lowest viscosity. High solids loading helps to reduce the shrinkage and related cracking possibilities during the sintering of green body, while low viscosity enhances the mold infiltration process and reduces defects due to infiltration. Figure 3(a) shows the viscosity of the ceramic slurry with 10D and 30D alumina powders with increasing solids loading at a fixed shear rate of 46 (1/s). Because of the low surface area of the 10D powder, a higher solids loading could be achieved compared with the 30D powder. High-purity 10D alumina powder was selected for this work. The alumina powder was already doped with 500 ppm MgO as a sintering aid.

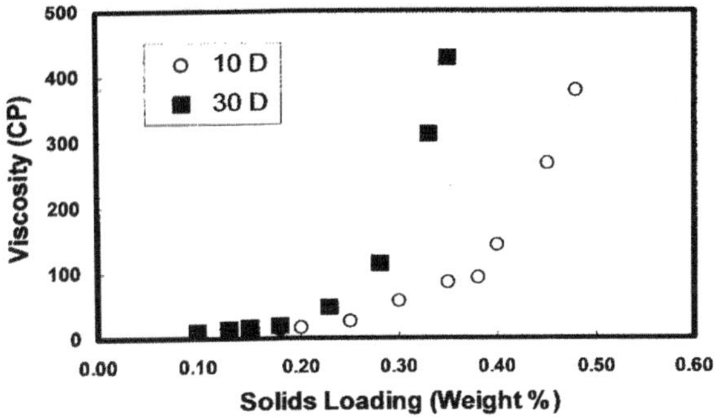

(a)

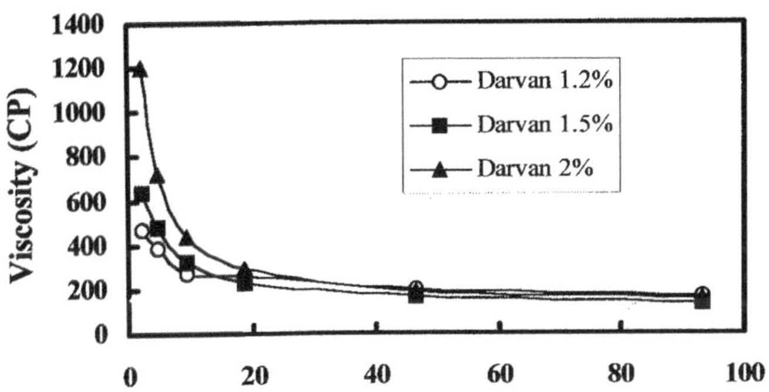

(b)

Fig. 3. (a) Effect of solids loading on the viscosity of 10D and 30D alumina ceramic powders. (b) Effect of dispersant amount on the viscosity of ceramic slurry with 10D.

Both slurry casting and gel casting processes were used to fabricate ceramic scaffolds. For the slurry casting process, 1-butanol (Fisher Scientific) was used as an antifoaming agent, Darvan 821A (R. T. Vanderbilt & Co., Norwalk, CT) was used as a dispersant, and B-1000 (Rohm and Haas, PA) was used as a binder. Ceramic powder, antifoaming agent, and dispersant were added to water and then ball-milled for 6 h in a polyethylene bottle. A Brookfield viscometer was used to determine the optimum weight percent of dispersant needed for the preparation of water-based ceramic slurry by measuring the viscosity at different shear rates for each solution. For the 10D alumina powder, Darvan amount 1.2 wt% of alumina powders was found to be optimum and beyond that dispersant increased the viscosity of the slurry as can be seen from Fig. 3(b). The required amount of binder was added to the mixture just before infiltration. Polymeric molds were then infiltrated with the ceramic slurry. The infiltrated molds were dried at room temperature for 2 to 3 days. The final slurry composition had 70.3 wt% alumina powder in water with 1.2 wt% Darvan 821 A, 1 wt% 1-butanol, and 10 wt% B-1000 binder.

For gel casting process, a thermosetting type of binder was used. First, water, acrylamide (Mallinkrodt), and *N,N'*-bisacrylamide (E. M. Science) were mixed well until a clear solution was formed. Alumina powder and Darvan 821A were added to the clear solution. The slurry was mixed for 2 h on a table-top ball-mill. Ammonium persulfate (E. M. Science) and tetramethylethylenediamine (J. T. Baker) were added to this solution and manually stirred for 1–2 min to achieve a homogeneous slurry. The solution was then poured into the polymeric mold, and subsequently the acrylamide polymerized. In our experience, for larger parts, the gel-casting approach was preferred because of fewer cracking problems during drying and sintering. The final gel composition had 77 wt% alumina in water with 2 wt% acrylamide and 1.2 wt% Darvan 821 A.

Binder removal and sintering of infiltrated molds were conducted in a Thermolyne high-temperature muffle furnace in a furnace air environment. A slower heating rate of 2°C/min was used up to 550°C to avoid cracking or distortion of the part due to binder removal. Above 550°C, samples were heated at 4°C/min. For the horse's knuckle, binder removal and sintering were completed in two steps. In the first step, structures were partially sintered to 1400°C in a bed of alumina setter powder (Alcoa A-14) and cooled to room temperature. The powder allowed the mold wax and processing aids to be wicked away while providing a structural support for the complex shaped objects. After partial sintering the brown structures were again fired to 1600°C for 3 h on a flat plate without any setter powder bed. For smaller samples with simple shapes, the binder removal and sintering were performed in one heating cycle without using any setter powders. Shrinkage was measured as a part of physical property measurement to understand the sintering behavior of these ceramics. Nonuniform shrinkage causes cracking and warping in the final product. Moreover, controlled shrinkage information can be used in the design stage to make necessary design modifications. Shrinkage also varies as a function of volume fraction porosity in these samples in which higher volume fraction porosity showed a lower amount of shrinkage.[15] For these porous alumina samples, linear shrinkage varied from 23% to 25%. Sintered density (d_{App}) for these samples was between 3.78 and 3.80 g/cm^3 (>95% theoretical density).

Figures 4(a) and (b) show the two halves of the alumina ceramic bone graft of the horse knuckle, which is a truncated build directly from the CAD file. It can be seen that the porosity in Fig. 4(a) is of uniform size and distribution (300 μm, 29 vol% porosity), but for Fig. 4(b), there is a gradient in porosity. There are three different types of porosity in the sample in Fig. 4(b), which more closely mimics the structure of real bones. The outer shell has a pore size of 300 μm with a volume fraction porosity of 29%. The inner regions are intended to loosely resemble the cancellous bone structure with a greater volume fraction porosity of 44% keeping the pore size constant at 300 μm. The center of the model is a complete void. All three regions of porosity are interconnected and continuous cell growth from outside to the inside is a viable option, if these scaffolds are implanted *in vivo*. The main advantage of this approach can be visualized from these two ceramic bone grafts. In this approach, any internal architecture or porosity can be added based on the patient's need by simply modifying the CAD file or the FDM tool-path. Moreover, any defects in the bone structure can be fixed simply by modifying the CAD file that was created from the CT scan. Figure 5 shows a picture of all three: the real bone, ABS polymer model fabricated via FDM, and porous alumina bone graft.

V. Biocompatibility Tests

The alumina powders that were used were of high-purity, medical-grade quality. The first step was to determine that the processing aids did not compromise the biocompatibility of the alumina. To confirm this, cytotoxicity and cell viability studies were performed. For the initial cytotoxicity studies, the PR1 cell line (rat pituitary tumor cell) was used. These cells were chosen because of their availability and aggressive nature of growth. The cells were seeded on sintered and crushed alumina samples. Results showed that the sintered alumina structures were nontoxic.[16]

The cell proliferation study was performed using a modified human osteoblast cell line (OPC1, Oregon Health Sciences Center).[17] These cells have a modified T-antigen that helps to grow more aggressively than normal human osteoblast cells. The cells were seeded on top of thin circular porous alumina disks 1 cm in diameter and 1 mm thick. The cells were cultured in a standard medium made of Dulbecco's modified Eagle's medium supplemented with 10% fetal bovine serum, bicarbonate buffer, 0.01*M*

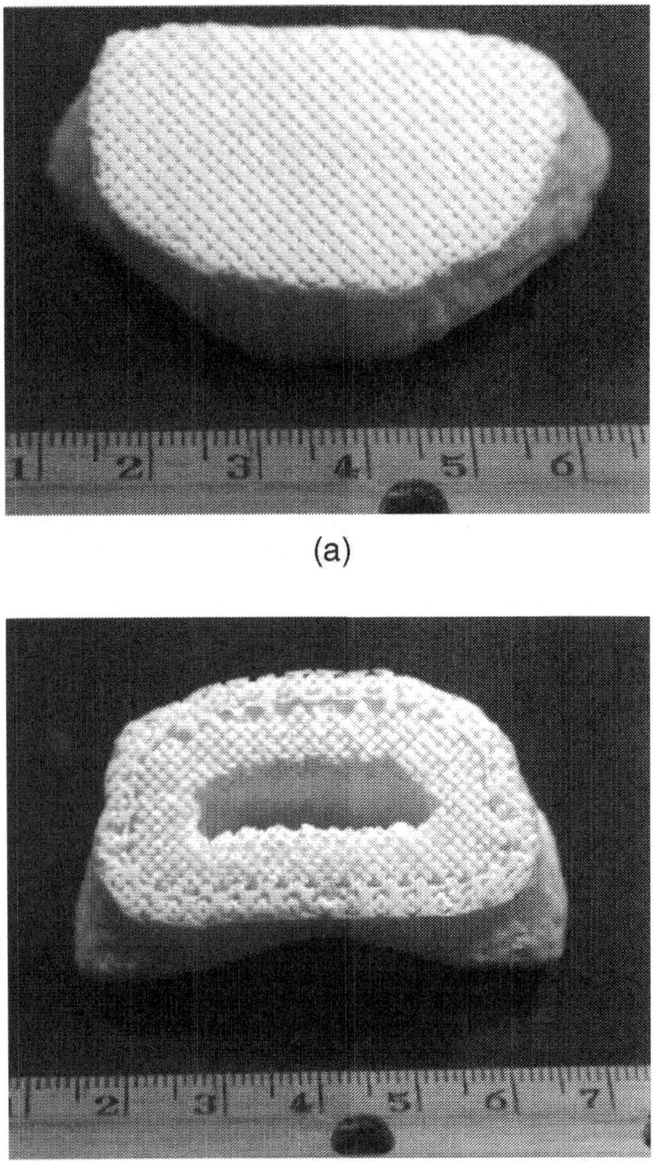

Fig. 4. Alumina ceramic bone grafts with (a) uniform and (b) gradient porosity.

Hepes buffer, 100 units/mL penicillin, and 100 mg/mL streptomycin. Early passage cells were cultured in the same medium supplemented with 5 ng/mL acidic fibroblast growth factor. The culture was incubated at 37°C in a humidified 5% CO_2 atmosphere. A colorimetric assay (MTT assay) was used to evaluate cell number at various times after seeding. This assay quantitates

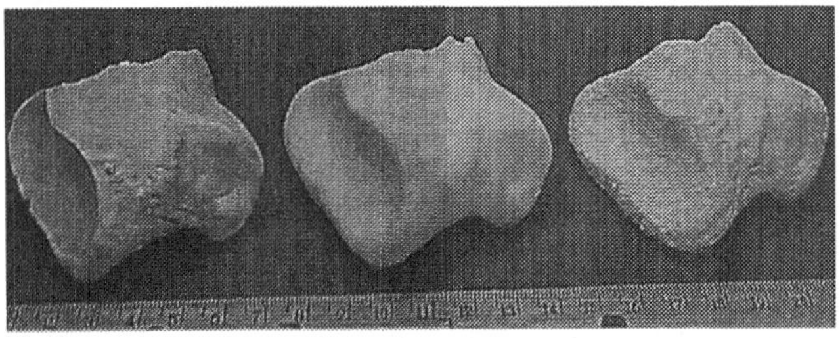

Fig. 5. From left to right, the original bone, the ABS bone model processed via FDM, and the porous alumina ceramic bone graft.

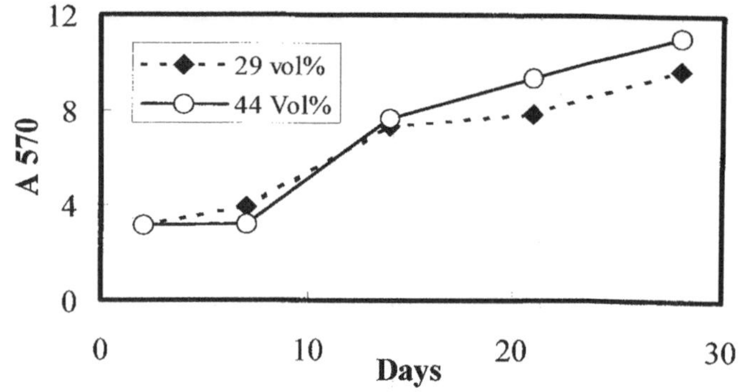

Fig. 6. Cell proliferation studies on porous alumina scaffolds using the OPC1 cell line.

the ability of mitochondrial dehydrogenases to metabolize 3-[4,5-dimethylthiazol-2-yl]-2,5-diphenyltetrazolium bromide to an insoluble formazan.[18] The amount of formazan is directly proportional to the total number of living cells. This enzyme assay produces a colored product, which is quantitated in a microplate reader at a wavelength of 570 nm. The higher the intensity in the microplate reader, the higher the number of living cells present on the scaffolds. The *in vitro* tests were repeated three times and then the average numbers were used for analysis. Figure 6 shows typical cell growth behavior after 28 days on porous alumina substrates having 29 and 44 vol% porosity with a pore size of 300 μm. In general, the results show that increasing pore volume had minor influence on cell density on these porous alumina scaffolds, though these results are sufficient to prove that the scaffolds are biocompatible. Figure 7 shows an optical micrograph of a 44 vol% scaffold after 28 days of OPC1 cell growth. It can be observed that OPC1 cells colonized very well on the ceramic surfaces during the 28 days. The matrix was originally white in color, but as the cells colonized the matrix with a monolayer, the color changed to gray.

VI. Mechanical Properties

Uniaxial compression tests were conducted with controlled porosity cylindrical alumina samples. Right cylindrical samples were fabricated via the indirect FDM process, 1 cm in diameter and 1.6 cm long. For each set of porosities, at least 20 samples were tested using a screw-driven Instron Model 4400 according to the ASTM standard C 1424-99. Samples with 29 vol% porosity with a pore size of 300 μm showed an average compressive

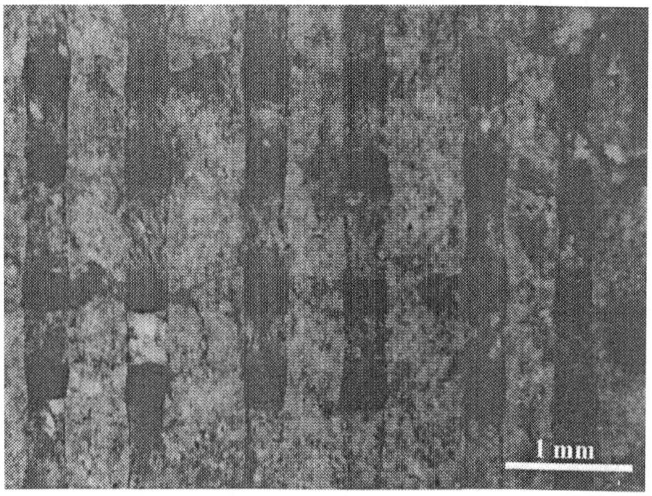

Fig. 7. Optical micrograph of 44 vol% alumina scaffold after 28 days of OPC1 cell growth.

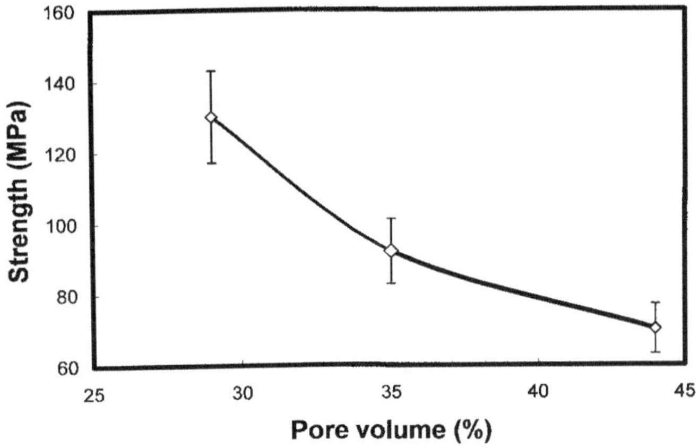

Fig. 8. Uniaxial compression strengths of porous alumina samples at a constant pore size of 300 μm.

strength of 130 ± 13 MPa, which is comparable to a typical human cortical bone. For samples with 44 vol% porosity with 480 μm pore size, the strength was reduced to 70 ± 14 MPa. Figure 8 shows the effect of volume fraction porosity on the compression strengths of porous alumina samples, where pore size was kept constant at 300 μm. It can be seen that increasing volume fraction porosity decreases the mechanical properties of these structures significantly. The failure trends followed the exponential equation proposed first by Ryshekewitch.[18] The equation was expressed as

$$\sigma = \sigma_0 \exp(-bP) \tag{1}$$

where σ is the stress of the porous structure in compression, σ_0 is the stress of nonporous structure, P describes volume fraction porosity, and b is an empirical constant. Ryshekewitch determined that the value of b varies between 6 to 9 for different loading conditions for zirconia and alumina ceramics. In our case, the average values for maximum compressive failure stress based on Fig. 8 for which the exponential in Eq. (1) is a good fit is given as

$$y = 508 \exp(-4.8P) \qquad (R^2 = 0.9921) \tag{2}$$

The experimental data showed similar behavior for nonrandom porous ceramic structures as proposed by the Ryshekewitch equation where compressive strength decreases as volume fraction porosity increases due to the increase in pore spacings. σ_0, the nonporous stress component, based on the above Ryshekewitch equation is 508 MPa. The value of P was found to be 4.8, which is lower than the reported values by Ryshekewitch. The higher values of b obtained by Ryshekewitch indicates that the strength should increase more as the volume fraction porosity decreases. The experimental results obtained in our case used controlled porosity structures with three-dimensionally interconnected porosity. The lower number of b may be due to the cumulative damage due to multiple pores and cracks through crack generation-linkage-propagation events. Further discussion of this subject can be found in Refs. 19 and 20.

VII. Conclusions

High-purity alumina ceramics were used to produce controlled-porosity bone grafts from CT scan data using the indirect FDM process. The CT scan data were first converted to a CAD file using commercial MIMICS software. The CAD file was then used to produce polymeric models as well as molds for ceramic prototypes. Both slurry casting and gel casting techniques were used to fabricate the ceramic parts. Biocompatibility studies proved that these bone grafts were nontoxic. Cell proliferation studies showed that the matrixes were biocompatible and volume fraction porosity had a minor influence on the cell growth. It was found that increasing porosity degraded the mechanical properties of these scaffolds.

Acknowledgments

We would like to acknowledge the experimental help from Rebekah Taylor, Raj Atisivan, Samar Kalita, Dr. Randy Kintner, and Travis Sonnett.

References

[1]L. L. Hench, "Bioceramics," *J. Am. Ceram. Soc.*, **81** [7] 1705–28 (1998).
[2]L. L. Hench, "Bioceramics: From Concepts to Clinic," *J. Am. Ceram. Soc.*, **74** [7] 1487–510 (1991).
[3]L. L. Hench and J. Wilson, *An Introduction to Bioceramics*. World Scientific, London, U.K., 1993.
[4]S. F. Hulbert, J. C. Bokros, L. L. Hench, J. Wilson, and G. Heimke, "Ceramics in Clinical Applications: Past, Present and Future"; pp. 189–213 in *High Tech Ceramics*. Edited by P. Vincenzini. Elsevier, Amsterdam, Netherlands, 1987.
[5]A. Ravaglioli and A. Krajewski, *Bioceramics: Materials, Properties, Applications*. Chapman and Hall, London, U.K., 1992.
[6]J. J. Klawitter and S. F. Hulbert, "Applications of Porous Ceramics for the Attachment of Load Bearing Orthopedic Applications," *J. Biomed. Mater. Res. Symp.*, **2**, 161 (1971).
[7]H. L. Marcus, J. J. Beaman, J. W. Barlow, D. L. Bourell, and R. H. Crawford (Eds.), Solid Freeform Fabrication Symposium Proceedings (University of Texas, Austin, TX), Vol. 1-12. University of Texas, Austin, TX, 1990–2001.
[8]M. L Griffith, T. Chu, W. Wagner, and J. W. Halloran, "Ceramic Stereolithography for Investment Casting and Biomedical Applications," *Solid Freeform Fabr. Symp. Proc.*, **6**, 31–38 (1996).
[9]R. Garg, R. K. Prud'homme, and I. A. Aksay, "Orthopedic Implants by Ceramic Stereolithography"; presented at the 100th Annual Meeting of the American Ceramic Society, Cincinnati, OH, May 2–6, 1998 (Bioceramics: Materials and Applications Symposium).
[10]A. Griffin, S. McMillian, C. Griffin, and K. Barton, "Bioceramic RP Materials for Medical Models," *Proc. Int. Conf. Rapid Prototyping, 7th*, 355–59 (1997).
[11]S. C. Danforth and A. Safari, Rutgers University, personal communication, 2000.
[12]C. Wivell, Materialise, Ann Arbor, MI, personal communication.
[13]T. M. G Chu, J. W. Halloran, S. J. Hollister, and S. E. Feinberg, "Hydroxyapatite with Designed Internal Architecture," *J. Mater. Sci.: Mater. Med.*, **12**, 471–78 (2001).
[14]S. Bose, S. Sugiura, and A. Bandyopadhyay, "Processing of Controlled Porosity Ceramic Structures via Fused Deposition Process," *Scr. Mater.*, **41** [9] 1009–14 (1999).
[15]S. Bose, J. Darsell, L. Hua, D. Sarkar, and A. Bandyopadhyay, "Processing, Biocompatibility and Biomechanical Testing of Porous Alumina Ceramics," *Ceram. Trans.*, **110**, 167–81 (1999).
[16]R. Atisivan, S. Bose, and A. Bandyopadhyay, "Effects of MgO Addition to Mullite Ceramics," *J. Am. Ceram. Soc.*, **84** [1] 221–23 (2001).
[17]S. R Winn, G. Randolph, H. Uludag, S. C. Wong, G. A. Hair, and J. O. Hollinger, "Establishing an Immortalized Human Osteoprecursor Cell Line: OPC1," *J. Bone Miner. Res.*, **14**, 1721–33 (1999).
[18]P. W. Sylvester, H. P. Birkenfeld, H. L. Hosick, and K. P. Briski, "Fatty Acid Modulation of Epidermal Growth Factor-Induced Mouse Mammary Epithelial Cell Proliferation *In Vitro*," *Exp. Cell Res.*, **214**, 145–53 (1994).
[19]R. Ryshkewitch, "Compression Strength of Porous Sintered Alumina and Zirconia," *J. Am. Ceram. Soc.*, **36** [2] 65–68 (1953).
[20]A. Hattiangadi and A. Bandyopadhyay, "Strength Degradation of Porous Ceramics Under Uniaxial Compressive Loading," *J. Am. Ceram. Soc.*, **83** [11] 2730–36 (2000). □

journal

J. Am. Ceram. Soc., 86 [8] 1440–42 (2003)

Preparation of Polymethylmethacrylate-Reinforced Functionally Graded Hydroxyapatite Composites

Masataka Ohgaki† and Kimihiro Yamashita*

Institute of Biomaterials and Bioengineering, Tokyo Medical and Dental University, 2-3-10, Kanda-surugadai, Chiyoda, Tokyo 101-0062, Japan

A functionally graded hybridization approach has been used in the formation of polymer-ceramic composites of polymethylmethacrylate (PMMA) and hydroxyapatite (HAp). HAp was successfully reinforced by sedimentary HAp distributions on a PMMA matrix using a centrifuge to avoid stress convergence on the interface. The stress-strain curves of the functionally graded PMMA-HAp composite showed sufficient mechanical strength with reduced brittleness. Scanning electron micrographs also showed evidence of exposed HAp on the surface of the composites.

I. Introduction

Hydroxyapatite (HAp) has the great advantage of being able to bond directly to living tissue *in vivo*;[1–4] furthermore, its ceramic forms exhibit osteoinductive properties.[5] However, fragility and poor mechanical properties of sintered HAp ceramics limit their application as artificial implants.[6] To overcome this inadequacy, hybridized biocomposites of bioceramics with metal or polymer have been developed for hard tissue engineering.[2,7,8] Several types of polymer/HAp composites have been produced as HAp-reinforced polymers.[9–13] However, the brittleness of HAp ceramics has not yet been ameliorated by HAp granule-dispersion in polymer or by conjugation of HAp and polymer. We have successfully reinforced HAp by hybridization of polymethylmethacrylate (PMMA). PMMA is extensively used in bone cements to fix load-bearing prosthetic components in total joint replacement surgery.[14] The long-term survival of cemented joint prostheses reportedly depends to a great extent on the strength of the PMMA bone cement.

In this work, functionally graded hybridization of HAp with PMMA (FGH HAp/PMMA) was effected to obtain both the bending strength and flexibility of PMMA and the biocompatility of HAp. The conditions of HAp/PMMA constitution for hybridization were found to govern the mechanical properties and biocompatibility.

II. Materials and Methods

(1) Synthesis of HAp Powder and PMMA Polymerization

Pure $CaCO_3$ powder (Wako Co. Ltd., Osaka, Japan) was decarbonated at 1100°C for 2 h, and the resultant CaO powder was hydrated with distilled water to $Ca(OH)_2$. A 0.6*M* H_3PO_4 solution (Wako Co. Ltd.) was added by drops to stirred 0.5*M* $Ca(OH)_2$ suspension, for a total Ca:P ratio of 10:6 at room temperature. The final pH value was adjusted to 9.0. After aging for 3 d, the resulting suspension was filtered by suction, then heated to 850°C for 2 h to calcinate. The structure of the product HAp powder was examined by X-ray powder diffraction (Model PW 1700, Philips, Eindhoven, Netherlands). To prepare the PMMA polymer, the bulk-polymerization method was used in this study, by which the viscosity of the reactant in PMMA polymerization could be controlled. Before the complexing with PMMA, HAp particles were exposed to NaOH solution. 100 g of methylmethacrylate (MMA) (Wako Co. Ltd.), 3 g of PMMA (Scientific Polymer Products, Ontario, NY) and 0.007 g of methacrylic acid (MA; Scientific Polymer Products) were put into the flask and mixed with stirring for ~8 h at 60°C under nitrogen gas atmosphere. The α-, α′-azobisisobutyronitrile (0.005 g) was used for the initiator in the polymerization process. The viscous PMMA fluid so obtained was transfused into a test tube and matured at 40°C to complete the polymerization. An outline of the process of preparation of HAp/PMMA composites is shown in Fig. 1. The low and high molecular weights of the obtained PMMA were measured by gel-permeation-chromatography (GPC; Models RID-6A and C-R7A, Shimadzu, Kyoto, Japan).

(2) Preparation of HAp-PMMA Composite and FGH HAp/PMMA

HAp-PMMA composites were prepared in advance of the functionally graded HAp/PMMA by homogeneous dispersion of HAp powders in the PMMA matrix. The HAp-PMMA composite was prepared by dispersion of 20 wt% HAp powder into the PMMA viscous fluid. The PMMA viscous-fluid-dispersed HAp was transfused into test tubes, then matured at 40°C to complete the polymerization.

Initially, most of the composites incurred breakage at the connective interface between HAp and polymer, because of poor conjugation at the interface. Next, a novel FGH HAp/PMMA was developed based on sedimentary HAp distributions, using a centrifuge to avoid stress convergence on the interface. MMA (100 g), PMMA (3 g), and MA (0.007 g) were mixed in a flask that was thermostatically controlled at 60°C, and α-, α′-azobisisobutyronitrile (0.005 g), as the polymerization initiator, was added by stirring. The viscosity of polymerized PMMA increased in the course of the polymerization process. The highly viscous PMMA resulting from 8 h of stirring was allowed to stand in an incubator at 40°C for 15 min, after which the HAp powder was added. The viscosity of the polymerizing PMMA fluid was exactly adjusted by an 8 h polymerization in order to prepare the FGH HAp/PMMA evaluated in this study. The viscous PMMA fluid, which was dispersed with 20 wt% HAp, was transfused into centrifuge tubes. The stratigraphic distributions of HAp and PMMA were gradually altered by the centrifuge, the graded ratio being dependent on the revolution rate and centrifuging time. A low-revolution rate with centrifuge for a short time caused no graded inclusion of HAp and PMMA. Conversely, a divisible and brittle interface between HAp

S. Deb—contributing editor

Manuscript No. 186992. Received September 6, 2002; approved March 3, 2003.
This work is partly supported by a Grant-in-Aid for Scientific Research from the Ministry of Education, Culture, Sports, Science and Technology of Japan. Contract grant number: (B)#14350457.

*Member, American Ceramic Society.
†Author to whom correspondence should be addressed. Fax: +81 3-5280-8005; e-mail: ohgaki.bcr@tmd.ac.jp

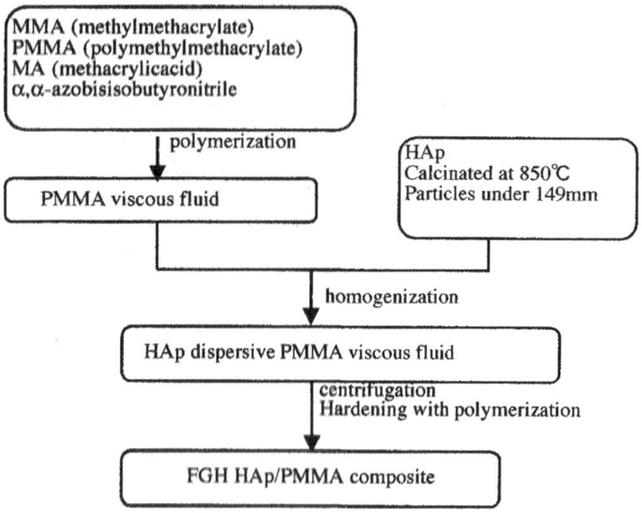

Fig. 1. Flow chart of preparation of HAp/PMMA composites.

and PMMA was formed by a high-revolution rate and the polymerized contraction. In this work, efficiently graded HAp/PMMA composite was obtained by centrifuging at 1000 rpm for 5 min. The HAp-PMMA gradient viscous products were completely polymerized at 40°C. The resulting HAp/PMMA composites were characterized by XRD and SEM.

(3) Flexural Strength Testing

To evaluate the effectiveness of the HAp/PMMA gradient composite materials, the mechanical strengths were determined. The mechanical properties of the HAp-dispersed composites and the gradient composites were measured by the three-point bending strength test with a universal testing machine (Model UUT 81–11, Ueshima, Tokyo, Japan). A condition of 15 mm span and at 1 mm/min cross-head speed was used for the three-point-bending test. The composite blocks were cut into test pieces, 20 mm × 3 mm × 2 mm in size, for the mechanical test. The test pieces were cut from every grade point of composition of the HAp/PMMA gradient composites. More than five tests pieces were used from each HAp-distribution condition. The maximum flexural stress was evaluated from the stress-strain curves.

III. Results and Discussion

Polymerized PMMA was colorless and transparent in appearance. Values of the number averaged molecular weight (M_n), the weight averaged molecular weight (M_w), and the Z-averaged molecular weight (M_z) of PMMA after fabrication are summarized in Table I. Because the values of ca. 280 000 for M_w and 610 000 for M_z were both far beyond the assay for molecular weight (5 to 300 000) for commercial PMMA, the polymerization of PMMA seemed to be perfectly completed in these experiments. As the multidispersibility value of M_w/M_n was limited to 2.3–2.7, versus 1.5–3.5 for commercial PMMA, this narrow distribution of molecular weight also suggested adequate polymerization of PMMA.

Table I. Molecular Weight of PMMA Obtained by GPC Measurement

Molecular Weight	M_n	M_w	M_z	M_w/M_n Dispersibility	M_z/M_w Dispersibility
Low	363	981	2.609	2.701	2.661
High	121,006	278,424	611,641	2.301	2.197

M_n: Number average molecular weight ($M_n = \Sigma$ NM/Σ N); M_w: Weight average molecular weight ($M_w = \Sigma$ NM^2/Σ N); M_z: Z average molecular weight ($M_z = \Sigma$ NM^3/Σ NM^2); M: molecular weight; N: number of polymer having M of molecular weight

In the HAp-powder-homogenized PMMA composites and the FGH HAp/PMMA that were obtained, HAp powders were well dispersed in every HAp-homogenized PMMA. XRD patterns of these samples are shown in Fig. 2. The crystallinity of HAp was confirmed with the typical XRD peaks in the FGH HAp/PMMA, in which the broad halo arose from amorphous PMMA. Figure 3 shows the prepared FGH HAp/PMMA and the microscopic observation of sections of the composites. For most polymer–ceramic composites, small openings or gaps are caused at the interface between the polymer and the ceramic sites on the section by the slice treatment. Close adhesion between HAp and PMMA was proved in the SEM photograph, because no disruption was observed at the interface of HAp and PMMA, in the sliced section. This HAp/PMMA adhesion coherency was attributed to polymerization contraction. To take advantage of this contraction, sufficient degassing of the viscous PMMA fluid was necessary before polymerization.

A gradient ratio of HAp/PMMA was effectively formed in FGH HAp/PMMA composites, as shown in Fig. 4. HAp contents were calculated from the densities measured on the sliced samples. At most locations within the FGH HAp/PMMA, there was a high content of PMMA, which would provide bending strength and flexibility, whereas one surface of the FGH HAp/PMMA had exposed HAp, which would have excellent biocompatibility.

The mechanical properties of the composite were evaluated by flexural strength testing. Elastic modurus for the test pieces of the each Hap-distribution condition were calculated by the results of a flexural strength test, shown in Fig. 5. Despite the inclusion of HAp powders into PMMA, there was not a big difference between the composites and PMMA in terms of flexural strength. It was suggested that stress did not concentrate on the interface between HAp and PMMA in the FGH HAp/PMMA. Therefore, this is considered to be a dynamic advantage of FGH HAp/PMMA as compared with the joint type composite. The stress-strain curves of FGH HAp/PMMA composite with 20 wt% of HAp content demonstrated enough strength under stress for medical application, along with the relaxation of brittleness and fragility (Fig. 6). This relaxation indicates bending and flexibility equivalent to PMMA, so that the brittleness observed in the HAp ceramic material is eliminated. As a result, the composite is

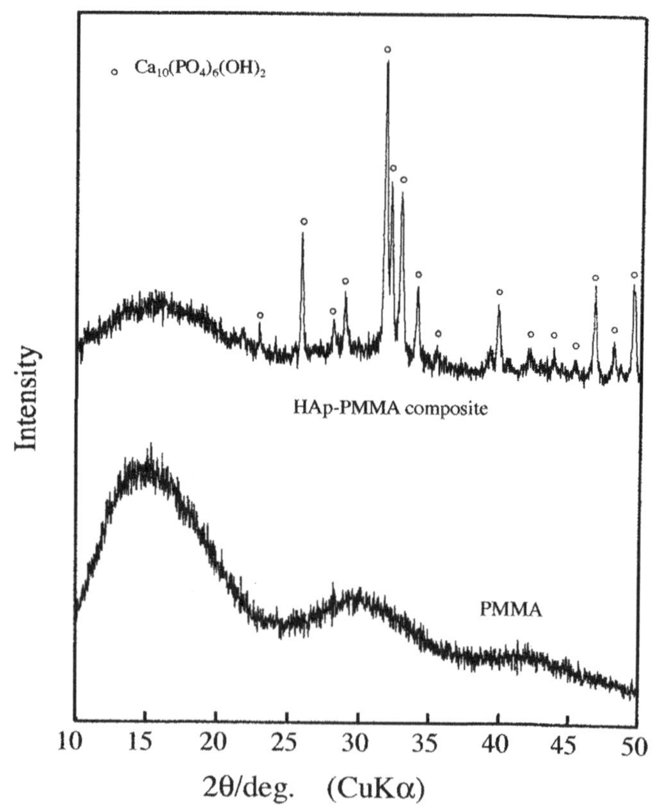

Fig. 2. XRD patterns of PMMA and HAp/PMMA composite.

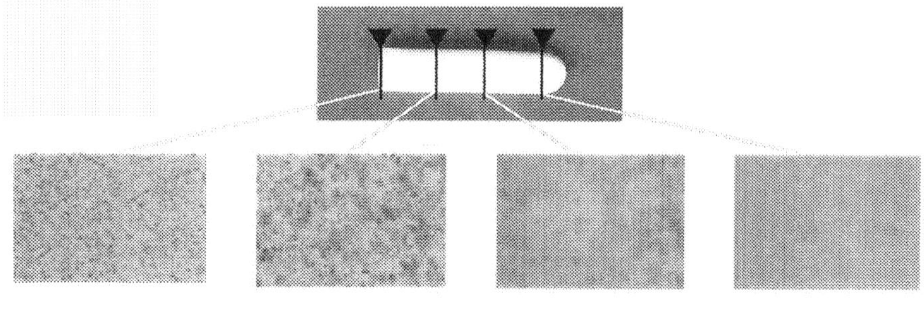

Fig. 3. Microscopic observation of FGH HAp/PMMA (upper) and the cross sections of HAp/PMMA composite (lower).

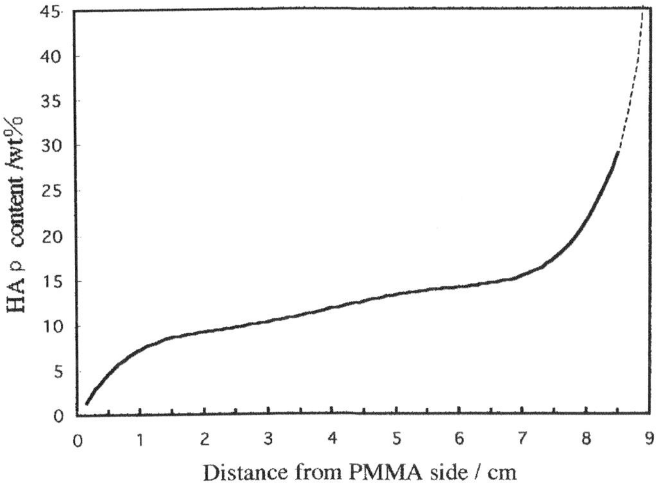

Fig. 4. Regional HAp contents versus distance from PMMA side of FGH HAp/PMMA composite.

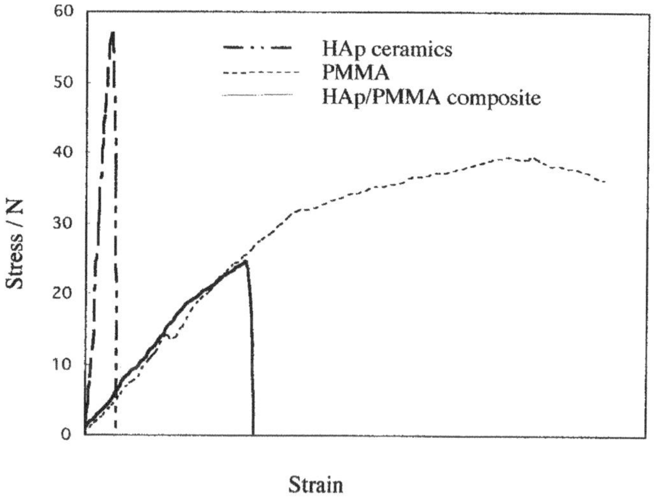

Fig. 6. Stress-strain curves of HAp/PMMA composites.

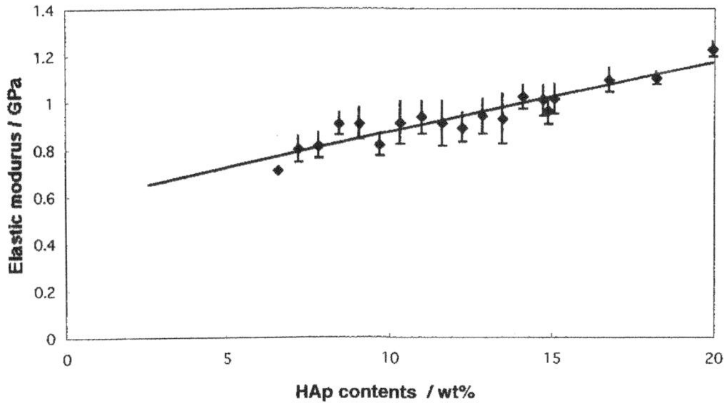

Fig. 5. Elastic modurus of HAp/PMMA gradient composite for the HAp contents.

expected to enjoy broad and variable medical application for the right material in the right place.

IV. Summary

HAp has been successfully reinforced by hybridization of functional PMMA by sedimentary HAp distribution via centrifuge, to avoid stress convergence at the interface. The functionally graded hybridization of HAp with PMMA (FGH HAp/PMMA) thus obtained was devised so as to preserve both the bending strength and flexibility of PMMA and the biocompatibility of HAp. The FGH HAp/PMMA is considered to provide a dynamic advantage over the joint type composite. The stress-strain curves of the FGH HAp/PMMA composite showed sufficient strength for medical application along with the relaxation of brittleness and fragility.

Acknowledgments

We thank Y. Kobori and T. Matsukura for their assistance in the measurement of XRD and IR.

References

[1]L. L. Hench and J. Wilson, *An Introduction to Bioceramics*; pp. 1–24. World Scientific, Singapore, 1993.

[2]L. L. Hench, "Bioceramics: From Concept to Clinic," *J. Am. Ceram. Soc.*, **74**, 1487–510 (1991).

[3]L. L. Hench and G. LaTorre, "Reaction Kinetics of Bioactive Ceramics, Part IV: Effect of Glass and Solution Composition" *Bioceramics*, **5**, 67–74 (1992).

[4]M. R. Filgueiras, G. LaTorre, and L. L. Hench, "Solution Effects on the Surface Reactions of a Bioactive Glass," *J. Biomed. Mater. Res.*, **27**, 445–53 (1993).

[5]G. Zambonin and M. Grano, "Biomaterials in Orthopedic Surgery: Effects of Different Hydroxyapatites and Demineralized Bone Matrix on Proliferation Rate and Bone Matrix Synthesis by Hymen Osteoblast," *Biomaterials*, **16**, 397–402 (1995).

[6]Y. K. Cheol and K. Sungmin, "Hydroxyapatite Formation on Bioactive Glass Coated Titanium," *Bioceramics*, **10**, 37–40 (1990).

[7]J. Li, B. Fartash, and L. Hermanson, "Hydroxyapatite-Alumina Composites and Bone-Bonding.," *Biomaterials*, **16**, 417–22 (1995).

[8]R. Labella, M. Barden, and S. Deb, "Novel Hydroxyapatite-Based Dental Composites," *Biomaterials*, **15**, 1197–200 (1994).

[9]W. Bonfielld, "Composites for Bone Replacement," *J. Biomed. Eng.*, **10**, 522–36 (1998).

[10]J. Huang, M. Wang, S. Best, K. E. Tanner, and W. Bonfield, "Evaluation of Bioglass® and Hydroxyapatite-Reinforced Poltethylene Composites after Aging in Simulated Body Fluid," *Bioceramics*, **11**, 165–68 (1998).

[11]W. Bonfield, *Materials Characteristics vs. in vivo Behaviour*; p. 137. Edited by P. Ducheyne P and J.E. Lemons. New York Academy of Science, New York, 1998.

[12]K. E. Tanner, C. Doyle, and W. Bonfield. "Clinical Implant Materials"; p. 149 in *Advances in Biomaterials*, 9, 1996.

[13]N. Ignjatovic, S. Tomic, M. Dakic, M. Miljkovic, M. Plavsic, and D. Uskokovic, "Synthesis and Properties of Hydroxyapatite/Poly-L-Lactide Composite Biomaterials," *Biomaterials*, **20**, 809–16 (1999).

[14]J. Charnley, *Acrylic Cement in Orthopedic Surgery*. Williams and Wilkins, Baltimore, Maryland, 1970. □

J. Am. Ceram. Soc., **86** [9] 1534–39 (2003)

Dispersing Behavior of Hydroxyapatite Powders Produced by Wet-Chemical Synthesis

Michele Pretto, Anna Luisa Costa, Elena Landi, Anna Tampieri, and Carmen Galassi

National Research Council, Institute of Science and Technology for Ceramics (CNR-ISTEC), I-48018 Faenza, Italy

Three hydroxyapatite powders with different surface properties were produced by wet-chemical synthesis and characterized. The electrokinetic properties of powders dispersed in water were investigated by electroacoustic spectroscopy measurements. The different surface reactivity (pH_{iep} and ζ potential versus pH curves) was related to the interplay of dissolution and adsorption of Ca^{2+} ions. With a view toward the preparation of porous bodies by sponge impregnation, the behavior of powder suspensions was studied. Four deflocculants were tested, and the optimum dispersing conditions for each powder were found. Anionic polyelectrolytes resulted in the best effective dispersing agent, with different optimum amounts added to the suspensions.

I. Introduction

Various biomedical applications are based on hydroxyapatite (HA) as a material for implants and bone regeneration, because of its excellent biocompatibility. Recently there has been an increasing demand for synthetic materials for bone replacement arising from the limited supply of autograft material and the risks associated with the use of allografts. HA is currently used in various forms, such as granules, coatings, and dense as well as porous bodies. Porous HA seems an ideal material for bone replacement as filler of both load-bearing and non-load-bearing osseous defects due to its potential to repair the site throughout a complete penetration of osseous tissue. Among the various processing routes, the impregnation of cellulosic sponges with HA powder suspension is one of the more effective for obtaining porous bodies with adequate dimensions and distribution of pores which mimics the morphology of spongy bone and favors the osteoconduction process.[1]

HA powder can be synthesized with several methods that result in a wide range of physicochemical characteristics (purity, stoichiometry, and morphology, etc.). Among those, the surface properties play a critical role in the dispersing behavior in water, which largely influences the final properties of materials produced by a slurry consolidation method. In fact, the control of the state of dispersion of the slurry is essential in improving performance during the impregnation step and the reliability of consolidated porous bodies.

The colloidal approach to powder processing is based on the control of the interparticle forces through the modification of the reactivity at the solid–liquid interface.[2–4] The flowing properties of the slurry will be consequently tailored so as to match the rheological response required under the processing conditions. This can be achieved through the optimization of the type and quantity of the dispersing agent, solid loading, and the particle size distribution and shape of the powder particles. The addition of polyelectrolytes as dispersants prevents the agglomeration of the suspended ceramic powder, as a consequence of electrosteric stabilization. The adsorption of charged polyelectrolytes increases repulsive interparticle forces either by an increase in the surface charge of the particle (electrostatic repulsion) or by the action of the polymeric chains that hinder approaching particles (steric repulsion).[5,6] Although direct surface force measurements (mainly based on atomic force microscopy) are known,[4,7,8] the observation of colloidal stability through rheological measurements represents the most diffuse indirect evaluation of interparticle forces. Nevertheless a better estimate of the electrostatic interaction can arise from the measurement of interfacial potential on which the electrostatic repulsion between particles depends. The surface electrical potential that can be measured is the ζ potential, defined as the electrical potential at the slipping plane. The ζ potential is located just around the surface, at the plane of the transition between zero and bulk fluidity. Its value is obtained from electrokinetic measurements[9] and is a result of surface charge compensation by ionic species adsorbed into the region closest to the solid surface (Stern layer, Gouy–Chapman–Stern–Grahame double-layer model).[10] For this reason the ζ potential provides useful information either about the surface potential or about the surface chemical environment. The measurement of ζ potential as a function of pH allows the identification of the pH at which the ζ potential is zero, termed pH_{iep} (isoelectric point). This provides further information about acid–base surface reactivity and the electrostatic degree of stabilization.

In this paper the properties of three HA powders, produced by wet-chemical synthesis, were analyzed. The dry-state properties and the water-based suspension behavior were investigated and related to study and optimize the dispersion state of the powders and to improve the performance of slurries for the cellulosic sponge impregnation in the production process of porous HA bodies for biomedical use.

II. Experimental Procedure

(1) *Materials and Methods*

HA powders were prepared by starting from $Ca(OH)_2$ (95 wt%, ACS reagent; $CaCO_3$, ≤3.0%; Fe, ≤0.05%; Mg and alkali salts, ≤1.0%; S compound, ≤0.1%; Aldrich) and H_3PO_4 (85 wt%; solution in water ACS reagent; Aldrich), both diluted in H_2O, following the reaction $5Ca(OH)_2 + 3H_3PO_4 \rightarrow Ca_5(PO_4)_3OH + 9H_2O$. The acid solution was added dropwise to the calcium hydroxide dispersion under proper temperature and stirring conditions. By varying the temperature of the process and the subsequent ripening time, it was possible to change the crystallinity degree of the product between 20% and 80%. Batches of powders with crystallinity degree $X_c \approx 20\%$ (powder L), 40% (powder M), and 80% (powder H) were prepared using a precipitation temperature of 35°, 70°, and 95°C, respectively. A ripening time of 2 h was used to produce HA powders with low and medium crystallinity degree, while the production process of a high-crystallinity powder involved 24 h of ripening. The precipitates were then washed with distilled water, filtered three times, and finally freeze-dried. The obtained powders were sieved at 400 and 150 μm.

J. A. Lewis—contributing editor

Manuscript No. 187488. Received September 4, 2001; approved April 9, 2003.

X-ray diffractometric analysis (Cu*K*α radiation, Miniflex Rigaku, Tokyo Japan) was used to determine the crystalline phases composition and the crystallinity degree of each powder. The specific surface area of the starting powders was evaluated by the BET method (Sorpty 1750, Carlo Erba, Milan, Italy). For particle size distribution measurement, the starting powders were analyzed by a sedigraph (Sedigraph 5100, Micromeritics, Norcross, GA) after ultrasonic dispersion for 10 min. To evaluate the Ca/P ratio, inductively coupled plasma–optical emission spectrometry (ICP-OES) analysis was performed (Liberty 200, Varian, Clayton South, Australia). IR analysis (FTIR 1750, Perkin-Elmer Instruments, Shelton, CT) was also performed to determine stoichiometry differences among the three powders, i.e., the presence of anions partially substituting PO_4^{3-} and/or OH^- groups. Morphologic evaluation of the powders was performed by SEM (Stereoscan 360, Leica, Cambridge, U.K.).

Four commercial deflocculants with different interaction with the ceramic surface were used: Calgon (**C**) (Riedel-de Haën, Seelze, Germany), Duramax D-3021 (**D1**), D-3005 (**D2**) (Rohm and Haas, Philadelphia, PA), and Tri Amino (**T**) (Angus Chemie GmbH, Ibbenbüren, Germany). Anionic polyelectrolyte dispersants enable preparation of HA suspensions with high powder concentration.[11–13] Deflocculant **C** (hexametaphosphate sodium salt) was selected to screen its affinity toward the HA powder surface, for the expected potential-determining role played by phosphate. Deflocculants **D1** and **D2** are ammonium salt solutions of polycarboxylate and polyacrylate with pH 7–8 and 6–7 and molecular weights of 2500 and 2400, respectively. Deflocculant **T** [tris(hydroxymethyl)aminomethane] is a cationic dispersant with a positively charged NH_3R^+ group and pH 10–11 when solubilized in water.

The ζ potential determination was performed with an electroacoustic technique using an electrokinetic sonic amplitude (ESA) measurement apparatus (Acoustosizer, Colloidal Dynamics, Sydney, Australia). All of the samples were prepared by ball milling the powders for 1 h into a $10^{-2}M$ KCl solution to maintain a constant ionic strength. A fixed concentration of 3 vol% solids was used, and the suspensions, placed in the measurement cell, were kept under constant stirring at 25°C. The aqueous dispersing behavior of HA powders with different crystallinity degree was investigated through the following measurements:

(A) *Potentiometric titration*: Automatic titration software was used to measure the ζ potential and conductivity as a function of pH between two fixed points: the starting point was the unadjusted pH (around 7) and the point of arrival was pH 4 or pH 12 for the acid or basic side of the titration curve, respectively; HNO_3 (1*M*) and KOH (1*M*) were used to adjust the pH. pH_{iep} was identified at the pH-axis crossing point.

(B) *Volumetric titration:* Automatic titration software was used to measure the ζ potential as a function of the deflocculant added, to determine the minimum amount of dispersant required to achieve the maximum ζ potential and to compare the dispersing power of the selected deflocculants. For titration a delay time of 2 min was set between two measurement points. The deflocculant concentration is expressed in terms of milligrams per square meter of the measured specific surface area to emphasize the interaction of dispersant with the ceramic powder surface.

III. Results and Discussion

(1) Characteristics of Dry Powders

HA powders, produced by controlling the temperature during the precipitation and the ripening time, presented three different values of crystallinity degree as follows: powder H = 80%, powder M = 40%, and powder L = 20%. The crystallinity degree, corresponding to the fraction of crystalline phase present in the examined volume, was evaluated by a method based on the progressive disappearance of the hollow between (112) and (300) reflections in the XRD spectrum, moving from high- to noncrystalline samples, as elsewhere reported. Moreover, XRD analysis of powders revealed no secondary phases besides HA. XRD spectra have been reported in a previous work.[12]

The powder morphology of sample L is reported in Fig. 1. Nanometric primary particles are agglomerated into micrometric aggregates. The particle size distributions reported in Fig. 2 are evidence that powders M and L are characterized by larger agglomerates formed of smaller primary particles in comparison with powder H, in which agglomerates are smaller but built by larger particles. These results are confirmed by specific surface area values corresponding to ≈115, 63, and 35 m^2/g for L, M, and H, respectively.

ICP analysis detects a Ca/P molar ratio of ≈1.66 for powder H and ≈1.69 for powders M and L (the stoichiometric one is 1.67).

FTIR spectra (Figs. 3(a–c)) provide evidence that the presence of a higher amount of HPO_4^{2-} and CO_3^{2-} groups in powders L and M with respect to powder H. The partial substitution of PO_4^{3-} with HPO_4^{2-} causes the formation of Ca-defective HA and can be inferred as responsible for a reduction of the theoretical Ca/P ratio.[14–17] Otherwise the partial substitution of PO_4^{3-} with CO_3^{2-} causes an increase in the Ca/P value so that the final Ca/P ratio is the result of the opposite effects of the HPO_4^{2-} and CO_3^{2-} groups, being as there are no secondary calcium phosphates' phases present in the powders.

The FTIR spectra reveal the presence of HPO_4^{2-} substituting PO_4^{3-} (1635 cm^{-1}), decreasing in the order M, L > H. The bands between 1435 and 1465 cm^{-1}, together with the absence of the peak at ≈1560 cm^{-1} show that the substitution of CO_3^{2-} occurs in the B position (PO_4^{3-} site),[18] and it is more pronounced in powders M and L, respectively.

On the contrary, the O–H stretch band around 3450 cm^{-1} is more accentuated in powder H, which shows small peaks for CO_3^{2-} and HPO_4^{2-}, and the associate broad peak, related to the hydration of the powder, is of minor importance for powder H with respect to M and L.

The thermogravimetric analysis provides evidence of the different contributions of the chemical substitutions in the three powders and confirms the FTIR data. The weight loss occurring at $T \leq 500°C$, about 7%, 4%, and 2% for powders L, M, and H, respectively, is due to the elimination of adsorbed water and CO_2, reflecting the different extents of the solvated surface, and secondarily to the condensation of HPO_4^{2-} ions, which involves H_2O elimination. A weight loss at $T \approx 800°C$ is assignable to the decarbonation of the carbonate apatite fraction, and it is higher for powder L. At $T \geq 800°C$ the weight loss is mainly due to dehydroxylation, which can extend over a wide range of temperature, up to and over 1400°C, when HA decomposition reactions also occur.[19,20]

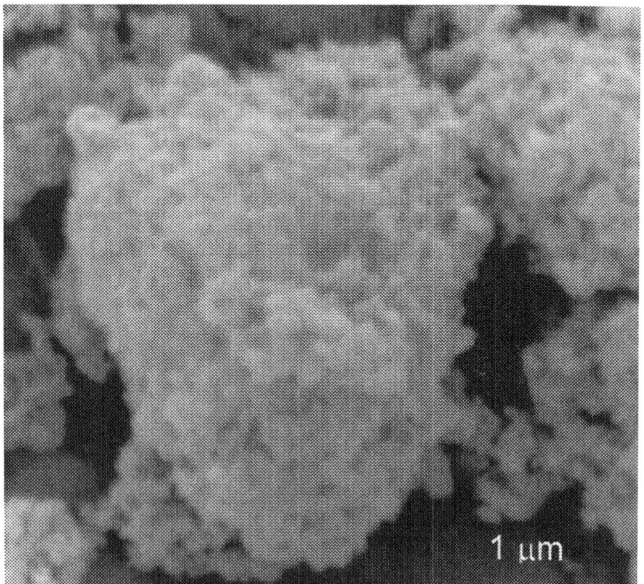

Fig. 1. SEM morphology of powder L.

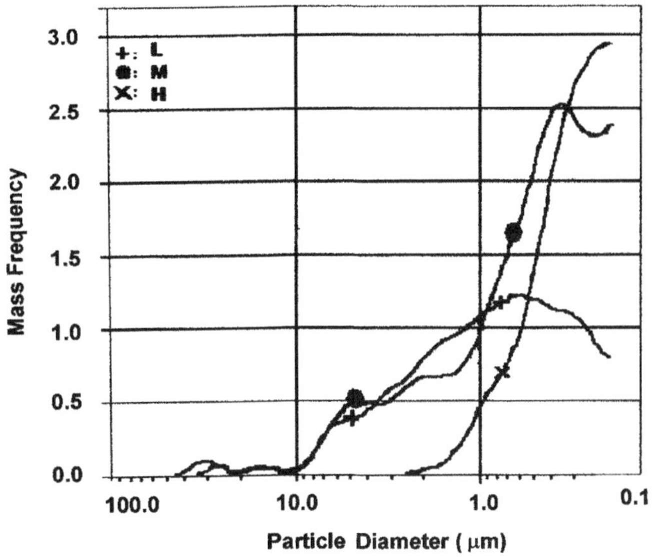

Fig. 2. Particle size distributions of powders L, M, and H.

(2) *Characteristics of Powders in Aqueous Medium*

(A) Solid–Water Interface Reactivity: The study of the behavior of HA powder in aqueous media gives information about its actual chemical reactivity in the biological environment because it is mainly based on aqueous salt solutions. For this purpose the solubility of HA in water has been extensively studied.[21] The stoichiometric dissolution of HA is very low ($pK_{sp} = 115$),[22] but nonstoichiometric dissolution due to the formation of surface complexes was demonstrated to occur and to cause phenomena of metastable equilibrium solubility.[23] In particular, a solid surface complex $Ca_2(HPO_4)(OH)_2$, formed by HA hydrolysis mechanism, controls the solubility equilibria, according to the following equations:[21,24]

$$Ca_{10}(PO_4)_6(OH)_2 + 6H_2O = 4Ca_2(HPO_4)(OH)_2 + 2Ca^{2+} + 2HPO_4^{2-} \quad (1)$$

$$4Ca_2(HPO_4)(OH)_2 = 8Ca^{2+} + 4HPO_4^{2-} + 8OH^- \quad (2)$$

The resulting nonstoichiometric Ca/P ratio in solution (1:1 for Eq. (1) or 2:1 for Eq. (2)) depends on which dissolution reaction prevails. If HA is prepared in water, the surface is, presumably, just covered with surface complex $Ca_2(HPO_4)(OH)_2$ and subjected either to the equilibrium shown in Eq. (2) or to adsorption phenomena of ionic species present in solution.[25] The formation of a surface layer arises from the nonstoichiometric dissolution exhibited by HA, and properties such as particle size, crystallinity degree, specific surface area, and solid loading strongly influence the change in composition of the saturated solution. Leaching experiments in a time scale of the electroacoustic measurements were conducted to check the Ca^{2+} content leached by the three powders without pH adjustments. The ICP analysis results, reported in Table I, provide evidence of an increasing concentration of calcium ions with increasing powder specific surface area, as expected by the increased content of the surface complex formed.

Generally speaking, the surface charge of apatite solids[26] is the result of pH and preferential dissolution or adsorption of calcium and phosphate ions, since H^+, OH^-, and lattice ions are the potential determining ions. The formation of surface complexes between potential-determining ions further complicates the estimation of ion activity product and surface potential. In Table II specific surface area values and mean particle size are summarized together with electrokinetic and electrochemical data of the dispersions measured before adjusting the pH (natural pH); the pH values of the isoelectric point, extracted from the curves of the ζ potential as a function of pH, are reported as well. The use of a

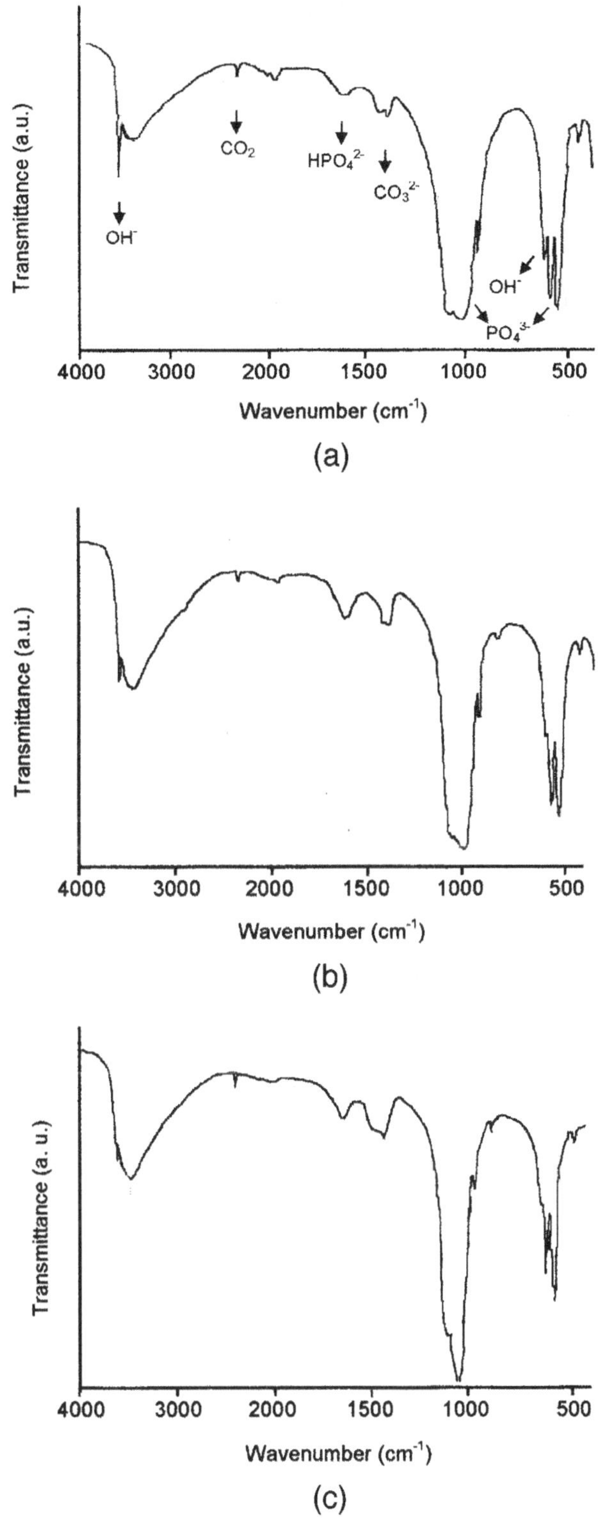

Fig. 3. FTIR spectra of powders (a) H, (b) M, and (c) L. The main absorption bands are indicated.

diluted electrolyte solution as the dispersing medium is necessary to ensure a constant ionic strength during acid or base addition. The natural pH of the HA powder suspensions is higher than pH 5.9 of a $10^{-2}M$ KCl solution as a consequence of basic hydrolysis of the surface in aqueous solution. The highest specific surface area of powder L, reflecting in the formation of the highest quantity of the $Ca_2(HPO_4)(OH)_2$ complex, provides a shift of the natural pH toward the most basic value. To evaluate the dissolution/adsorption effects, the conductivity of the suspension of the

Table I. ICP AES Analysis (Ca, 317.93 nm)

Powder	Ca^{II} (mg/L)	Ca^{II} (wt%)†
H	2.2	0.006
M	4.0	0.010
L	5.3	0.013

†Referred to the weight of powder.

Table II. Some Properties of Hydroxyapatite Powders and Suspensions

Powder	Ssa (m^2/g)	D50 (μm)	Natural pH	Cond. (S/m)	ζ potential (mV)	pH_{iep}
L	115	0.45	8.4	0.11	+5.4	8.9
M	63	0.29	6.7	0.11	+3.0	7.0
H	35	0.16	6.8	0.12	+1.7	7.1

three powders was compared with the conductivity of the surrounding medium ($10^{-2}M$ KCl), titrated in the same conditions and reported in Fig. 4. The pronounced conductivity increase arises from HA dissolution effects that occur at about pH 6 for powders H and M and at about pH 8 for the more soluble powder L. The higher content of CO_3^{2-} groups in powder L accounts for the increase in the conductivity at more basic pH as the dissolution of carbonate occurs at pH around 8. The ζ-potential measurements as a function of pH are reported in Fig. 5. The slightly positive ζ potential exhibited by the three powders at natural pH is due to a prevailing adsorption of Ca^{2+} ions with respect to HPO_4^{2-}. In the acidic side of the curve the powders are positively charged, and the ζ-potential values are comparable until pH 6. The establishment of a cationic specific adsorption determines a shift of the pH_{iep} of powder L toward basic pH. This strong shift (about pH_{iep} 9) can be due either to the higher content of Ca^{2+} ions, leached from the surface complex, or to the presence of CO_3^{2-} groups that show a stronger affinity for Ca^{2+} ions. The shift of pH_{iep} is not evident for powders H and M that show about pH_{iep} 7, close to the values reported in the literature.[13,27] In the basic side of the titration curve the absolute value of the ζ potential seems to be related to the Ca^{2+} concentration in the solution. In fact, above pH_{iep}, the absolute value of the ζ potential is smaller, with a higher content of Ca^{2+} in solution (the ζ potential at pH 12 is −30, −23, and −16 mV for H, M, and L powders, respectively).

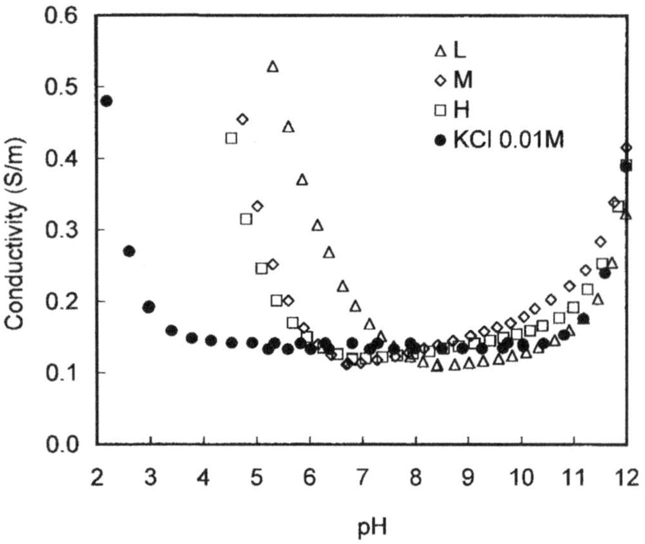

Fig. 4. Conductivity of the dispersions of powders L, M, and H and of the $10^{-2}M$ KCl solution as a function of pH.

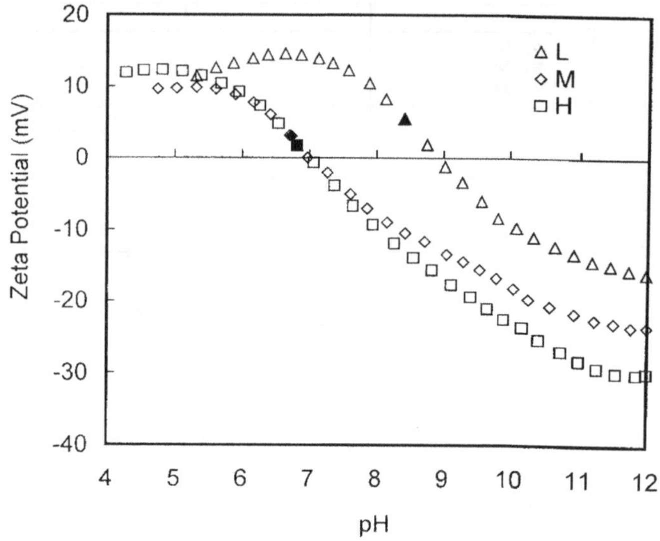

Fig. 5. ζ potential versus pH of the dispersions of powders L, M, and H. The solid mark shows the starting ζ potential and pH.

(B) Effect of the Dispersants: The ζ-potential and conductivity values versus the amount of dispersants, for powder H, are plotted in Fig. 6. All the dispersants studied increase the value of the negative ζ potential. The surface is negatively charged already by the adsorption of a small amount of anionic dispersants. Further addition of dispersant increases the ζ potential until a constant value is reached (the maximum or final ζ potential value) corresponding to a complete particle coverage by the dispersant

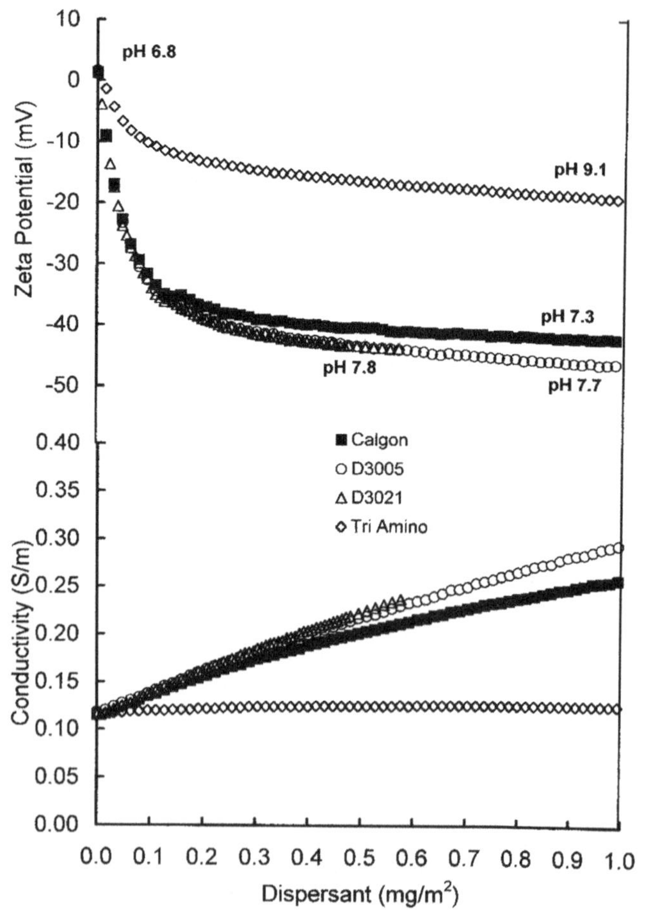

Fig. 6. ζ potential and conductivity versus the amount of dispersant added, for powder H.

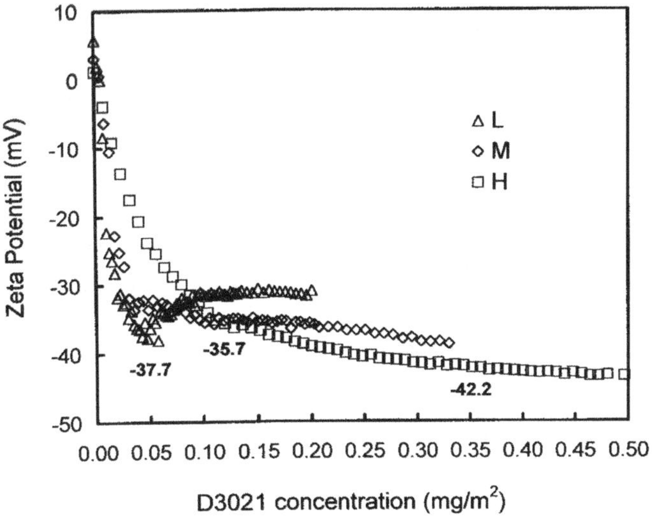

Fig. 7. ζ potential of powders L, M, and H versus the amount of deflocculant D3021 (in $10^{-2}M$ KCl) (the initial and final pH values are reported in Table III).

(optimum amount of dispersant). The cationic dispersant does not result in an increase in the positive surface potential, but it still results in a negatively charged surface as it undergoes a basic hydrolysis (the pH increases from 7 to 9). Consequently the modification of the surface potential can be attributed to the preferential adsorption of OH^- ions (the ζ potential reaches the value of −18 mV, as in the case of the pH titration reported in Fig. 5) with respect to the cationic amino groups. OH^- adsorption compensates for the increase of ionic concentration, and the conductivity remains constant.

The conductivity increase during the titration with the anionic dispersant can be attributed either to the replacement of bivalent Ca^{2+} and HPO_4^{2-} ions bonded to the surface by NH_4^+ and polycarboxylate anions or to the increase of the concentration of dispersant into the suspension after powder coverage. The replacement mechanism was confirmed in a study regarding the adsorption of polyacrylic acids and their sodium salts on HA,[28] where it was detected that the maximum concentration of calcium or phosphate ions released in the presence of polyacrylate was higher than that released in water. Nevertheless the absence of a one-to-one ratio between the amount of dispersant adsorbed and the amount of calcium and phosphate ions released to the solution was ascribed to competitive mechanisms such as the complexation of calcium ions by polyacrylate matrix. The ionic environment and its contribution to the conductivity is further complicated by the basic hydrolysis of polyacrylate, which justifies the increase of pH during the titration, and by nonstoichiometric solubility equilibria involving the surface. The ζ potential of powders L, M, and H versus the amount of dispersants D3005 and D3021 are reported in Figs. 7 and 8, respectively. These dispersants were chosen on the basis of the results reported in Fig. 6, being the most effective in increasing the absolute value of the ζ potential for the three powders. The titration curves of powders H and M, shown in Figs. 7 and 8, decrease monotonically until a plateau value is reached. Powder L shows a minimum in the titration curve, corresponding to the maximum value of negative ζ potential. Some data extrapolated from these curves are summarized in Table III. The optimum amount of dispersant reported corresponds to the value of the ζ potential above which further variation is negligible. The optimum amount of dispersant is inversely proportional to the values of the specific surface area of the powders, the lowest amount being adsorbed on the powder with the highest specific surface area in both cases. A possible explanation can be given by taking into account the different dissolution and readsorption mechanisms involving the surface complexes that govern the solid–water interface reactivity. In particular, it can be considered that Ca^{2+} ions adsorbed on the three powders in different amounts can interfere with the dispersant anchorage. Powder H, covered by the lower amount of Ca^{2+} ions, shows higher affinity with the dispersant, thus reaching the highest final value of the ζ potential. The effect of the Ca^{2+} ions concentration on the ζ potential was checked by repeating the same titration reported in Fig. 7, for powder H, with the addition of a Ca^{2+} amount equal to that spontaneously leached by the surface in water (0.006 wt%, as reported in Table I). The lower value of the ζ potential reached at the end of the titration in the presence of a double amount of Ca^{2+} ions, as shown in Fig. 9, confirms the above-mentioned hypothesis.

From comparison of the ζ-potential curves versus the amount of dispersant (Figs. 7 and 8), deflocculant D3021 is determined to be the more effective dispersant for all powders, giving higher ζ-potential values for the same amount used; moreover, the increase in final the ζ potential obtained with D3005 is negligible with respect to the bigger amount used.

Following these results several slurries, with variable powder concentration, were prepared, with D3021 being selected as the dispersant in the amounts of 0.35, 0.11, and 0.05 mg/m^2, for powders H, M, and L, respectively. Such slurries were tested in the impregnation process of cellulosic sponges, giving good results with respect to the possibility of modulating the pore size and distribution, and the crystallinity degree of the fired porous bodies.

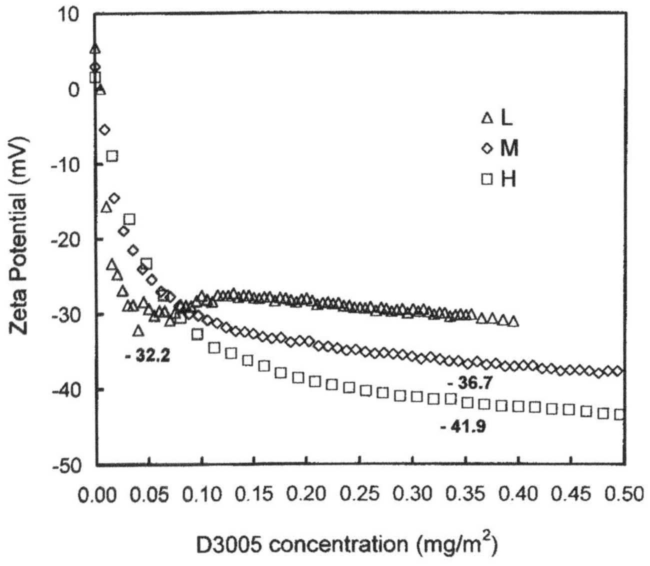

Fig. 8. ζ potential of powders L, M, and H versus the amount of deflocculant D3005 (in $10^{-2}M$ KCl) (the initial and final pH values are reported in Table III).

Table III. Initial and Final Characteristics of HA Suspensions with Two Deflocculants

	Dispersant† (mg/m^2)		pH			ζ potential (mV)			
				Final		Initial		Final	
Powder	D3021	D3005	Initial	D3021	D3005	D3021	D3005	D3021	D3005
L	0.05	0.04	8.4	8.8	8.9	+5.8	+5.5	−37.7	−32.1
M	0.11	0.35	6.7	7.4	7.7	+3.1	+3.0	−35.7	−36.7
H	0.35	0.35	6.8	7.8	7.7	+1.2	+1.6	−42.2	−41.9

†Optimum amount.

IV. Conclusions

This study confirmed that the surface reactivity of HA powder produced by precipitation is very complex in either the dry or the wet state and strongly dependent on the processing parameters

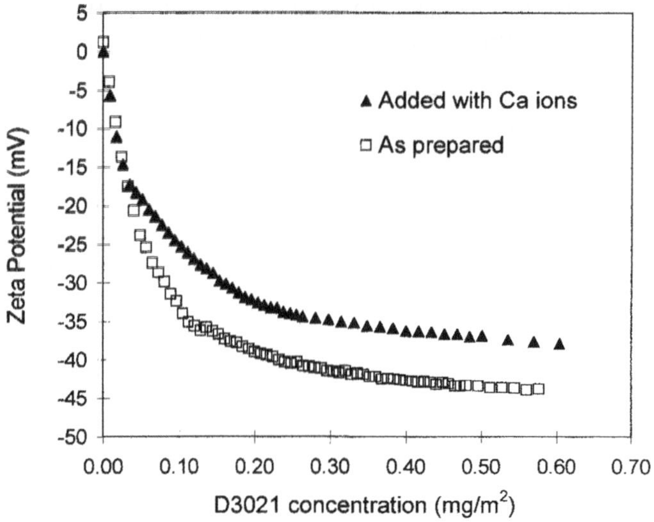

Fig. 9. ζ potential of powder H as prepared and added with Ca ions versus the amount of deflocculant D3021 (in $10^{-2}M$ KCl).

during the synthesis route. The conductivity and ζ-potential measurements as a function of pH, conducted to investigate the complex surface chemical reactivity in water, provided evidence that the formation of a surface complex promotes the interplay of dissolution and readsorption equilibria, the former governed by the specific surface area and the latter determining the resulting surface potential. The presence of different amounts of HPO_4^{2-} and CO_3^{2-} groups on the three powders is confirmed by FTIR and thermal analyses.

The ζ-potential measurements as a function of the amounts of the different dispersants added determined the best dispersing condition (type and quantity of dispersant), which reflected the three powders' differences in terms of the surface specific area and chemistry. The different interactions with the most effective anionic electrolyte was attributed to the dissolution/adsorption effects of Ca^{2+} ions, although a thorough study of the adsorption mechanism involved was outside of the aim of this work.

These results optimized the preparation of slurries for each powder and consequently improved the performance of cellulosic sponges impregnation in the production of fired porous bodies of HA, with variable characteristics of porosity degree, pore size, and distribution, or characterized by a gradient of porosity and/or crystallinity, which is a very important goal in view of the biomedical application as bone substitute.

References

[1]A. Tampieri, G. Celotti, S. Sprio, A. Delcogliano, and S. Franzese, "Porosity-Graded Hydroxyapatite Ceramics to Replace Natural Bone," *Biomaterials*, **22**, 1365–70 (2001).

[2]F. F. Lange, "Powder Processing Science and Technology for Increased Reliability," *J. Am. Ceram. Soc.*, **72** [1] 3–15 (1989).

[3]R. G. Horn, "Surface Forces and Their Action in Ceramic Materials," *J. Am. Ceram. Soc.*, **73** [5] 1117–35 (1990).

[4]W. M. Sigmund, N. S. Bell, and L. Bergström, "Novel Powder-Processing Methods for Advanced Ceramics," *J. Am. Ceram. Soc.*, **83** [7] 1557–74 (2000).

[5]J. N. Israelachvili, *Intermolecular and Surface Forces*; pp. 288–311. Academic Press, London, U.K., 1985.

[6]B. Vincent, "The Stability of Solid/Liquid Dispersions in the Presence of Polymers"; pp. 149–62 in *Solid/Liquid Dispersions*. Edited by Th. F. Tadros. Academic Press, London, U.K., 1987.

[7]W. A. Ducker, T. J. Senden, and R. M. Pashley, "Direct Measurement of Colloidal Forces Using an Atomic Force Microscope," *Nature (London)*, **353**, 239–41 (1991).

[8]W. A. Ducker, T. J. Senden, and R. M. Pashley, "Measurements of Forces in Liquids Using a Force Microscope," *Langmuir*, **8**, 1831–36 (1992).

[9]J. H. Adair, J. A. Casey, and S. Venigalla (Eds.), *Handbook on Characterization Techniques for the Solid-Solution Interface*. American Ceramic Society, Westerville, OH, 1993.

[10]J. Lyklema, "Structure of the Solid/Liquid Interface and the Electrical Double Layer"; pp. 63–90 in *Solid/Liquid Dispersions*. Edited by Th. F. Tadros. Academic Press, London, U.K., 1987.

[11]F. Lelièvre, D. Bernache-Assolant, and T. Chartier, "Influence of Powder Characteristics on the Rheological Behaviour of Hydroxyapatite Slurries," *J. Mater. Sci.: Mater. Med.*, **7**, 489–94 (1996).

[12]S. Guicciardi, C. Galassi, E. Landi, A. Tampieri, K. Satou, and G. Pezzotti, "Rheological Characteristics of Slurry Controlling the Microstructure and the Compressive Strength Behavior of Biomimetic Hydroxyapatite," *J. Mater. Res.*, **16**, 163–70 (2001).

[13]L. M. Rodríguez-Lorenzo, M. Vallet-Regí, and J. M. F. Ferreira, "Colloidal Processing of Hydroxyapatite," *Biomaterials*, **22**, 1847–52 (2001).

[14]J. Zhou, X. Zhang, J. Chen, S. Zeng and K. De Groot, "High Temperature Characteristics of Synthetic Hydroxyapatite," *J. Mater. Sci.: Mater. Med.*, **4**, 83–85 (1993).

[15]Y. Han, K. Xu, J. Lu, and Z. Wu, "The Structural Characteristics and Mechanical Behaviors of Nonstoichiometric Apatite Coatings Sintered in Air Atmosphere," *J. Biomed. Mater. Res.*, **45**, 198–203 (1999).

[16]K. Kamiya, T. Yoko, K. Tanaka, and Y. Fujiyama, "Growth of Fibrous Hydroxyapatite by the Hydrolysis of Brushite," *J. Mater. Sci.*, **24**, 827–32 (1989).

[17]A. Tampieri, G. Celotti, S. Sprio, and C. Mingazzini, "Characteristics of Synthetic Hydroxyapatites and Attempts to Improve Their Thermal Stability," *Mater. Chem. Phys.*, **64**, 54–61 (2000).

[18]Y. Suetsugu, I. Shimoya, and J. Tanaka, "Configuration of Carbonate Ions in Apatite Structure Determined by Polarized Infrared Spectroscopy," *J. Am. Ceram. Soc.*, **81** [3] 746–48 (1998).

[19]Z. Zyman, Y. Cao, and X. Zhang, "Periodic Crystallization Effect in the Surface Layer of Coatings During Plasma Spraying of Hydroxyapatite," *Biomaterials*, **14**, 1140–44 (1993).

[20]C. K. Wang, C. P. Ju, and J. H. Chern Lin, "Effect of Doped Bioactive Glass on Structure and Properties of Sintered Hydroxyapatite," *Mater. Chem. Phys.*, **53**, 138–49 (1998).

[21]T. S. B. Narasaraju and D. E. Phebe, "Review of Some Physico-Chemical Aspects of Hydroxylapatite," *J. Mater. Sci.*, **31**, 1–21 (1996).

[22]S. Chander and D. Fuerstenau, "Solubility and Interfacial Properties of Hydroxyapatite: A Review"; pp. 29–49 in *Adsorption on and Surface Chemistry of Hydroxyapatite*. Edited by D. N. Misra. Plenum Press, New York, 1984.

[23]A. Chettry, Z. Wang, J. Hsu, J. L. Fox, A. A. Baig, A. M. Barry, H. Zhuang, M. Otsuka, and W. I. Higuchi, "Metastable Equilibrium Solubility Distribution of Carbonated Apatite as a Function of Solution Composition," *J. Colloid Interface Sci.*, **218**, 57–67 (1999).

[24]H. M. Rootare, V. R. Deitz, and F. G. Carpenter, "Solubility Product Phenomena in Hydroxyapatite–Water Systems," *J. Colloid Sci.*, **17**, 179–206 (1962).

[25]V. K. La Mer, "The Solubility Behavior of Hydroxyapatite," *J. Phys. Chem.*, **66**, 973–78 (1962).

[26]P. Somasundaran and Y. H. C. Wang "Surface Chemical Characteristics and Adsorption Properties of Apatite"; pp. 129–49 in *Adsorption on and Surface Chemistry of Hydroxyapatite*. Edited by D. N. Misra. Plenum Press, New York, 1984.

[27]R. K. Mishra, S. Chander, and D. W. Fuerstenau, "Effect of Ionic Surfactans on the Electrophoretic Mobility of Hydroxyapatite," *Colloids Surf.*, **1**, 105–19 (1980).

[28]D. N. Misra, "Adsorption of Polyacrylic Acids and Their Sodium Salts on Hydroxyapatite: Effect of Relative Molar Mass," *J. Colloid Interface Sci.*, **181**, 289–96 (1996). □

J. Am. Ceram. Soc., 85 [2] 401–407 (2002)

Improving the Durability of a Biomedical-Grade Zirconia Ceramic by the Addition of Silica

Laurent Gremillard, Jerome Chevalier, Thierry Epicier, and Gilbert Fantozzi

Department of Metallurgy and Physical Properties of Materials, Associate Research Unit 5510, National Institute of Applied Sciences, 69621 Villeurbanne Cedex, France

The lifetime of tetragonal zirconia ceramic implants is controlled by their resistance to slow crack growth and low-temperature degradation (LTD). A decrease of the grain size is often proposed to decrease the effect of LTD on zirconia; however, this decrease also reduces the resistance to crack propagation. An alternative approach is reported here; such an approach consists of introducing a silica glass phase only at triple grain junctions, without changing the grain size. The addition of a small amount of silica (0.5 wt%) decreases the internal stresses, which improves the resistance to LTD without affecting the resistance to crack propagation. These results are discussed from a microstructural standpoint.

I. Introduction

Ceramic materials are now becoming a competitive alternative to the common metal–polyethylene or metal–metal joint prosthesis devices in orthopedic surgery, because they strongly reduce the amount of wear debris.[1] Alumina became very popular in the 1980s, but fracture problems have been reported in the literature.[2,3] Then, zirconia ceramics were introduced in orthopedics in the early 1990s, to solve the problem of fracture of ceramic femoral heads. Indeed, tetragonal zirconia ceramics that have been stabilized with yttria (so-called Y-TZP) exhibit high toughness (K_{IC}) (up to 7 MPa·m$^{1/2}$) and strength (up to 2 GPa). Such values are due to both small grain size and a phase-transformation toughening mechanism. Currently, more than 350 000 zirconia femoral heads have been implanted, with good clinical success.[4]

Zirconia ceramics can exist as two polymorphs at room temperature: a tetragonal, metastable phase (the *t*-phase, which can be obtained using stabilizers such as yttrium or cerium oxides), and a monoclinic, stable phase (the *m*-phase). A cubic phase exists in zirconia with higher concentrations of stabilizers. The *t*-phase is generally obtained after sintering yttria-stabilized tetragonal zirconia polycrystals (the so-called Y-TZP) ceramics that have 2–3 mol% Y_2O_3; however, this phase can transform to the *m*-phase, for example, if energy is added into the environment by elastic or chemical stimuli.

When considering a given ceramic for orthopedic prostheses, one must focus on its resistance to slow crack growth (SCG). This phenomenon occurs at stress intensity factors (K_I) less than the toughness K_{IC}, because of stress-assisted corrosion by water molecules,[5–7] which may be located at the origin of an implant fracture.[8] It is illustrated by plotting the crack-propagation speed V versus the stress intensity factor K_I (V–K_I diagrams). These diagrams generally exhibit three stages:[5–7] in stage I (lowest K_I values), the crack speed is limited by the reaction rate between the water molecules and the chemical bonds of the ceramic. In stage II, the speed is limited by the diffusion of corrosive species toward the crack tip (where the reaction occurs). Stage III (the highest K_I values) represents fast fracture under vacuum conditions (essentially independent of the environment). A threshold below which no propagation occurs defines a "safety factor" for the use of bioceramics; such a threshold has been clearly observed in tetragonal zirconia ceramics.[9] TZP has also been shown to exhibit good resistance to SCG,[9] because the overall V–K_I diagram of TZP is shifted toward higher K_I, compared to that of alumina.[10] Indeed, during propagation, stress concentrations at the crack tip provoke a local tetragonal to monoclinic (*t*–*m*) transformation. This transformation is accompanied by a volume increase of ~4%, which creates compressive stresses at the crack tip that act to reduce the crack driving force. The coarser the grain size, the greater the grain transformability and, consequently, the greater the transformation toughening. Thus, increasing the grain size improves the resistance to SCG.[6] At the same time, increasing the grain size decreases the stability of tetragonal zirconia, thus favoring the isothermal transformation of tetragonal grains to the *m*-phase at the surface of zirconia. This mechanism is known as low-temperature degradation (LTD).[11] The volume increase associated with the *t*–*m* transformation induces a microcracking and an increase of the surface roughness. Such an increase of roughness with time may increase the wear rate.[12] The different experimental features of the LTD in TZP are as follows:[13–16]

(1) The transformation is slow at room temperature and shows a maximum rate at ~200°–300°C.

(2) The transformation is accelerated in humid media (in presence of water or water vapor).

(3) The transformation starts on the surface and extends into the bulk.

Different mechanisms have been proposed to explain the aging phenomenon. In all models, the roles of the water molecule and internal stresses are emphasized.[13–17] However, the real mechanism has not been identified yet. A recent investigation has shown that the transformation occurs via a nucleation and growth mechanism.[16] Observations have shown that the LTD begins via the transformation of one or a few grains. Then, the transformation propagates from the initially transformed grains to their neighbors, because of the formation of stresses and microcracks around them (the growth step of the nucleation–growth aging kinetics). Increasing the grain size of zirconia ceramics decreases their stability; therefore, the LTD is even more important when the grain size is coarse.[18] Some authors have emphasized the key role of internal stresses on LTD. Indeed, high internal stresses[17] should increase the transformation rate. However, no experimental evidence for the real influence of residual stresses on LTD rates has been established.

It is expected that a period of 25 years *in vivo* is necessary to induce consequent damage due to LTD of a sample surface.[19] This time period is long enough for the case of modern orthopedic implants, which have an average lifetime of 10 years. However, considering an aging population and a growing demand for

P. F. Becher—contributing editor

Manuscript No. 187847. Received March 19, 2001; approved October 15, 2001.

implants with a lifetime of >30 years, LTD must be delayed for the new generation of prostheses (for example, ceramic–ceramic couples). Thus, our goal has been to increase the resistance of zirconia ceramics to isothermal transformation without affecting their good resistance to SCG. Increasing the grain size is not appropriate, because it has a contradictory role on crack propagation and isothermal transformation. Here, we have chosen to modify the microstructure of zirconia ceramics by adding small and controlled quantities (e.g., 0.5 wt%) of silica. The resistances to LTD and SCG of doped and undoped materials have been characterized. Stress measurements were also conducted via X-ray diffraction (XRD) analysis to investigate the role of silica addition on internal stresses, and then on LTD.

II. Experimental Procedure

(1) *Materials*

The starting powder was an ultrapure powder (Tosoh, Tokyo, Japan), stabilized in the tetragonal phase with 3 mol% of yttria (3Y-TZP), and with <200 ppm of total impurities (<60 ppm SiO_2). The materials were processed using a slip-casting method; all slurries had a solids content of 80 wt% (the dispersing additive was "Acrylon" PROX B 03, Protex/Synthron, Levallois Perret, France). To obtain zirconia ceramics with a silica content of 0.5 wt%, colloidal silica (Ludox HS40, Aldrich Chemical Co., Milwaukee, WI) was added to one slurry. The different slurries were placed into plaster molds to eliminate water and form green compacts 40 mm × 20 mm × 5 mm in size. Then, the green compacts were dried at room temperature in air for 7 d. Organic compounds were removed by heating at 600°C (at a heating rate of 15°C/h). Compacts were sintered at 1450°C for 5 h in air (at a heating and cooling rate of 300°C/h) to achieve grain sizes of ~0.6 μm (measured by scanning electron microscopy (SEM), according to the ASTM E112 standard). The addition of small quantities of silica did not induce any variation of the grain size; therefore, all the batches present the same overall microstructure, except for the silica content. In the following, the zirconia ceramic without any addition of silica will be called "Z-S0" and the ceramic that has been doped with 0.5 wt% of silica will be called "Z-S05."

(2) *Aging*

LTD was quantified by monitoring the monoclinic content (X_m) on the surface of the material versus aging time. X_m was measured using an XRD technique and calculated from the Garvie–Nicholson equation.[20]

Samples were initially polished with diamond pastes to a 1 μm finish, to achieve a smooth surface (roughness of 2–3 nm, as measured using optical interferometry (Phase Shift Technology®, ADE Phase Shift, Tucson, AZ)) and remove all surface stresses due to machining. The monoclinic phase was undetectable before the aging tests.

Tests were conducted in steam, at a temperature of 134°C, under a pressure of 2 bars (~0.2 MPa). A period of 1 h in this treatment has been shown to be representative of four years *in vivo*.[19] Monoclinic content measurements were performed periodically (every 3 h). The surfaces of the aged samples were examined using the optical interferometer and by optical microscopy with Nomarski contrast, to emphasize any change of the surface topology.

(3) *Subcritical Crack Growth*

SCG was measured using double-torsion tests. This technique has been described elsewhere.[5,21,22] The procedure allows crack speeds of 10^{-11}–10^{-3} m/s to be measured as a function of the stresses at the crack tip (K_I). The samples were polished with diamond pastes to a 3 μm finish and heated at 1250°C before testing to remove residual stresses.

(4) *Microstructures*

Microstructures were observed using transmission electron microscopy (TEM). Samples were cut to a thickness of 100 μm, then ground to 10 μm with a dimpler, and finally ion-milled to electron transparency with argon gas. Glass phases at triple junctions were observed using a "diffuse dark-field method"[23] (Model 200 CX, JEOL, Tokyo, Japan). Grain-boundary observations were performed using high-resolution electron microscopy (Model 2010F, JEOL) (the resolution limit was better than 0.12 nm). Nanoprobe or sub-nanoprobe analysis (energy-dispersive X-ray spectroscopy (EDX) and electron energy loss spectroscopy (EELS)) was also performed on the same instrument.

(5) *Internal Stresses*

Internal stresses were measured using XRD, with the Williamson–Hall method, as described in detail by Warren.[24] The X-ray penetration depth in zirconia ceramics is ~5 μm;[25] therefore, our measurements are representative of the surface stress state. From Bragg's law (Eq. (1)),

$$2d \sin \theta = \lambda \tag{1}$$

where d is the inter-reticular distance, θ the diffraction angle, and λ the wavelength of X-rays, the following relation (Eq. (2)) can be inferred:[24]

$$\beta\left(\frac{\cos \theta}{\lambda}\right) = \frac{1}{T} + \epsilon\left(\frac{\sin \theta}{\lambda}\right) \tag{2}$$

In this equation, β represents the width of peaks corrected using the instrumental width, T the particle size, and ε the deformation ($\beta = \Delta\theta/\theta$ and $\epsilon = \Delta d/d$). Hence, plotting $\beta \cos \theta$ versus $\sin \theta$ for all the peaks of the diffractogram should produce a straight line of slope ε. In the present work, approximately twenty peaks with different (*hkl*) values were used, thus giving average information on the lattice distortion. Therefore, this method should be considered to be a semiquantitative evaluation of internal strains, but one which will allow for good comparison between batches.

III. Results

Figure 1 shows the crack speed V versus the stress intensity factor K_I for doped and undoped zirconia ceramics. Both curves present three stages, in agreement with the stress-corrosion model and previous experimental results.[6] A threshold below which no propagation occurs (K_{I0}) was measured in the two batches. The fracture toughness (K_{IC}) was deduced from Fig. 1, using the K_I value needed to propagate the crack at a speed of $V > 1$ mm/s. The two V–K_I curves are similar and the K_{I0} and K_{IC} values are equivalent for both the Z-S0 and Z-S05 materials. This observation shows that silica addition does not necessary promote crack propagation, contrary to the commonly accepted idea.

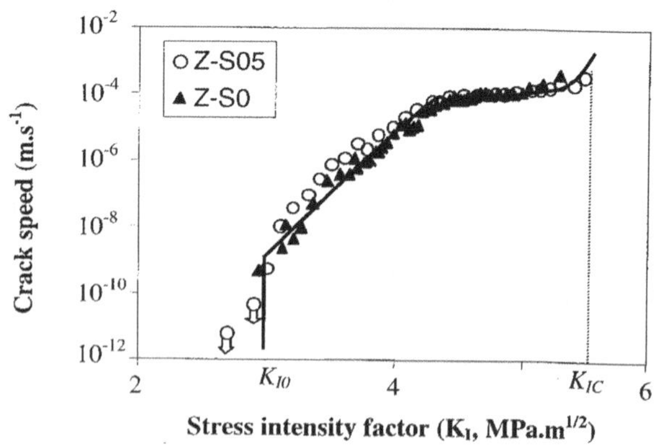

Fig. 1. Plot of crack rate versus stress intensity factor K_I for pure and 0.5-wt%-SiO_2-doped 3Y-TZP, showing that the resistance to crack propagation is not affected by the presence of small quantities of SiO_2. Arrows pointing downward indicate that no crack propagation could be measured at this point.

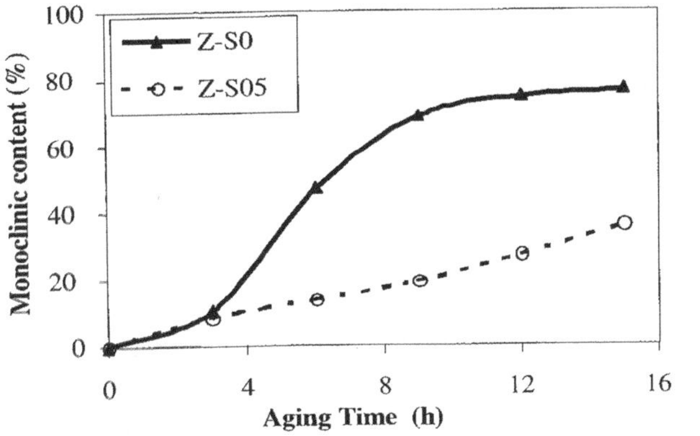

Fig. 2. Aging kinetics of pure and doped 3Y-TZP, showing that the resistance to low-temperature degradation is much better in the SiO_2-doped material.

Inversely, the resistance to LTD is highly improved by the addition of silica (see Fig. 2). The amount of *m*-phase in the Z-S0 batch increases as time increases, following a sigmoidal behavior (acceleration, then apparent saturation of the transformation), representing a nucleation-and-growth mechanism already analyzed in this material.[16] LTD begins via the transformation of one or a few grains. Then, the transformation propagates from the initially transformed grains to their neighbors, because of the apparition of stresses and microcracks around them (the growth step of the nucleation–growth aging kinetic). The maximum transformation (~75%) is attained after 15 h in a humid atmosphere at 134°C for the Z-S0 batch (these conditions represent ~60 years *in vivo*). In contrast, the amount of *m*-phase in the Z-S05 material only slightly increases, following an almost-constant rate variation with time. For example, after 15 h, only 30% of the Z-S05 material has transformed. This constant rate variation should traduce a transformation kinetic via randomly dispersed nucleation only:[26] there is a random transformation of grains with time, but no propagation to the neighbors. Figure 3 shows micrographs of the surface of both batches after 6 h of aging, taken using optical microscopy (Model Axiophot, Zeiss, Karlsruhe, Germany) with Nomarski contrast (the indents visible at the corners are marks used to locate the zone). The relief is much more important in the Z-S0 batch than in the Z-S05 batch, which traduces a higher surface roughening, due to surface transformation. Another clue is brought by the images and roughness measurements that have been obtained using optical interferometry. Indeed, as shown on Fig. 4, after 2 or 3 h in an autoclave, the Z-S0 material shows a typical image of transformation via the nucleation and growth of monoclinic nuclei[16] (transformation spots are observed from small surface uplifts, which appear brighter on the images), whereas the Z-S05 batch only presents few and small transformed spots (which are almost not visible in the micrographs). This observation confirms that, even if both materials may present a nucleation of monoclinic phase, only the undoped material undergoes a growth of monoclinic nuclei. Figure 5 shows the roughness of both materials, relative to time, over a range of 0–6 h of treatment. An increasing roughening of the surface can be measured in the Z-S0 material from 2 h of steam treatment (~8 years *in vivo*), whereas the roughness remains on the order of 3 nm for the ZS-05 material, even after 6 h (~24 years *in vivo*).

X-ray measurements of the lattice distortions (or internal stresses) were performed on undoped samples and samples that were doped with 0.5 wt% silica. They show that the addition of silica reduces the internal stresses (see Fig. 6): they may be twice as large in the Z-S0 material than in the Z-S05 material (mean least-squares fitting of the Williamson–Hall plot leads to a mean deformation of 0.5% for the Z-S0 material and 0.35% for the Z-S05 material). This finding clearly indicates that a small amount of silica significantly decreases the internal stresses in zirconia.

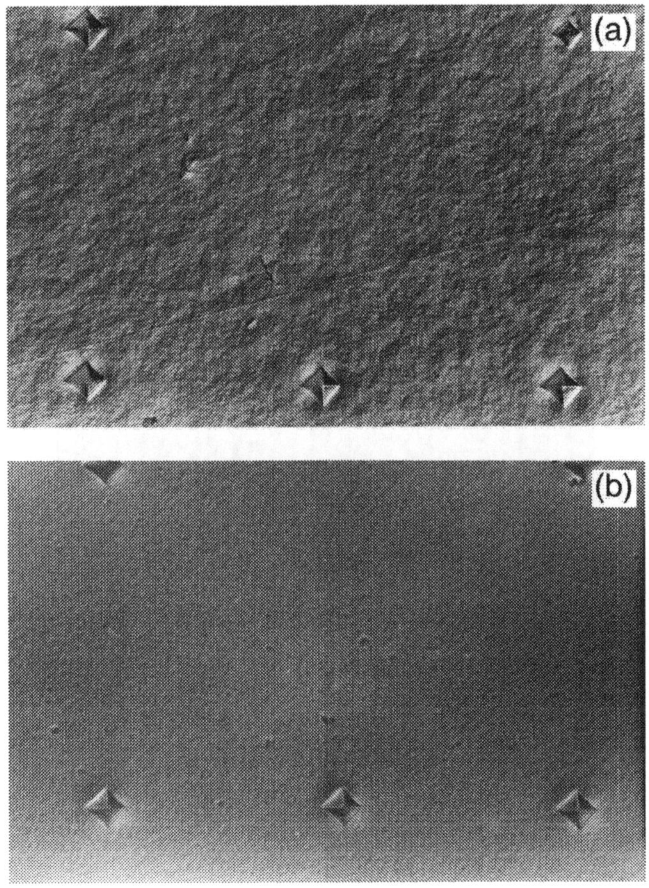

Fig. 3. Optical micrographs, with Nomarski contrast, of pure TZP (top) and silica-doped TZP (bottom) after 6 h in an autoclave; the roughness of Z-S0 is much more notable.

Conventional TEM work shows a clear difference between the microstructures of both materials. Figure 7 shows that the grains are generally faceted and have sharp angles in the Z-S0 material, whereas the grains are much more rounded in the Z-S05 material. High-resolution transmission electron microscopy (HRTEM) observations of the silica-doped samples (see Fig. 8) show that a glassy phase is observed at some triple junctions (Fig. 8(a)); however, no continuous noncrystalline film could ever be observed at the grain boundaries (see, for example, Fig. 8(b)), among the more than thirty edge-on grain boundaries that have been studied.

EELS analysis confirms the chemical nature of the glassy pockets (i.e., silica; see Fig. 8(c)) and the absence of any detectable amount of silicon in or near the grain boundaries (Fig. 8(c)). The presence of Si^{4+} ions at the grain boundaries also could have been detected by a shift of the O peak;[27] this situation was not observed.

IV. Discussion

The decrease of internal stresses when silica glass is added was expected by different authors:[28–30] cooling stresses (presumably from an anisotropic thermal expansion of the tetragonal phase) are relaxed, thanks to the presence of a viscous amorphous phase at high temperatures, and the presence of vitreous phase at triple junctions makes grains rounder (see Fig. 7(b)) and, thus, reduces the stress concentrations at the grain corners.

During LTD, the nucleation phenomenon of the *m*-phase seems to operate in both the Z-S0 and Z-S05 materials. Then, the *t*–*m* transformation rate remains constant in the Z-S05

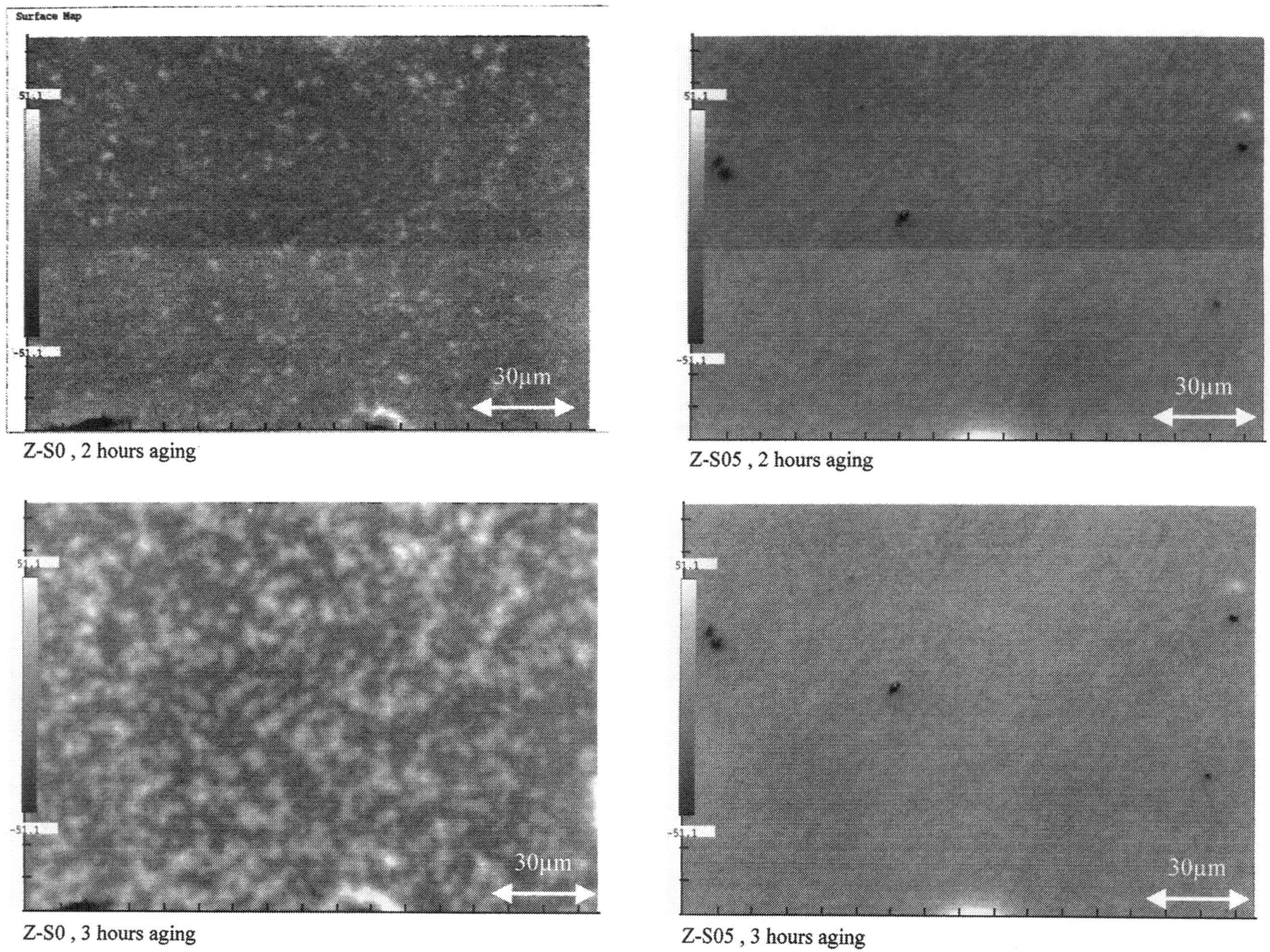

Fig. 4. Optical interferometry micrographs of Z-S0 material (left) and Z-S05 material (right) after 2 h (top row) and 3 h (bottom row) in an autoclave. Monoclinic spots are visible as the brighter areas.

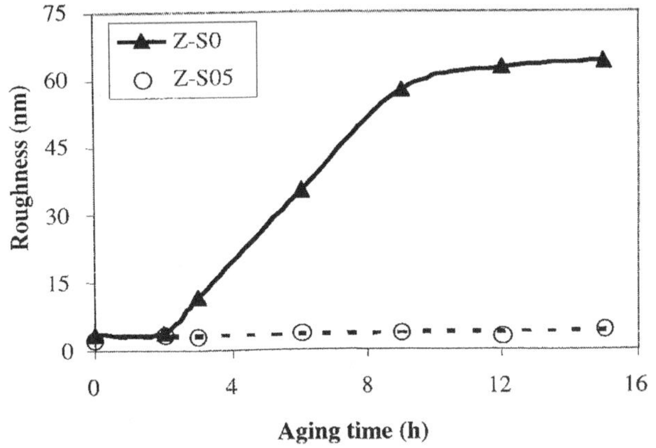

Fig. 5. Plot of roughness versus aging time, showing the roughening effect on pure 3Y-TZP (filled triangles); this effect is not visible in SiO_2-doped 3Y-TZP (open circles).

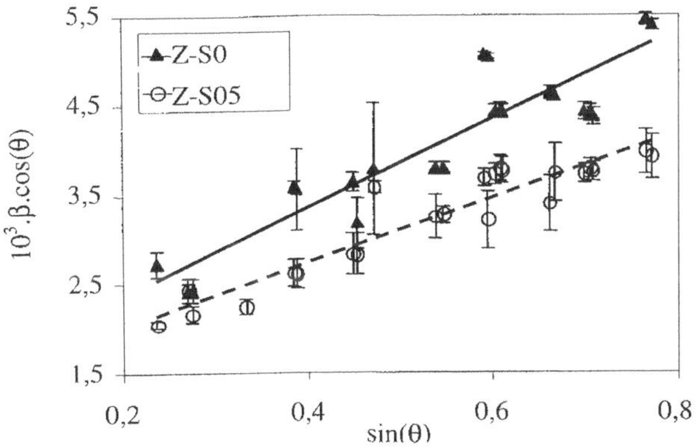

Fig. 6. Williamson–Hall plot of (▲) pure and (○) doped 3Y-TZP, showing that Z-S0 material exhibits more internal stresses that Z-S05 material.

material, whereas a significant acceleration in this rate is observed in the Z-S0 material. This condition is due to the growth of monoclinic nuclei in the Z-S0 material: monoclinic nuclei continue to appear and existing nuclei grow, as a consequence of the surrounding stresses and microcracking. In contrast, in the Z-S05 batch, only the apparition of new nuclei is observed, and no growth at all occurs with these nuclei. This concept is confirmed by the micrographs in Figs. 3 and 4. Note that nucleation of the monoclinic phase does not increase the roughness significantly: it is easy to calculate that, for one transformed grain (diameter of ~0.5 μm), a volume increase of 4% should yield a linear elongation of ~6 nm. This result is the case for the Z-S05 material, where the roughness does not change significantly, relative to aging duration. In contrast, a transformation of several grains is much more significant for the roughness: the size expansion of transformed aggregates can attain a value of 50 nm,[16] and such a roughness is easily visible using optical interferometry. This observation explains why nucleation and growth leads to a roughening of the surface in the case of the ZS-0 material (35 nm after 6 h, i.e., 24 years *in vivo*, which is still a very low roughness for a femoral head). Interestingly, optical interferometry observations revealed a difference between the Z-S0 and Z-S05 materials, even after short aging times, not in terms of roughness (which is not enough sensitive to the initial stage of transformation), but in terms of the number of small uplifts that appear with time. This observation indicates that the growth of nuclei is reduced in the Z-S05 material and the nucleation rate seems to be slower.

The internal stresses seem to be important for LTD. Indeed, Z-S05 material exhibits much less internal stress than does Z-S0 material (see Fig. 7), and its LTD behavior is much better. The presence of internal stresses probably facilitates the growth of monoclinic nuclei: the elastic energy they provide can add to that produced by the deformation around monoclinic nuclei, which is sufficient to extend the transformation to neighboring grains. Thus, a reduction of the internal stresses clearly limits the nuclei growth. In contrast, the internal stresses seem to have no significant influence on SCG. SCG is ruled by the fracture of crack-tip bonds and by the transformation toughening mechanism. SEM observations of the crack paths in Y-TZP[5,6] show that the fracture of these materials is purely intergranular. The HRTEM observations clearly show the absence of a continuous noncrystalline film at the grain boundaries. Hence, the grain

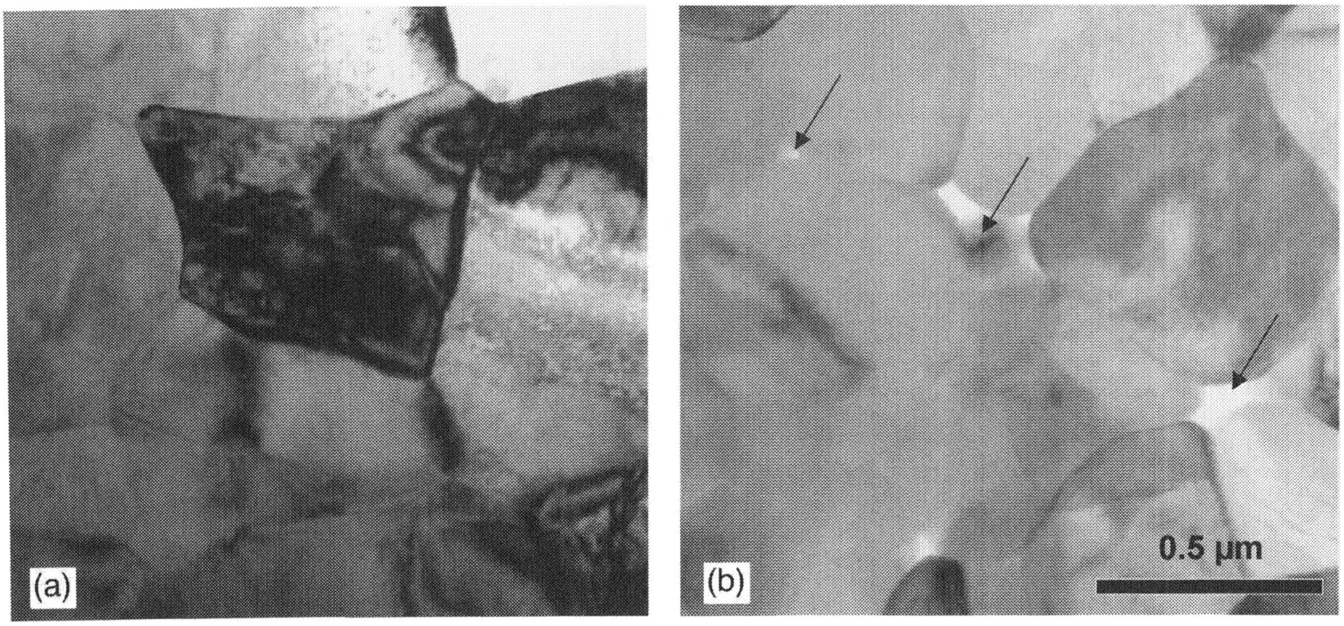

Fig. 7. Conventional TEM micrographs of (a) Z-S0 and (b) Z-S05 material, showing faceted, strained grains for Z-S0 material and round grains with small amorphous pockets (see arrows) for Z-S05 material.

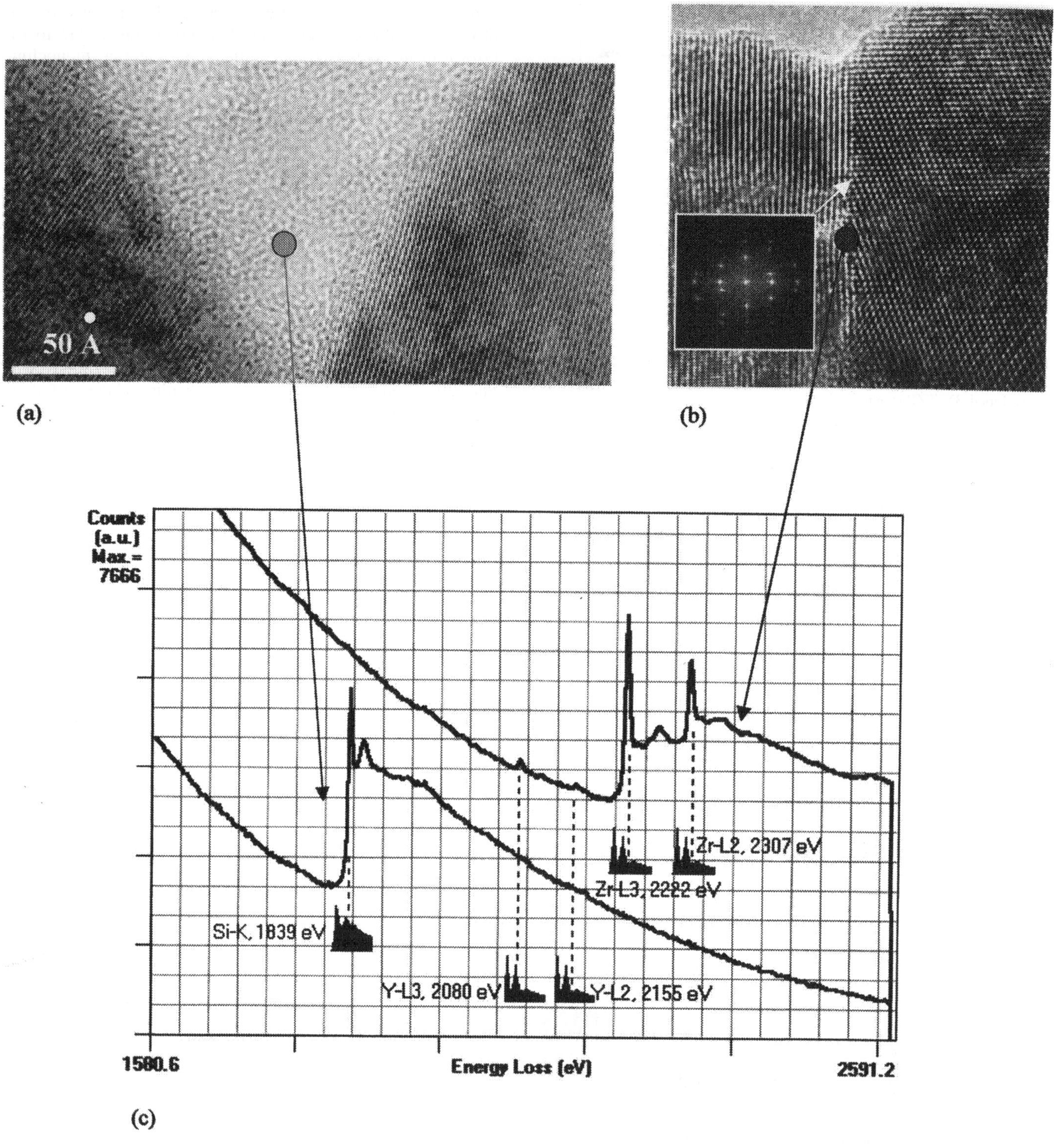

Fig. 8. HRTEM micrographs of Z-S05 material, showing that (a) a glassy phase is present at triple junctions and (b) there is no glass layer at the grain boundaries. Figure 8(c) shows EELS results that correspond to Figs. 8(a) and (b), as indicated (electron-probe diameter of 1 nm).

boundaries in the Z-S0 and Z-S05 materials are composed of Zr—O and Y—O bonds and, thus, are identical in both batches. One could have expected that the internal (cooling) stresses affect the phase-transformation reinforcement. However, these cooling stresses are very localized (nanometer scale); thus, they bring only a negligible elastic energy, in comparison with the energy needed to transform a large zone. Then, the phase-transformation reinforcement (micrometer scale) is not affected by the cooling stresses. In addition, because the grain sizes are identical in both materials, the reinforcements are also identical. These two features ("clean" grain boundaries and the same reinforcement in both materials) explain the equivalent crack resistance of the Z-S0 and Z-S05 materials.

V. Conclusion

The evolutions of slow crack growth and low-temperature degradation (LTD) in 3-mol%-yttria-doped tetragonal zirconia polycrystalline (3Y-TZP) ceramics that are doped with a small amount of silica have been characterized. The addition of small amounts of silica was shown to improve the resistance to aging greatly, without affecting the crack-propagation resistance. On one hand, the presence of a glassy phase at triple junctions acts to reduce the internal stresses and, thus, increases the resistance to LTD. On the other hand, the constant grain size and the glass-free grain boundaries can explain the constant crack-propagation resistance.

Acknowledgments

The authors thank Bernard Cales and Franceline Villermaux (Norton Desmarquest Fine Ceramics) for their helpful scientific contribution and for their financial support to this study. The Consortium Lyonnais de Microscopie Electronique (CLYME) is acknowledged for the use of the JEOL 2010F high-resolution electron microscope.

References

[1]H. McKellop and B. Lu, "Friction, Lubrication and Wear of Polyethylene/Metal and Polyethylene/Ceramic Hip Prostheses on a Joint Simulator"; p. 118 in *Transactions of the 4th World Biomaterials Congress* (Berlin, Germany, 1992). Society for Biomaterials, Minneapolis, MN.

[2]R. J. Michaud and S. Y. Rashad, "Spontaneous Fracture of the Ceramic Ball in a Ceramic–Polyethylene Total Hip Arthroplasty," *J. Arthroplasty*, **10**, 863–67 (1995).

[3]E. W. Fritsch and M. Gleitz, "Ceramic Femoral Head Fracture in Total Hip Arthroplasty," *Clin. Orthop. Relat. Res.*, **328**, 129–36 (1996).

[4]B., Cales, "15 Years Experience in Zirconia Hip Joint Heads: The Main Characteristics, Advantages and Recommendations for Use"; in *Proceedings of the 6th Biomaterials Congress: Workshop on Zirconia Femoral Heads for THPs* (Kamuela, HI, May 16, 2000). Society of Biomaterials, Minneapolis, MN, 2000.

[5]J. Chevalier, "Slow Crack Growth Behavior of 3Y-TZP Biomedical Ceramics"; Ph.D. Thesis. INSA de Lyon, Lyon, France, 1996.

[6]J. Chevalier, C. Olagnon, and G. Fantozzi, "Subcritical Crack Propagation in 3Y-TZP Ceramics," *J. Am. Ceram. Soc.*, **82** [11] 3129–38 (1999).

[7]B. Lawn, *Fracture of Brittle Solids*, 2nd Ed. Cambridge University Press, Oxford, U.K., 1993.

[8]G. Willmann, "Ceramic Femoral Heads for Total Hip Arthroplasty," *Adv. Eng. Mater.*, **2**, 114–22 (2000).

[9]J. Chevalier, C. Olagnon, G. Fantozzi, and B. Cales, "Subcritical Crack Growth and Thresholds in a 3Y-TZP Ceramic under Static and Cyclic Loading Conditions," *Ceram. Int.*, **23**, 263–66 (1997).

[10]J. Chevalier, A. H. De Aza, G. Fantozzi, M. Schehl, and R. Torrecillas, "Extending the Lifetime of Ceramic Orthopaedic Implants," *Adv. Mater.*, **12** [21] 1619–21 (2000).

[11]H. G. Lu and S. Y. Chen, "Low Temperature Aging of t-ZrO_2 Polycrystals with 3 mol% Y_2O_3," *J. Am. Ceram. Soc.*, **70** [8] 537–41 (1987).

[12]V. Saiko, "Wear of Polyethylene Acetabular Cups against Zirconia Femoral Heads Studied with a Hip Joint Simulator," *Wear*, **176**, 207–12 (1994).

[13]M. Yoshimura, T. Noma, K. Kawabata, and S. Sōmiya, "Role of H_2O on the Degradation Process of Y-TZP," *J. Mater. Sci. Lett.*, **6**, 465–67 (1987).

[14]M. Hirano, "Inhibition of Low Temperature Degradation of Tetragonal Zirconia Ceramics—A Review," *Br. Ceram. Trans. J.*, **91**, 139–47 (1992).

[15]E. Lilley, "Review of Low Temperature Degradation in Y-TZPs"; pp. 387–406 in Ceramic Transactions, Vol. 10, *Corrosion and Corrosive Degradation of Ceramics*. Edited by R. E. Tressler and M. McNallen. American Ceramic Society, Westerville, OH, 1990.

[16]J. Chevalier, B. Cales, and J. M. Drouin, "Low Temperature Aging of Y-TZP Ceramics," *J. Am. Ceram. Soc.*, **82** [8] 2150–54 (1999).

[17]S. Schmauder and H. Schubert, "Significance of Internal Stresses for the Martensitic Transformation in Yttria-Stabilized Tetragonal Zirconia Polycrystals during Degradation," *J. Am. Ceram. Soc.*, **69** [7] 534–40 (1986).

[18]J.-F. Li and R. Watanabe, "Phase Transformation in Y_2O_3-Partially-Stabilized ZrO_2 Polycrystals of Various Grain Sizes during Low-Temperature Aging in Water," *J. Am. Ceram. Soc.*, **81** [10] 2687–91 (1998).

[19]J. Chevalier, J. M. Drouin, and B. Cales, "Low Temperature Aging Behavior of Zirconia Hip Joint Heads"; pp. 135–38 in *Bioceramics*, Vol. 10, Proceeding of the 10th International Symposium on Ceramics in Medicine (Paris, France, Oct. 5–9, 1997). International Society of Ceramics in Medicine, San Bernadino, CA.

[20]R. C. Garvie and P. S. Nicholson, "Phase Analysis in Zirconia Systems," *J. Am. Ceram. Soc.*, **55** [6] 303–305 (1972).

[21]D. P. Willams and A. G. Evans, "A Simple Method for Studying Slow Crack Growth," *J. Test. Eval.*, **1** [4] 264–67 (1973).

[22]J. Chevalier, M. Saadaoui, C. Olagnon, and G. Fantozzi, "Double-Torsion Testing a 3Y-TZP Ceramic," *Ceram. Int.*, **22**, 171–77 (1996).

[23]M. K. Cinibulk, H. J. Kleebe, and M. Rühle, "Quantitative Comparison of TEM Techniques for Determining Amorphous Intergranular Film Thickness," *J. Am. Ceram. Soc.*, **76** [2] 426–32 (1993).

[24]B. E. Warren, *X-ray Diffraction*. Addison-Wesley, New York, 1969.

[25]J. Emsley, *The Elements*; 2nd Ed. Oxford University Press, Oxford, U.K., 1991.

[26]J. W. Christian, *The Theory of Transformations in Metals and Alloys*, 2nd Ed.; pp. 1–19. Pergamon Press, Oxford, U.K., 1965.

[27]Y. Ikuhara, P. Thavorniti, and T. Sakuma, "Solute Segregation at Grain Boundaries in Superplastic SiO_2-Doped TZP," *Acta Mater.*, **45** [12] 5275–84 (1997).

[28]M. L. Mecartney, "Influence of an Amorphous Second Phase on the Properties of Yttria-Stabilized Tetragonal Zirconia Polycrystals (Y-TZP)," *J. Am. Ceram. Soc.*, **70** [1] 54–58 (1987).

[29]Y. J. Lin, P. Angelini, and M. L. Mecartney, "Microstructural and Chemical Influence of Silicate Grain-Boundary Phases in Yttria-Stabilized Zirconia," *J. Am. Ceram. Soc.*, **73** [9] 2728–35 (1990).

[30]L. Gremillard, T. Epicier, J. Chevalier, and G. Fantozzi, "Microstructural Study of Silica Doped Zirconia Ceramics," *Acta Mater.*, **48** [18/19] 4647–52 (2000). □

J. Am. Ceram. Soc., 85 [2] 493–95 (2002)

Transparent Hydroxyapatite Ceramics through Gelcasting and Low-Temperature Sintering

Harikrishna Varma, Sekhara Pillai Vijayan, and Sivadasan Suresh Babu

Biomedical Technology Wing, Sree Chitra Tirunal Institute for Medical Sciences and Technology (SCTIMST), Poojapura, Thiruvananthapuram 695012, India

Transparent hydroxyapatite (HAP) was prepared by sintering gel-cast powder compacts at 1000°C for 2 h; the resultant HAP material was studied using X-ray diffractometry, transmission electron microscopy, scanning electron microscopy, and microhardness measurement. Nanoscale HAP crystallites were prepared using a precipitation method that involved calcium nitrate and ammonium dihydrogen orthophosphate solutions; the preparation was conducted at a temperature of 0°C. The precipitate was gel-cast and sintered at 1000°C in the form of a transparent ceramic that had a uniform grain size of 250 μm. The maximum Vickers microhardness obtained for a sample sintered at 1000°C was 6.57 GPa. The sintering behavior of gel-cast samples prepared from high-temperature-precipitated HAP was compared with that of material prepared at 0°C.

I. Introduction

SYNTHETIC calcium phosphates, especially calcium hydroxyapatite (HAP, $Ca_{10}(PO_4)_6(OH)_2$), have been used in the medical field as bone substitute implant material for the last three decades.[1,2] This implementation is made possible mainly because of their similarity, chemically and structurally, to the mineral portion of human hard tissue. Although these materials are highly biocompatible, their use is limited to non-load-bearing applications, because of their poor mechanical strength.[3] Various chemical methods have been developed for the synthesis of phase-pure HAP powders.[4] Usually, these powders are synthesized by adding a phosphate solution to a calcium salt solution, both of which are kept at high pH. The precipitation temperature has a direct effect on the nature and size of the HAP particles formed.[5] Also, crystallite size decreases to the submicrometer level with decreasing precipitation temperature.[6] If such particles can be properly processed, dense and uniform sintered ceramics can be produced under lower sintering conditions. In the present work, a transparent, fine-grained and high-density ceramic has been obtained by sintering green HAP blocks that were produced through low-temperature synthesis and gelcasting. The effect of sintering temperature on the hardness of these gel-cast samples is discussed.

II. Experimental Procedure

Aqueous ammoniated calcium nitrate ($Ca(NO_3)_2$) solution and ammoniated ammonium dihydrogen orthophosphate ($NH_4H_2PO_4$) solutions (pH 10.00) were prepared in stoichiometric ratio for the formation of $Ca_{10}(PO_4)_6(OH)_2$ (HAP). Both solutions were cooled to 0°C via storage in a deep freezer. Then, the calcium nitrate solution was placed in a beaker, kept in a freezing-mixture bath, and thoroughly stirred. The ammonium dihydrogen orthophosphate solution was added dropwise into the above-mentioned calcium nitrate solution, using a separating funnel. The system was further stirred for another hour after completion of the precipitation. The precipitate was kept in the mother liquor for 24 h before washing with distilled water, using a high-speed centrifuge. The thoroughly washed precipitate was made into a cake form by pouring the precipitate suspension into a Büchner funnel. The filter cake was removed and dried in a humidity-controlled atmosphere at 24°C for 30 d (this specimen is hereafter referenced as sample A). In another experiment, the precipitation reaction was conducted at 80°C and the precipitate was formed into dried filter cakes using the same processing steps that were described previously (this specimen is hereafter referenced as sample B). The dried samples were sintered in a high-temperature furnace at 1000°–1200°C a rate of heating of 8°C/min. The soaking time was maintained at 2 h in all the cases that were studied.

The density of the sintered samples was determined using the Archimedes method. X-ray diffraction (XRD) patterns of the gel-cast sample were taken with an X-ray diffractometer (Model D5005, Siemens, Karlsruhe, Germany), using Cu$K\alpha$ radiation. The morphology of the precipitated particle was observed using transmission electron microscopy (TEM) (Model H600, Hitachi, Tokyo, Japan). The morphology of the fracture surface was observed using scanning electron microscopy (SEM) (Model S2400, Hitachi). Analysis of the calcium and phosphorus content was performed, using ethylenediaminetetraacetic acid (EDTA) titration and spectrophotometry, respectively. Microhardness was measured (Model HMV2000, Shimadzu) using a Vickers indenter.

III. Results

Figure 1 shows the transparent nature of sample A sintered at 1000°C for 2 h. The sample was slightly bluish in color, which might be due to the presence of a trace of Mn ions in the calcium nitrate reagent. Figures 2(a) and (b) show XRD patterns of the gel-cast samples (samples A and B, respectively). The peaks obtained for sample A are broader compared to those for sample B. The X-ray line-broadening study, based on the Scherrer method,[7] showed that the primary crystallite size of sample A is ~35 nm. TEM micrographs of the two previously mentioned HAP powders are shown in Figs. 3(a) and (b). These micrographs show that the crystallite size of sample A is 30–50 nm, whereas sample B consists of acicular particles >100 nm in size.

When the above-described powders were subjected to gelcasting and drying for 30 d, green densities of 30% and 37% of the theoretical density were obtained for samples A and B, respectively. These specimens were thinned to disks with a thickness of 3 mm before they were subjected to sintering studies.

Figure 4 shows a plot of density versus sintering temperature of the gel-cast samples A and B. Disks produced from sample A attained densities as high as 98% of the theoretical density (3.16 g/cm^3) when sintered at 1000°C. These samples were transparent.

T. B. Troczynski—contributing editor

Manuscript No. 188314. Received August 21, 2000; approved February 14, 2001.

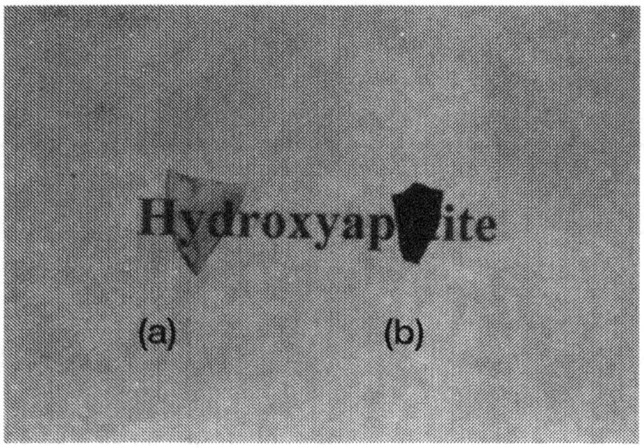

Fig. 1. Photograph showing HAP (a) precipitated at 0°C and sintered at 1000°C and (b) precipitated at 80°C and sintered at 1000°C.

Reduced transparency was observed as the sintering temperature was increased. Sample B attained >98% of the theoretical density only at 1100°C. None of the sintered disks prepared from sample B exhibited any transparency.

SEM micrographs of the polished and etched surfaces of disks of samples A and B after sintering at 1000°C are shown in Figs. 5(a) and (b). Sample A sintered at 1000°C has a uniform microstructure and the grain size is ~250 nm. Very little intergranular porosity is observed in this microstructure. The microstructure of sample B at 1000°C is composed of grains >500 nm in size with intergranular porosity (Fig. 5(b)). A higher sintering temperature was required to densify the green disks of sample B completely.

Figure 6 shows the variation of the Vickers's microhardness (H_V) of samples A and B sintered at various sintering temperatures. The sintered disks of sample A exhibited high H_V values. When the sintering temperature attained a value of 1100°C, a decrease in the H_V value was observed. In the case of sample B, the maximum microhardness was obtained at 1100°C and stabilized at similar H_V values with further increases in the sintering temperature. The H_V value of sample B is lower than that of sample A in all the cases studied, except that at 1200°C.

IV. Discussion

The precipitation temperature of HAP has a major role in determining the nature and size of the basic crystallites that are formed. In the present work, nanoscale crystallites were obtained by maintaining a preparation temperature of ≤0°C. Interestingly, the crystallite size is more regular in the case of low-temperature-derived sample A, whereas the particles in sample B appear to be acicular and have a high aspect ratio. This observation may be due to the preferential *c*-axis-oriented growth of hexagonal HAP crystallites at elevated temperatures.

The processing of nanoscale particles is generally difficult. In the present case, the gelcasting method could be effectively used to obtain uniform green bodies. Even though the green densities obtained in the present method are lower than that of samples prepared via usual pressure-compaction techniques described elsewhere (which are normally 50% of the theoretical value),[8,9] the

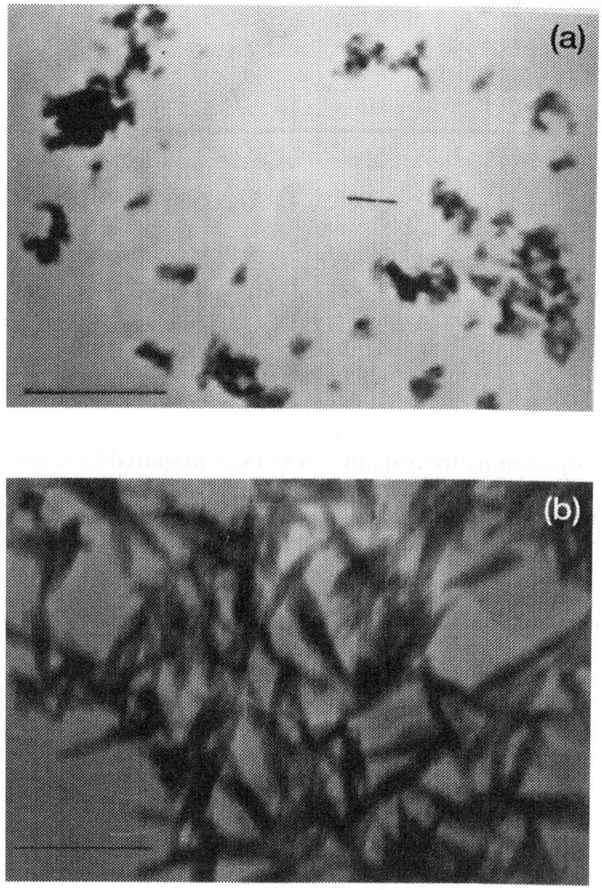

Fig. 3. TEM micrographs of samples (a) A and (b) B. (Bar = 100 nm in each micrograph.)

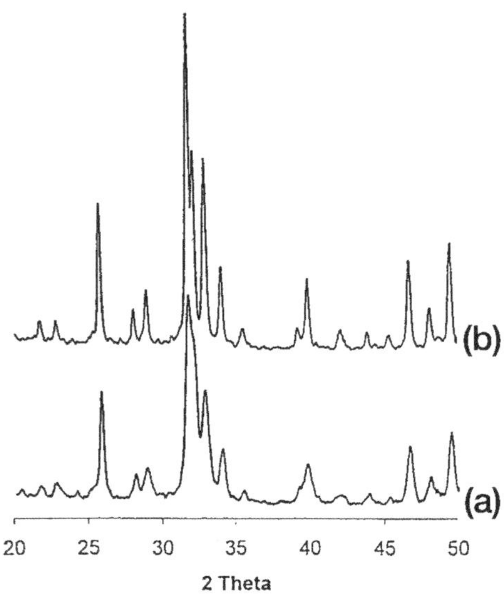

Fig. 2. XRD patterns of HAP gel-cast samples (samples (a) A and (b) B).

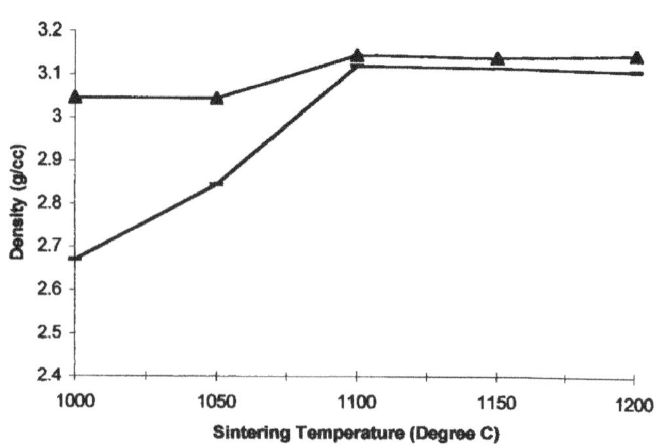

Fig. 4. Plot of density versus sintering temperature ((▲) sample A and (■) sample B).

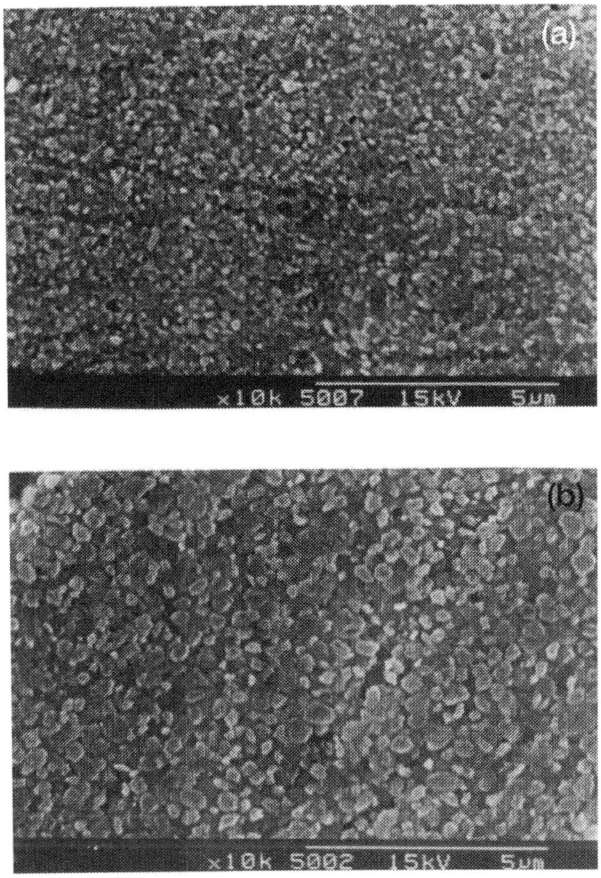

Fig. 5. SEM micrographs of samples (a) A and (b) B, each sintered at 1000°C.

uniform packing of the crystallites seems to impart better sintering characteristics. The increased densification behavior of sample A may be due to the uniform packing of the crystallites; their increased surface area characteristics may also have a positive effect on densification. The transparent nature of these samples is also due to the sintered grain structure being composed of grains <250 nm in size. It is well-known that, to obtain a good transparent polycrystalline ceramic, the grain size should be preferably smaller than the wavelength of light, as observed in other systems.[10] The high microhardness of sample A could be attributed to its smaller grain size. A decrease in the H_V values of high-temperature-derived samples is expected, because of the exaggerated grain growth and the possible liquid-phase formation that results from the segregation of impurity ions at the grain boundaries.

V. Conclusions

Nanoscale hydroxyapatite particles can be processed effectively using a gelcasting technique. The gel-cast specimens could be

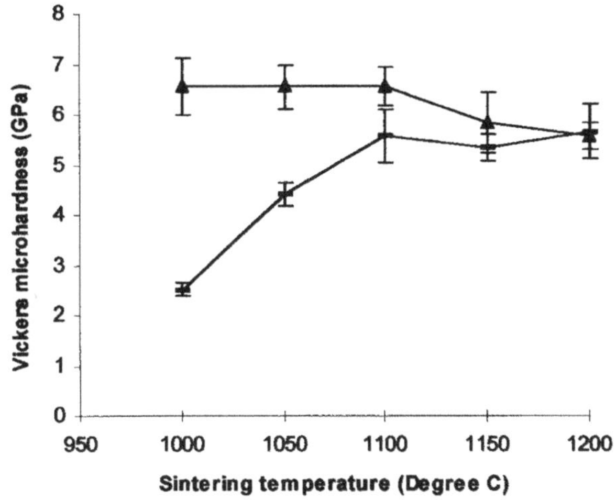

Fig. 6. Plot of Vickers microhardness (H_V) versus sintering temperature ((▲) sample A and (■) sample B).

sintered to >98% of the theoretical density at a lower temperature (1000°C). These samples were transparent, and the microstructure showed that they were composed of grains 200–250 nm in size. The high microhardness values obtained for these samples are expected, because of their smaller grain size and cleaner grain-boundary characteristics.

Acknowledgment

The authors wish to thank the Director of SCTIMST for giving permission to publish this work.

References

[1]M. Jarcho, "Calcium Phosphate Ceramics as Hard Tissue Prosthetics," *Clin. Orthop. Relat. Res.*, **157**, 257–78 (1981).

[2]L. L. Hench and J. Wilson (eds.), *An Introduction to Bioceramics*, Advanced Series in Ceramics, Vol. I. World Scientific, Singapore, 1993.

[3]A. Tampieri, G. Celotti, F. Szontagh, and E. Landi," Sintering and Characterization of HA and TCP Bioceramics with Control of Strength and Phase Purity," *J. Mater. Sci.: Mater. Med.*, **8**, 29–37 (1997).

[4]R. Z. LeGeros and J. P. LeGeros, "Dense Hydroxyapatite"; see Ref. 2, pp. 139–80.

[5]Y. Yubao, C. P. A. T. Klein, J. De Wijn, S. Van Der Meer, and K. De Groot, "Shape Change and Phase Transition of Needlelike Non-stoichiometric Apatite Crystals," *J. Mater. Sci.: Mater. Med.*, **5**, 263–68 (1994).

[6]Y. Yubao, J. De Wijn, C. P. A. T. Klein, S. Van Der Meer, and K. De Groot, "Preparation and Characterization of Nanograde Osteoapatitelike Rod Crystals," *J. Mater. Sci.: Mater. Med.*, **5**, 252–55 (1994).

[7]M. N. Rahaman, *Ceramic Processing and Sintering*. Marcel Dekker, New York, 1995.

[8]H. K. Varma and R. Sivakumar, "Preparation and Characterization of Free Flowing Hydroxyapatite Powders," *Phosphorus Res. Bull.*, **6**, 35–38 (1996).

[9]H. K. Varma and R. Sivakumar, "Dense Hydroxyapatite through Gelcasting Technique," *Mater. Lett.*, **29**, 57–61 (1996).

[10]B. E. Yoldas, "Alumina Gels that Form Porous Transparent Al_2O_3," *J. Mater. Sci.*, **10**, 1856–60 (1975). □

journal

J. Am. Ceram. Soc., **85** [3] 517–22 (2002)

Biomimetic Hydroxyapatite Coating on Metal Implants

Pamela Habibovic,[†] Florence Barrère,[†,‡] Clemens A. van Blitterswijk,[†,‡] Klaas de Groot,[†,§] and Pierre Layrolle*,[†,¶]

IsoTis NV, Professor Bronkhorstlaan 10, 3720 MB Bilthoven, The Netherlands

iBME, Twente University, The Netherlands

Biomaterial Research Group, Leiden University, The Netherlands

The combination of the high mechanical strength of metals with the osteoconductive properties of calcium phosphates make hydroxyapatite coatings on titanium implants widely used in orthopedic surgery. However, the most popular coating method, plasma spraying, exhibits some important drawbacks: the inability to cover porous implants and to incorporate biologically active agents, delamination, and particle release. The aim of this study was to elaborate a dense, strong, and thick calcium-phosphate coating on titanium and porous-tantalum implants using a two-step biomimetic procedure. In the first step, the implants were soaked in a solution that was 5 times more concentrated than regular simulated body fluid (SBF-A solution). A thin but uniform amorphous calcium-phosphate coating was deposited on the metal. Then, the implants were immersed in the SBF-B solution, which had a similar composition as the SBF-A solution, but with decreased contents of crystal growth inhibitors (i.e., Mg^{2+} and HCO_3^-). This resulted in the fast precipitation of a 30 μm thick crystalline calcium-phosphate coating. The pH of the SBF-B solution and the thickness of the crystalline coating layer were studied as a function of time. The Fourier transform infrared spectra and X-ray diffraction patterns showed that this new coating closely resembles bone mineral. Our biomimetic coating should facilitate rapid bone formation around the implant, reducing therewith the patient's recovery time after surgery.

I. Introduction

PLASMA sprayed coatings, mainly hydroxyapatite (HA), on titanium alloy (Ti6Al4V) prostheses have been widely used in orthopedic surgery to reconstruct hip and knee joints. Earlier investigations have shown that these coatings can successfully enhance clinical success to a <2% failure rate after 10 years.[1] Despite excellent clinical performances, the plasma-spray process is limited by intrinsic drawbacks. For instance, this line-of-sight process takes place at high temperatures. The process is, therefore, limited to thermally stable phases such as HA, and the incorporation of growth factors that stimulate bone healing is impossible. Moreover, this process cannot provide even coatings on porous metal surfaces.

Recently, other techniques have been studied to improve the quality of coatings, such as electrophoretic deposition,[2] sputter deposition,[3] and sol–gel.[4] Nevertheless, the deposition of apatite coatings from simulated body fluids (SBFs) offers the most promising alternative to plasma spraying and other coating methods. The biomimetic approach has four main advantages: (i) it is a low-temperature process applicable to any heat-sensitive substrate including polymers;[5] (ii) it forms bonelike apatite crystals having high bioactivity and good resorption characteristics;[6] (iii) it is evenly deposited on, or even into, porous or complex implant geometries;[7] and (iv) it can incorporate bone-growth-stimulating factors.

This biomimetic approach consists of soaking metal implants in simulated body fluids at a physiologic temperature and pH. Apatite coatings have successfully been formed by the immersion of chemically pretreated substrates such as glasses, metals, and polymers in metastable SBFs.[8–10] Although SBF mimics the inorganic composition, pH, and temperature of human blood plasma, it is unknown whether these conditions are optimal for a coating process. Indeed, a thin apatite layer has previously been obtained on pretreated substrates by using long immersion time (i.e., 7–14 days) with a daily refreshment of SBFs.[11–13] The difficulty results from the metastability of SBF. The process requires replenishment and a constant pH to maintain supersaturation for apatite crystal growth. As a result of the low solubility product of HA and the limited concentration range for the metastable phase, this operation is extremely difficult and might lead to local precipitation or uneven coatings. Such an intricate and long process can hardly be applicable in the coating prostheses industry.

This paper describes a new biomimetic route for coating titanium alloy and porous tantalum with uniform and thick HA layers in a few hours. Thereby, no chemical pretreatment of the substrate is needed. Our process takes advantage of the higher solubility of calcium phosphate in acidic conditions and its precipitation at a neutral pH. A weak gaseous acid, CO_2, is used to decrease the pH, allowing much higher ionic concentrations for SBFs. While CO_2 gas is naturally released from the solution, the pH and, therewith, saturation, are slowly and uniformly increased. Therefore, carbonate-containing HA crystals precipitate on the implants.

II. Experimental Procedure

(1) Materials

The biomimetic coatings were applied on two different materials: Ti6Al4V plates (20 mm × 20 mm × 1 mm; Smitfort Staal BV, Zwijndrecht, The Netherlands) and porous tantalum cylinders. The adhesion strength of the coating is dependent on the mechanical interlock of the biomimetic HA coating and the implant surface.[14,15] For optimal coating, an average surface roughness of 3.5 μm is required. This surface roughness on the Ti6Al4V plates was obtained via grit blasting, using corundum particles with a particle size of 595–841 μm under a pressure of 4 bar (Stratec Medical, Obendorf, Switzerland).

The porous tantalum implants were manufactured by chemical vapor infiltration of pure tantalum onto a highly porous vitreous

N. P. Padture—contributing editor

Manuscript No. 187738. Received April 30, 2001; approved October 26, 2001.

*Member, American Ceramic Society.
†IsoTis NV.
‡iBME, Twente University.
§Biomaterial Research Group, Leiden University.
¶Author to whom correspondence should be addressed (E-mail address: pierre.layrolle@isotis.com).

Table I. Inorganic Composition of Human Blood Plasma (HBP), Simulated Body Fluid (SBF), and Coating Solutions SBF-A and SBF-B

Component	Ion concentration (m*M*)							
	Na^+	K^+	Ca^{2+}	Mg^{2+}	Cl^-	HPO_4^{2-}	HCO_3^-	SO_4^{2-}
HBP	142.0	5.0	2.5	1.5	103.0	1.0	27.0	0.5
SBF	142.0	5.0	2.5	1.5	148.8	1.0	4.2	0.5
SBF-A	714.8		12.5	7.5	723.8	5.0	21.0	
SBF-B	704.2		12.5	1.5	711.8	5.0	10.5	

carbon skeleton (Implex Corp., Allendale, NJ). The porosity of the structure was ~75%, and the average size of the interconnected pores was 450 μm. Before coating, the implants were ultrasonically cleaned for 15 min in acetone, ethanol (70%), and demineralized water.

(2) Coating Solutions

The coating process consisted of two steps. In the first step, the heterogeneous nucleation of a thin and amorphous calcium phosphate layer on the metal surface was obtained. During the second step, the growth of a thick and crystallized apatite coating on the implants was favored because of the lower Mg^{2+} and HCO_3^- contents.

The SBF-A and SBF-B solutions (Table I) were prepared according to Kokubo's SBF solution,[16] excluding the TRIS-buffer, K^+ ions, and SO_4^{2-} ions. In the first-step solution, the SBF-A was 5 times more concentrated in NaCl, $MgCl_2{\cdot}6H_2O$, $CaCl_2{\cdot}2H_2O$, $Na_2HPO_4{\cdot}2H_2O$, and $NaHCO_3$ than Kokubo's SBF solution. The SBF-B solution had the same composition as the SBF-A solution but, as explained earlier, the contents of inhibitors of crystal growth (i.e., Mg^{2+} and HCO_3^- were lower (Table I)). All salts (reagent grade; Merck, Darmstadt, Germany) were precisely weighed (±0.01 g) and dissolved in demineralized water under a supply of CO_2 gas at a flow of 650 L/min for 20 min and stirring at a speed of 250 rounds per minute (rpm).

The pH evolution was studied as a function of time in coating the SBF-A and SBF-B solutions. As a reference, the pH development in time was studied in a solution containing NaCl at a concentration of 683 m*M* in demineralized water.

(3) Coating Process

All experiments were performed in a 7L bioreactor (Applikon Dependable Instruments, Schiedam, The Netherlands) (Fig. 1).

The implants were first soaked in a SBF-A solution for 24 h to seed the metal surface with calcium phosphate nuclei. During this process, the temperature was kept at 37°C and the solution was stirred at 250 rpm. To exchange CO_2 gas from the solution with air, a top aeration at a flow of 450 mL/min was performed. Moreover, air was added through the solution (500 mL/min flow) after the pH had reached a value of 7.1. At the end of the process, the coated samples were cleaned with demineralized water and dried in air overnight. Then, the implants were soaked for another 48 h in a SBF-B solution under crystal growth conditions. The temperature was maintained at 50°C and the stirring speed at 250 rpm. The same aeration system was used as described above. During this process, two samples were removed from the solution after 1, 2, 3, 4, 5, 6, 7, 8, 24, and 48 h. Finally, the coated samples were cleaned with demineralized water and dried in air overnight. At the end of both processes, the solutions were filtered through Whatman filter paper No. 5 (Whatman, Inc., Clifton, NJ). The precipitate was collected and dried at 50°C overnight.

(4) Chemical and Structural Characterization of the Coatings

All samples were first investigated macroscopically. After gold-sputtering, the coated samples were observed microscopically using an environmental scanning electronic microscope apparatus equipped with a field-emission gun (ESEM-FEG; Model XL-30, Philips, Eindhoven, The Netherlands) at an accelerating voltage of 10 keV, coupled with energy-dispersive X-ray analysis (EDAX) to check for any calcium-phosphate coating. The thickness of the coating was determined using an Eddy-current (electromagnetic) test method (Electrophysic Minitest 2100, Radiometer, Copenhagen, Denmark).[17] Both coating and precipitate were investigated by Fourier transform infrared spectroscopy (FTIR; Model Spectrum 1000, Perkin–Elmer Analytical Instruments, Norwalk, CT) and X-ray diffraction (XRD; Miniflex goniometer, Rigaku, Tokyo, Japan). X-rays were produced by a monochromatic source (Cu*K*α, λ = 1.54 Å, 30 kV, 15 mA). All the XRD patterns were recorded at the same conditions (scan range: 2θ = 3.00°–60.00°; scan speed: 2.00°/min; scan step: 0.02°). The crystallinity of the coating[18] and the calcium phosphate ratio[19] were determined. Both coatings and precipitate have similar FTIR spectra and XRD patterns. For convenience, analyses were performed on the precipitate.

III. Results

(1) pH Study

Comparing the pH curves versus time in the NaCl reference solution and the SBF-A and SBF-B solutions, it was observed that the initial pH of the NaCl reference was significantly lower (3.7) than the initial pH values of the SBF-A and SBF-B solutions (5.8 and 5.7, respectively). The end pH of the NaCl reference (6.6) after 24 h was lower as well (pH_{end} SBF-A = 8.3; pH_{end} SBF-B = 7.9). Moreover, the pH of the NaCl reference and SBF-A solution increased progressively from the beginning to the end of the process, while during the process in the SBF-B solution, a drop in the pH was observed.

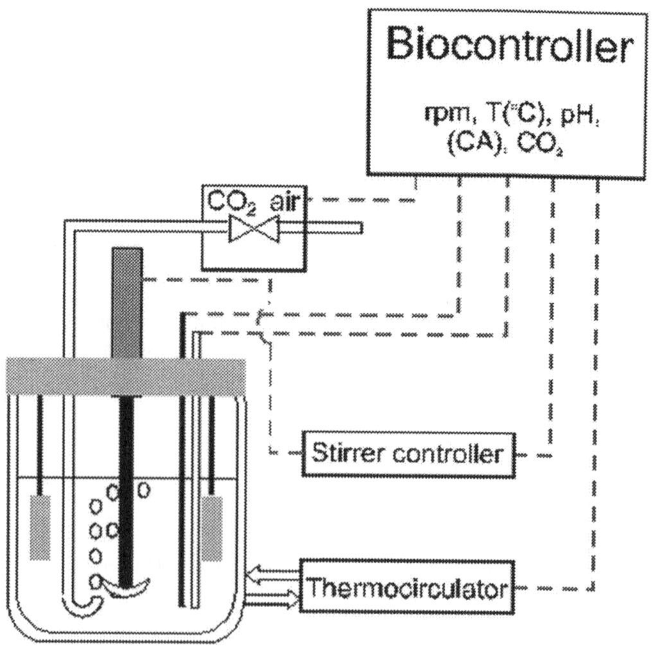

Fig. 1. Bioreactor for biomimetic coating of the metal implants.

(2) Coating Process

After 24 h of soaking in the SBF-A solution, the implants were covered with a calcium phosphate film with a thickness of ~3 μm. The ESEM photographs showed that this calcium phosphate layer was uniformly deposited on the Ti6Al4V surface (Fig. 2(a)). The coating was dense and consisted of globules. This thin coating exhibited some cracks, probably formed during the drying process of the coated samples. The EDAX spectrum (not shown) indicated calcium and phosphate peaks, with minute contents of magnesium and sodium. Small peaks of the Ti6Al4V substrate were also detected. The FTIR spectrum of the precipitate and coating (Fig. 3(a)) showed featureless phosphate and carbonate bands. Intense and broad bands assigned to oxygen-hydrogen stretching and bonding were observed at 3435 and 1642 cm^{-1}, respectively. Moreover, three bands at 868, 1432, and 1499 cm^{-1} corresponded to the CO_3 groups. Finally, the one-component bands at 560 and 1045 cm^{-1} showed the presence of PO_4. This FTIR spectrum is characteristic of carbonated amorphous calcium phosphate. The XRD pattern of the SBF-A precipitate (Fig. 4(a)) corroborates the FTIR results, showing only the halo characteristic of an amorphous phase.

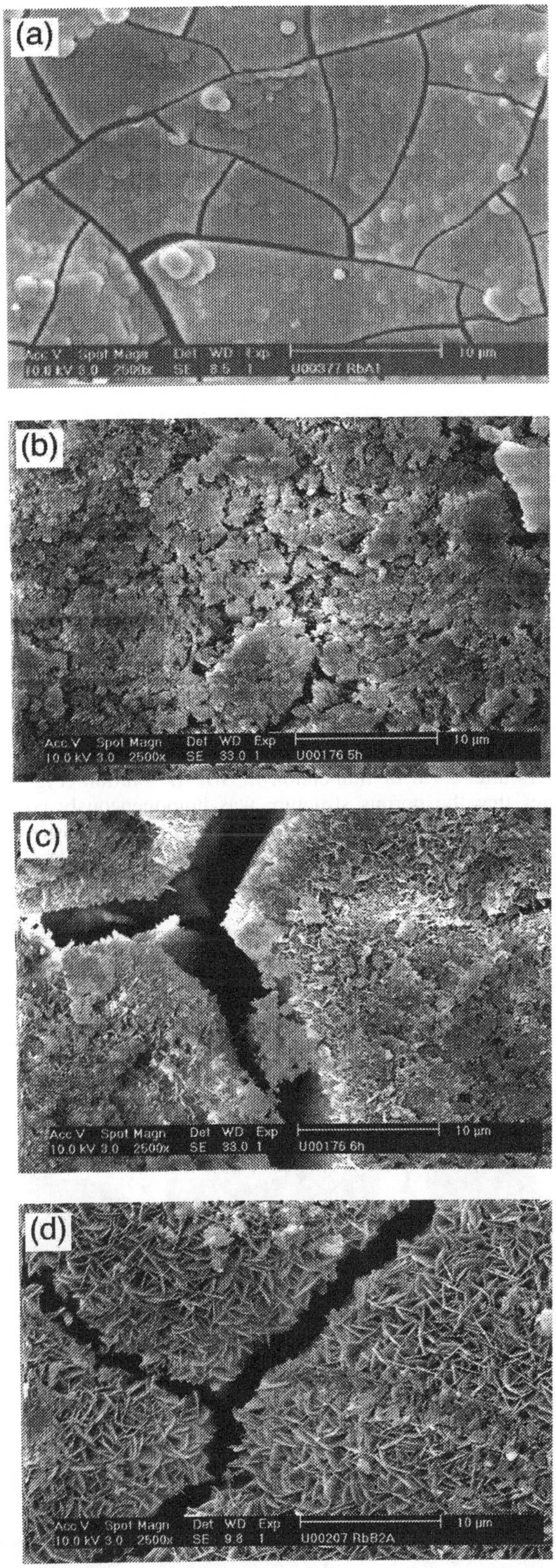

Fig. 2. ESEM photographs (magnification 2500×) of (a) SBF-A coating, (b) SBF-B coating after 5 h, (c) SBF-B coating after 6 h, and (d) SBF-B coating after 24 h on a Ti6Al4V plate.

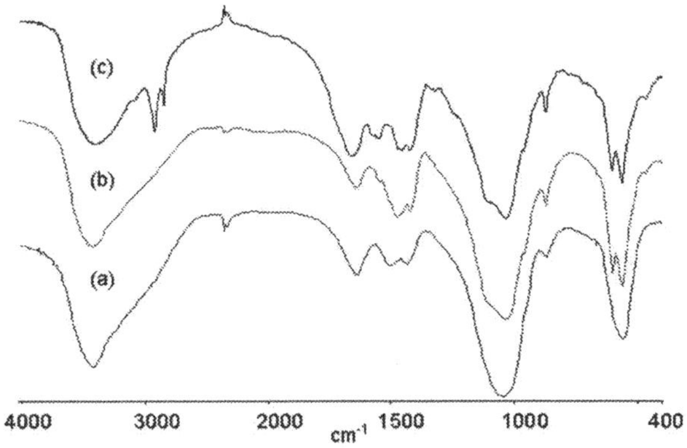

Fig. 3. Infrared spectra of (a) SBF-A coating, (b) SBF-B coating, and (c) bone.

The immersion process in the SBF-B solution was used to develop a second coating layer on the seeded Ti6Al4V surface resulting from the first coating process. During the immersion process in the SBF-B solution, the pH and coating thickness development were studied (Fig. 5). The pH of the solution at the beginning of the process stabilized at 5.7. During the first 4 h of the process, the pH increased progressively until a value of 6.2. Then, after 4 h, a drop of 0.4 pH units occurred. After this drop, the pH started increasing again, and reached a value of 8.2 after 24 h. The pH elaboration of the solution was followed until 48 h, and the final pH was 8.9.

During the first 4 h of the process, the solution remained clear, and the thickness of the second coating layer grew very slowly (i.e., ≤1.5 μm/h). During the drop in the pH, the precipitation occurred in the solution. After the pH drop, the coating thickness started increasing significantly with the rise in pH. Between 5 and 6 h of the immersion, the coating thickness grew to ~30 μm, after which it remained constant up to 48 h of soaking.

The ESEM photographs of the titanium implants after 5 and 6 h of immersion (Figs. 2(b) and (c)) show many differences. After 5 h, the metal was covered with loose calcium phosphate

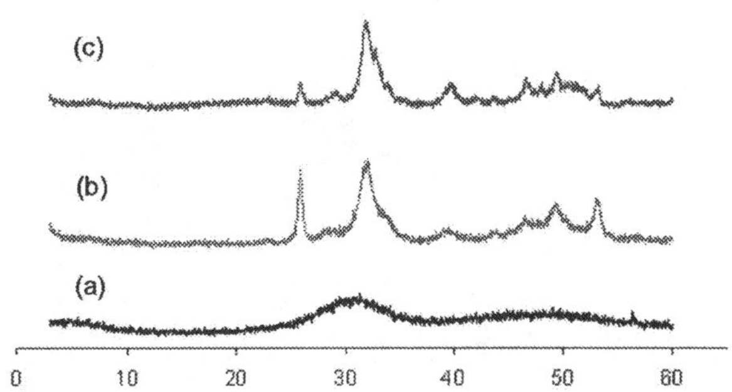

Fig. 4. XRD patterns of (a) SBF-A coating, (b) SBF-B coating, and (c) bone.

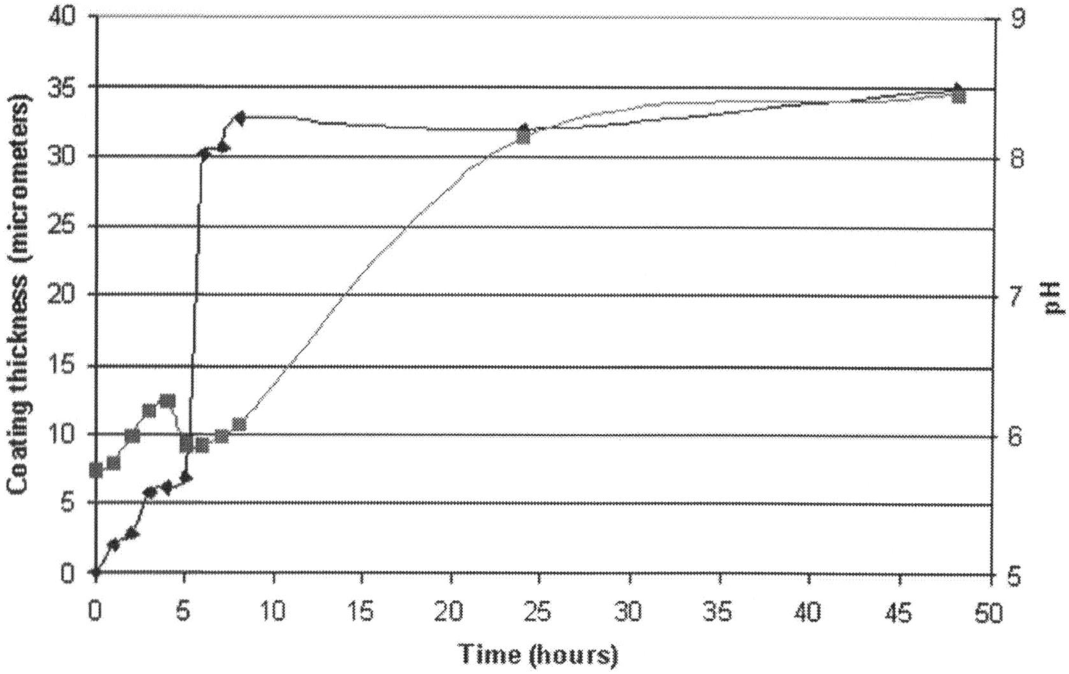

Fig. 5. (■) pH and (◆) coating thickness versus immersion time in SBF-B solution.

particles. The surface looked rough, without any visible crystals, and the thickness of the calcium phosphate layer was locally different. After 6 h of immersion, the coating thickness was 30 μm. In this case, the entire metal surface was homogeneously covered with a well-formed, bluish coating consisting of globules with some tiny crystals. The coating contained many wide cracks. After 24 h of soaking, the thickness of the coating did not change significantly in comparison to the coating after 6 h of soaking. However, the coating looked more homogeneous and denser (Fig. 2(d)), the cracks were much narrower, and the surface consisted of well-formed crystals 1–3 μm in size.

As explained earlier, the EDAX spectrum of the coating from the SBF-A solution showed high calcium and phosphate peaks, and lower magnesium, sodium, and titanium peaks. The EDAX spectrum of the coating after 5 h of soaking in the SBF-B solution showed lower calcium and phosphate peaks and a higher titanium peak, suggesting partial dissolution of the amorphous coating. The magnesium peak was also lower, indicating a difference in the amount of magnesium ions in the coating obtained from the SBF-A and SBF-B solutions. After 6 h of soaking in the SBF-B solution, an increase in phosphate and calcium peaks and a decrease in titanium peaks corroborated the growth of the coating. Finally, the EDAX spectrum of the coating after 24 h of soaking showed very high calcium and phosphate peaks, while the titanium peak was not visible anymore.

The ESEM photograph of the surface of porous tantalum cylinders after 24 h of immersion in SBF-B solution (Fig. 6(a)) indicates that the porous structure was homogeneously covered with a crystalline calcium-phosphate coating. On the cross-sectional surface (Fig. 6(b)), a coating was also visible on the inside of the implant. All pores were well-coated with a thick calcium phosphate layer.

The FTIR spectrum of the precipitate from the SBF-B solution, gathered between 400 and 4000 cm^{-1} (Fig. 3(b)), exhibited the characteristics of a carbonated apatite type A-B. The bands at 3435 and 1640 cm^{-1} corresponded to the oxygen-hydrogen groups. CO_3 group bands were observed at 1493, 1417, and 872 cm^{-1}, whereas bands at 1061, 599, and

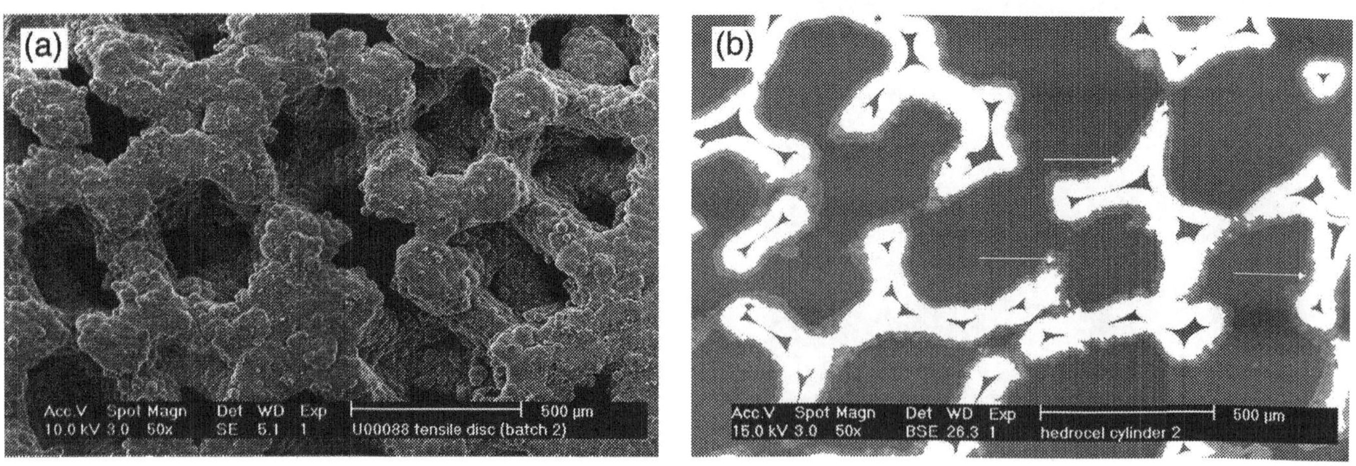

Fig. 6. ESEM photographs (magnification 50×) of (a) SBF-B coating on the surface and (b) cross section of porous tantalum cylinders; white arrows indicate the coating.

563 cm^{-1} were assigned to PO_4/HPO_4 groups. The XRD pattern exhibited broad diffraction lines (Fig. 4(b)). The position and intensities of these diffraction lines indicated an apatitic structure. The peak at $2\theta = 32.1°$ corresponded to the overlapping of (211), (112), (300), and (202) diffraction peaks. Moreover, the peak at $2\theta = 25.8°$, corresponding to the (002) diffraction plane, indicated that the SBF-B precipitate consisted of small apatitic crystals. The crystals had a size of 2–3 μm. The crystallinity of the precipitate was 75%, and its calcium phosphate ratio was 1.67.

Previously published results[20] showed that the final apatite coating is well-adhered to the Ti6Al4V substrate, and that no coating delamination or spalls were observed during the scratch test.

IV. Discussion

The results of the experiments show that highly-concentrated solutions can be obtained by the addition of the mildly acidic gas, CO_2. It is, namely, well-known that the solubility of calcium phosphate salts increases with the decrease of pH.[21] Dissolution of CO_2 gas results in a pH decrease caused by the formation of carbonic acid H_2CO_3 (reaction (1)), after which the acid immediately dissociates in the HCO_3^- and CO_3^{2-} species (reactions (2) and (3)).

$$CO_2 + H_2O \leftrightarrow H_2CO_3 \tag{1}$$

$$H_2CO_3 + H_2O \leftrightarrow HCO_3^- + H_3O^+ \tag{2}$$

$$HCO_3^- + H_2O \leftrightarrow CO_3^{2-} + H_3O^+ \tag{3}$$

When CO_2 gas gradually releases from the solutions, the pH slowly increases again. In the case of the NaCl reference, the pH increases progressively from the start to finish of the process, slowly approaching the pH of water (6.5). The presence of HCO_3^- and HPO_4^{2-} ions in SBF solutions, together with the CO_2 and HCO_3^- ions that are formed during the dissolution of CO_2 gas (reactions (2) and (3)), leads to the formation of a buffered solution. This might explain the fact that the initial pH values of the SBF-A and SBF-B solutions were higher than that of the NaCl reference. During the processes in the SBF-B solution, a drop in the pH was observed simultaneously with the start of precipitation in the solution. This drop of the pH may be explained by the start of the precipitation of the crystalline phase, according to reaction (4).

$$10Ca^{2+} + 6PO_4^{3-} + 2OH^- \leftrightarrow Ca_{10}(PO_4)_6(OH)_2 \tag{4}$$

Because of the decreased amount of OH^- ions in the solution, a pH drop was observed. After precipitation, CO_2 gas continued to release from the solution and, therefore, the pH increased progressively until the end of the process.

In the SBF-A solution, more HCO_3^- species were present in comparison with the SBF-B solution (Table I). Therefore, the buffering capacity of the CO_2/HCO_3^- couple was higher. This might explain a slightly higher initial pH and the absence of pH drop during the process in the SBF-A solution, in comparison with the process in the SBF-B solution.

Another factor that may influence the pH evolution during the coating process is the amount of the NaCl species, i.e., the ionic strength of the solution.[22] The rate of the CO_2 release from the solution is higher in the case of low ionic strength, followed by a higher pH increase. This causes an early and sudden precipitation in the solution. Consequently, the supersaturation of the solution is markedly lowered, and less ionic species' are available in the solution for the calcium phosphate nucleation on the substrate. Moreover, there is a relation between the calcium phosphate concentration and the pH at which precipitation occurs: the lower the concentration, the higher the precipitation pH.[21]

As was previously described, a 3 μm thick amorphous layer of carbonated calcium phosphate was obtained on the metal sample by immersion in the SBF-A solution. *In vivo* experiments performed by our group (unpublished results) showed that this amorphous coating was too thin to be able to enhance osteointegration of the implants. Moreover, earlier *in vitro* dissolution experiments[23] showed that, at both an acidic and neutral pH, amorphous carbonated calcium phosphate dissolves markedly faster than other calcium-phosphate coatings (i.e., octacalcium phosphate (OCP), carbonated apatite (CAp), and HA).

According to the literature and our experience, a coating that successfully enhances osteointegration of metal implants needs to be thick and crystallized enough to accommodate the bone healing process. Preliminary experiments were performed in order to grow a crystalline coating on a metal surface without immersion in the SBF-A solution. By immersing cleaned Ti6Al4V directly into the SBF-B solution, a loose and nonuniform layer was obtained, which shows the relevance of amorphous precoating. That is why our biomimetic coating consists of two steps.

Immersion of the implants in a SBF-A solution is necessary for seeding the metal surface with calcium phosphate nuclei. During this nucleation process, calcium phosphate seeds are precipitated in the solution and on the metal surface. Some of these nuclei can dissolve in the solution and some can expand in size. Homogeneous nucleation (precipitation) occurs spontaneously in the solution and can proceed if other seeds form in the meantime. Heterogeneous nucleation, on the other hand, takes place on the metal surface. Both, homogenous and heterogeneous nucleation are in competition during the process in the SBF-B solution. However, nuclei are energetically more stable on the seeded metal surface than in the solution. It is, therefore, essential to provide the metal surface with a thin and uniform primer calcium phosphate layer for subsequent growth of the final coating. The kinetics of the process in the SBF-A solution were reported in detail by Barrère *et al.*[24]

After reaching their critical size, seeds can start growing into crystals. The nucleation and growth kinetics of the crystal depend on the temperature, pH, composition, and saturation of the solution. Calcium and phosphate ions are responsible for the formation of the calcium phosphate layer on the metal surface, while magnesium and carbonate ions favor heterogeneous nucleation rather than crystal growth. As is given in Table I, the SBF-B solution has the same composition as the SBF-A solution, but the contents of Mg^{2+} and HCO_3^- ions are lower. Resulting from lower amounts of these so-called crystal growth inhibitors,[25–32] a crystalline apatite phase is formed and a drop in the pH is observed at the start of precipitation by immersion in the SBF-B solution. Moreover, a smaller amount of HCO_3^- ions, compared to the SBF-A solution, decreases the buffering capacity of the CO_2/HCO_3^- couple and, thereby, variations in the pH can be observed. With a lower amount of Mg^{2+} in the SBF-B solution, the calcium phosphate precipitation is accelerated, and the growing coat becomes more crystallized. Earlier research[33–36] proved that crystal growth from a supersaturated solution occurs quickly. This can explain the fact that, within 1 h, the coating thickness grows by 25 μm. Because of precipitation and crystal growth, the amount of calcium and phosphate in the solution decreases. One hour after the start of precipitation, the contents of the calcium and phosphate are too low for further growth. Between the end point of crystal growth and the end of the process, there is equilibrium between the amount of calcium and the amount of phosphate in the coating and in the solution. However, the coating might dissolve and reprecipitate onto surface, resulting in a more homogeneous and denser coating at the end of the process.

As mentioned previously, dense adherent film is formed because of the heterogeneous nucleation on the metal surface. However, it is very difficult to prevent loose precipitate in the solution from sticking to the metal surface. This means that both phenomena contribute to film growth, but to a different extent.

There is a difference in the calcium/phosphate ratio between natural calcified tissues (enamel, dentine, and bone) and the biomimetic coatings. The calcium/phosphate ratio of the natural calcified tissues is ~1.60, depending on many parameters such as age, sex, bone sites, etc.[37] The biomimetic coating has a calcium/

phosphate ratio of 1.67 ± 0.02, as determined after calcination at 1000°C by XRD and FTIR. In the case of the biomimetic coating, small amounts of magnesium and sodium can substitute for calcium in the HA lattice, lowering the calcium/phosphate ratio. However, carbonate is able to substitute for phosphate, which results in the transformation of HA into CAp, and increases the calcium/phosphate ratio. Because the second effect is much stronger, the overall effect is a higher calcium/phosphate ratio compared to bone.

The FTIR spectra (Fig. 3) and the XRD patterns (Fig. 4) show the similarities in composition and structure between our biomimetic coating and bone. An earlier report of an experiment with osteoclast-enriched mouse bone marrow cell cultures on different coatings[6] showed that numerous resorption lacunae, characteristic of osteoclastic resorption, were found on carbonated apatite after cell culture. In the case of OCP coating, no pits could be found. The obtained results indicated that biomimetic calcium-phosphate coatings are easily resorbed by osteoclasts *in vitro*. This phenomenon corresponds to full integration into the human body of biomimetically coated implants. On the contrary, conventional plasma-sprayed coatings may delaminate and release large sintered particles that are not easily degraded by cells.[38] The last results might indicate that our biomimetic coatings are markedly more bioactive than plasma-sprayed coatings. However, additional *in vivo* research is necessary to confirm these expectations.

V. Conclusion

The formation of thick and homogeneous calcium-phosphate coatings on Ti6Al4V implants and porous tantalum substrates is possible by using a biomimetic method consisting of two steps. By this method, the coating is produced within a few hours and without any chemical pretreatment. The first step of the process results in the formation of a thin amorphous coating, which finally leads to the fast precipitation of a 30 ± 10 μm thick dense calcium-phosphate coating in the second step of the process. The formation of this coating is strongly related to the Mg^{2+} content. The evolution of the pH during the coating process is dependent on the ionic strength of the solution (i.e., the amount of NaCl), and the amount of HCO_3^- ions, which, together with the present CO_2, buffer the solution. The final coating closely resembles bone mineral. The biomimetic coating applied on dense and porous orthopedic implants should enhance bone apposition and bone ingrowth, leading to the fast and stable osteointegration of prostheses.

References

[1]L. I. Havelin, L. B. Engesaeter, B. Espehaug, O. Furnes, S. A. Lie, and S. E. Vollset, "The Norwegian Arthroplasy Register, 11 Years and 73,000 Arthroplasties," *Acta Orthop. Scand.*, **71** [4] 337–53 (2000).

[2]P. Ducheyne, W. van Raemdonck, J. C. Heughebaert, and M. Heughebaert, "Structural Analysis of Hydroxyapatite Coatings on Titanium," *Biomaterials*, **7** [2] 97–103 (1986).

[3]J. L. Ong, L. C. Lucas, W. R. Lacefield, and E. D. Rigney, "Structure, Solubility and Bond Strength of Thin Calcium Phosphate Coatings Produced by Beam Sputter Deposition," *Biomaterials*, **13** [4] 249–54 (1992).

[4]B. Ben-Nissan, C. S. Chai, and K. A. Gross, "Effect of Solution Aging on Sol-Gel Hydroxyapatite Coatings," *Bioceramics*, **10**, 175–78 (1997).

[5]C. Du, P. Klasens, R. E. de Haan, J. Bezemer, F. Z. Cui, K. de Groot, and P. Layrolle, "Biomimetic Calcium Phosphate Coatings on PolyActive® 1000/70/30," *J. Biomed. Mater. Res.*, **59**, 535–46 (2002).

[6]S. Leeuwenburgh, P. Layrolle, F. Barrère, J. Schoonman, C. A. van Blitterswijk, and K. de Groot, "Osteoclastic Resorption of Biomimetic Calcium Phosphate Coatings *In Vitro*," *J. Biomed. Mater. Res.*, **56**, 208–15 (2001).

[7]P. Layrolle, C. van der Valk, R. Dalmeijer, C.A. van Blitterswijk, and K. de Groot, "Biomimetic Calcium Phosphate Coatings and Their Biological Performances," *Bioceramics*, **13**, 391–94 (2001).

[8]H. B. Wen, J. G. C. Wolke, J. R. de Wijn, F. Z. Cui, and K. de Groot, "Fast Precipitation of Calcium Phosphate Layers on Titanium Induced by Simple Chemical Treatment," *Biomaterials*, **18**, 1471–78 (1997).

[9]H. M. Kim, F. Miyaji, T. Kokubo, and T. Nakamura, "Preparation of Bioactive Ti and its Alloys via Simple Chemical Surface Treatment," *J. Biomed. Mater. Res.*, **32**, 409–17 (1996).

[10]S. Yamada, T. Nakamura, T. Kokubo, M. Oka, and T. Yamamura, "Osteoclastic Resorption of Apatite Formed on Apatite- and Wollastonite-Containing Glass-Ceramic by a Simulated Body Fluid," *J. Biomed. Mater. Res.*, **28**, 1357–63 (1994).

[11]P. Li, I. Kangasniemi, K. de Groot, and T. Kokubo, "Bonelike Hydroxyapatite, Induction by a Gel-Derived Titania on a Titanium Substrate," *J. Am. Ceram. Soc.*, **77**, 1307–12 (1994).

[12]T. Peltola, M. Patsi, H. Rahiala, I. Kangasniemi, and A. Yli-Urpo, "Calcium Phosphate Induction by Sol-Gel-Derived Titania Coatings on Titanium Substrates *In Vitro*," *J. Biomed. Mater. Res.*, **41**, 504–10 (1998).

[13]P. Li and P. Ducheyne, "Quasi-Biological Apatite Film Induced by Titanium in a Simulated Body Fluid," *J. Biomed. Mater. Res.*, **41**, 341–48 (1998).

[14]E. Leitao, M. A. Barbosa, and K. de Groot, "Influence of Substrate Material and Surface Finishing on the Morphology of the Calcium-Phosphate Coating," *J. Biomed. Mater. Res.*, **36**, 85–90 (1987).

[15]K. A. Thomas and S. D. Cook, "An Evaluation of Variables Influencing Implant Fixation by Direct Bone Apposition," *J. Biomed. Mater. Res.*, **19**, 875–901 (1985).

[16]T. Kokubo, H. Kushitani, S. Sakka, T. Kitsugi, and T. Yamamuro, "Solutions Able to Reproduce *In Vivo* Surface-Structure Changes in Bioactive Glass-Ceramics A-W3," *J. Biomed. Mater. Res.*, **24**, 721–34 (1990).

[17]"Standard Practice for Measuring Coating Thickness by Magnetic-Field or EDDY-Current (Electromagnetic) Test Methods," ASTM Designation E 376. *1996 Book of ASTM Standards.* American Society for Testing and Materials, West Conshohocken, PA.

[18]J. S. Flach, L. A. Shimp, C. A. van Blitterswijk, and K. de Groot, "A Calibrated Method for Crystallinity Determination of Hydroxylapatite Coatings"; in *Characterization and Performance of Calcium Phosphate Coatings for Implants*, ASTM Special Technical Publication 1196. Edited by E. Horowitz and J. E. Perr. American Society for Testing Materials, West Conshohocken, PA, 1994.

[19]"Determination Quantitative du Rapport Ca/P de Phosphates de Calcium"; Paper No. 94-066 in *Materiaux pour Implants Chirurgicaux.* Association Française de Normalisation (ANFOR), Paris, France, 1998.

[20]F. Barrère, P. Layrolle, C.A. van Blitterswijk, and K. de Groot, "Physical and Chemical Characteristics of Plasma-Sprayed and Biomimetic Apatite Coating," *Bioceramics*, **12**, 125–28 (1999).

[21]J. C. Elliot, *Structure and Chemistry of the Apatites and Other Calcium Orthophosphates*; p. 4. Elsevier, Amsterdam, The Netherlands, 1994.

[22]F. Barrère, P. Layrolle, C.A. van Blitterswijk, and K. de Groot, "Influence of NaCl and HCO_3 on the Biomimetic Ca-P Coating Process from SBFx5 Solution," *Biomaterials*, in press.

[23]F. Barrère, M. Stigter, P. Layrolle, C.A. van Blitterswijk, and K. de Groot, "*In Vitro* Dissolution of Various Calcium-Phosphates Coatings on Ti6Al4V," *Bioceramics*, **13**, 67–70 (2000).

[24]F. Barrère, P. Layrolle, C.A. van Blitterswijk, and K. de Groot, "Fast Formation of Biomimetic Ca-P Coatings on Ti6Al4V," *Mater. Res. Soc. Symp. Proc.*, **599**, 135–40 (2000).

[25]H. Newesely, "Changes in Crystal Types of Low Solubility Calcium Phosphates in Presence of Accompanying Ions," *Arch. Oral Biol.*, **6** [Special Supplement] 174–80 (1961).

[26]B. Tomazic, M. Tomson, and G. H. Nancollas, "Growth of Calcium Phosphates on Hydroxyapatite Crystals: The Effect of Magnesium," *Arch. Oral Biol.*, **20**, 803–808 (1975).

[27]M. H. Salimi, J. C. Heughbaert, and G. H. Nancollas, "Crystal Growth of Calcium Phosphates in the Presence of Magnesium Ions," *Langmuir*, **1**, 119–22 (1985).

[28]E. D. Eanes and S. L. Rattner, "The Effect of Magnesium on Apatite Formation in Seeded Supersaturated Solutions at pH = 7.4," *J. Dent. Res.*, **60** [9] 1719–23 (1980).

[29]A. L. Boskey and A. S. Posner, "Magnesium Stabilization of Amorphous Calcium Phosphate: A Kinetic Study," *Mater. Res. Bull.*, **9**, 907–16 (1974).

[30]G. H. Nancollas, B. Tomazic, and M. Tomson, "The Precipitation of Calcium Phosphate in the Presence of Magnesium," *Croatia Chemica Acta*, **48**, 431–38 (1976).

[31]N. S. Chikerur, M. S. Tung, and W. E. Brown, "A Mechanism for Incorporation of Carbonate into Apatite," *Calcif. Tissue Int.*, **32**, 55–62 (1980).

[32]B. N. Bachara and H. R. A. Fisher, "The Effect of Some Inhibitors on the Nucleation and Crystal Growth of Apatite," *Calcif. Tissue Res.*, **3**, 348–57 (1969).

[33]H. Füredi-Milhofer, L. Brecevic, and B. Purgaric, "Crystal Growth and Phase Transformation in the Precipitation of Calcium Phosphates," *Faraday Discuss. Chem. Soc.*, **61**, 184–90 (1976).

[34]P. Koutsoukos, Z. Amjad, M. B. Tomson, and G. H. Nancollas, "Crystallization of Calcium Phosphates: A Constant Composition Study," *J. Am. Chem. Soc.*, **102** [5] 1553–57 (1980).

[35]M. J. J. M. van Kemenade and P. L. de Bruyn, "A Kinetic Study of Precipitation from Supersaturated Calcium Phosphate Solutions," *J. Colloid Interface Sci.*, **118**, 564–85 (1987).

[36]G. T. Kohman, "Precipitation of Crystals from Solution"; pp. 152–62 in *The Art and Science of Growing Crystals.* Edited by J. Gilman. Wiley, London, U.K., 1963.

[37]R. LeGeros, *Calcium Phosphates in Oral Biology and Medicine*; pp. 109–27. Karger, Basel, Switzerland, 1991.

[38]J. D. de Bruijn, J. S. Flach, H. Leenders, J. van den Brink, and C.A. van Blitterswijk, "Degradation and Interface Characteristics of Plasma-Sprayed Coatings with Different Crystallinities," *Bioceramics*, **5**, 291–98 (1992). □

journal

J. Am. Ceram. Soc., 85 [4] 800–806 (2002)

Effects of Yttria-Stabilized Zirconia on Plasma-Sprayed Hydroxyapatite/Yttria-Stabilized Zirconia Composite Coatings

Lei Fu,*,† Khiam Aik Khor,‡ and Joo Peng Lim

School of Mechanical and Production Engineering, Nanyang Technological University, Singapore 639798

The low bonding strength between hydroxyapatite (HA) and the metal substrate interface of plasma-sprayed HA coating has been a point of potential weakness in its application as a biomedical prosthesis. In the present study, yttria-stabilized (8 wt%) zirconia (YSZ) has been used to enhance the mechanical properties of HA coatings. The effects of YSZ additions (in the range 10–50 wt%) on the phase composition, microstructure, bond strength, elastic modulus, and fracture toughness of plasma-sprayed HA/YSZ composite coatings have been studied. The results indicated that decomposition of HA during plasma spraying was reduced significantly with the addition of zirconia. The higher the zirconia content, the lower the amount of calcium oxide, tricalcium phosphate, and tetracalcium phosphate formed in the coatings. In addition, there was a trace of calcium zirconate formed when less than 30 wt% zirconia was present. A solid solution of HA mixed with YSZ formed during plasma spraying; however, the amount of unmelted particles increased as the zirconia increased. The mechanical properties of the HA/YSZ composite coatings, such as bond strength, elastic modulus, and fracture toughness, increased significantly as the contents of zirconia increased.

I. Introduction

Hydroxyapatite (HA), $Ca_{10}(PO_4)_6(OH)_2$, is a bioceramic material with favorable osteoconductive and bioactive properties that promote rapid bone formation and strong biological fixation to bony tissues.[1–3] However, HA is a brittle and relatively weak ceramic. The poor mechanical properties limited HA to use only in nonload-bearing areas of the human body. To extend the applications of HA, some tough but bioinert ceramics such as TiO_2, Al_2O_3, and ZrO_2 were used to form bioactive ceramic composites for improved mechanical performances.[4–8]

Hydroxyapatite coating sprayed on a metal substrate is an attractive alternative for obtaining an implant that can be used in tensile load-bearing applications. The plasma-spraying technique is the most popular method to make HA coatings.[9,10] The application of plasma-sprayed HA-coated implants has increased significantly in recent years because of the advantages, *i.e.*, increased tolerance of surgical inaccuracies,[11,12] fast fixation of the implants in bone,[13] firm implant–bone attachment,[14] and protection of surrounding bone against metal ion release from metallic implants.[15] It is always desirable that an HA coating stays on the surface of an implant in a biological environment as long as possible. However, the bond strength of an HA-coating/metal-substrate interface has been the point of potential weakness in prosthesis because it is limited by the strength of hydroxyapatite, porosity, inclusions in the lamellar structure of the coating, and the residual stress in the coating. Recent research[16] has shown that the mechanical properties of HA coatings can be improved by the addition of yttria-stabilized zirconia (YSZ; 5–10 wt%). *In vitro* test results[17] indicate that the dissolution rate of HA/YSZ composite coatings is slower than that of HA coatings, and the bonding strength of HA/YSZ coating is superior to that of HA coatings. In our study, 10, 30, and 50 wt% YSZ, respectively, have been added to the HA to improve the mechanical properties of the coatings. The effects of YSZ on the phase composition, microstructure, bond strength, elastic modulus, and fracture toughness of the HA/YSZ composite coatings have been investigated.

II. Materials and Methods

(1) *Powders and Specimen Preparations*

Hydroxyapatite and 8 wt% yttria-stabilized zirconia were obtained commercially (Plasmalloy from Miller Thermal, Inc., Appleton, WI) with average particle sizes of 34 and 30 μm, respectively. The HA particles were spherical in shape, whereas the ZrO_2 particles were angular. Both powders had a purity of 99% and were 100% crystalline. To study the effects of ZrO_2 on HA coatings, the powders of ZrO_2 and HA were mechanically ball milled together in three weight proportions, *i.e.*, 10, 30, and 50 wt% of ZrO_2, for 3 h at 100 rpm in a planetary ball mill (Model Pulverisette-5, Fritsch GmbH, Albisheim, Germany). The particle-size distribution was obtained after milling using a laser particle sizer (Model Analysette 22 Compact, Fritsch). The particle-size distribution of the ball-milled HA/YSZ mixture powders is shown in Fig. 1. Figure 2 illustrates the particle morphology of the ball-milled powders. The mixed powders exhibit a sponge-like texture forming agglomerates. The mean particle size of the ball milled powders is 13.6 μm. Figure 3 shows the X-ray diffraction (XRD) results of HA/YSZ powders after ball milling.

The substrates used for the coatings were Ti–6Al–4V. Two shapes were used, one in plate form for microstructure and phase analyses, the other in cylindrical form for bond strength measurements. All were sand-blasted using SiC particles to roughen the surface and then ultrasonically cleaned. A 100 kW net energy computerized control plasma system coupled with a six-axis robot unit (Model SG-100, Praxair Surface Technologies, Danbury, CT) was used to ensure repeatability of the plasma-spraying process. The arc current of plasma was 1000 A. The plasma working gas was a mixture of argon and helium. The gas flow rates were 1.70 and 1.10 m^3/h, respectively. The powder feed rate was 10 g/min, and the spray distance was 10 cm.

(2) *Material Characterization*

The phase analysis was conducted using an X-ray diffractometer (Model MPD 1880, Philips, Eindhoven, Netherlands) with Ni-filtered Cu$K\alpha$ radiation at 40 kV and 30 mA. A 2θ range from 20°–80° was covered at a step size of 0.02°/min. Scanning electron microscopy (SEM; Model JSM-5600LV, JEOL, Tokyo,

J. L. Smialek—contributing editor

Manuscript No. 189151. Received August 19, 1999; approved July 16, 2001.
Financially support by National Science and Technology Board (NSTB) and Ministry of Education of Singapore.
*Member, American Ceramic Society.
†Current address: Dept. of Materials Science and Engineering, Northwestern University, Evanston, IL 60208.
‡Author to whom correspondence should be addressed.

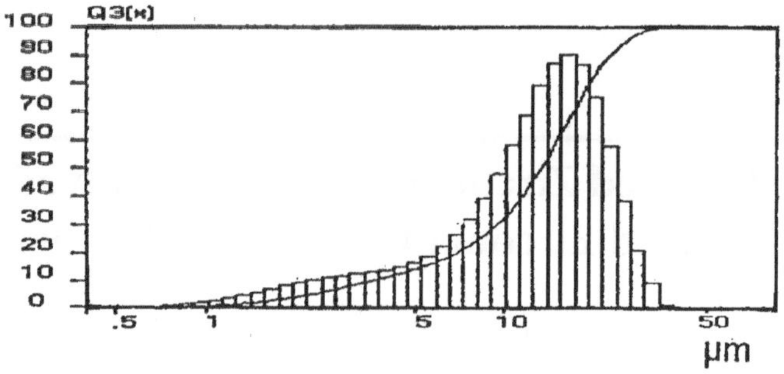

Fig. 1. Particle-size distribution of the ball-milled HA/YSZ mixture powders.

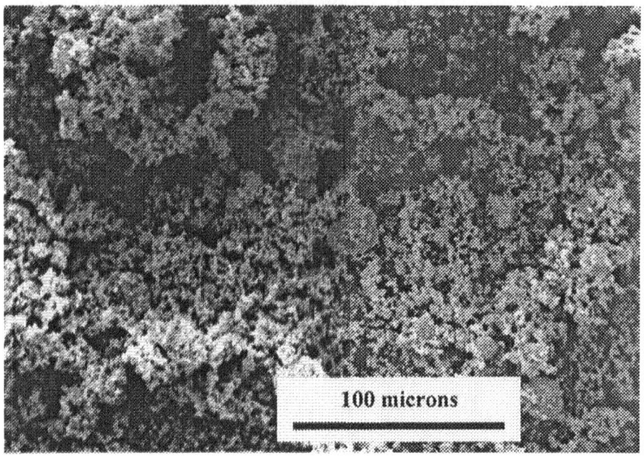

Fig. 2. Particle morphology of the as-milled composite powders.

Japan) equipped with an energy-dispersive X-ray unit was used to study the microstructure characteristics and the elemental analysis of the composite coatings.

A 2.54 cm diameter rod of titanium alloy was used for the measurement of the bond strength of the coatings per ASTM International standard C-633. For specimen preparation, one rod was sand-blasted and plasma sprayed with an HA/YSZ coating of 150 μm thickness. The coupling rod was also sand-blasted, glued with thermoplastic, and then joined under pressure in a fixture to the rod with HA/YSZ composite coating. The couples, cured at 98°C for an hour, were subjected to the tensile tests. A universal test machine (Model 5569, Instron, Canton, MA) was used to determine the tensile-bond strength of the coatings. The maximum force at full speed was 25 kN. The maximum speed at full load was 250 mm/min. For each testing material, five samples were used, and the bond strength data are reported as the average values.

The micro-hardness of the coating was determined using a micro-hardness tester (Model MHT, CSEM, Neuchâtel, Switzerland). The cross-sectional surface of the coating was used as the testing surface. The mean value of ten indentations was taken from the same coating. The Young's modulus of the coatings was obtained during the indentation of the coatings. The software, provided by the micro-hardness tester, calculated the Young's modulus in accordance with the relation from Oliver *et al.*[18] The fracture toughness, K_{IC}, of the composite coating can be calculated using[19,20]

$$K_{IC} = 0.016\left(\frac{E}{H}\right)^{0.5}\left(\frac{P}{C^{1.5}}\right) \quad (1)$$

where E is theYoung's modulus (in units of MPa), H is the Vickers's hardness (also in units of MPa), P is the load (in units of kg-f), and C is the sum of the half diagonal of the Vickers's indent and crack length (given in millimeters). The fracture toughness value and the Young's modulus were also the average of ten indentations.

III. Results and Discussion

(1) *Effects on the Phase Composition of HA/YSZ Composite Coatings*

Figure 4 shows the XRD patterns of the as-sprayed coatings obtained at an arc current of 1000 A: (a) XRD pattern with 10 wt% ZrO_2 addition, (b) pattern with 30 wt% ZrO_2 addition, (c) 50 wt% ZrO_2 addition. Referring to the XRD patterns, the coating with 50 wt% ZrO_2 consisted of ZrO_2, HA, amorphous phase, and a trace of CaO; at 30 wt% ZrO_2, the main phases were ZrO_2, HA, and amorphous phase with a small amount of CaO, $Ca_3(PO_4)_2$ (TCP), $Ca_4P_2O_9$ (TTCP), and a trace of $CaZrO_3$; at 10 wt% ZrO_2, the phase compositions were ZrO_2, HA, CaO, TCP, and TTCP with a small amount of $CaZrO_3$. Tetragonal zirconia remained stable during plasma spraying. No other zirconia phase appeared after plasma spraying.

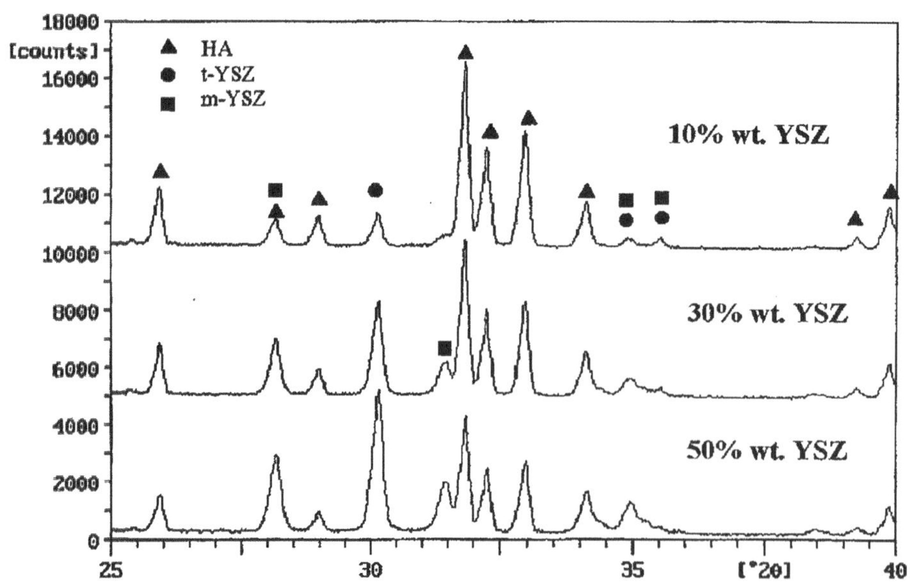

Fig. 3. XRD patterns of the HA/YSZ powders after ball milling.

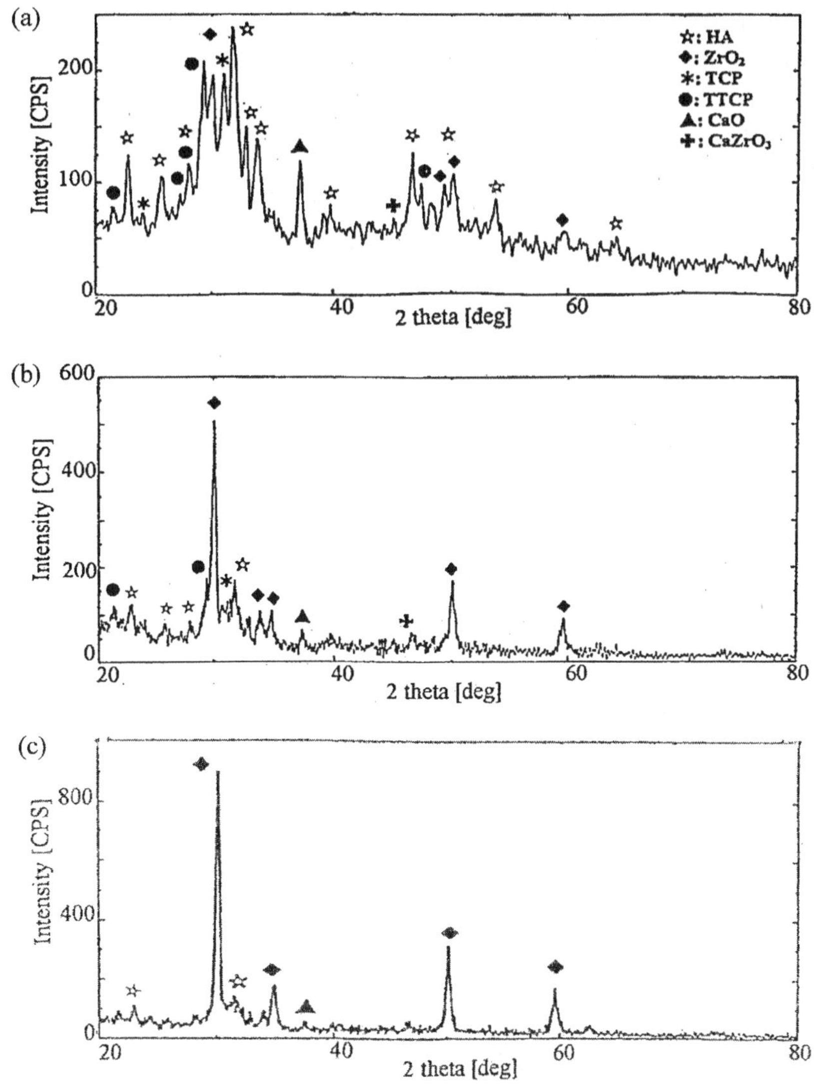

Fig. 4. XRD patterns of as-sprayed coatings obtained at an arc current of 1000 A (HA: $Ca_{10}(PO_4)_6(OH)_2$, ZrO_2: tetragonal zirconia, TCP: $Ca_3(PO_4)_2$, TTCP: $Ca_4P_2O_9$). (a) 10 wt% ZrO_2, (b) 30 wt% ZrO_2, (c) 50 wt% ZrO_2.

The experimental results showed that the addition of ZrO_2 reduced the presence of CaO detected by XRD after plasma spraying. There was a small amount (Fig. 4(c)) of CaO formed with the addition of 50 wt% ZrO_2. The coatings with 10 wt% ZrO_2 consisted of a considerable amount of CaO (Fig. 4(a)), *i.e.*, at the same plasma-spraying parameters, the more ZrO_2 added, the less the amount of CaO formed. Figure 4 also indicates that the addition of ZrO_2 decreases the formation of TTCP and TCP significantly. There was none or a trace amount of TCP; TTCP formed with specimens containing 50 wt% zirconia; and more TCP and TTCP formed in the coatings containing 10 wt% zirconia. The amount of TCP and TTCP increased with decreasing amounts of zirconia. XRD patterns showed that $CaZrO_3$ formed with the addition of 10 wt% zirconia, whereas there was no trace of $CaZrO_3$ in the composite coating containing 50 wt% zirconia. This indicates that increasing the content of zirconia results in decreasing the formation of $CaZrO_3$ in the coatings.

Investigating hot pressed and hot isostatic pressed bulk ZrO_2/HA composite at 1050°C, Ioku *et al.*[21] found that the CaO in HA diffuses into ZrO_2 to cause the tetragonal ZrO_2 to transform into cubic ZrO_2. The loss of CaO will then accelerate the decomposition of HA into β-TCP at >800°C. The reaction of their study is as follows:

$$\text{Y-ZrO}_2(\text{t}) + \text{Ca}_{10}(\text{PO}_4)_6(\text{OH})_2 \rightarrow \text{CaO doped Y-ZrO}_2(\text{c}) + 3\beta\text{-Ca}_3(\text{PO}_4)_2 + \text{H}_2\text{O} \quad (2)$$

Tamari *et al.*[22] hot pressed bulk materials at 1300°–1400°C and also found the transformation of tetragonal ZrO_2 into cubic ZrO_2 phase after sintering; however, α-TCP was the decomposition product rather than β-TCP. The following reactions occurred simultaneously:

$$\text{Ca}_{10}(\text{PO}_4)_6(\text{OH})_2 \rightarrow 3\alpha\text{-Ca}_3(\text{PO}_4)_2 + \text{CaO} + \text{H}_2\text{O} \quad (3)$$

$$\text{ZrO}_2(\text{t}) + \text{CaO} \rightarrow \text{CaO-doped ZrO}_2(\text{c}) \quad (4)$$

Wu and Yeh[23] indicated that HA will decompose into β-TCP, CaO, and ZrO_2 will further react with CaO to produce a new phase of $CaZrO_3$. Chang *et al.*[24] studied plasma spraying of YSZ-reinforced HA composite coatings. The maximum zirconia addition in their study was 10 wt%. The result showed that ZrO_2 reacted with CaO in HA to form $CaZrO_3$ and accelerated HA decomposition to α-TCP and TTCP during plasma spraying. The reactions were assumed as

$$\text{Ca}_{10}(\text{PO}_4)_6(\text{OH})_2 + \text{ZrO}_2 \rightarrow \text{CaO-poor Ca}_{10}(\text{PO}_4)_6(\text{OH})_2 + \text{CaZrO}_3 + \text{H}_2\text{O} \quad (5)$$

$$\text{CaO-poor Ca}_{10}(\text{PO}_4)_6(\text{OH})_2 \rightarrow \alpha\text{-Ca}_3(\text{PO}_4)_2 + \text{Ca}_4\text{P}_2\text{O}_9 + \text{H}_2\text{O} \quad (6)$$

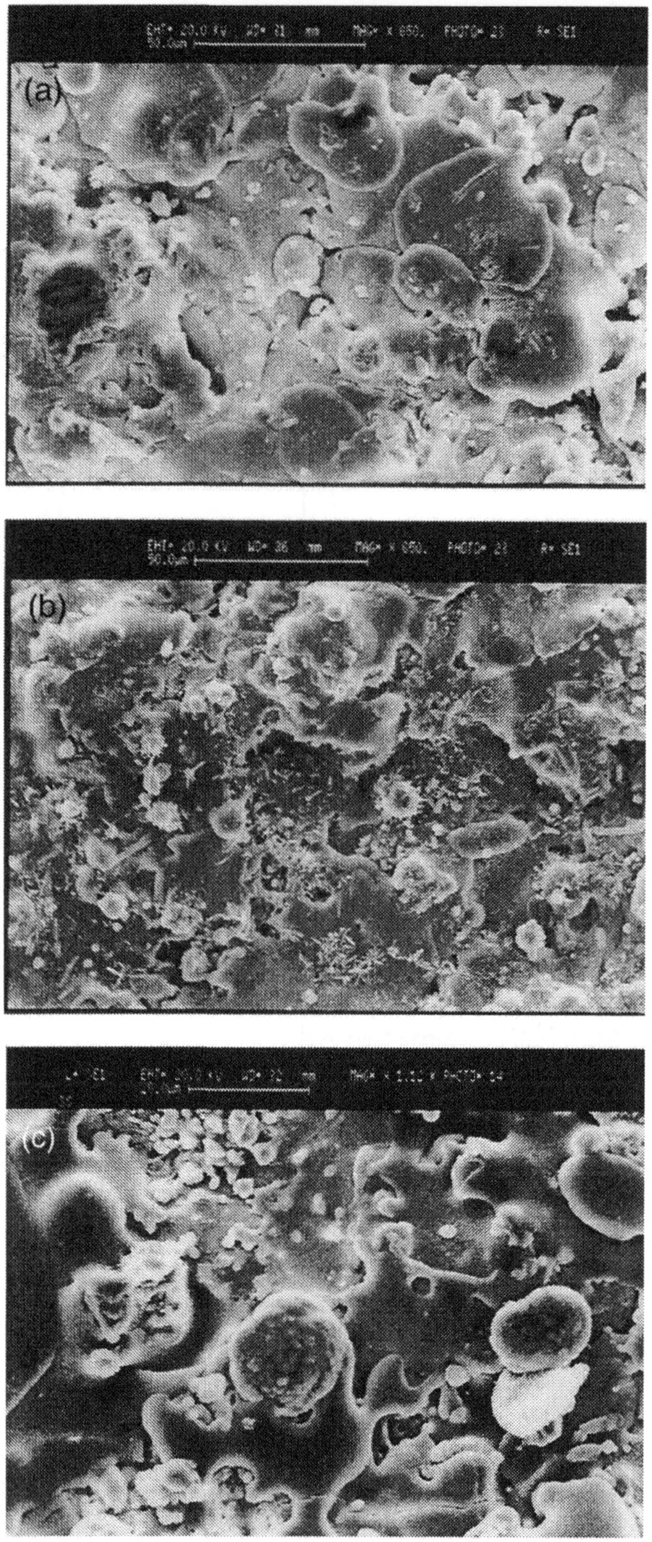

Fig. 5. Surface morphologies measured by SEM of plasma-sprayed HA/YSZ composite coatings. (a) 10 wt% ZrO_2, (b) 30 wt% ZrO_2, (c) 50 wt% ZrO_2.

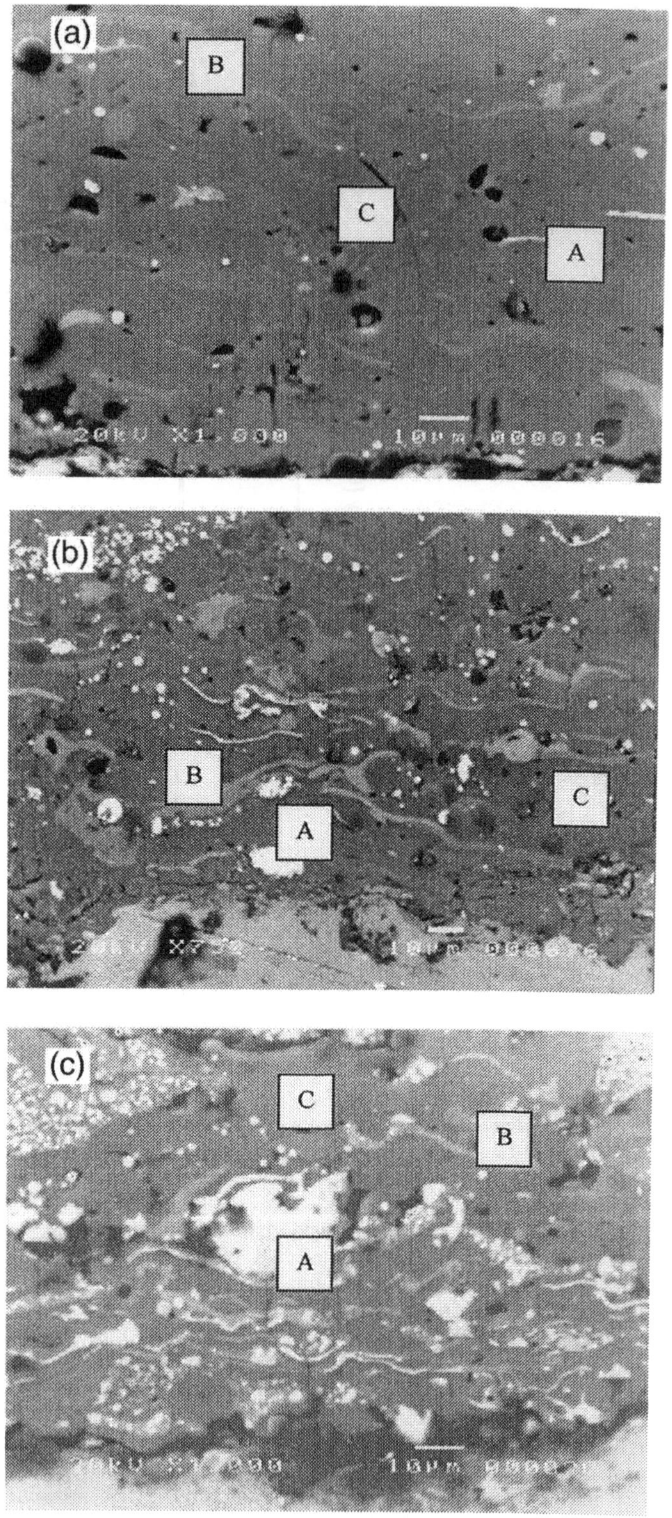

Fig. 6. Cross-sectional microstructures of HA/YSZ composite coatings. (a) 10 wt% ZrO_2, (b) 30 wt% ZrO_2, (c) 50 wt% ZrO_2.

Direct reaction between HA and ZrO_2 was also assumed to occur during plasma spraying:

$$Ca_{10}(PO_4)_6(OH)_2 + ZrO_2 \rightarrow \alpha\text{-}Ca_3(PO_4)_2 + CaZrO_3 + H_2O \quad (7)$$

In contrast to the previous works[19–21] and plasma-sprayed HA coatings with <10 wt% zirconia,[24] the present study of plasma spraying HA/YSZ composite coatings with zirconia addition in the range of 10–50 wt% found that CaO, α-TCP, and the TTCP phase in the coatings could be reduced by increasing the amount of zirconia. Meanwhile, some $CaZrO_3$ appeared in the coatings with the addition of less zirconia. We assumed that two steps had taken place during plasma spraying: The first was that the Ca dissolved into the zirconia to form a solid solution. This dissolution caused the crystalline HA to transform into an amorphous phase. The second step was that HA decomposed to form CaO, which reacted with ZrO_2 to form $CaZrO_3$, TCP, and TTCP. The first step played

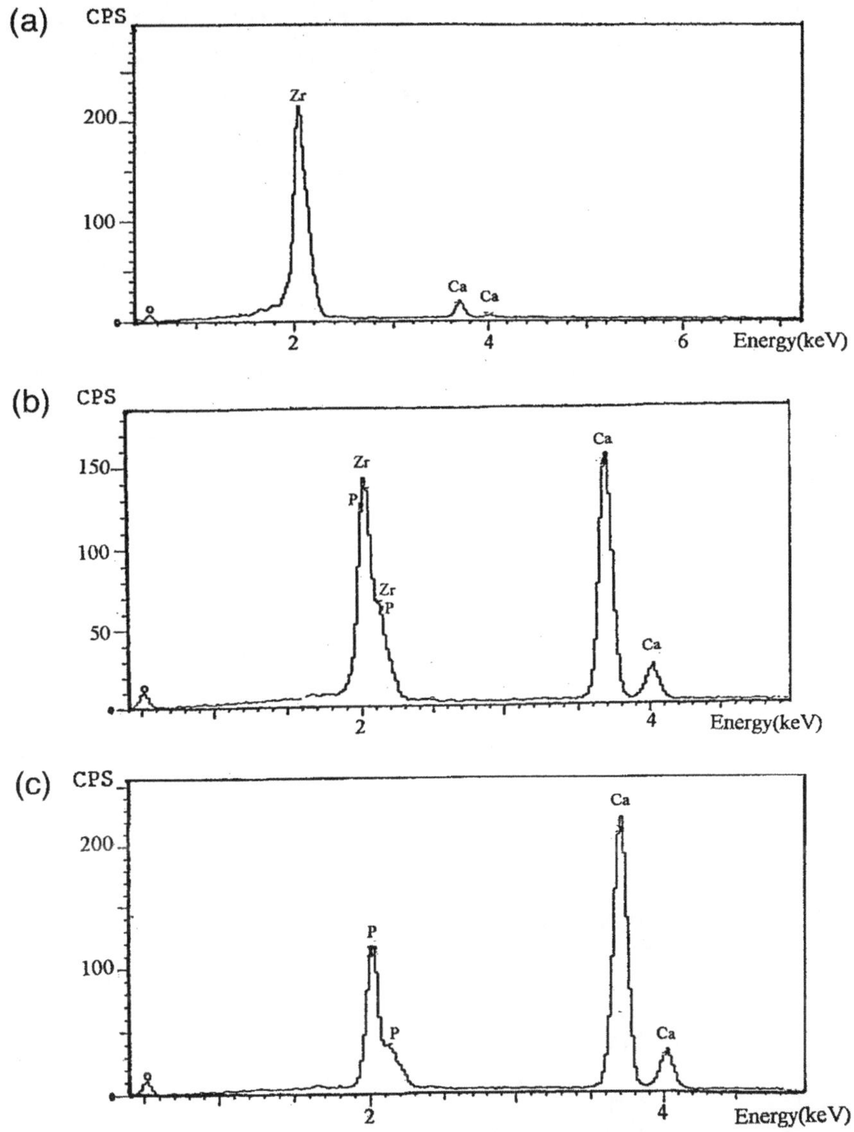

Fig. 7. Elemental analysis as measured by EDX (30 wt% ZrO_2 sample). (a) Region A (white region), (b) Region B (gray region), (c) Region C) (dark region).

an important role in plasma spraying. Because the particles' resident time in the high-temperature plasma was quite short, there was insufficient time for the HA to decompose after the Ca dissolution in zirconia. The higher the amount of zirconia addition, the greater the dissolution of HA. At the same time, more crystalline HA transformed to amorphous calcium phosphate. $CaZrO_3$ formation came from the reaction between CaO and ZrO_2 instead of the direct reaction between HA and ZrO_2. This can be inferred from the XRD results of the coatings with different amounts of zirconia (Fig. 4). If $CaZrO_3$ came from the direct reaction between HA and ZrO_2, $CaZrO_3$ should be formed more at 50 wt% zirconia, and the amount of $CaZrO_3$ in 50 wt% zirconia should be higher than that in 10 wt% zirconia. In fact, no $CaZrO_3$ formed with the addition of 50 wt% zirconia, and more $CaZrO_3$ appeared in coatings containing 10 wt% zirconia along with more content of CaO formation.

With the addition of zirconia, the additional reactions besides the HA decomposition occurring during plasma spraying are assumed to be

$$Ca_{10}(PO_4)_6(OH)_2 + ZrO_2 \rightarrow Ca_{10}(PO_4)_6O\text{-doped } ZrO_2 + H_2O \quad (8)$$

$$CaO + ZrO_2 \rightarrow CaZrO_3 \quad (9)$$

Equation (8) plays an important role in the reaction during plasma spraying when more zirconia was added to HA. Equation (9) occurs at a lower content of zirconia.

(2) *Effects on the Microstructure of HA/YSZ*

The surface morphologies of plasma-sprayed HA/YSZ composite coatings are shown in Fig. 5. The HA/YSZ composite coatings contain more unmelted small particles with increasing amounts of zirconia. The SEM cross-sectional microstructure in Fig. 6 (back-scattering electron images) shows the addition of zirconia causes an increase in porosity of the coatings. The rationale of higher porosity and more unmelted particles of ZrO_2-added coatings is supposed to be caused by either the higher melting point of ZrO_2 (2680°C) or the lower thermal conductivity (~1 W/mK), while the melting point of HA is ~1670°C. As the content of ZrO_2 increases, the heat of the plasma flame might be insufficient to melt the ZrO_2 powders completely. If the zirconia is melted completely with the use of higher power levels, it will cause more hydroxyapatite to decompose into CaO and other calcium phosphates. The CaO is an undesirable phase in the medical implants.

It can be seen from Fig. 6 that the solid solution with different gradient gray regions formed with the zirconia addition. The

Table I. Mechanical Properties of HA/YSZ Composite Coatings

ZrO_2 content (wt%)	Young's modulus (GPa)	Fracture toughness ($MPa{\cdot}m^{1/2}$)	Tensile bond strength (MPa)
0			19.36 ± 1.48
10	34.93 ± 2.14	0.92 ± 0.02	22.47 ± 2.31
30	40.36 ± 2.49	1.12 ± 0.02	27.32 ± 1.73
50	44.50 ± 3.73	1.50 ± 0.03	32.15 ± 2.54

higher the content of zirconia, the more the formation of the solid solution. The solid solution formed during plasma spraying, whereas the molten zirconia mixed with different content of molten HA to form the gray regions.The solid solution mixture of HA and zirconia improved the mechanical properties of the composite coatings. Figure 7 shows the EDX element analysis results from white region to dark region. It identified that the white region where the main elements are zirconium and oxygen represents zirconia; the dark region containing the elements of calcium, phosphorous, and oxygen represents the hydroxyapatite; and the gray region with elements of calcium, phosphorous, zirconium, and oxygen represents the solid solution of HA/ZrO_2.

(3) Effects on the Mechanical Properties

The effects of the additions of zirconia on the mechanical properties of HA/YSZ coatings such as tensile-bond strength, fracture toughness, and Young's modulus are shown in Table I. The coatings in Table I are sprayed at the same processing parameters.

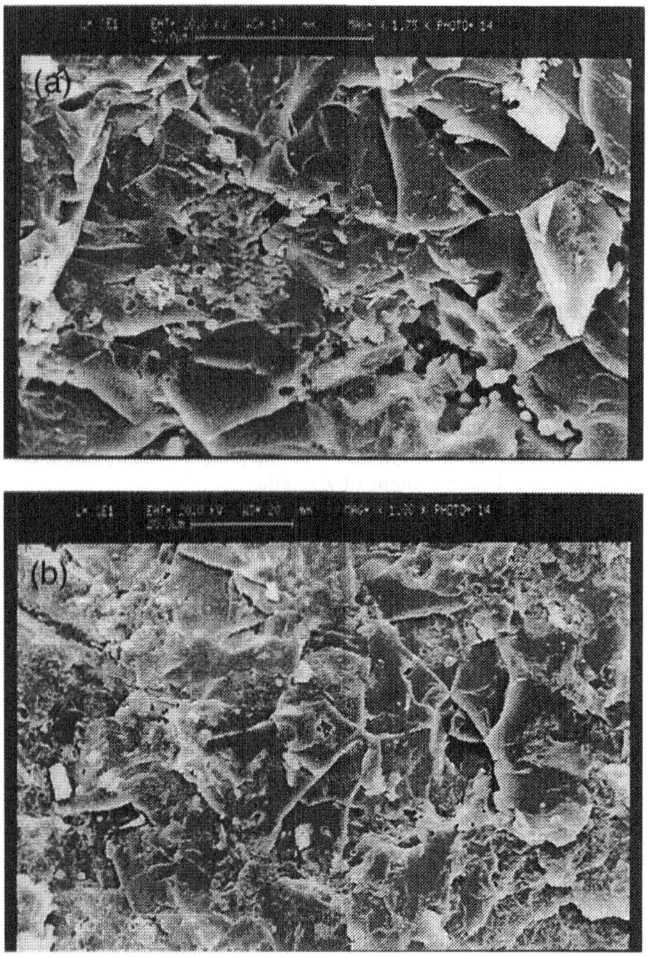

Fig. 8. Fracture surface morphologies after bond strength test. (a) 10 wt% ZrO_2, (b) 50 wt% ZrO_2.

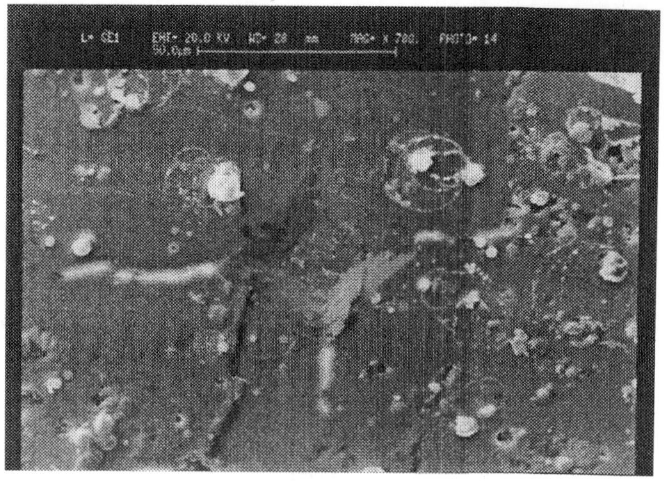

Fig. 9. Vickers's indent and induced microcracks in 10 wt% ZrO_2 composite coating.

HA coating shows the lowest bond strength, and 50 wt% zirconia composite coating shows the highest bond strength. The bond strength of the composite coating has been improved by the addition of zirconia and increases with an increase in zirconia content. The tensile fracture surface of the composite coating was investigated by SEM (Fig. 8), which showed that the failure during tensile tests occurred at the coating layer, instead of the interface between the substrate and coating. There is a different amount of unmelted zirconia particles for the coatings with different zirconia additions at the fracture surface, and the amount of unmelted zirconia particles increases with the addition of more zirconia. The molten state of the coating with 10 wt% ZrO_2 is better than that with 50 wt% ZrO_2. This is consistent with the results discussed in the effects on the microstructure, which identifies that the unmelted particles will be the potential weakness of the HA/YSZ composite coatings. The molten state of the zirconia should be improved as much as possible to achieve higher bond strength of the coatings. It can be deduced from the tensile fracture surface that the bond strength of the composite coating at the interface of substrate and coating is higher than the values shown in Table I.

Figure 9 shows a typical Vickers's indent in a 10 wt% zirconia composite coating. The microcracks induced by the indentation load were observed by SEM. The length of each microcrack (the flaring line from the square corner) can be measured, and the average length of the indent can be obtained and used to calculate the fracture toughness according to the formula (Eq. (1)). The relationship between the fracture toughness and zirconia content, the Young's modulus, and zirconia content is also shown in Table I. It can be inferred that the fracture toughness and the Young's modulus of the composite coatings increased with the zirconia content. The more zirconia added, the higher the fracture toughness and Young's modulus achieved.

The results of the bond strength, the fracture toughness, and the Young's modulus of HA/YSZ composite coatings show that the mechanical properties of the composite coatings can be improved by the addition of zirconia, although there are more unmelted particles in the coatings with higher zirconia contents, indicating that the positive effect of toughening by zirconia outweighs the negative effect of increased porosity and unmelted zirconia particles. The molten state of the zirconia powders plays an important role in the improvement of the mechanical properties of HA/YSZ composite coatings.

IV. Conclusions

Studies have been made of the effects of yttria-stabilized zirconia on the phase composition, microstructure, mechanical properties such as bond strength, fracture toughness, and Young's modulus of HA/ZrO_2 composite coatings. The main phases of as-sprayed coatings were hydroxyapatite, tetragonal ZrO_2, and CaO, TCP, TTCP, or $CaZrO_3$, depending on the zirconia content. The results indicated that the content of phases CaO, TCP, and TTCP decreased with increasing amounts of zirconia from 10–50 wt%. Some ZrO_2 reacted with CaO decomposed from the HA with <30 wt% zirconia to form $CaZrO_3$. Tetragonal ZrO_2 remained stable during the plasma spraying. Some HA mixed with the zirconia to form solid solution during plasma spraying. The amounts of unmelted zirconia particles and the porosity of the composite coating increased with increasing amounts of zirconia. The mechanical properties of HA/ZrO_2 composite coatings such as bond strength, fracture toughness, and Young's modulus have been improved significantly with the increase of zirconia. All the failure of the bond strength tests occurred at the coating layer, instead of at the interface of the substrate and coating. The fracture surface indicated that the molten state of zirconia particles plays an important role in increasing the mechanical properties of the HA/YSZ composite coatings. The advantageous effects of toughening outweigh the adverse effect of increased porosity and unmelted particles associated with the incorporation of ZrO_2.

References

[1]K. A. Khor and P. Cheang, "Effects of Powder Feedstock on Thermal Sprayed Hydroxyapatite Coatings"; pp. 147–52, *Proceedings of the 7th National Thermal Spray Conference*, June 20–24, Boston, MA. Edited by C.C Berndt and S. Sampath. ASM International, Materials Park, OH, 1994.

[2]L. Erick, F. Thomas, and K. Michael, "Production of Biocompatible Coatings of Hydroxyapatite and Flourapatite"; *Thermal Spray Technology*, pp. 337–43. Edited by D. L. Houck. ASM International, Materials Park, OH, 1989.

[3]A. Osaka, Y. Miura, K. Takeuchi, M. Asada, and K. Takahashi, "Calcium Hydroxyapatite Prepared from Calcium Hydroxide and Othorphosphoric Acid," *J. Mater. Sci.: Mater. Med.*, **2**, 51–55 (1991).

[4]V. V. Silva and R. Z. Domingues, "Hydroxyapatite-Zirconia Composites Prepared by Precipitation Method," *J. Mater. Sci.: Mater. Med.*, **8**, 907–10 (1997).

[5]J. Li, H. Liao, and L. Hermansson, "Sintering of Partially-Stabilized Zirconia and Partially-Stabilized-Hydroxyapatite Composites by Hot Isostatic Pressing and Pressureless Sintering," *Biomaterials*, **17**, 1787–90 (1996).

[6]H. X. Ji and P. M. Marquis, "Sintering Behavior of Hydroxyapatite Reinforced with 20 wt % Al_2O_3," *J. Mater. Sci.: Mater. Med.*, **28**, 1940–45 (1993).

[7]H. X. Ji and P. M. Marquis, "Preparation and Characterization of Al_2O_3 Reinforced Hydroxyapatite," *Biomaterials*, **13** [11] 744–48 (1992).

[8]A. Ravaglioli and A. Krajewski, *Bioceramics: Materials, Properties and Applications*. Chapman and Hall, New York,1992.

[9]J. F. Kay, T. S. Goles, and R. L. Riley, "Hydroxyapatite Coated Subperiosteal Dental Implants: Design Rationale and Clinical Experience," *J. Prosthet. Dent.*, **58**, 339–43 (1987).

[10]K. de Groot, R. Gesink, C. P. A. T. Klein, and P. Serekian, "Plasma-Sprayed Coatings of Hydroxyapatite," *J. Biomed. Mater. Res.*, **21**, 1375–81 (1987).

[11]J. F. Kay and T. C. May, "Stable HA Coatings for Non-Precision Implant Placements"; pp. 302, *Proceedings of Fourth World Biomaterials Congress*. Berlin, Germany, April 24–28, 1992.

[12]J. A. Jansen, J. P. C. M. Van de Waerdan, J. G. C. Wolke, K. de Groot, "Histologic Evaluation of the Osseous Adaptation to Titanium and Hydroxyapatite-Coated Titanium Implants," *J. Biomed Mater. Res.*, **25**, 972–89 (1991).

[13]S. D. Cook, K. A. Thomas, J. F. Kay, and M. Jarcho, "Hydroxyapatite-Coated Titanium for Orthopaedic Implant Application," *Clin. Orthop.*, **232**, 225–43 (1988).

[14]W. J. A. Dhert, C. Klein, J. Wolke, and K. de Groot, "A Mechanical Investigation of Fluorapatite, Magnestium Whitlockite and Hydroxyapatite Plasma Sprayed Coatings in Goats," *J. Biomed. Mater. Res.*, **25**, 1183–1200 (1991).

[15]P. Ducheyne, J. Cuckler, S. Radin, and E. Nazar, *CRC Handbook of Bioactive Ceramics*; pp. 123–31. Edited by T. Yamamuro, L. L. Hench, and J. Wilson. CRC Press, Boca Raton, FL, 1990.

[16]E. Chang, W. J. Chang, B. C. Wang, and C. Y. Yang, "Plasma Spraying of Zirconia Reinforced Hydroxyapatite Composite on Titanium Part I: Phase, Microstructure and Bonding Strength," *J. Mater. Sci.: Mater. Med.*, **8**, 193–200 (1997).

[17]E. Chang, W. J. Chang, B. C. Wang, and C. Y. Yang, "Plasma Spraying of Zirconia Reinforced Hydroxyapatite Composite Coatings on Titanium, Part II: Dissolution Behavior in Simulated Body Fluid and Bonding Degradation," *J. Mater. Sci.: Mater. Med.*, **8**, 201–11 (1997).

[18]W. C. Oliver and G. M. Pharr, "An Improvement Technique for Determining Hardness and Elastic Modulus Using Load and Depth Displacement Sensing Indentation Experiments," *J. Mater. Res.*, **7** [6] 1564–83 (1992).

[19]G. R Anstis, P. Chantikul, B. R. Lawn, and D. B. Marshall, "A Critical Evaluation of Indentation Techniques for Measuring Fracture Toughness: Indirect Crack Measurement," *J. Am. Ceram. Soc.*, **64**, 533–38 (1981).

[20]G. K. Beshish, C. W. Florey, F. J. Worzala, and W. J. Lenling, "Fracture Toughness of Thermal Spray Ceramic Coatings Determined by Indentation Technique," *J. Therm. Spray Tech.*, **2**, 1–6 (1993).

[21]K. Ioku, S. Somiya, and M. Yoshimura, "Hydroxyapatite Ceramics with Tetragonal Zirconia Particle Dispersion Prepared by HIP Post-Sintering," *J. Ceram. Soc. Jpn.*, **99**, 13–20 (1991).

[22]N. Tamari, M. Mouri, and I. Kondo, "Mechanical Properties and Existing Phases of Composite Ceramics Obtained by Sintering of a Mixture of Hydroxyapatite and Zirconia," *J. Jpn. Ceram. Soc.*, **95**, 806–809 (1987).

[23]J. M. Wu and T. S. Yeh, "Sintering of Hydroxylapatite-Zirconia Composite Materials," *J. Mater. Sci.*, **23**, 3771–77 (1988). □

J. Am. Ceram. Soc., **85** [5] 1318–20 (2002)

Preparation of a Bioactive Poly(methyl methacrylate)/Silica Nanocomposite

Sang-Hoon Rhee*,†

Korea Research Institute of Chemical Technology, Daejeon 305-600, Korea

Je-Yong Choi

Kyungpook National University, Daegu 700-422, Korea

The nanocomposite of a poly(methyl methacrylate)/silica containing calcium salt was synthesized through the sol–gel method. Methyl methacrylate was co-polymerized with 3-(trimethoxysilyl)propyl methacrylate and then co-condensed with tetraethyl orthosilicate and calcium nitrate tetrahydrate. Low crystalline hydroxycarbonate apatite was successfully formed on the surface after soaking in simulated body fluid for 1 week at 36.5°C. This study demonstrates that this nanocomposite may be used as a bioactive bone substitute or filler for poly(methyl methacrylate) bone cement.

I. Introduction

Poly(methyl methacrylate) (PMMA) is a representative material used as a bone cement because of its self-hardening property and excellent mechanical properties compared with other polymers. However, the application is almost restricted to bone cement because of its bio-inertness; no chemical or biological bonding occurs at the interface between the PMMA and bone, causing wear debris of PMMA from repeated interfacial movement.[1] This causes osteolysis and subsequent loosening of an implant.[2]

Many researchers, therefore, have attempted to give osteoconductivity to the PMMA bone cement by introducing bioactive ceramic fillers.[3–7] However, the interfacial strength between bioactive ceramic filler and the PMMA is of concern because of the lack of adhesion between the two phases, resulting in an early failure at the interface. In addition, the size of the ceramic filler used for this purpose is several tens of micrometers, so its distribution in the composite is inhomogeneous and exposure to the surface becomes small. This reduces the osteoconducting ability of PMMA with ceramic filler.

The improvement of the adhesion between the ceramic fillers and the PMMA could be achieved using a silane coupling agent;[5,6] however, the increase of bioactive ceramic fillers exposed on the surface could not be achieved through this method. Therefore, if the nanometer-sized bioactive ceramics can be dispersed homogeneously and bonded covalently to the PMMA at the molecular level, all problems are likely to be solved.

In the present investigation, a PMMA/silica nanocomposite made via the sol–gel reaction with methylmethacrylate (MMA), tetraethyl orthosilicate (TEOS), and 3-(trimethoxysilyl)propyl methacrylate (MSMA) as a coupling agent was re-examined with the main focus on its use as a bioactive bone substitute. Because of its superior mechanical properties of the nanocomposite, applications as a biomaterial have already been reported; there have been feasibility tests as filler for PMMA bone cement[8] and resin for dental applications.[9,10] However, these studies were not aimed at giving and using bioactivity, but simply using its superior mechanical properties to single PMMA.

In this study, a PMMA/silica nanocomposite was designed to produce the low crystalline hydroxy carbonate apatite (HCA) on its surface in the simulated body fluid (SBF) using the silanol group as a nucleation site and calcium salt as a promoter for the nucleation of HCA via the increase of ionic activity product.

II. Experimental Procedure

The trimethoxysilyl functionalized polymethylmethacrylate was prepared by free radical polymerization of 3-(trimethoxysilyl)propyl methacrylate (MSMA) with methyl methacrylate (MMA) using benzoyl peroxide (BPO) as an initiator.[11] The content of MSMA in the copolymer was 20 mol%. The MMA and MSMA were mixed for 1 h using dry toluene as a solvent. The BPO (0.01 mol%) was added to the solution and, subsequently, free radical polymerization was performed at 70°C. After mixing for 24 h, the copolymer was purified via repeated precipitation in dry hexane. Hereafter, the poly(methylmethacrylate-co-3-(trimethoxysilyl)propyl methacrylate) will be referred to as PMCM.

The PMCM was hydrolyzed and co-condensed with tetraethyl orthosilicate (TEOS) with HCl as a catalyst to yield hybrid sol–gel material. The TEOS solution was prepared by mixing tetrahydrofuran (THF), water, and calcium nitrate tetrahydrate (CNT) for 1 h. The molar ratio of TEOS:water:HCl:CNT was 1:3:0.01:0.15. Hereafter, this solution will be referred to as solution T. The PMCM powder was dissolved in the THF with a concentration of 20 wt%. Hereafter, this solution will be referred to as solution P. Solutions T and P were mixed for 1 h at room temperature and then poured into a Teflon mold. The gel was slowly dried for 1 week and then dried again under vacuum at 30°C for 48 h. The pure PMMA was also made for comparison through the free radical polymerization with the same method described. Hereafter, the pure PMMA and the PMMA/silica nanocomposite will be referred to as specimens P and S, respectively.

The test of the bioactivity was performed in the SBF[12] that has almost the same ion concentrations as human blood plasma.[13] Disk-shaped specimens (10 mm in diameter × 1 mm thick) were soaked in 30 mL of the SBF at 36.5°C for 1 week. After soaking, the specimens were removed from the fluid and gently rinsed with ion-exchanged distilled water and then dried at room temperature.

S. Sakka—contributing editor

Manuscript No. 187606. Received August 20, 2001; approved December 27, 2001.
This work was supported by the Intellectual Bio-interface Engineering Center (IBEC) of the Korea Science and Engineering Foundation (KOSEF) of the Korean government.

*Member, American Ceramic Society.
†Author to whom correspondence should be addressed.

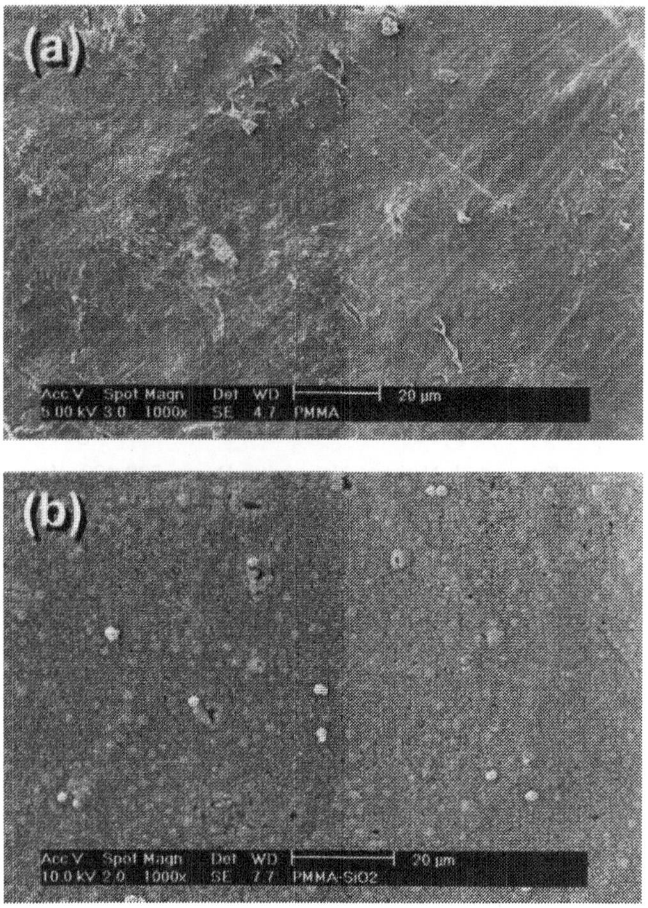

Fig. 1. Microstructures of specimens (a) P and (b) S after soaking in simulated body fluids at 36.5°C for one week.

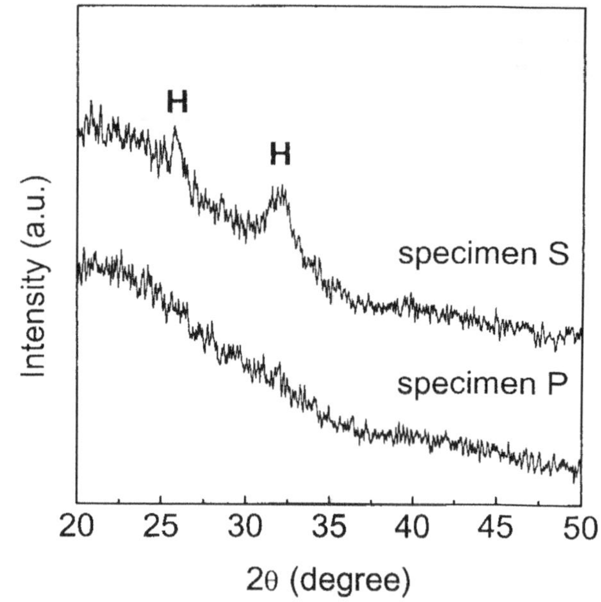

Fig. 2. Thin-film XRD results for specimens P and S after soaking in the simulated body fluids at 36.5°C for one week.

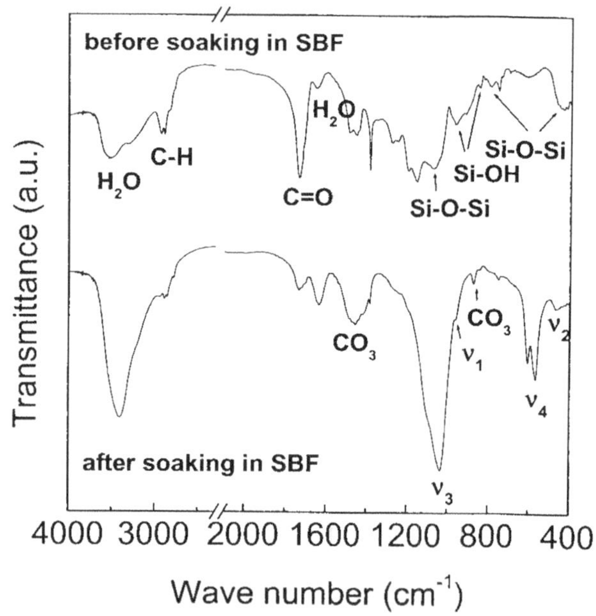

Fig. 3. FT-IR transmission spectra for specimen S before and after soaking in simulated body fluids at 36.5°C for one week.

The surface microstructures and crystal phase formed on the specimens were analyzed by field emission scanning electron microscopy (FE-SEM; XL30S, Philips Electron Optics, Eindhoven, The Netherlands) and thin film X-ray diffractometry (TF-XRD), respectively, with an angle of 1° to the direction of the incident X-ray beam. For infrared spectroscopy measurements, the pulverized specimens were diluted with 100-fold KBr powder (Spectra Tech, Shelton, CT) and the background noise was corrected with pure KBr data. The ionic concentrations of calcium, phosphorous, and silicon in the SBF were measured with inductively coupled plasma atomic emission spectroscopy (Ultima-C, Jovin-Yvon, Yvon, France) after soaking specimen S for 1 week.

III. Results and Discussions

Figure 1 shows the microstructures of specimens P and S after soaking in the SBF at 36.5°C for 1 week. A relatively rough surface with some cracks, which is believed to have resulted from the swelling of the PMMA, was observed in specimen P. However, a low crystalline HCA layer as described later was observed to form on the surface of specimen S.

Figure 2 shows the TF-XRD profiles measured for specimens P and S after soaking in the SBF at 36.5°C for 1 week. No specific peaks assigned to apatite were observed in specimen P, while two apatite peaks, denoted by "H," were observed in specimen S. Because the apatite peaks were comparatively broader than a normal apatite, it was inferred that the grown apatite crystals had low crystallinity.

Figure 3 shows the FT-IR spectra measured for specimen S before and after soaking in the SBF. The Si–O–Si band was observed at 1075, 791, 434 cm^{-1}, and the Si–OH band was observed at 960 and 845 cm^{-1} before soaking in the SBF.[14] The asymmetrical stretching (ν_3) and bending (ν_4) modes of the PO_4 ion were detected at ~1039, 602, and 564 cm^{-1}, respectively, after soaking in the SBF for 1 week. The symmetric stretching modes (ν_1 and ν_2) of the PO_4 ion were also found at ~960 and 462 cm^{-1}, respectively. Further, two stretching modes and an out-of-plane mode of CO_3 ion were also observed at ~1456, 1419, and 876 cm^{-1}, respectively. This means that the PO_4 sites of the apatite structure, i.e., B-site, were partly substituted by carbonate ions.

The initial ionic concentrations of calcium, phosphorus, and silicon in the SBF were 100.20, 30.94, and 0.00 ppm, respectively. However, these concentrations became 123.33 ± 2.31, 4.31 ± 0.07, and 15.27 ± 0.06 ppm, respectively, after soaking for 1 week. The increase of ionic concentrations of calcium and silicon after soaking originated from their release from specimen S, while the decrease of ionic concentration of phosphorous might be the result of the formation of the HCA layer (Figs. 1(b) and 2).

From the above results, it can be presumed that the formation of the HCA layer is critically dependent on the silanol group and the release of calcium ion from the nanocomposite, because the HCA was not formed in the pure PMMA (Figs. 1(a) and 2). For an explanation of the nucleation and growth of the HCA layer observed in this work, the nucleation model of bioglass[2] or bioglass ceramics[15] is quite appropriate.

When the PMMA/silica nanocomposite containing calcium salt is soaked into the SBF, calcium ion is dissolved into the SBF and it produces the silanol group on the surface by exchange of the Ca^{2+} ion combined with the Si–O^- group in the sample with H_3O^+ ion in the SBF. In addition, the release of Ca^{2+} ions increases ionic activity product of apatite in the SBF, so it promotes the nucleation of HCA on the silanol group.[16] Once the apatite nuclei are formed, they grow spontaneously because the SBF itself has already been supersaturated with respect to apatite.[17] The mechanical and biological assays of this nanocomposite are under investigation and will be published in the near future.

IV. Conclusions

The nanocomposite of poly(methyl methacrylate)/silica was synthesized via the sol–gel method. Its bioactivity was assessed using the SBF and low crystalline HCA was successfully formed on its surface after soaking for 1 week at 36.5°C. The formation mechanism of the low crystalline HCA was similar to that on the bioglass. This nanocomposite is likely to be useful for a bone substitute or filler for PMMA bone cement because of its bioactivity.

References

[1]G. Lewis, "Properties of Acrylic Bone Cement: State of the Art Review," *J. Biomed. Mater. Res., Appl. Biomater.*, **38**, 155–82 (1997).

[2]L. L. Hench, "Bioceramics," *J. Am. Ceram. Soc.*, **81** [7] 1705–28 (1998).

[3]W. F. Mousa, M. Kobayashi, S. Shinzato, M. Kamimura, S. Yoshihara, I. A. Zeineldin, and T. Nakamura, "Biological and Mechanical Properties of Commercial PMMA Bone Cements Containing AW–GC Filler"; pp. 545–48 in *Bioceramics*, Vol. 12. Edited by H. Ohgushi, G. W. Hastings, and T. Yoshikawa. World Scientific Publishing Co. Pte., Ltd., Nara, Japan, 1999.

[4]W. Hennig, B. A. Blencke, H. Brömer, K. K. Deutscher, A. Gross, and W. Ege, "Investigations with Bioactivated Polymethylmethacrylate," *J. Biomed. Mater. Res.*, **13**, 89–99 (1979).

[5]J. T. Heikkilä, A. J. Aho, I. Kangasniemi, and A. Yli-Upro, "Polymethylmethacrylate Composites: Disturbed Bone Formation at the Surface of Bioactive Glass and Hydroxyapatite," *Biomaterials*, **17**, 1755–60 (1996).

[6]W. F. Mousa, M. Kobayashi, S. Shinzato, M. Kamimura, M. Neo, S. Yoshihara, and T. Nakamura, "Biological and Mechanical Properties of PMMA-based Bioactive Bone Cement," *Biomaterials*, **21**, 2137–46 (2000).

[7]J. C. Behiri, M. Braden, S. Khorasani, D. Wiwattanadate, and W. Bonfiled, "Advanced Bone Cement for Long-Term Orthopedic Implantations"; pp. 301–307 in *Bioceramics*, Vol. 4. Edited by W. Bonfield, G. W. Hastings, and K. E. Tanner. Elsevier Science, London, U.K., 1991.

[8]J.-M. Yang, C.-S. Lu, Y.-G. Hsu, and C.-H. Shih, "Mechanical Properties of Acrylic Bone Cement Containing PMMA–SiO_2 Hybrid Sol–Gel Material," *J. Biomed. Mater. Res., Appl. Biomater.*, **38**, 143–54 (1997).

[9]Y. Wei and D. Jin, "A New Class of Organic-Inorganic Hybrid Dental Materials," *Polym. Prepr.*, **38** [2] 122–23 (1997).

[10]P. P. Paul, S. F. Timmons, and W. J. Machowski, "Organic-Inorganic Hybrid Dental Restorative Composites," *Polym. Prepr.*, **38**[2] 124, (1997).

[11]Y. Wei, D. Yang, and R. Bakthavatchalam, "Thermal Stability and Hardness of New Polyacrylate–SiO_2 Hybrid Sol–Gel Materials," *Mater. Lett.*, **13**, 261–66 (1992).

[12]T. Kokubo, H. Kushitani, S. Sakka, T. Kitusgi, and T. Yamamuro, "Solutions Able to Reproduce in Vivo Surface-Structure Changes in Bioactive Glass-Ceramic A-W," *J. Biomed. Mater. Res.*, **24**, 721–34 (1990).

[13]J. Gamble, *Chemical Anatomy, Physiology and Pathology of Extracellular Fluid*, 6th Ed.; pp.1–15. Harvard University Press, Cambridge, MA, 1967.

[14]X. Li and T. A. King, "Spectroscopic Studies of Sol–Gel-Derived Organically Modified Silicates," *J. Non-Cryst. Solids*, **204**, 235–42 (1996).

[15]T. Kokubo, H. Kushitani, C. Ohtsuki, S. Sakka, and T. Yamamuro, "Chemical Reaction of Bioactive Glass and Glass-Ceramics with a Simulated Body Fluid," *J. Mater. Sci. Mater. Med.*, **3**, 79–83 (1992).

[16]T. Kokubo, "Surface Chemistry of Bioactive Glass-Ceramics," *J. Non-Cryst. Solids*, **120**, 138–51 (1990).

[17]W. F. Neuman and M. W. Neuman, *The Chemical Dynamics of Bone Mineral*; p. 34. University of Chicago, Chicago, IL, 1958. □

journal

J. Am. Ceram. Soc., **85** [6] 1634–36 (2002)

Reaction Sintering and Mechanical Properties of Hydroxyapatite–Zirconia Composites with Calcium Fluoride Additions

Hae-Won Kim, Young-Hag Koh, Byung-Ho Yoon, and Hyoun-Ee Kim*

School of Materials Science and Engineering, Seoul National University, Seoul 151-742, Korea

The effects of calcium fluoride (CaF_2) additions on the densification and mechanical properties of hydroxyapatite–zirconia composites (HA–ZrO_2) were investigated. When small amount of CaF_2 was added, the density of the composites was markedly enhanced. The reactions of HA with CaF_2, which led to the formation of fluorapatite (FA), were attributed to the observed improvements in densification. When HA–20-vol%-ZrO_2 composites were sintered, with the addition of 5 vol% of CaF_2, in air at 1300°C, the density of the specimen approached 98% of the theoretical value. The flexural strength and fracture toughness of the composites were also improved, as a result of the enhanced densification.

I. Introduction

Hydroxyapatite (HA, $Ca_{10}(PO_4)_6(OH)_2$) ceramics have been widely used as substitute materials for human bone and teeth, because of their excellent biocompatibility.[1–3] However, their relatively low strength and fracture toughness have restricted wider applications. To overcome this limitation, reinforcing agents have been introduced, in the form of particles, platelets, and fibers, to form HA-based composites. Zirconia (ZrO_2) is one of the most widely used reinforcing agents, because of its superb strength and fracture toughness. However, when zirconia (ZrO_2) is added to HA, the temperature at which HA decomposes to tricalcium phosphate (TCP, $Ca_3(PO_4)_2$) is reduced, resulting in a detrimental effect on the densification and mechanical properties of the sintered bodies.[4]

Much effort has been exerted to overcome the reaction between HA and ZrO_2. Sintering in a wet atmosphere[5] or the addition of ZrO_2 particles coated with Al_2O_3[6] each has been effective in suppressing the reaction. However, in most cases, hot-pressing[6,7] or hot isostatic pressing (HIP)[4,8] processes, which have many technical and economic problems associated with them, still are necessary to obtain HA–ZrO_2 composites with high densities.

Even though fluorapatite (FA, $Ca_{10}(PO_4)_6F_2$) is known to have greater thermal and chemical stability than HA,[9–11] only a limited amount of research has been conducted on the sintering behavior and mechanical properties of FA and FA-based composites.[12] In this study, the stability of HA–ZrO_2 composites was determined to be enhanced by the formation of FA during the sintering process. This FA was formed via the addition of small amounts of CaF_2 to the HA–20-vol%-ZrO_2 system and sintering in air. The effect of these additions on the FA formation, densification, and mechanical properties of the HA–ZrO_2 composites was investigated.

N. Claussen—contributing editor

Manuscript No. 187572. Received July 20, 2001; approved February 25, 2002.
*Member, American Ceramic Society.

II. Experimental Procedures

High-purity HA (Alfa Aesar Co., Ward Hill, MA) and ZrO_2 (3Y-TZP, Tosho Co., Tokyo, Japan) powders were used to fabricate HA–20-vol%-ZrO_2 composites. CaF_2 in a range of concentrations (up to 10 vol%) was added, and the mixed powders were milled in ethanol for 24 h, using ZrO_2 balls as media. After milling, the mixtures were dried in a rotary vacuum evaporator, passed through a 70-mesh screen, cold isostatically pressed (CIPed) at 300 MPa, and then sintered in air at various temperatures (900°–1500°C) for 1 h. The heating rate was 10°C/min, and the cooling rate was normal furnace cooling.

The apparent porosity was measured using the Archimedes method. The microstructure of the specimens was observed via scanning electron microscopy (SEM) after the specimens were polished with diamond slurries down to a 1 μm finish. The composition of the specimens was characterized using X-ray diffraction (XRD) patterns. Lattice parameters were calculated from the XRD results that were obtained, using silicon standard powder, to investigate the structural changes that occur during the sintering process. The specimens for mechanical testing were machined into a bar shape with dimensions of 3 mm × 4 mm × 25 mm and polished with diamond slurries. The flexural strength was determined using a four-point flexural configuration with a crosshead speed of 0.5 mm/min, with inner and outer spans of 10 and 20 mm, respectively. The fracture toughness of the specimens was determined by the indentation-strength (I-S) method.[13] After the polished surface was indented with a Vickers indenter at a load of 49 N for 15 s, the fracture strength was measured using the previously mentioned four-point flexural configuration.

III. Results and Discussion

The densification behavior of the HA–20-vol%-ZrO_2 composites was markedly improved by small additions of CaF_2. Some typical microstructures of the specimens after sintering are shown in Fig. 1. When the composite was sintered in air at 1350°C for 1 h without CaF_2, the specimen exhibited poor densification, as shown in Fig. 1(A). However, when a small amount (5 vol%) of CaF_2 was added to the composite, the specimen displayed almost full density, as clearly illustrated in Fig. 1(B). The effect of CaF_2 on the densification of the HA–ZrO_2 composite is quantitatively shown in Fig. 2. Without CaF_2, the apparent porosity of the composite after sintering at 1350°C was >30%. Even though densification of the composite began to occur actively at temperatures of >1400°C, HA was seriously degraded through decomposition to TCP, as will be discussed later. However, the addition of CaF_2 allowed the HA–ZrO_2 body to attain full densification; moreover, the densification temperature steadily decreased as the amounts of CaF_2 increased.

The role of CaF_2 in the HA–ZrO_2 composites was analyzed using XRD patterns, as shown in Fig. 3. When the composite without any CaF_2 was sintered at temperatures of >1100°C, strong β-TCP and $CaZrO_3$ peaks were observed, at the expense of HA

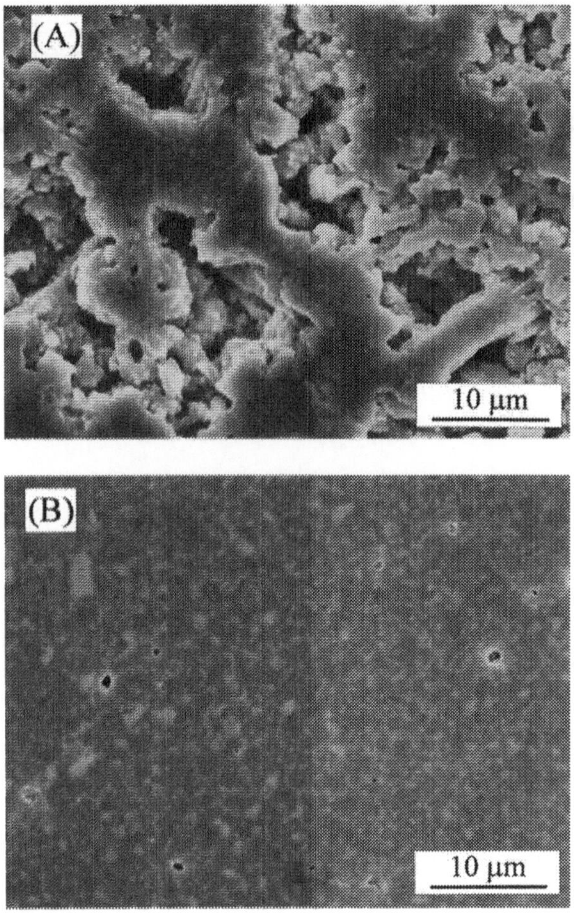

Fig. 1. SEM images showing the microstructure evolution of HA–20-vol%-ZrO_2 composites after sintering at 1350°C for 1 h (A) without CaF_2 and (B) with 5 vol% of CaF_2.

peaks (see pattern "(A)" in Fig. 3), which suggests extensive decomposition of HA to β-TCP:[4,6]

$$Ca_{10}(PO_4)_6(OH)_2 + t\text{-}ZrO_2 \rightleftarrows 3Ca_3(PO_4)_2 + 2H_2O + CaZrO_3/c\text{-}ZrO_2 \quad (1)$$

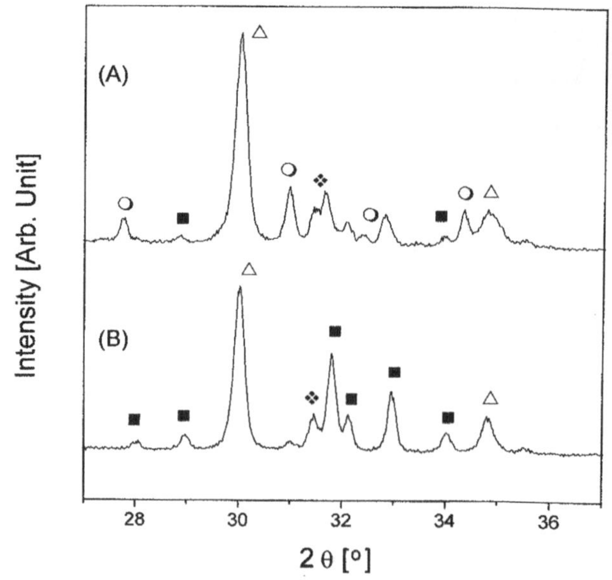

Fig. 3. XRD patterns of HA–20-vol%-ZrO_2 composites after sintering at 1150°C for 1 h without CaF_2 (pattern "(A)") and with 5 vol% of CaF_2 (pattern "(B)"). (Legend is as follows: (■) HA, (△) ZrO_2, (❖) $CaZrO_3$, and (○) β-TCP.)

This equation indicates that, in addition to the formation of TCP and water vapor, the Ca ions in the HA diffused into the tetragonal ZrO_2 (t-ZrO_2) to form $CaZrO_3$ and cubic ZrO_2 (c-ZrO_2). In contrast, when 5 vol% of CaF_2 was added to the composite (pattern "(B)" in Fig. 3), a negligible amount of TCP was detected. However, $CaZrO_3$ and c-ZrO_2 were still observed and no CaF_2 peaks were observed. Therefore, the $CaZrO_3$ or c-ZrO_2 are presumed to originate from the CaF_2 rather than from the HA.

These XRD patterns suggest that, when CaF_2 is added to the HA–ZrO_2 systems, the F ions are thought to react with HA to form a fluorapatite (FA) in a manner whereby some of the OH ions in the HA are substituted with the F ions in the CaF_2. This substitution could alter the HA lattice parameters, because HA and FA form a solid solution over a wide range. The variations in lattice parameters calculated from the XRD patterns are shown in Fig. 4. As the CaF_2 contents in the composite increased, the ***a***-axis lattice constant decreased remarkably whereas that of the ***c***-axis

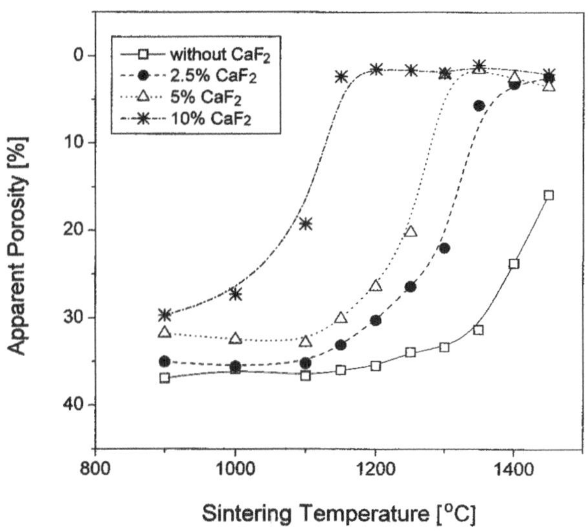

Fig. 2. Apparent porosity of HA–20-vol%-ZrO_2 composites after sintering at various temperatures for 1 h (*) with 10 vol% of CaF_2, (△) with 5 vol% of CaF_2, (●) with 2.5 vol% of CaF_2, and (□) without CaF_2.

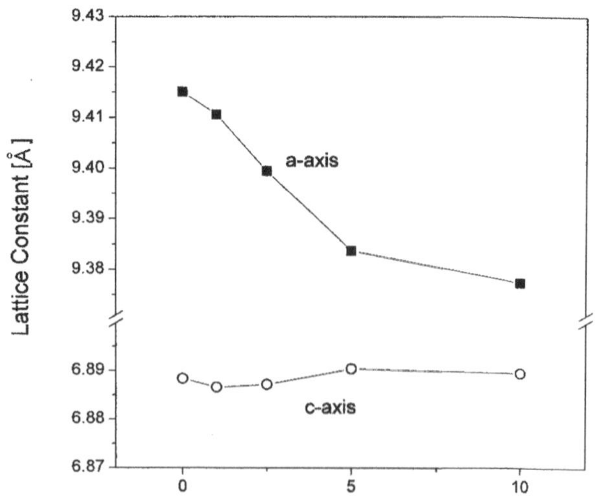

Fig. 4. Changes in the HA lattice constants ((■) ***a***-axis and (○) ***c***-axis), as a function of CaF_2 addition, after sintering at 1150°C for 1 h.

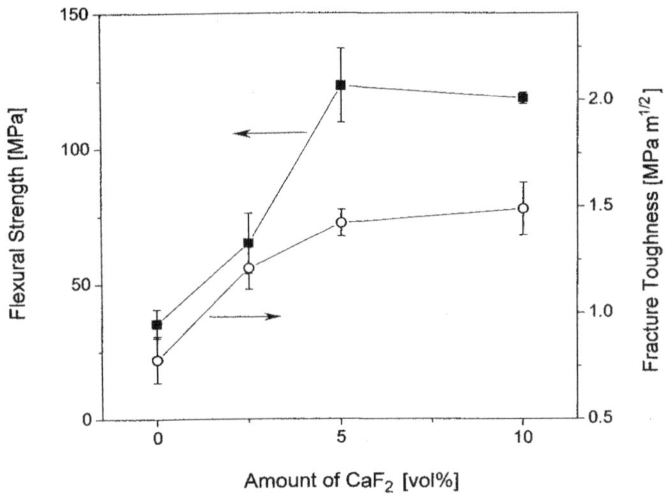

Fig. 5. (■) Flexural strength and (○) fracture toughness of HA–20-vol%-ZrO_2 composites after sintering at 1350°C for 1 h with the addition of different amounts of CaF_2.

increased slightly. These results concur with those made by Legeros *et al.*,[14] who reported that the substitution of F^- ions for OH^- ions in HA causes a contraction in the ***a***-axis without any significant effect on the ***c***-axis.

The improvements in sinterability and microstructure had a strong influence on the mechanical properties of the HA–ZrO_2 composites. The flexural strength and fracture toughness of the HA–ZrO_2 composites, versus the amount of added CaF_2, are shown in Fig. 5. When the composite without any CaF_2 was sintered at 1350°C, the mechanical properties were not particularly high: it had a strength of just 35 MPa and a fracture toughness of only 0.7 MPa·m$^{1/2}$. Interestingly, these values are very close to those of pure HA that has been sintered in air.[2] However, the mechanical properties were markedly enhanced by adding 5 vol% of CaF_2 to the composites; strength and fracture values of 130 MPa and 1.5 MPa·m$^{1/2}$, respectively, were observed. These improved mechanical properties were attributed to the reduction in porosity that resulted from the addition of CaF_2. In this case, even though the reinforcing capability of the ZrO_2 was somewhat reduced because of the transformation to the cubic phase, it nevertheless acted as a reinforcing agent for the HA. In reality, several reports on the reinforcing effect of c-ZrO_2 on other ceramics have been made.[15,16] Microstructural refinement with the incorporation of ZrO_2 is another possible reason for the observed improvements in mechanical properties.[17] This pressurelessly sintered HA–ZrO_2 composite with improved mechanical properties is a promising material for biomedical usages. Moreover, the use of c-ZrO_2 might be advantageous over the tetragonal phase, because of the possible aging phenomenon of t-ZrO_2 in a physiologic environment.[18]

IV. Summary and Conclusions

The sinterability of the hydroxyapatite–zirconia (HA–ZrO_2) composite was significantly improved by the addition of small amounts of CaF_2. When 5 vol% of CaF_2 was added to HA–20-vol%-ZrO_2 composite and sintered in air at 1300°C, the density of the resultant composite was >98% of the theoretical density. The formation of fluorapatite (FA) during the sintering process was attributed to the improvements in sinterability. The mechanical properties (flexural strength and fracture toughness) of the composites were also enhanced, as a result of the density improvement.

References

[1]L. L. Hench and E. C. Ethridge, *Biomaterials: An Interfacial Approach*. Academic Press, New York, 1982.

[2]W. Suchanek and M. Yoshimura, "Processing and Properties of Hydroxyapatite-Based Biomaterials for Use as Hard Tissue Replacement Implant," *J. Mater. Res.*, **13** [1] 94–117 (1998).

[3]R. Z. Legeros, "Apatites in Biological Systems," *Prog. Cryst. Growth Charact.*, **4**, 1–45 (1981).

[4]J. Li, H. Liao and L. Hermansson, "Sintering of Partially-Stabilized Zirconia and Partially-Stabilized Zirconia–Hydroxyapatite Composites by Hot Isostatic Pressing and Pressureless Sintering," *Biomaterials*, **17**, 1787–90 (1996).

[5]J. A. Delgado, "Zirconia-Toughened Hydroxyapatite Ceramic Obtained by Wet Sintering," *J. Mater. Sci.: Mater. Med.*, **10**, 715–19 (1999).

[6]Y.-M. Kong, S. Kim, H.-E. Kim, and I.-S. Lee, "Reinforcement of Hydroxyapatite Bioceramic by Addition of ZrO_2 Coated with Al_2O_3," *J. Am. Ceram. Soc.*, **82** [11] 2963–68 (1999).

[7]J. Li, L. Hermansson, and R. Soremark, "High-Strength Biofunctional Zirconia: Mechanical Properties and Static Fatigue Behavior of Zirconia–Apatite Composites," *J. Mater. Sci.: Mater. Med.*, **4**, 50–54 (1993).

[8]M. Takaki, M. Mochida, N. Uchida, K. Saito, and L. Uematsu, "Filter Cake Forming and Hot Isostatic Pressing for TZP-Dispersed Hydroxyapatite Composite," *J. Mater. Sci.: Mater. Med.*, **3**, 199–203 (1992).

[9]R. Z. Legeros, L. M. Silverstone, G. Daculsi, and L. M. Kerebel, "*In Vitro* Caries-like Lesion Formation in F-containing Tooth Enamel," *J. Dent. Res.*, **62**, 138–44 (1983).

[10]G. S. Ingram, and P. F. Nash, "A Mechanism for the Anticaries Action of Fluoride," *Caries Res.*, **14**, 298–303 (1980).

[11]E. C. Moreno, M. Kresak, and R. T. Zahradnik, "Fluoridated Hydroxyapatite Solubility and Caries Formation," *Nature (London)*, **247**, 64–65 (1974).

[12]F. B. Ayed, J. Bouaziz, and K. Bouzouita, "Pressureless Sintering of Fluorapatite under Oxygen Atmosphere," *J. Eur. Ceram. Soc.*, **20**, 1069–76 (2000).

[13]P. Chantilkul, G. R. Anstis, B. R. Lawn, and D. B. Marshall, "A Critical Evaluation of Indentation Techniques for Measuring Fracture Toughness: II, Strength Method," *J. Am. Ceram. Soc.*, **64** [9] 539–43 (1981).

[14]R. Z. Legeros, *Calcium Phosphates in Oral Biology and Medicine: Monographs in Oral Science*; Vol. 15. Edited by H. M. Myers. S. Karger, Basel, Switzerland, 1991.

[15]K. Shobu, T. Watanabe, J. Drennan, R. H. J. Hannink, and M. V. Swain, "Toughening Mechanisms and Microstructures of TiB_2-ZrO_2 Composites"; pp. 1091–99 in Advances in Ceramics, Vol. 24B, *Science and Technology of Zirconia III*. Edited by S. Sōmiya, N. Yamamoto, and H. Hanagida. American Ceramic Society, Westerville, OH, 1988.

[16]L. Donzel and S. G. Roberts, "Microstructure and Mechanical Properties of Cubic Zirconia (8YSZ)/SiC Nanocomposites," *J. Eur. Ceram. Soc.*, **20**, 2457–62 (2000).

[17]R. W. Rice, "Microstructure Dependence of Mechanical Behavior"; pp. 199–381 in *Treatise on Materials Science and Technology*, Vol. 11. Edited by R. K. MacCrone. Academic Press, New York, 1977.

[18]I. Thompson and R. D. Rawlings, "Mechanical Behaviour of Zirconia and Zirconia-Toughened Alumina in a Simulated Body Environment," *Biomaterials*, **11** [7] 505–508 (1990). □

IV. Summary and Conclusions

The sinterability of the hydroxyapatite–zirconia (HA–ZrO_2) composite was significantly improved by the addition of small amounts of CaF_2. When [illegible] vol% of CaF_2 was added to HA–20 vol% ZrO_2 composite and sintered at 1300°C, the density of the resulting composite was ~98% of the theoretical density. The [illegible]

[illegible]

journal

J. Am. Ceram. Soc., **85** [7] 1738–44 (2002)

Formation and Properties of Hydroxyapatite–Calcium Poly(vinyl phosphonate) Composites

Yaser E. Greish* and Paul W. Brown*

Intercollege Materials Research Laboratory, Pennsylvania State University, University Park, Pennsylvania 16802

Ceramic–polymer composites composed of hydroxyapatite ($Ca_{10}(PO_4)_6(OH)_2$, HAp) and calcium poly(vinyl phosphonate) salt were prepared by warm-pressing powder mixtures of tetracalcium phosphate ($Ca_4(PO_4)_2O$, TetCP) and poly(vinyl phosphonic acid) (PVPA) at a weight ratio of 3.5:1. The effects of temperature (to 300°C), pressure (to 690 kpsi), or compaction time (to 1 h) on the extent of conversion were studied using X-ray diffraction, Fourier transform infrared spectroscopy, differential scanning calorimetry, and scanning electron microscopy coupled with energy dispersive spectroscopy. The conversion of TetCP to HAp and formation of the calcium poly(vinyl phosphonate) salt was enhanced at higher temperature, pressure, and/or longer compaction time. Mechanical property determinations showed both the tensile strengths and elastic moduli continuously increase with increasing temperature, pressure, and compaction time. However, the glass transition temperature values of the composites were only minimally higher than that of the unreacted polymer.

I. Introduction

Hard tissues, such as bones and teeth, are natural ceramic-polymer composites composed of hydroxyapatite (HAp) and collagen.[1] A variety of ceramic–polymer composites is used as hard tissue analogues. For example, composites produced by reactions between acidic polyelectrolytes and zinc oxide or basic glasses[2] are used in dentistry. However, neither of the constituents in these composites is biologically familiar. An alternative approach is to produce composites of synthetic HAp and biomedical polymers.[3] In some preparations, HAp acts as a reinforcing phase for the polyacid salt matix.[4] Composites of this type are expected to exhibit properties that may closely approximate those of hard tissues.[4]

There are several classes of biomedical polymers. One of these is polyelectrolytes, such as poly(carboxylic acid)s, and poly(phosphonic acid)s. Poly(carboxylic acid)s are widely used as constituents in dental restorative materials because they appear to form both a molecular and mechanical bond with native tooth materials.[5] Their adherence to enamel and dentin is believed to result either from strong ionic bonds between their carboxylate groups and the apatite surface or from the displacement of the phosphate groups on the apatite surface by carboxylate groups.[6] Similarly, it has been found that phosphonate ions can exchange with the phosphate ions on hydroxyapatite crystals.[7] For example, ^{32}P-polyphosphonated polyethylene forms a strong, practically irreversible, insoluble monolayer on tooth enamel surface[8]; this suggests that polymeric compounds carrying multiple phosphonate ions have high affinities for HAp surfaces because the polymer can simultaneously attach itself to many sites.[9] Poly(vinyl phosphonic acid) (PVPA) solutions have also been used to prepare dental cements by mixing with aluminosilicate glasses.[10] This polyacid attacks the glass-releasing calcium and aluminum ions, which then react with the polyanions forming their corresponding poly(vinyl phosphonate) salts.[11]

HAp can be produced at low temperatures by cement-like reactions of acidic and basic calcium phosphates. Because tetracalcium phosphate ($Ca_4(PO_4)_2O$, TetCP) is the only calcium phosphate more basic than HAp,[12,13] there are various HAp preparation techniques that use TetCP as a starting material.[14–17] Greish and Brown demonstrated that TetCP (Ca/P = 2.00) undergoes a solid-state hydrolysis reaction in the presence of a poly(acrylic-*co*-itaconic) (CoP).[18] The reaction initiates with the attack of the TetCP surfaces by protons released from the polymer, releasing Ca^{2+} ions in turn. COO^- groups on the polymer are then neutralized by the Ca^{2+} ions forming a cross-linked calcium polyalkenoate salt.[18] Formation of the salt is accompanied by formation of HAp, according to Eq. (1):

$$2CoP + 3Ca_4(PO_4)_2O \rightarrow 2Ca\text{-}CoP + Ca_{10}(PO_4)_6(OH)_2 \quad (1)$$

Similar reactions occur when PVPA is used as the polyacid.[19,20] In this case, the reaction products formed were found to depend on the stoichiometry of the starting materials.[20] At low TetCP/PVPA weight ratios, reaction products contained anhydrous dicalcium phosphate (DCPA) in addition to the HAp and the calcium polyphosphonate salt. DCPA forms according to Eq. (2):[20]

$$Ca_4(PO_4)_2O + PVPA \rightarrow Ca\text{-}PVPA + CaHPO_4 + [Ca_{10}(PO_4)_6(OH)_2] + \sim\tfrac{1}{2}H_2O \quad (2)$$

Subsequently, the DCPA reacts with residual TetCP forming HAp according to Eq. (3).[20]

$$(2 + x)CaHPO_4 + 2Ca_4(PO_4)_2O \rightarrow Ca_{10}(PO_4)_6(OH)_2 + xCaHPO_4 \quad (3)$$

Our prior study showed the mechanical properties of these composites to be inferior to those of the HAp-calcium poly(acrylate) composites.[19] This was attributed to the high proportion of polymer compared with that of the copolymer in the HAp-calcium poly(acrylate) composites because DCPA formed.[18] Alternatively, reaction takes place in the same manner as in Eq. (1) at TetCP/PVPA weight ratios ≥1.5:1 forming the calcium poly(vinyl phosphonate) salt and HAp,[20] according to Eq. (4):

$$2PVPA + 3Ca_4(PO_4)_2O \rightarrow 2Ca\text{-}PVPA + Ca_{10}(PO_4)_6(OH)_2 \quad (4)$$

The objective of the present study is to investigate the effect of temperature, pressure, and/or time on composite formation by the acid-base solid-state reaction between TetCP and PVPA (at a TetCP:PVPA ratio of 3.5:1 by weight).[21–23] Composite compositions were characterized using X-ray diffraction (XRD) and

A. Jagota—contributing editor

Manuscript No. 188226. Received October 3, 2000; approved August 9, 2001.
This work was supported by the National Science Foundation, under Grant No. NSF DMR 9510272.

*Member, American Ceramic Society.

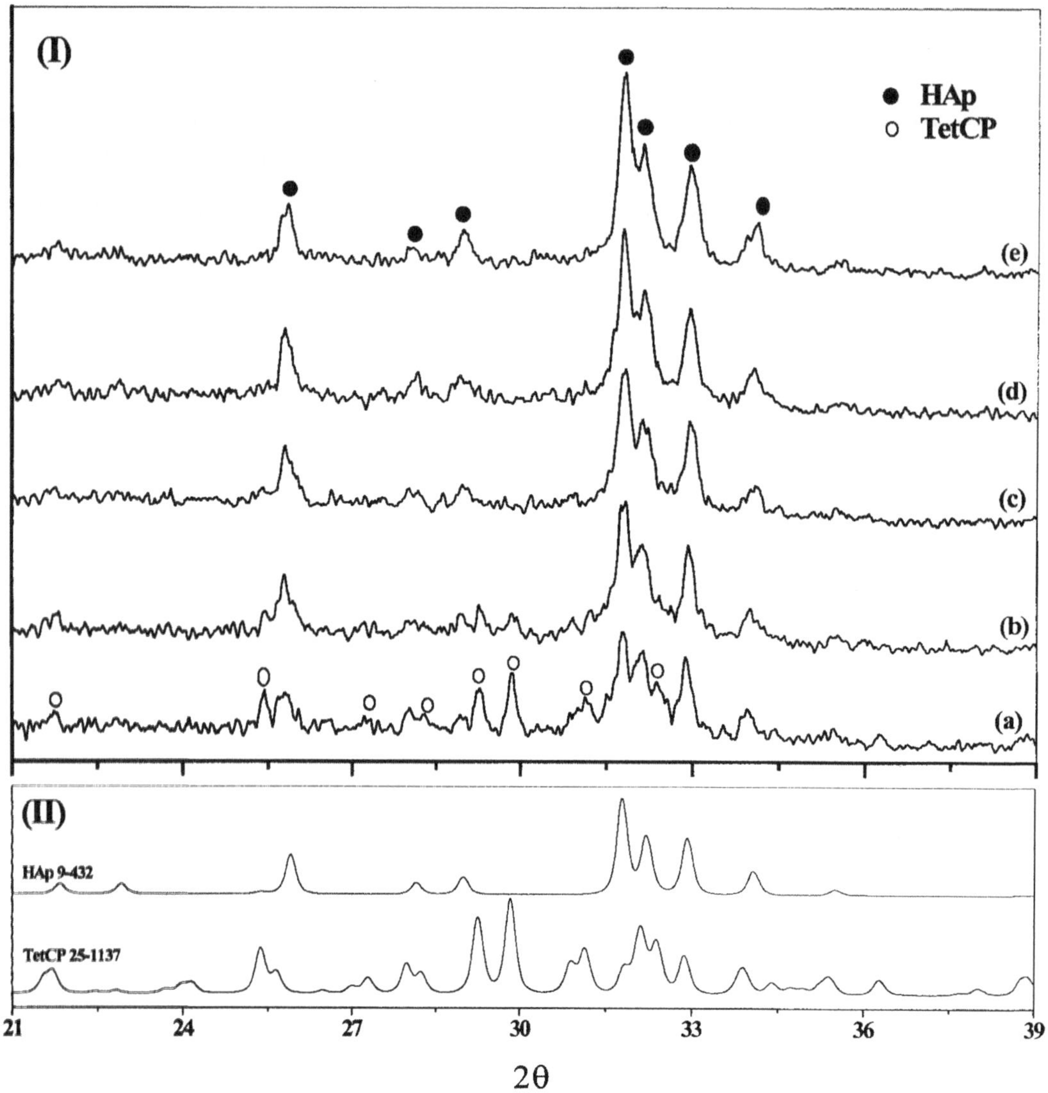

Fig. 1. XRD patterns of "I" samples warm-pressed for 30 min at 552 MPa and (a) 200°C, (b) 225°C, (c) 250°C, (d) 275°C, and (e) 300°C, and "II" standard HAp and TetCP samples.

Fourier-transform infrared spectroscopy (FT-IR). Thermal stabilities were determined by differential scanning calorimetry (DSC). Both fracture strengths and elastic moduli were measured. Microstructures of fractured surfaces were observed by scanning electron microscopy, coupled with energy-dispersive spectroscopy (SEM-EDS).

II. Materials and Methods

(1) Synthesis of $Ca_4(PO_4)_2O$

$CaCO_3$ (OSRAM Sylvania, Towanda, PA) and $Ca(H_2PO_4)_2 \cdot H_2O$ (MCPM) (FMC Corp., Philadelphia, PA) powders were mixed in a molar ratio of 3:1 and milled in n-heptane for 16 h. The resultant slurry was filtered and dried at room temperature for 24 h. The powder mixture was then fired at 1310°C for 2 h and rapidly quenched to room temperature. The fired product was ground by mortar and pestle, milled in a mill (Sweco, Nivelles, Belgium) for 24 h, then assessed for $Ca_4(PO_4)_2O$ (TetCP) phase purity using XRD and FT-IR. TetCP powder was stored under vacuum to avoid reaction with ambient moisture. Particle size of the powder was ~4 μm, as measured by a laser diffraction particle size and distribution analyzer (Malvern Instruments, Inc., Malvern, U.K.).

(2) Poly(vinyl phosphonic acid)

PVPA (molecular weight ≈ 2000) (PolyScience, Inc., Niles, IL) was also maintained under vacuum to avoid its hydration. The glass transition temperature (T_g) of the polymer was found to be ~242°C as determined by DSC (TA Instruments, Newcastle, DE) at a heating rate of 1°/min. Particle size of the powder was ~2.5 μm, as measured by SEM.

(3) Composite Formation

TetCP and PVPA powders in a TetCP:PVPA ratio of 3.5:1 (by weight) were thoroughly mixed with a mortar and pestle, then placed in a stainless steel mold with a 0.5-inch-diameter cavity. The mold was wrapped with heating tape (Thermolyne Brisk Heat, Dubuque, IA), and the powders were warm-pressed at temperatures (up to 300°C), pressures (up to 690 kpsi) and times (up to 1 h) using a Carver warm-press. During the heating process, pressure was released five or six times before the maximum temperature was attained to expel the water vapor produced during reaction. At the end of each experiment, the assembly was permitted to cool to room temperature at the maximum pressure of the experiment. The composites were removed and ground using a mortar and pestle to be characterized for their compositions. Disk-shaped samples prepared by the same method were used for mechanical properties measurements.

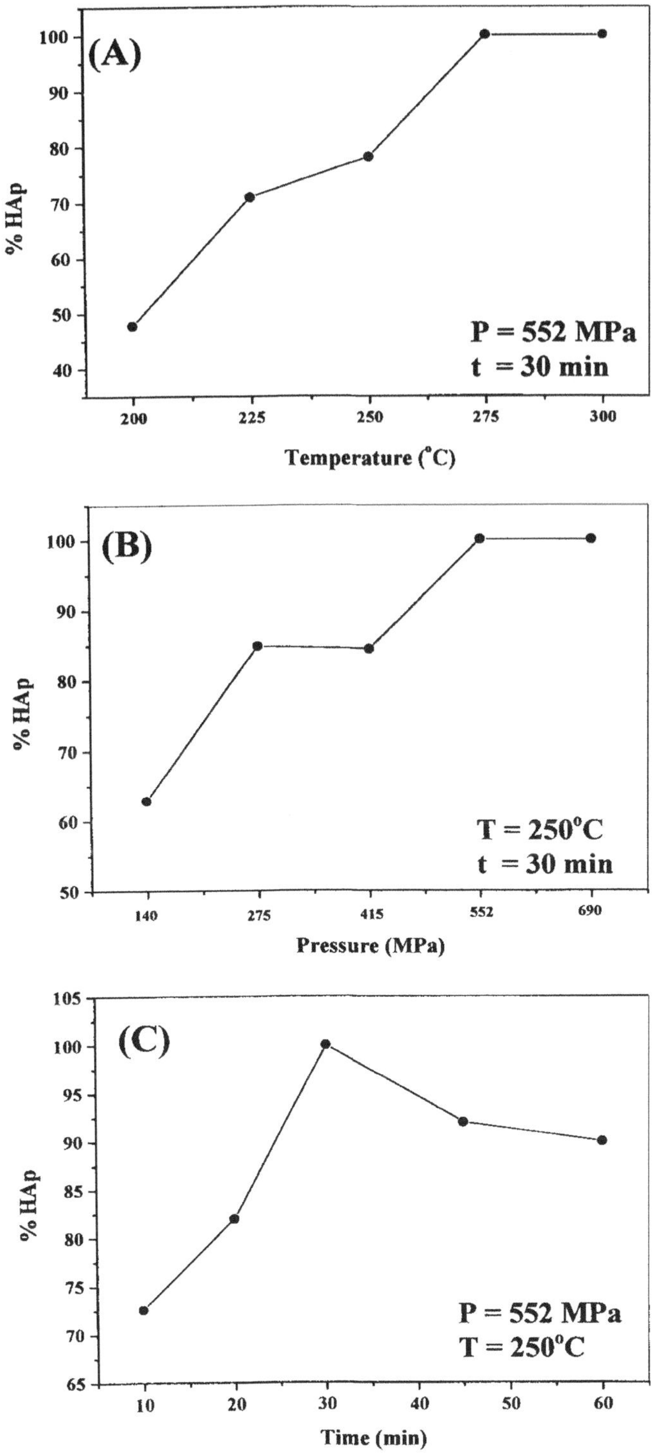

Fig. 2. Percentage of HAp in composites prepared at different (A) temperatures, (B) pressures, and (C) times.

(4) *Composite Characterization*

XRD analyses were performed using an automated diffractometer (Scintag, Inc., Sunnyvale, CA) at a step size of 0.02°, scan rate of 4°/min, and a scan range from 20°–40° 2θ. In patterns where TetCP was observed, the extent of conversion of TetCP to HAp was estimated using the following relationship[24]

$$\%\ \text{HAp} = \left(\frac{I_{\text{HAp}}}{I_{\text{HAp}} + I_{\text{TetCP}}}\right) \times 100 \tag{5}$$

where I_{HAp} corresponds to the intensity of its 002 peak at $2\theta = 25.9°$; I_{TetCP} corresponds to the intensity of its 200 peak at $2\theta = 25.4°$.

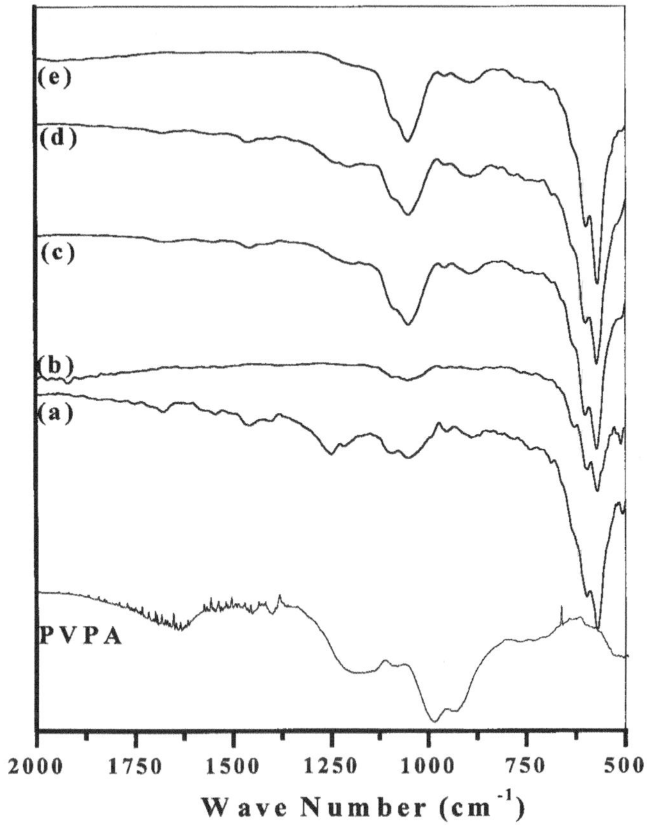

Fig. 3. FT-IR spectra of samples warm pressed for 30 min at 250°C and (a) 140, (b) 275, (c) 415, (d) 552, and (e) 690 MPa.

A single-beam infrared spectrometer (Model MB100, Bornem/Hartmann & Braun, Quebec City, Canada) was used, and spectra were obtained over the wavenumber range of 400-4000 cm^{-1} at a resolution of 3 cm^{-1}. The potassium bromide (KBr; spectroscopic grade, Aldrich Chemical, Milwaukee, WI) drifts technique was used with a KBr/sample ratio of 100/1.

Microstructures of the fractured surfaces were examined using a dual-stage SEM (Model XL-20, Philips, Eindhoven, The Netherlands).

(5) *Measurement of Mechanical Properties*

The fracture strengths of the composites were determined by diametral compression[25] using an automated Instron machine at a crosshead speed of 0.05 cm/min. A right circular disk is compressed diametrically between two flat plates, and the maximum tensile stress is developed normal to the loading direction across the loading diameter. The maximum tensile strength, which occurs on the daimetral plane between loading points, is given by $\sigma = 2P/(Dt)$, where P is the load, D the specimen diameter, and t the thickness. A fabric pad was inserted between the hard plates and the specimen to reduce the compressive stresses at the loading lines.

Elastic moduli were measured using the sound velocity technique[26] where a disk-shaped sample is placed between two ceramic transducers connected to a 150 MHz oscilloscope (Model 2445B, Tektronix, Beaverton, OR). The velocity of a transmitted ultrasonic wave is related to the elastic modulus by the following equation:

$$E = V^2\rho_t\left[\frac{(1+\nu)(1-2\nu)}{(1-\nu)}\right] \tag{6}$$

where V is the sound wave velocity (equal to the thickness of the sample divided by the transit time), ν the Poisson's ratio (taken as 0.294, calculated from the rule of mixtures of the components in

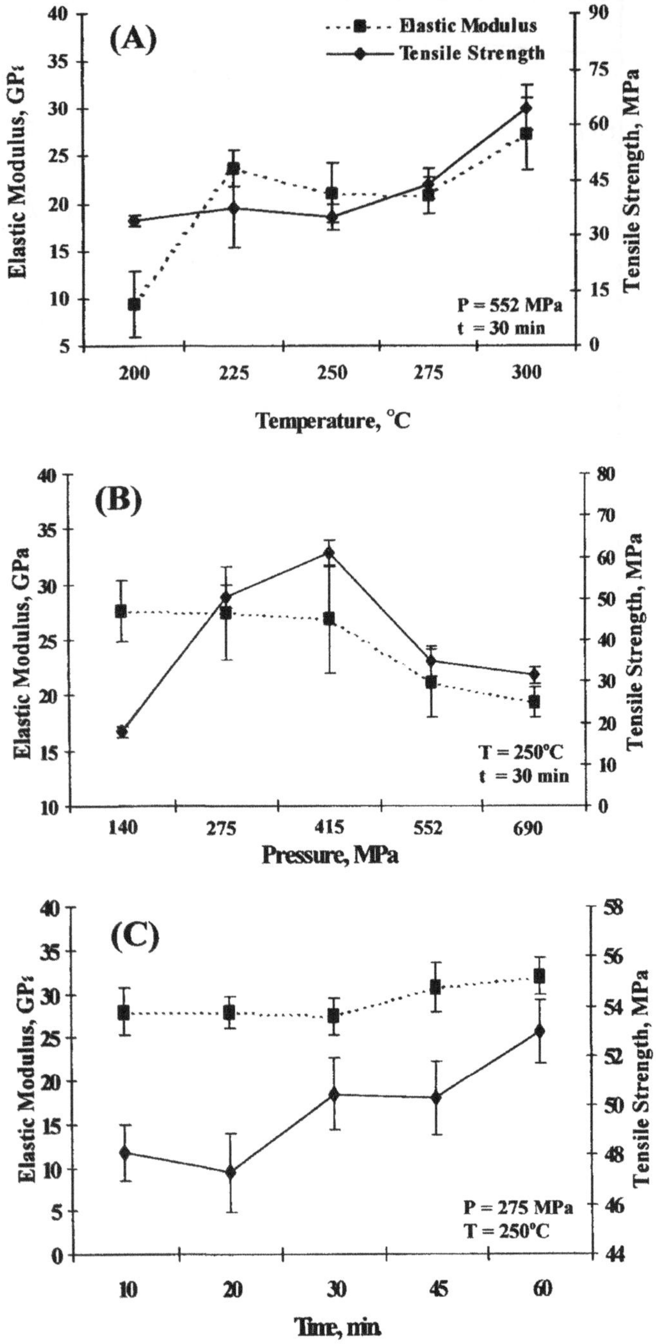

Fig. 4. Tensile strength and elastic modulus of composites prepared at different (A) temperatures, (B) pressures, and (C) times.

the composite), and ρ_t the true density (as measured by a liquid penetration technique, similar to ASTM C 373–88 method[27] using xylene instead of water. The values reported are based on the average of five determinations of tensile strength and elastic modulus.

III. Results and Discussion

(1) Composite Compositions

Figure 1 shows the XRD patterns of the products after warm pressing a 3.5:1 weight ratio TetCP–PVPA powder mixture at 200°C for 30 min at 550 MPa. The peaks at 25.5°, 29.3°, 29.9°, 31.2°, and 32.5° 2θ indicate the presence of unreacted TetCP. Only minor proportions of HAp were observed (peaks at 25.8°, 31.8°, 32.9°, and 34.2°) indicating an incomplete conversion. After

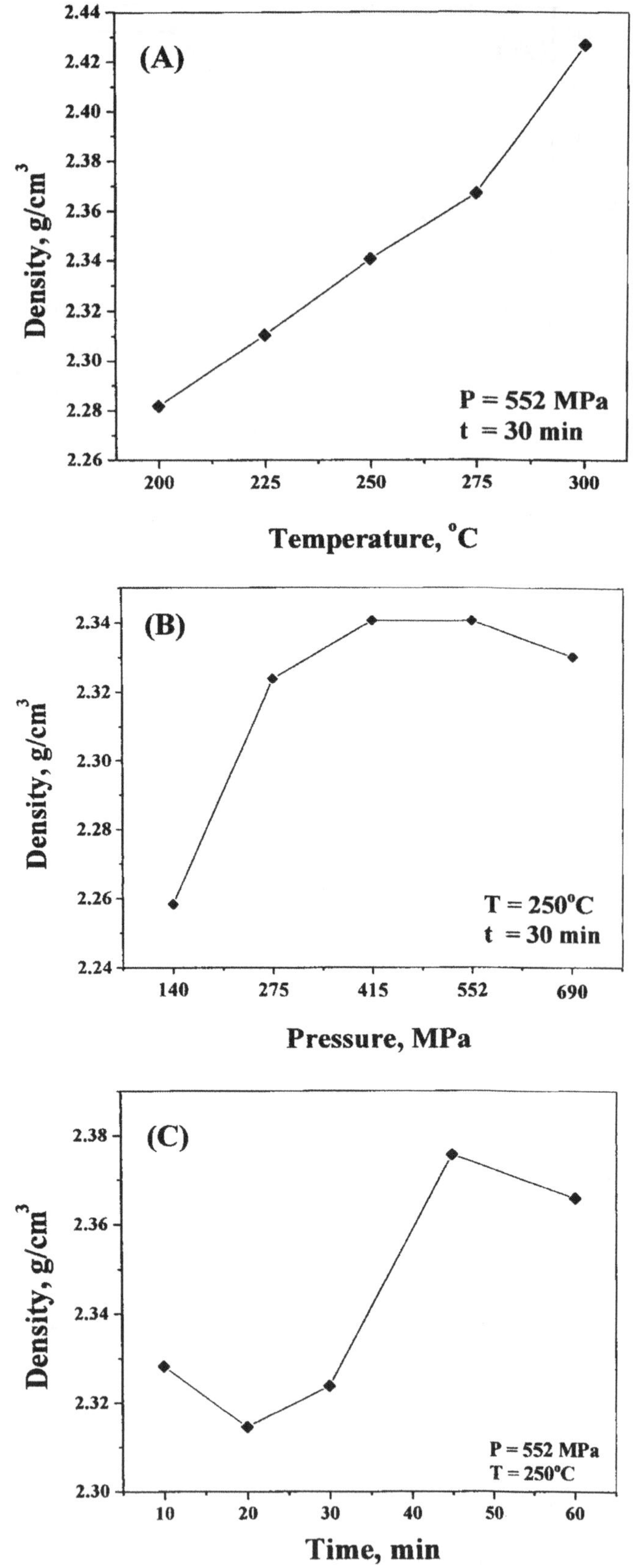

Fig. 5. Density of composites prepared at different (A) temperatures, (B) pressures, and (C) times.

processing at 225°C, the presence of these HAp peaks indicates it to be the primary crystalline phase. At compaction temperatures >225°C, the amount of HAp formed increased, indicating the more extensive conversion of TetCP. This is in accord with the findings that the T_g of the polymer is ~250°C. This is also in

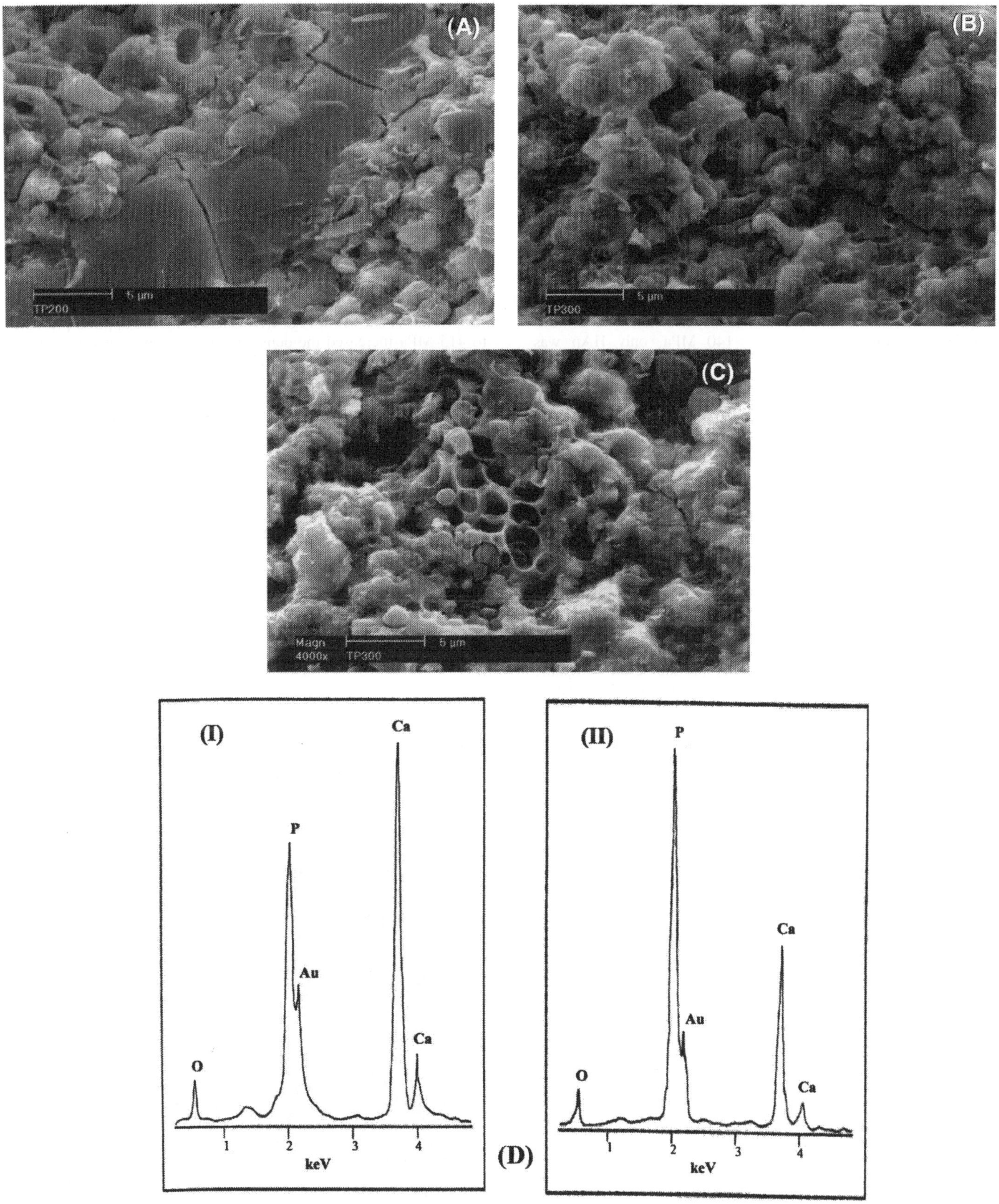

Fig. 6. SEM micrographs of composites prepared for 30 min at 552 MPa and (A) 200°C, (B) 300°C, and (C) 300°C (different area). Figure 6(D) shows the EDS spectra of two different spots in the sample shown in Fig. 6(C).

accord with our previous results[20] where HAp was the main phase formed at this TetCP:PVPA ratio when samples were warm-pressed at 300°C and the same compaction pressure and time. The current XRD results show that HAp can be formed as the only phase in samples pressed at 250°C and 550 MPa.

Figure 2(A) illustrates the increase in the proportion of HAp with increasing temperature when composites were pressed at 552 MPa for 30 min. This illustrates a large enhancement in the rate of reaction as temperature approaches the T_g of the polymer. Figure 2(A) also shows the maximum extent of conversion was achieved after heating at temperatures >250°C. The determination of the T_g values of these composites by DSC showed only a 13°C (to 255°C) increase with calcium poly(phosphonate) salt formation. In contrast, our previous results[19] showed that a mixture of HAp and unreacted TetCP was formed at 250°C and 275 MPa in samples containing a TetCP:PVPA ratio of 1.5:1. This may be attributed to the low content of TetCP and the lower compaction pressure in these samples. This confirms that the higher the TetCP:PVPA ratio is, the higher the rate of conversion of TetCP to HAp would be under the same pressing conditions. However, the difference in the compaction pressure is also expected to play an important role in this reaction.

Building on these results, samples were warm-pressed for 30 min at 250°C and various pressures. Figure 2(B) illustrates the extent of HAp formation depending on the compaction pressure. Pressing at 140 MPa, resulted in the coexistence of TetCP and HAp, thus indicating this pressure to be insufficient to achieve complete reaction. At pressures >140 MPa, only HAp was observed.

Figure 3 compares the FT-IR spectra of samples pressed for 30 min at 250°C at pressures of 140, 275, 415, 552, and 690 MPa with that of neat PVPA. The bands at 938 and 987 cm^{-1} (assigned to the symmetric and asymmetric vibrations of P=O of the polymer, respectively) moved to 892 and 955 cm^{-1}, respectively with lower absorption intensities.[28] This behavior was observed in all samples and indicates salt formation.[28] The presence of an absorption band at 1190 cm^{-1} in all spectra indicates the presence of bonds in these salts with P=O character.[28] Salt formation was confirmed by the presence of a new band at 1051 cm^{-1}, which is assigned to the poly(phosphonate) salt;[28] this results from the interaction between the calcium ions with the phosphonate ions of the polymer. The existence of the PO_4^{3-} absorption band for either TetCP or HAp in the range of 1090–960 cm^{-1} indicates an overlap occurs between this band and that of the salt. The presence of two strong absorption bands at 576 and 594 cm^{-1} is the result of apatite formation.[29] The increased resolution of these two bands as well as the band at 1051 cm^{-1} with increasing compaction pressure indicates the presence of HAp in these samples.[10] As previously discussed, the increase in T_g caused by salt formation was only ~13°C.

To study the effect of increasing the compaction time on the formation of HAp, samples were warm-pressed at 250°C and 275 MPa for up to 1 h. The effect of increasing the warm-pressing time on the conversion of TetCP to HAp is shown in Fig. 2(C). TetCP was observed in samples processed for 10 and 20 min. Although there was some variability in the maximum extent of conversion at this TetCP:PVPA ratio, approximately complete conversion was achieved after 30 min of warm-pressing. This variability is associated with the retention of minor amounts of TetCP in samples compacted for longer times. As with the other processing conditions described, the T_g values of these composites were ~255°C.

Regardless of the processing conditions used to prepare these composites, DCPA was not observed. This is in contrast to the observation of DCPA in composites produced using low TetCP:PVPA ratios.[20]

(2) *Composites Properties and Microstructure*

Figure 4(A) shows the tensile strength and elastic modulus values of composites prepared for 30 min at 552 MPa and different temperatures. Both the tensile strengths and the elastic moduli of the composites increased with compaction temperature. This is attributed to increased conversion of TetCP to HAp and the concurrent formation of the calcium poly(vinyl phosphonate) salt. Formation of these products increased the densities of the composites as shown in Figs. 5(A) and 6. The micrographs in Fig. 6 show the gradual increase in density with temperature. The calcium poly(phosphonate) salt exhibited two microstructural features. Figure 6(A) shows the unreacted polymer at 200°C as featureless zones within which cracks developed during the mechanical testing. At 300°C, the calcium poly(phosphonate) salt developed a porous structure. Such a structure was uncommon at 200°C. Compaction at 300°C also resulted in the maximum extent of conversion of TetCP to HAp, a structure with the highest density, as shown in Fig. 6(B) and, consequently, the highest mechanical properties among these samples. The tensile strength and elastic modulus achieved after pressing at 300°C were ~65 MPa and ~27 GPa, respectively. Figure 6(D) shows the elemental analysis of the products of a composite warm-pressed at 300°C. Two spots (labeled "I" and "II") in the micrograph shown in Fig. 6(C) were analyzed by EDS. Both composites contained calcium, phosphorus, and oxygen. However, the relative intensities of the calcium and phosphorus varied. The Ca/P ratio for (I) is higher than for (II), indicating the latter to be the calcium poly(phosphonate) salt.

The effect of increasing the compaction pressure on the mechanical properties of these composites when processed at 250°C for 30 min is shown in Fig. 4(B). Increasing the applied pressure to 415 MPa increased the densities of the composites. Commensurately, the tensile strengths of these composites also increased. Compaction at higher pressures did not result in additional densification, as shown in Figs. 5(B), 7(A), and 7(B). Rather, the densities decreased and accompanied decreases in the mechanical properties. Tensile strength and elastic modulus values of composites warm pressed at 415 MPa were ~61 MPa and ~27 GPa, respectively.

Figure 4(C) shows the mechanical properties of composites prepared at 275 MPa and 250°C for different times. These results are in accordance with the XRD findings and the density results shown in Fig. 5(C). The incomplete conversion of TetCP to HAp after 10 and 20 min of warm-pressing resulted in less-dense bodies and consequently lower mechanical properties. As the compaction time was increased, density increased and the mechanical properties improved. The highest values for the tensile strength and

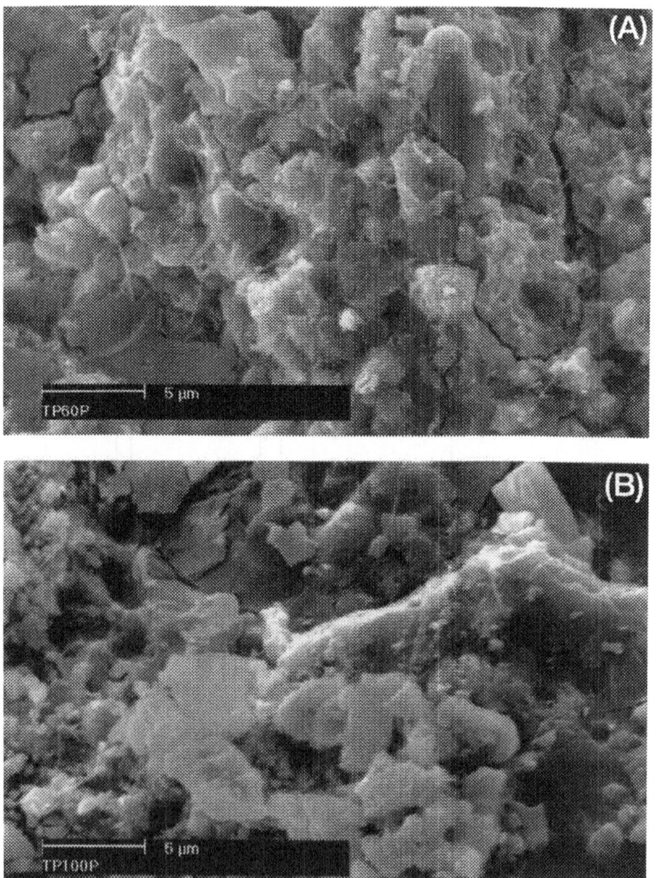

Fig. 7. SEM micrographs of samples warm-pressed for 30 min at 250°C and (A) 415 and (B) 690 MPa.

elastic modulus, respectively, were ~53 MPa and ~32 GPa and these were achieved after 60 min warm-pressing. The tensile strength values of the current composites are lower than those of long bones (121–149 MPa),[30] but in the range of those reported for dentine (29.6–105.5 MPa)[31] and higher than that reported for enamel (10.3 MPa).[32] On the other hand, tensile strength values are higher than those of similar composites such as HAp-calcium poly(carboxylate) (23–86 MPa),[18] zinc poly(carboxylate) (6.92–15.5 MPa)[33] and glass isonomer (2.2–14.2 MPa).[34] Elastic moduli of the current composites are higher than long bone (17.2–18.6 GPa)[30] and dentine (0.26–14.7 GPa)[31] but lower than those of enamel (84.1–130 GPa).[35] Compared with similar composites, the current composites have similar elastic moduli to HAp-calcium poly(carboxylate) composites (19–39 GPa)[18] but higher values than zinc poly(carboxylate) composites (2.4–4.4 GPa)[36,37] and glass isonomer cements (1.1–4.7 GPa).[38,39]

IV. Conclusions

The effects of temperature, pressure, and time on the formation of hydroxyapatite–calcium poly(vinyl phosphonate) composites were studied. The extent of hydroxyapatite formation increased with increasing temperature or pressure as observed by X-ray diffraction and Fourier transform infrared spectroscopy. Tensile strengths and elastic moduli of these composites increased with increasing compaction temperature or time. By increasing the compaction pressure, these properties also increased attaining 415 MPa then decreased. Composites showed T_g values minimally higher than that of the polymer.

References

[1]J. F. Shackelford, "Related Biological Materials" (Ch. 4) in Advanced Ceramics, Vol. 1, *Bioceramics*; p. 25. Gordon and Breach Science Publishers, New York, 1999.

[2]K. S. Tenhuisen and P. W. Brown, "Effects of Citric and Acetic Acids on the Formation of Ca-deficient Hydroxyapatite at 38°C," *J. Mater. Sci.: Mater. Med.*, **5**, 291–98 (1994).

[3]W. Bonfield, "Design of Bioactive Ceramic-Polymer Composites"; pp. 299–303 in *An Introduction to Bioceramics*. Edited by L. L. Hench and J. Wilson. World Scientific Advanced, River Edge, NJ, 1993.

[4]P. W. Brown, C. Durucan, and Y. E. Greish, "The Formation of Hydroxyapatite and Hydroxyapatite-Based Composites"; pp 161–64 in *Bioceramics*, Vol. 11. Edited by R. Z. LeGeros and J. P. LeGeros. World Scientific Publishing Co. Ltd., Singapore, 1998.

[5]A. D. Wilson, "Alumino-Silicate Polyacrylic Acid and Related Cements," *Br. Polym. J.*, **6**, 165–79 (1974).

[6]J. W. McLean and A. D. Wilson,"The Clinical Development of the Glass-Ionomer Cements, I: Formulations and Properties," *Aust. Dent. J.*, **22**, 31–36 (1974).

[7]R. F. Sognnaes, J. H. Shaw, and R. Bogorogh, "Radiotracer Studies on Bone, Cementum, Dentin, and Enamel of Rhesus Monkeys," *Am. J. Physiol.*, **180**, 408–20 (1955).

[8]M. Anbar and G. A. St. John, "Adsorption of Polyphosphonated Polyethylene in Enamel of Teeth," *J. Dent. Res.*, **3**, 778 (1971).

[9]M. Anbar and E. P. Farley, "Potential Use of Organic Polyphosphonates as Adhesives in the Restoration of Teeth," *J. Dent. Res.*, **33** [4] 879–88 (1974).

[10]A. D. Wilson and J. W. Nicholson, "Acid-Base Cements: Their Biomedical and Industrial Applications"; p. 310 in *Chemistry of Solid State Materials*, Vol. 3. Cambridge University Press, Cambridge, U.K., 1993.

[11]J. Ellis and A. D. Wilson, "Phosphonated Cements: A New Class of Dental Materials," *J. Mater. Sci. Lett.*, **9**, 1058–60 (1990).

[12]R. I. Martin and P. W. Brown, "Hydration of Tetracalcium Phosphate," *Adv. Cem. Res.*, **5** [19] 119–25 (1993).

[13]C. S. Reed, K. S. Tenhuisen, P. W. Brown, and H. R. Allcock, "Thermal Stability and Compressive Strength of Calcium-Deficient HAp-poly[bis(carboxylatophenoxy) phosphazene] Composites," *Chem. Mater.*, **8**, 440–47 (1996).

[14]W. E. Brown and L. C. Chow, "A New Calcium Phosphate, Water-Setting Cement"; pp. 353–79 in *Cement Research Progress*. Edited by P. W. Brown. American Ceramic Society, Columbus, OH, 1986.

[15]M. T. Fulmer, R. I. Martin, and P. W. Brown, "Formation of Hydroxyapatite at Near Physiological Temperature," *J. Mater. Sci.: Mater. Med.*, **3**, 299–305 (1992).

[16]P. W. Brown and M. T. Fulmer, "The Kinetics of Hydroxyapatite Formation at Low Temperature," *J. Am. Ceram. Soc.*, **74**, 934–40 (1991).

[17]P. W. Brown, N. Hocker, and S. Hoyle, "Variations in Solution Chemistry during Low Temperature Formation of Hydroxyapatite," *J. Am. Ceram. Soc.*, **74**, 1848–54 (1991).

[18]Y. E. Greish and P. W. Brown, "Hydrolysis of Tetracalcium Phosphate in the Presence of Poly(alkenoic acids)," *J. Mater. Res.*, **14** [12] 4637–42 (1999).

[19]Y. E. Greish and P. W. Brown, "Preparation and Characterization of Calcium Phosphate–Poly(vinyl phosphonic acid) Composites," *J. Mater. Sci.: Mater. Med.*, in press.

[20]Y. E. Greish and P. W. Brown, "Chemically Formed HAp–Ca Poly(vinyl phosphonate) Composites," *Biomaterials*, in press.

[21]W. E. Fitzgerald and L. E. Nielsen, "Viscoelastic Properties of the Salts of Some Polymeric Acids," *Proc. R. Soc. London A*, **282**, 137–46 (1964).

[22]J. E. Fields and L. E. Nielsen, "Dynamic Mechanical Properties of Some Polymeric Acid Zinc Salts," *J. Appl. Polym. Sci.*, **12**, 1041–51 (1968).

[23]L. E. Nielsen, "The Mechanical and Other Physical Properties of Polyelectrolyte Salts in Solid Sate," *Polym. Eng. Sci.*, **9** [5] 356–59 (1969).

[24]Y. Matsuya, S. Matsuya, J. M. Antonuccil, S. Takagi, L. C. Chow, A. Akash, and A. Akamine, "Mechanical Strength of Various Types of Calcium Phosphate Cements"; presented at the International Symposium on Advanced Materials with Biomedical Applications, National Institute of Standards and Technology, Gaithersburg, MD, June 7–8, 1999.

[25]M. B. Thomas, R. H. Doremus, M. Jarcho, and R. L. Salsbury, "Dense Hydroxyapatite: Fatigue, and Fracture Strength after Various Treatments from Diametral Tests," *J. Mater. Sci.*, **15**, 891–94 (1980).

[26]D. J. Green, "Elastic Behavior" (Ch. 2) in *An Introduction to the Mechanical Properties of Ceramics*; p. 63. Cambridge University, Cambridge, U.K., 1998.

[27] "Standard Test Method for Water Absorption, Bulk Density, Apparent Porosity, and Apparent Specific Gravity of Fired Whitware Products," ASTM Designation C 373–88. *1988 Book of ASTM Standards*. American Society for Standards and Testing Materials, West Conshohocken, PA.

[28]J. Ellis and A. D. Wilson, "A Study of the Cements Formed between Metal Oxides and Poly(vinyl phosphonic acid)," *Polym. Int.*, **24**, 224–28 (1991).

[29]M. P. Ginebra, E. Fernandez, E. A. P. DeMayer, R. M. H. Verbeeck, M. G. Boltong, J. Ginebra, F. C. M. Driessens, and J. A. Planell, "Setting Reaction and Hardening of an Apatitic Calcium Phosphate Cement," *J. Dent. Res.*, **76** [4] 905–12 (1997).

[30]N. R. Boeree, J. Dove, J. J. Copper, J. Knowles, and G. W. Hastings, "Development of a Degradable Composite for Orthopaedic Use: Mechanical Evaluation of an Hydroxyapatite-Polyhydroxybutyrate Composite Material," *Biomaterials*, **14**, 793–96 (1993).

[31]H. Sano, B. Ciucchi, W. G. Matthews, and D. H. Pashley, "Tensile Properties of Mineralized and Demineralized Human and Bovine Dentin," *J. Dent. Res.*, **73**, 1205–11 (1994).

[32]R. L. Bowen and M. S. Rodriquez, "Tensile Strength and Modulus of Elasticity of Tooth Sucture and Several Restorative Materials," *J. Am. Dent. Assoc.*, **64** [3] 378–87 (1962).

[33]J. A. Barton Jr., G. M. Brauer, J. M. Antonucci, and M. J. Raney, "Reinforced Polycarboxylate Cements," *J. Dent. Res.*, **54** [2] 310–23 (1975).

[34]G. Eliades and G. Palaghias, "*In Vitro* Characterization of Visible Light-Cured Glass Ionomer Liners," *Dent. Mater*, **9**, 198–203 (1993).

[35]H. H. Moroi, K. Okimoto, R. Moroi, and Y. Terada, "Numeric Approach to the Biomechanical Analysis of Thermal Effects in Coated Implants," *Int. J. Prosthodont.*, **6**, 564–72 (1993).

[36]J. M. Powers, J. W. Farah, and R. G. Craig, "Modulus of Elasticity and Strength Properties of Dental Cements," *J. Am. Dent. Assoc.*, **92** [3] 588–91 (1976).

[37]G. Oilo and S. Espevik, "Kompresjonsstyrke og Deformering hos Dentale Sementer," *Nor. Tannlaegeforen Tid.*, **88** [11] 500–503 (1978).

[38]L. E. Tam, E. Pulver, D. McComb, and D. C. Smith, "Physical Properties of Calcium Hydroxide and Glass-Ionomer Base and Lining Materials," *Dent. Mater.*, **5**, 145–49 (1989).

[39]L. E. Tam, E. Pulver, D. McComb, and D. C. Smith, "Physical Properties of Proprietary Light-Cured Lining Materials," *Oper. Dent.*, **16**, 210–17 (1991). □

J. Am. Ceram. Soc., 85 [10] 2578–80 (2002)

journal

Fabrication of Macrochannelled-Hydroxyapatite Bioceramic by a Coextrusion Process

Young-Hag Koh,*,† Hae-Won Kim,* and Hyoun-Ee Kim*

School of Materials Science and Engineering, Seoul National University, Seoul, 151–742, Korea

John W. Halloran*

Materials Science and Engineering Department, University of Michigan, Ann Arbor, Michigan 48109-2136

A coextrusion process was used to fabricate macrochannelled hydroxyapatite (HA). To improve the powder characteristics, the HA powder was calcined at 900°C in air for 1 h. A feedrod composed of HA (shell) and carbon black (core) was coextruded at 120°C through a symmetric 8:1 square reduction die. After the first coextrusion, the individual pieces were bundled, warm-pressed, and then coextruded again. After removing the binder, the billet was sintered at 1350°C for 1h in air. Uniform, 27 vol% macrochannels with a diameter of 270 μm were formed in the dense HA through removal of the carbon black. The compressive strength of the test specimens was strongly dependent on the macrochannel direction due to the stress concentrations related to the macrochannel geometry.

I. Introduction

Hydroxyapatite (HA, $Ca_{10}(PO_4)_6(OH)_2$) has been regarded as a promising biomaterial due to its high biocompatibility, good bioaffinity and osteoconduction, and its crystallographic and chemical similarity to the human bone.[1–5] When HA materials are used as implants, they are slowly replaced by the host bone, forming a direct bond with the neighboring bone structure. Recently, the fabrication of bioceramics with porous configurations has attracted particular attention because a porous network allows tissue infiltration, which in turn enhances implant-tissue attachment.[6–8] However, conventional pore forming methods, such as the hydrothermal exchange process,[9] the pyrolysis of organic particles,[10–13] and polyurethane sponge techniques,[13] have shown limited control over the pore geometry. As a result, these porous HA bodies have a wide range of porosity and pore sizes with a much smaller interconnecting fenestration. Hence, the optimal pore geometry for osteoconduction is not yet fully understood.

In this study, a new method for manufacturing uniformly macrochannelled-HA materials using a coextrusion process was developed.[14] The effect of calcination of HA powder on providing a thermoplastic/HA blend was also investigated. Sintered macrochannelled-HA samples were analyzed by X-ray diffraction (XRD) and optical microscopy. In addition, the compressive strengths of the sintered samples were measured both perpendicular and parallel to the macrochannel direction.

G. Hilmas—contributing editor

Manuscript No. 187164. Received February 5, 2002; approved June 21, 2002.
*Member, American Ceramic Society.
†Now with University of Michigan, Ann Arbor, MI.

II. Experimental Procedure

Commercially available $Ca_{10}(PO_4)_6(OH)_2$ (HA) (Sigma-Aldrich Co., Milwaukee, WI) powder was used as the ceramic material. The HA powder was calcined at 900°C for 1 h in air to improve the powder characteristics. After calcination, the changes in the size and crystallinity were monitored by BET and XRD, respectively. The as-received and calcined HA powders with 1 wt% stearic acid (Sigma-Aldrich Co.) as a dispersant were ball-milled in ethanol for 24 h using alumina balls as media. The mixture was then dried in an oven at 80°C for 24 h. Carbon black powder (Cabot Black Pearls BP-120; Cabot Corp., Boston, MA) was used as a fugitive material.

Ethylene ethyl acrylate (EEA 6182; Union Carbide, Danbury, CT) and Acryloid B67 (Rohm and Haas, Philadelphia, PA) resins were used as binders and fused at 105°C in a heated shear mixer (PlastiCorder PL 2100 Electronic Torque Rheometer; C. W. Brabender, South Hackensack, NJ). Powder (HA or carbon black) was then gradually added to the melt. Agents (heavy mineral oil (Witco, Petrolia, PA), polyethylene glycol (PEG 1000, Acros Organics, NJ, USA), and stearic acid) were added as processing aids to ensure a consistent apparent viscosity value (~3000 Pa·s). Once compounded, the HA thermoplastic compound was warm-pressed into a 38mm square mold and cored for the insertion of a carbon black thermoplastic compound, which was fabricated using a 22mm cylindrical die. The assembly of HA and carbon black was warm-pressed at 160°C with 10 MPa to create a multicomponent feedrod for the coextrusion (Fig. 1(A)). The initial feedrod was extruded through a symmetric 8:1 square reduction die using a piston extruder (Bradford Small Scale Extrusion Unit; Bradford University Research, Ltd., West Yorkshire, U.K.) at 120°C at a rate of 3 mm/min (Fig. 1(B)). After coextrusion, the individual pieces were bundled and uniaxially warm-pressed at 160°C and 10 MPa pressure to create the second feedrod. After a second coextrusion, the initial repeat unit had undergone a total size reduction by a factor of 64 (Fig. 1(C)).

The green billet was heat-treated in a two-stage process (binder-burnout and sintering). Binder burnout was performed in an alumina tube furnace with a slow heating rate up to 700°C in flowing air to prevent defects, such as bloating and cracks. The resulting billets were then sintered at temperatures ranging from 1250°C to 1400°C for 1 h in air. The sintered macrochannelled-HA body was sliced into dimensions of 3 mm × 3 mm × 3 mm with a diamond saw to produce the specimens for measuring the compressive strength. All surfaces were polished down to 30 μm with a resin bonded diamond wheel. The compressive strengths were measured both normal and parallel to the macrochannel directions. Five specimens were tested for each experimental condition. In addition, the sintered body was analyzed using optical microscopy and XRD analysis.

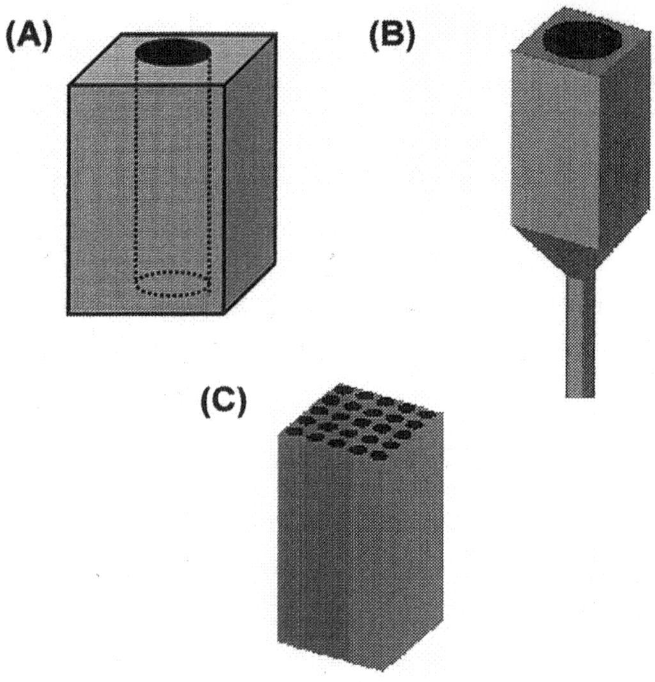

Fig. 1. Schematic of (A) the initial feedrod, composed of HA (shell) and carbon black (core), (B) coextrusion, and (C) second extrudate.

III. Results and Discussion

The shear-mixing behaviors of the as-received and calcined HA powders were observed by measuring the viscosity versus the ceramic content, as shown in Fig. 2. When more than 35 vol% of the as-received HA powder was added to the melted binder (EEA), the viscosity did not change (Fig. 2(A)). This suggested an inhomogeneous mixing behavior. However, when the calcined powder was mixed with the binder, the ceramic volume fraction could be increased to above 50 vol% with homogeneous mixing (Fig. 2(B)).

The viscosity of the ceramic-polymer mixtures is strongly dependent on the powder characteristics, such as the specific surface area, the particle shape and the extent of agglomeration.[15] After calcination, the specific surface area was notably reduced from 63 m^2/g to 16 m^2/g due to the growth of particles by partial sintering. The primary particle of the as-received HA powder was extremely small and severely agglomerated. In general, such agglomerates are known to be difficult to disperse due to their small particle size and their surface charge state. However, the calcined HA powder had soft agglomerates that could be readily separated through subsequent ball milling. Therefore, an improved shear-mixing behavior of the calcined HA powder was mainly due to the reduction in the specific surface area and the removal of hard agglomerates.

To investigate the sinterability of HA, the extruded HA samples were sintered at temperatures ranging from 1250°C to 1400°C for 1h in air. The relative density increased with increasing sintering temperature up to 1350°C, but decreased at 1400°C. The decrease in density was related to the formation of β-tricalcium phosphate (β-TCP, $Ca_3(PO_4)_2$) through HA decomposition. The formation of β-TCP was observed clearly by XRD analyses, as shown in Fig. 3. Up to 1350°C, the XRD patterns were unchanged with only HA peaks (Fig. 3(A)). However, after sintering at 1400°C, a β-TCP peak was also detected along with the HA peaks (Fig. 3(B)). When HA is sintered at high temperature, β-TCP is formed in a favorable manner with CaO, leaving pores in the sintered body due to the following reaction mechanism:

$$Ca_{10}(PO_4)_6(OH)_2(s) \rightarrow 3Ca_3(PO_4)_2(s) + CaO(s) + H_2O(g) \quad (1)$$

Moreover, the starting temperature of β-TCP formation (>1350°C) increased when using the calcined powder, indicating that the improved powder characteristic also increased the thermal stability of HA.

Uniform macrochannels were formed on the densified HA body, as shown in Fig. 4, by the removal of carbon black after thermal treatment. The macrochannel fraction and size were ~27 vol% and ~270 μm, respectively, as described in Table I. No defects, such as bloating, cracks or pores were observed. The compressive strength of the macrochannelled HA was strongly dependent on the macrochannel direction, as described in Table I. The compressive strength of the samples parallel to the macrochannel direction was much higher than that of samples normal to the macrochannel direction by a factor of ~1.8. This anisotropy was attributed to the characteristics of the macrochannelled structure, such as the stress concentration factors and the defects associated with coextrusion processing. The stress concentration factor is ~3 for a spherical cavity,[16] suggesting that the material can be fractured more easily. In other words, when a stress is applied to the normal direction of the macrochannel, cracks

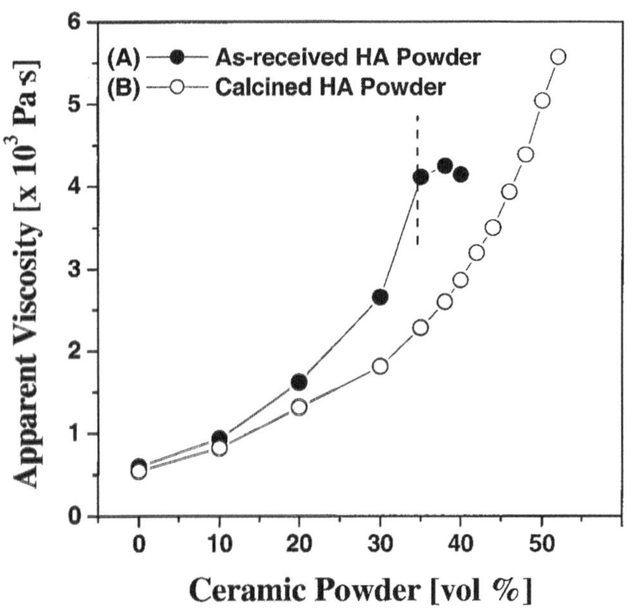

Fig. 2. Apparent viscosity of the thermoplastic compounds using (A) as-received and (B) calcined HA powder, as a function of the powder content.

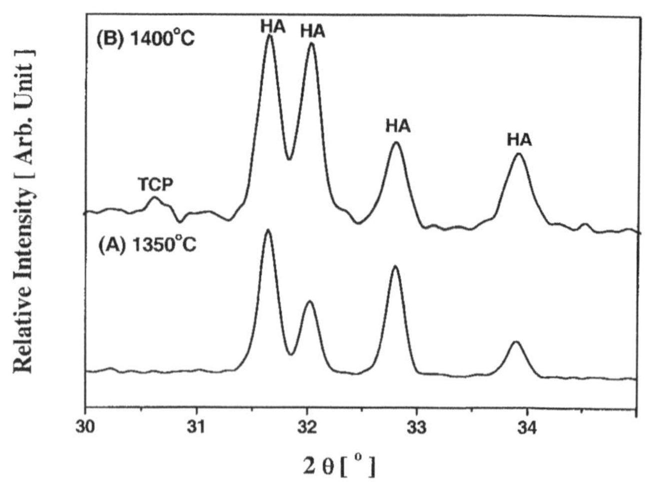

Fig. 3. XRD patterns of a HA extrudate sintered (A) at 1350°C and (B) at 1400°C for 1 h in air.

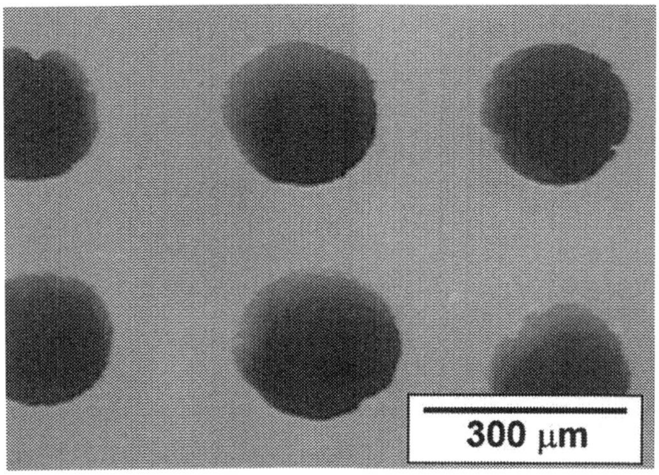

Fig. 4. Optical micrograph of the cross section of the macrochannelled HA.

Table I. Summarized Properties of the Macrochannelled-HA

Sample	Macro-channel fraction (vol%)	Macro-channel size (μm)	Compressive strength (MPa)	
			Parallel	Normal
Macro-channelled-HA	27 ± 0.7	270 ± 11	240 ± 32	132 ± 11

generate more easily around the macrochannels, leading to a lower stress-retaining capability.

IV. Summary and Conclusions

A biocompatible macrochannelled hydroxyapatite was fabricated using coextrusion. An initial feedrod, a compound of HA (shell) and carbon black (core), was coextruded twice through a symmetric 8:1 square reduction die at 120°C. This produced an extrudate with a cross section identical to that of the initial feedrod but with a 64:1 reduction in size. After binder burnout and sintering, the body was composed of dense HA containing a uniform array of 270 micrometer diameter, smooth pore channels occupying 27% of its volume. A maximum compressive strength (240 ± 32 MPa) was observed for the sample parallel to the macrochannel direction.

References

[1]L. L. Hench, "Bioceramics: From Concept to Clinic," *J. Am. Ceram. Soc.*, **74** [7] 1487–510 (1991).

[2]R. Z. Legeros, "Apatites in Biological Systems," *Prog. Cryst. Growth Charact.*, **4**, 1–45 (1981).

[3]R. Z. LeGeros and J. P. Legeros, "Dense Hydroxyapatite"; pp.139–80 in *An Introduction to Bioceramics*, Advanced Series in Ceramics, Vol. 1. Edited by L. L. Hench and J. Wilson. World Scientific, Singapore, 1993.

[4]C. Lavernia and J. M. Schoenung, "Calcium Phosphate Ceramics as Bone Substitutes," *Am. Ceram. Soc. Bull.*, **70** [1] 95–100 (1991).

[5]T. S. B. Narasaraju and D. E. Phebe, "Review: Some Physicochemical Aspects of Hydroxyapatite," *J. Mater. Sci.*, **31** [1] 1–21 (1996).

[6]M. Jarcho, "Calcium Phosphate Ceramics as Hard Tissue Prosthetics," *Clin. Orthop. Relat. Res.*, **157**, 259–78 (1981).

[7]H. M. Rosen, "Porous, Block HA as an Interpositional Bone Graft Substitute in Orthognatic Surgery," *Plast. Reconstr. Surg.*, **83**, 985–90 (1989).

[8]N. Passuti, G. Daculsi, J. M. Rogez, S. Martin, and J. V. Bainvel, "Macroporous Calcium Phosphate Ceramic Performance in Human Spine Fusion," *Clin. Orthop. Relat. Res.*, **248**, 169–76 (1989).

[9]D. M. Roy and S. K. Linnehan, "HA Formed from Coral Skeletal Carbonate by Hydrothermal Exchange," *Nature (London)*, **247**, 220–22 (1974).

[10]D.-M. Liu, "Fabrication and Characterization of Porous Hydroxyapatite Granules," *Biomaterials*, **17**, 1955–57 (1996).

[11]M. Fabbri, G. C. Celotti, and A. Ravaglioli, "Granulates Based on Calcium Phosphate with Controlled Morphology and Porosity for Medical Applications: Physico-Chem. Parameters and Production Technique," *Biomaterials*, **15**, 474–77 (1994).

[12]D.-M. Liu, "Control of Pore Geometry on Influencing the Mechanical Property of Porous Hydroxyapatite," *J. Mater. Sci. Lett.*, **15**, 419–21 (1996).

[13]A. Slosarczyk, "Highly Porous Hydroxyapatite Material," *Powder Metall. Int.*, **21**, 24–25 (1989).

[14]A. T. Crumm, "Microfabrication by Coextrusion"; Ph. D Thesis. University of Michigan, Ann Arbor, MI, 2000.

[15]H. Barnes, J. Hutton, and K. Walters, "Rheology of Suspensions"; pp. 115–39 in *An Introduction to Rheology*. Edited by H. Barnes. Elsevier, New York, 1989.

[16]B. Lawn, *Fracture of Brittle Solids*; Ch. 1. Cambridge University Press, Cambridge, U.K., 1993. □

(shell) and carbon black (core), was coextruded twice through a symmetric X-square reduction die at 120°C. This produced an extrudate with a cross section identical to that of the initial feedrod but with a [illegible] reduction in size. [illegible]

References

[illegible]

journal

J. Am. Ceram. Soc., 85 [11] 2771–77 (2002)

Effect of Silicon Substitution on the Sintering and Microstructure of Hydroxyapatite

Iain R. Gibson,† Serena M. Best,‡ and William Bonfield‡

IRC in Biomedical Materials, Queen Mary, University of London, London, E1 4NS, United Kingdom

The substitution of between 0 and 1.6 wt% silicon (Si-HA) in hydroxyapatite (HA) inhibited densification at low temperatures (1000°–1150°C), with these effects being more significant as the level of silicon substitution was increased. For higher sintering temperatures (1200°–1300°C), the sintered densities of HA and Si-HA compositions were comparable. Examination of the ceramic microstructures by scanning electron microscopy (SEM) showed that silicon substitution also inhibited grain growth at higher sintering temperatures (1200°–1300°C). The negative effect of silicon substitution on the sintering of HA at low temperatures (1000°–1150°C) was reflected in the hardness values of the ceramics. However, for higher sintering temperatures, e.g., 1300°C, where sintered densities were comparable, the hardness values of Si-HA compositions were equal to or greater than that of HA, reflecting the smaller grain sizes observed for the former.

I. Introduction

SYNTHETIC hydroxyapatite (HA), $Ca_{10}(PO_4)_6(OH)_2$, is used extensively as a ceramic medical implant material as it has a chemical and phase composition comparable to the inorganic component of bone. Although HA has the ability to allow new bone to form along its surface, the number of medical applications of HA are limited for the following reasons: relatively low fracture strength and toughness,[1] remodeling in the body over a long time period,[2] and a relatively slow rate of osseointegration.[3] A number of approaches have been developed to improve the mechanical properties of HA biomaterials, which include producing a polyethylene–HA composite,[4] the addition of a second, high-strength ceramic phase, such as yttria-doped zirconia (Y-TZP),[5] or the addition of a glass-reinforcing phase, e.g., a $CaO–P_2O_5$ glass.[6] An established and simple method of improving the rate of remodeling of an HA implant is to introduce appreciable levels of a more resorbable calcium phosphate phase, such as β-tricalcium phosphate (TCP).[7] The current and very popular approach to speeding up the rate of osseointegratiion of HA implants is to incorporate biological entities, such as growth factors, proteins, and cells, onto the surface of the HA implant.[8]

Another approach to improving the biological properties of HA is to adjust its chemical composition to more closely approximate that of bone mineral. The most common example of this is the substitution of carbonate ions into the HA structure[9,10] such that the product contains between 3 and 8 wt% carbonate, which is similar to the levels detected in bone mineral.[11] Studies have shown that this type of substitution can increase the solubility of HA[12,13] and also enhance the proliferation of human osteoblast cells *in vitro*.[14] Other ions, which are found in bone mineral, have been substituted into the HA structure, such as magnesium,[15] fluorine,[16] and sodium,[17] although their role on the biological performance of HA has not been clearly established.

We have recently developed a novel substituted HA, where silicon, or silicate, ions are substituted for phosphorus, or phosphate ions.[18,19] Silicon is incorporated in a controlled manner at levels of up to 2 wt%, which allows the phase composition to remain as HA, with no secondary phases such as TCP or CaO being formed. Preliminary studies on these new silicon-substituted HA ceramics have indicated that they have an enhanced *in vitro* biological response compared with stoichiometric HA.[20] These initial results provide insight into the potential benefits of silicon substitution to the biological properties of HA. Based on the results of numerous studies of the effect of carbonate substitution on the physical properties of HA ceramics, such as the degree of densification and the sintered microstructure,[21–23] it is reasonable to expect that the substitution of even low levels of silicon, or silicate, ions into HA will also influence the densification and grain growth characteristics of the materials.

The aim of the present study was to determine the effect of silicon substitution on the physical properties of HA. A range of silicon-substituted HA compositions have been prepared and processed so that they all exhibit similar powder properties and these compositions have been sintered over a range of temperatures. Sintered densities and microstructures were studied and the mechanical properties of the resulting ceramics were assessed by measuring their Vickers hardness values.

II. Experimental Procedure

Stoichiometric HA and a series of silicon-substituted HAs, containing 0.4, 0.8, and 1.6 wt% silicon, were prepared according to an aqueous precipitation method described elsewhere.[18,19] The resulting precipitate was filtered, dried overnight at 80°C, and then ground to a fine powder. The powder was subsequently ball-milled, using a porcelain mill pot with alumina milling balls, for 1 h. The powder was then removed from the mill pot and passed through a series of sieves; as a result of this process, the maximum particle size of the final powder that was used in this study was less than 75 μm.

Compacts were produced by pressing uniaxially 1 g of processed powder, in a 16 mm diameter steel die, at 200 MPa. The powder compacts were sintered in a furnace at temperatures between 1000° and 1300°C, at 50°C intervals, for 2 h, with heating and cooling rates of 2.5° and 10°/min, respectively.

The particle size distribution and mean particle size of the different processed powders were measured using a Malvern Mastersizer X (Malvern Instruments, Malvern, U.K.). The specific surface area of the powders was determined by the Brunauer–Emmett–Teller (BET) method (Micromeretics Gemini II 2370 surface area analyzer, Micromeretics, Ltd., U.K.).

S. C. Danforth—contributing editor

Manuscript No. 187736. Received April 30, 2001; approved August 13, 2002.
Supported by the Engineering and Physical Sciences Research Council (EPSRC), U.K., under Grants No. GR/L39919/01 and GR/J67284/01.

†Now with the Department of Biomedical Science, Institute of Medical Sciences, University of Aberdeen, Foresterhill, Aberdeen, AB25 2ZD, United Kingdom.
‡Now with the Department of Materials Science and Metallurgy, University of Cambridge, Cambridge, CB2 3QZ, United Kingdom.

The Ca, P, and Si contents of the samples were determined by X-ray fluorescence (XRF) spectroscopy (Philips PW1606 spectrometer), the carbon contents by C–H–N analysis (Control Equipment Corp. Model 240 XA CHN elemental analyzer), and the phase composition of the sintered samples was determined by X-ray diffraction (XRD) (Siemens D5000 diffractometer, Siemens GmbH, Germany) using Cu$K\alpha$ radiation. From the X-ray diffraction data the average crystallite size of the as-precipitated powders was calculated using the Scherrer formula. The peak width of the (002) reflection was used in the calculations, and silicon was used as a reference material.

The thermal behavior of the HA and Si-HA compositions was determined by differential thermal analysis (DTA), (Seteram Labsys DTA/DSC 1600, Seteram, France) at a heating rate of 10°C/min to 1500°C in an air atmosphere.

The green and sintered densities of the HA and Si-HA ceramics were obtained from the measurement of the geometric dimensions and the sample mass for low-density samples (<95% of the theoretical density) and by the water immersion method for high-density samples (>95%); for low-density samples, the water immersion method allows water to enter the pores, resulting in false values of the sample density. For each sintering condition, three compacts were sintered and the average value of sintered density was determined. All densities were quoted as a percentage of the theoretical density of HA,[24] 3.156 $g{\cdot}cm^{-3}$.

The microstructures of the sintered HA ceramics were studied using scanning electron microscopy (JEOL 6300 SEM, JEOL, Japan). One surface of the specimen was polished to a 10 μm finish, and then etched in 10% phosphoric acid for 10 s. Before examination, the specimens were coated with a thin layer of gold to prevent charging in the microscope. The grain sizes were determined using the intercept method,[26] with the measurement of ~200 grains per micrograph. The activation energy (E_A) for grain growth was calculated by plotting ln (grain size) versus (sintering temperature, K)$^{-1}$ and determining the gradient, which corresponded to $E_A \times R$, the gas constant, as described by Barralet *et al.*[22]

The Vickers hardness, H_v, of sintered specimens was determined using a microhardness indenter (Shimadzu, Japan). A 500 g load was applied for 10 s to produce an indent. The average diagonal length of the indent was measured and this was repeated 5 times for each sample. The Vickers hardness, H_v, was calculated from the method described in the ASTM E384.[26]

III. Results

The results of particle size analysis (PSA) and the specific surface area analysis (BET) of the HA and Si-HA powders after milling and sieving (<75 μm) are presented in Table I. The standard power processing steps used for all materials resulted in similar particle size distributions, indicated by the comparable values of *d*(0.1), *d*(0.5), and *d*(0.9), and average particle sizes, regardless of the level of silicon substitution. The specific surface areas of the different powders were comparable, although the two compositions with the highest silicon contents (HA-0.8Si and HA-1.6Si) had slightly higher values than the pure HA and the lowest silicon content sample (HA-0.4Si) (Table I). The crystallite size of the primary particles of the different compositions, calculated from the X-ray diffraction data using the Scherrer equation, are also listed in Table I. Increasing the Si content of the substituted HA did not appear to have a significant effect on the crystallite size. It should be noted, however, that this method gives an average crystal length and that using the (002) peak from the diffraction data will result in a dimension along the *c*-axis of the crystal, rather than an overall dimension of the crystal in three dimensions.

The measured chemical compositions of the different HA and Si-HA samples are presented in Table II. As described previously,[18] the composition of the reaction mixture was calculated on the basis that one silicon, or silicate, ion substituted for one phosphorus, or phosphate ion. This means that the calculated Ca/(P + Si) molar ratio should be 1.67, which corresponds to the Ca/P molar ratio of stoichiometric HA. The measured compositions of the HA and Si-HA samples, presented in Table II, agree with this substitution mechanism. Carbon was present in all as-precipitated samples and this was in part due to the adsorption/incorporation of carbonate ions from solution; this carbon was lost on sintering. It was noted that the carbon level increased as the level of silicon substitution increased.

X-ray diffraction patterns of sintered samples of HA and Si-HA (HA-1.6Si, containing the highest silicon content of 1.6 wt%) are shown in Fig. 1, for a sintering temperature of 1200°C. All compositions produced a diffraction pattern that matched the standard for HA,[24] and no secondary phases, such as CaO or $Ca_3(PO_4)_2$ (TCP), were observed for any of the different levels of silicon substitution. The same result was observed for all of the sintering temperatures (1000° to 1300°C) used in this study, with no evidence of phase decomposition for any of the compositions.

Differential thermal analysis (DTA) data of stoichiometric HA and silicon-substituted HA (HA-0.8Si) heated to 1500°C at 10°C/min are presented in Fig. 2. No endothermic peaks were observed that corresponded to the melting of any phase. The endotherm at ~1450°C corresponds to the decomposition of HA to other calcium phosphate phases, namely tricalcium phosphate and tetracalcium phosphate. It should be noted that the silicon substitution did not appear to alter the temperature of this decomposition endotherm.

The green densities of samples varied between 1.71 $g{\cdot}cm^{-3}$ (54%) to 1.80 $g{\cdot}cm^{-3}$ (57%), with no direct correlation between the Si content and the green densities. The effect of silicon substitution on the densification of HA is illustrated in Fig. 3. At low sintering temperatures (1000° to 1150°C) the silicon substitution had a significant effect, with the sintered density obtained for any given temperature decreasing as the level of silicon substitution increased. This effect was most noticeable at the lowest sintering temperature used in this study and, as the sintering temperature was increased, the negative effect of the silicon substitution on the sintered density became less. For example, for a sintering temperature of 1050°C, stoichiometric HA sintered to a relatively high density of 93% of the theoretical density, whereas the 0.4, 0.8, and 1.6 wt% Si-HA samples sintered to only 78%, 73%, and 62%, respectively. This trend continued until a sintering temperature of 1200°C was used; at this temperature comparable densities of ~94%–96% of the theoretical density were achieved for all samples. As the sintering temperature was increased to 1300°C, there was no significant difference between the sintered densities of stoichiometric HA and any of the Si-HA compositions.

Table I. Results of Particle Size Analysis of HA and Si-HA Powders†

Si (wt%)	*d*(0.1) (μm)	*d*(0.5) (μm)	*d*(0.9) (μm)	Average (μm)	Specific surface area (m^2/g)	Crystallite size (nm)
0	2	22	65	29	75	26
0.4	3	23	63	29	78	24
0.8	2	23	66	30	87	25
1.6	2	21	61	26	87	24

†*d*(0.1), *d*(0.5), and *d*(0.9) refer to the measured particle size, or diameter, of 10%, 50%, and 90% of the powder particles. The specific surface area (from BET measurement) and crystallite size (from X-ray diffraction data using the Scherrer formula) of the different compositions are also included.

Table II. Results of Chemical Analysis of HA and Si-HA Compositions Using X-ray Fluorescence

Si (wt%)		Ca/P molar ratio	Ca/(P + Si) molar ratio	C (measured) (wt%)
Calcd	Measured			
0	0	1.68	1.68	0.34
0.4	0.38	1.71	1.68	0.47
0.8	0.76	1.75	1.67	0.77
1.6	1.69	1.83	1.68	1.17

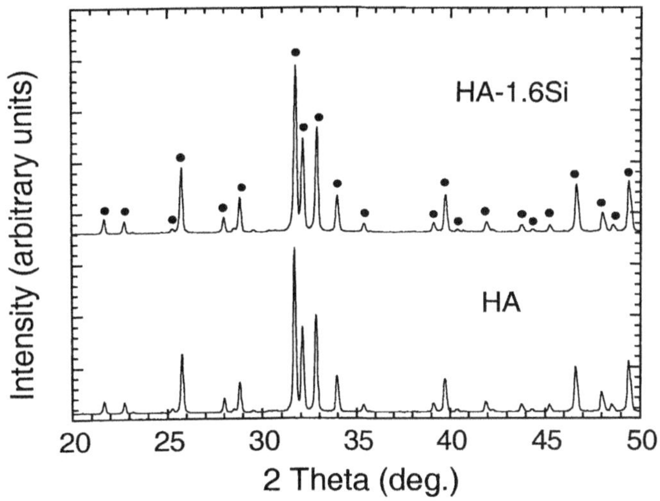

Fig. 1. X-ray diffraction patterns of stoichiometric HA and silicon-substituted HA (1.6 wt% Si) sintered at 1200°C.

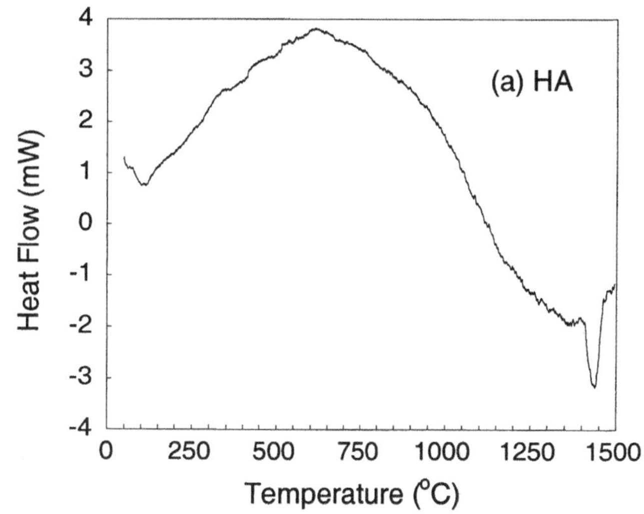

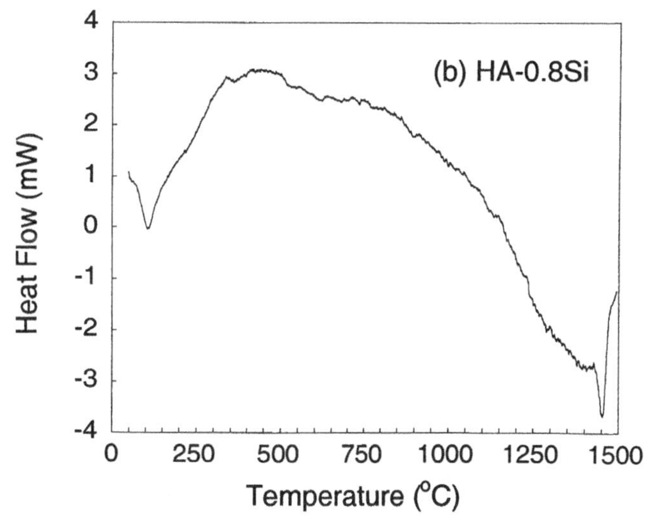

Fig. 2. Differential thermal analysis (DTA) data of (a) stoichiometric HA and (b) silicon-substituted HA (HA-0.8Si) heated to 1500°C at 10°C/min, showing the absence of any melting endotherms. The endotherm at ~1450°C corresponds to the decomposition of HA to other calcium phosphate phases.

The effect of silicon substitution on the sintered microstructure of HA ceramics was studied using scanning electron microscopy (SEM); a representative selection are presented in Figs. 4(a,b), showing HA and Si-HA samples sintered at 1200°C. At 1000°C, the microstructure of the HA sample indicated the initial sintering of a powder compact where necks were beginning to form between submicrometer particles (data not shown). In some areas, agglomerates of HA particles started to sinter together, forming dense areas between 2 and 10 μm in size. By contrast the Si-HA samples did not appear to have reached the same stage of sintering, with the microstructure resembling that of an unsintered powder compact.

At 1200°C, the HA sample had a grain size which was significantly greater than that observed for the Si-HA samples, and this was most noticeable for the highest silicon content of 1.6 wt% (Fig. 4(d)). All of the Si-HA samples had a unimodal grain size of between 0.5 and 1 μm, whereas stoichiometric HA had a bimodal grain size with an average grain size of 1–2 and 5 μm. Although the average grain size of Si-HA samples was much smaller than for HA at 1200°C, it must be noticed that at this temperature the Si-HA samples still had appreciable levels of microporosity in the microstructure, whereas the HA sample was near full density at 1200°C. At a higher sintering temperature of 1300°C (data not shown) all samples showed an increase in grain size, but the HA sample continued to have the largest grain size of all samples. At 1300°C, the Si-HA samples produced a bimodal distribution of grain sizes, with microstructures that were comparable to the stoichiometric HA at 1200°C (Fig. 4(a)).

Using the micrographs of the microstructures of samples sintered between 1000° and 1300°C, the activation energies of grain growth for HA and Si-HA samples were calculated. The calculated activation energy for HA was 141 kJ·mol^{-1}, whereas the 0.4, 0.8, and 1.6 wt% Si-HA samples produced values of 205, 183, 187 kJ·mol^{-1}, respectively (the correlation coefficients of the linear plots of ln (grain size) vs (sintering temperature, K)$^{-1}$ were 0.99, 0.97, 0.97, and 0.99, respectively, and the ±SD of ~10 kJ·mol^{-1} for all samples). There is a clear difference between the grain growth kinetics of the stoichiometric HA sample and the Si-substituted HAs, with the substitution of silicon into the HA lattice resulting in an increase in the activation energy.

The effect of silicon substitution on the Vickers hardness, H_v, of ceramic test specimens sintered at temperatures between 1000° and 1300°C is illustrated in Fig. 5. For a sintering temperature of 1000°C, the HA sample had a hardness of ~240 H_v, whereas all the Si-HA samples had values of ~80–100 H_v. This large difference in hardness can be related to the significant differences observed for the sintered densities of the HA and Si-HA samples at 1000°C, as observed in Fig. 3. Increasing the sintering temperature from 1000° to 1300°C resulted in a small but steady increase in Vickers hardness of the stoichiometric HA, reaching a value of ~350 H_v for the highest sintering temperature. Increasing the sintering temperature of the Si-HA samples resulted in more significant changes in the hardness values. The 0.4 and 0.8 wt% Si-HA compositions had higher hardness values than HA when sintered at 1100°C, and at 1200°C all Si-HA compositions had higher hardness values, with the 1.6 wt% Si-HA sample having the highest value of ~600 H_v. From Fig. 3, all of the Si-HA samples had lower sintered densities than HA at 1100° and 1200°C. However, although the densities were lower, it was noted from SEM investigation that the Si-HA samples had smaller grain sizes than HA at these temperatures (Figs. 4(a–d)).

The hardnesses of samples sintered at 1300°C were comparable, although the sample containing the highest level of silicon, 1.6 wt% Si-HA, still had a high value of ~560 H_v. Sintering at 1300°C resulted in comparable sintered densities for all HA and Si-HA samples. Also, SEM analysis revealed that the grain sizes of the 0.4, 0.8 wt% Si-HA and HA samples were more comparable than at lower sintering temperatures although the 1.6 wt% Si-HA sample still had a significantly smaller grain size than the other samples sintered at 1300°C.

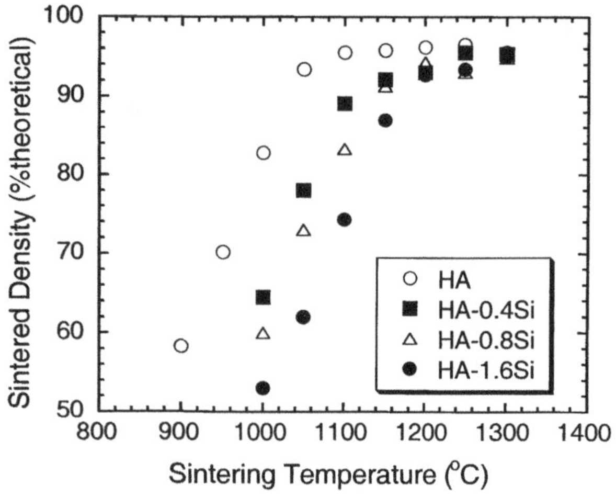

Fig. 3. Effect of silicon substitution and sintering temperature on the sintered density (expressed as a percentage of the theoretical density) of hydroxyapatite.

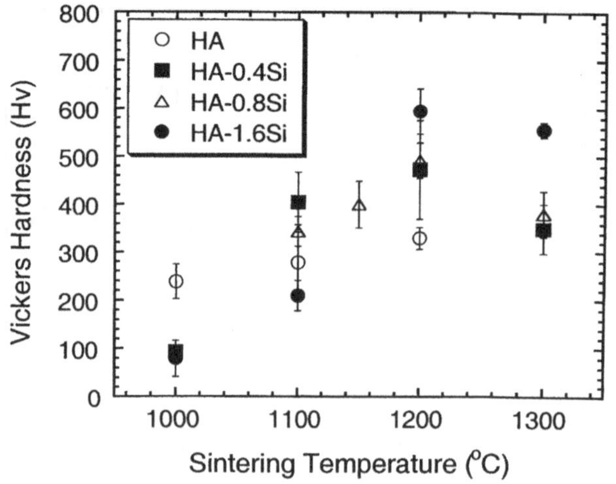

Fig. 5. Effect of silicon substitution and sintering temperature on the Vickers hardness (H_v) of hydroxyapatite ceramics, sintered between 1000° and 1300°C.

IV. Discussion

To assess the effect of changes in the chemical composition on the sintering behavior of an HA powder, it is essential to limit other properties, such as powder particle size[27] and phase composition,[28] that can affect the sintering process. Using standard powder synthesis and processing steps,[29] HA and Si-HA powders were prepared with similar average crystallite sizes, particle sizes, and particle size distributions (Table I). The specific surface areas of the different powders showed only a small variation with varying silicon substitution. A study by Patel *et al.*[30] showed that, in processing HA powders similar to the one used in this study, varying the specific surface area by calcination did not affect the sintering process and final sintered density. By controlling the chemical composition of the reactants,[19] the sintered HA and Si-HA specimens in this study always presented a phase composition of pure HA, with no secondary phases such as CaO or TCP present. Phase purity is a significant point, as Royer *et al.*

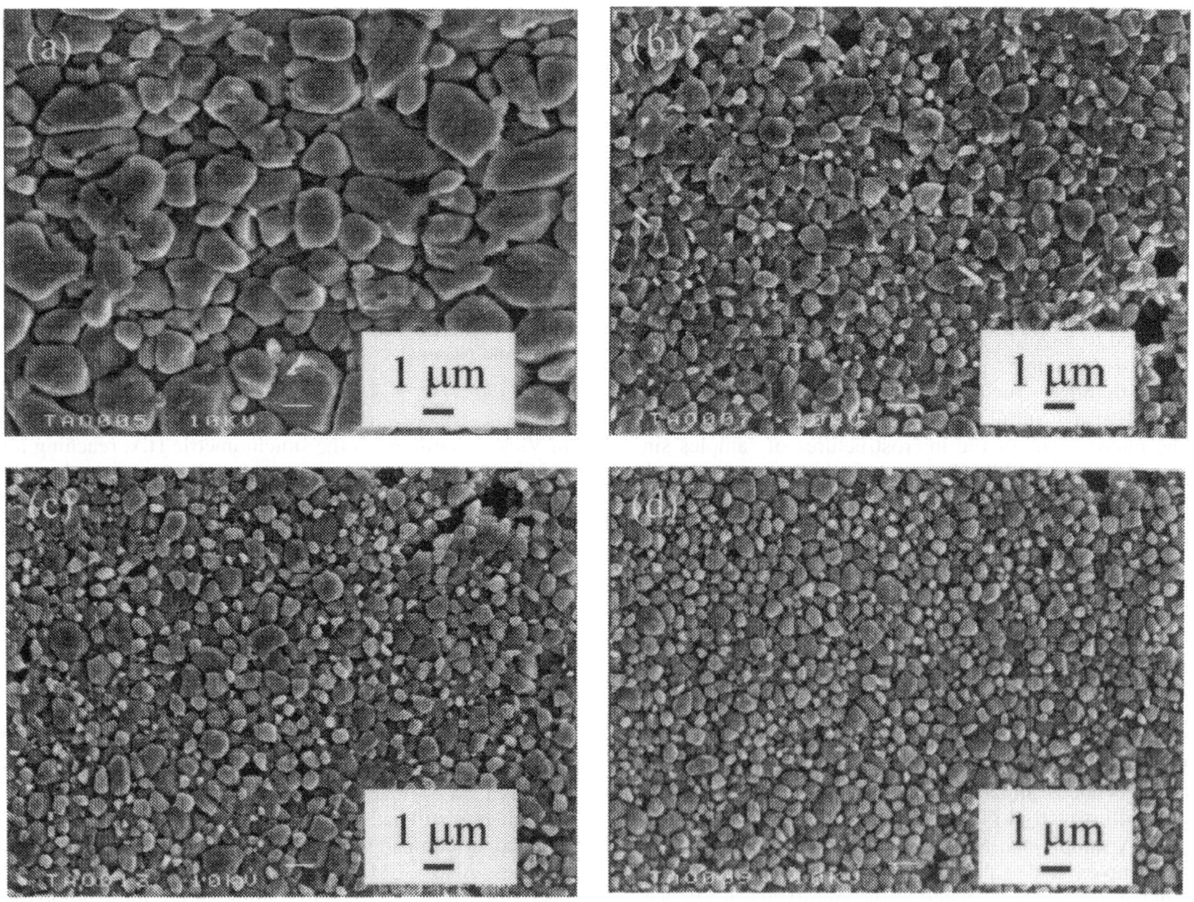

Fig. 4. Scanning electron microscopy (SEM) images showing the effect of silicon substitution on the microstructures of sintered ceramics of (a) HA, (b) HA-0.4Si, (c) HA-0.8Si, and (d) HA-1.6Si sintered at 1200°C.

illustrated that secondary phases such as CaO or TCP retard densification of HA.[28]

Silicon substitution had a very clear effect on the densification process of HA, as illustrated in Fig. 3. Although the silicon substitution does not appear to affect the sintered density that can be achieved at high temperatures, such as 1300°C, it does appear to have an effect on the sintering process. This was demonstrated clearly by the low sintered densities obtained for Si-HA compositions at low temperatures, and by he fact that the lowest densities were obtained for the highest level of silicon substitution. The silicon substitution was also shown to have a clear effect on the grain size of the sintered ceramics; for any given sintering temperature, the Si-HA ceramics had a smaller grain size than the stoichiometric HA ceramic. This was demonstrated further by the different values calculated for the activation energy of grain growth for HA (141 $kJ \cdot mol^{-1}$) and the Si-HA samples (183–205 $kJ \cdot mol^{-1}$). This value for HA was comparable to values calculated by Barralet *et al.*[22] from literature data for various HA samples, ranging from 126 to 147 $kJ \cdot mol^{-1}$, but all of the calculated values for HA and Si-HA were lower than the value reported by Cihlar *et al.*[31] (215 $kJ \cdot mol^{-1}$) for grain growth of sintered injection-molded HA ceramics.

The role that the silicon substitution is playing on the sintering process of HA can be determined by considering the effect that sintering additives have on HA[32,33] and the effect that other ionic substitutions have on the sintering/densification of HA.[21–23,34] A comprehensive study by Suchanek *et al.*[32] reported the effects of a range of sintering additives on the sintering of HA. Sintering additives, or aids, should be clearly separated from ionic substitutions in that they are typically a discrete second phase in the ceramic, as opposed to an ionic species that enters the crystal structure. Sintering aids that are used to enhance the densification are typically compounds with low melting points that promote liquid-phase sintering; examples highlighted by Suchanek *et al.* were Na_2CO_3, KCl, and $Na_2Si_2O_5$, all of which have melting points lower than 1000°C. The sintering behavior of Si-HA observed in Fig. 3 may initially suggest that such a mechanism is occurring, as the densities are significantly lower than HA at low temperatures, but achieve comparable densities at higher temperatures. The fact that silicon is being substituted into HA may suggest that it could be feasible that the silicon is actually forming a secondary phase which would behave as a sintering aid. Chemical characterization, such as XRD analysis, has shown, however, that the sintered Si-HA does not contain any secondary crystalline phases. The substitution mechanism proposed elsewhere by the authors illustrated that the silicon substitution requires a decrease in the level of hydroxyl groups and this was found experimentally, along with linear changes in the lattice parameters with increasing Si contents.[19] Further evidence against the presence of a secondary silicon-containing phase that may act as a sintering aid is presented by thermal analysis of the Si-HA compared with stoichiometric HA (Fig. 2). Heating the HA and Si-HA samples in a DTA under conditions comparable to those of the sintering regime showed that there was no difference between the samples, with no endothermic peaks observed that would correspond to the melting of a secondary phase, resulting in liquid-phase sintering. Thermal analysis of HA with different sintering aids, e.g., Na_2O, CaF_2, SiO_2, by Kanazawa *et al.*[33] showed strong endothermic peaks in the DTA corresponding to the melting of the sintering aid. Finally, from the composition of the Si-HA samples presented in Table II, if any secondary phase was possible it would probably be a calcium silicate phase, which has a melting point in the region of 1400°C.

Chemical analysis of the samples did reveal that an increasing level of carbon was present in the as-precipitated samples (Table II) as the level of silicon substitution was increased. Aqueous precipitation of HA at high pH usually results in some level of carbonate adsorption/incorporation, and this carbonate is normally lost on sintering. The Si-HA samples had significantly more carbon present than the stoichiometric HA, and this may be due to the presence of acetate groups that would have remained from the silicon acetate precursor. Although C–H–N analysis again showed that no carbon remained in the Si-HA samples after sintering, it is possible that the burnout of the carbonaceous material affected the sintering process.

Considering the effect of other ionic substitutions on the sintering/densification of HA powders may provide a clearer insight into the behavior observed with silicon substitution in the present study. The sintering of carbonate-substituted HA, where carbonate groups substitute for phosphate (B-type) groups or phosphate and hydroxyl (AB-type) groups, has been reported extensively.[21–23,35] All of these studies reported that the carbonate substitution has the effect of drastically reducing the sintering temperature required to achieve near-full density by an order of 200°–400°C, compared with HA. The carbonate substitution also has the effect of reducing the grain size of the final ceramic,[22] although it is not clear whether this is a direct effect of carbonate substitution controlling grain growth or just a factor of using reduced sintering temperatures compared with stoichiometric HA. The mechanism that describes the enhanced sintering of these B-type and AB-type CO_3-substituted HA materials has not been reported extensively, but it is probably a combined factor of increased vacancy concentration due to the substitutions and the use of a CO_2/H_2O sintering atmosphere.

In contrast, however, where carbonate substitutes for only hydroxyl groups, A-type, Doi *et al.*[35] reported that there was no difference in the sintering behavior compared with stoichiometric HA. A study by Senamaud *et al.*[34] showed that substitution of fluoride ions for hydroxyl ions in HA has the effect of reducing the sintered density of the resulting ceramic, compared with stoichiometric HA. The authors took care to control the surface areas of the different HA and F-HA powders so that before sintering they all exhibited the same physical powder properties, thereby limiting the variables that could be affecting the sintered densities. From their results and their previous studies, the authors concluded that the fluoride ions interact with the hydroxyl ions, thereby limiting the mobility of OH groups that are instrumental in the densification of HA. Both A-type carbonate substitution and fluoride substitution do not generate the same number of vacancies as the B-type or AB-type carbonate substitutions and this may contribute to these results.

In the present study, the silicon substitution has been described previously by the following mechanism:[19]

$$Ca_{10}(PO_4)_{6-x}(SiO_4)_x(OH)_{2-x} \quad (1)$$

Here, silicon, or silicate, substitutes for phosphate with the concomitant loss of a hydroxyl group, observed by Fourier transform infrared spectroscopy,[19] to maintain charge balance. The above mechanism means that vacancies are introduced on the hydroxyl site as the level of silicon substitution is increased, but no cation vacancies are introduced. It may be the case that the hydroxyl groups in the Si-HA interact more strongly with the calcium or silicate groups compared with HA, and as the number of hydroxyl groups decreases as the silicon substitution increases[19] then this effect becomes more significant. This theory would correlate to the findings of Senamaud *et al.* with F-HA.[34] It could be envisaged that when a high enough sintering temperature is reached, the mobility of the hydroxyl groups in Si-HA is improved and the sintering process begins to match that of HA.

Another significant difference that should be highlighted between the Si-HA in this study and AB- or B-type CO_3–HA materials is that the former is not sintered in a non-air atmosphere, i.e., CO_2, that may take part directly in the sintering process, which is clearly an advantage in the latter two materials.

The silicon substitution affected the grain size of the sintered ceramics and this was most noticeable for sintering temperatures of 1200° and 1300°C where the HA and Si-HA samples had comparable sintered densities. The silicon substitution resulted in a smaller grain size compared with stoichiometric HA, and this was demonstrated very clearly by comparing the microstructure of HA with that of the Si-HA sample with the highest level of silicon substitution (Figs. 4(a–d)). From Fig. 3 it is clear that the stoichiometric HA achieved near-full density at 1100° to 1150°C, so by 1300°C a significant amount of grain growth was probably possible. In contrast the Si-HA did not achieve a comparable density until temperatures of 1250°–1300°C so, as the sintering process was probably only nearing completion at this temperature, grain growth had probably not commenced. The silicon substitution appeared to have the effect of inhibiting grain growth of HA to some degree, as observed from the higher activation energy, without affecting the sintered density of ceramic specimens prepared at 1200° to 1300°C.

The differences that were observed in the sintered densities at low sintering temperatures (1000°–1100°C) and the grain sizes at high sintering temperatures (1200°–1300°C) were reflected in the hardness values of the different materials (Fig. 5). Stoichiometric HA showed a gradual increase in hardness as the sintering temperature was increased and this can be related to an increase in density.[36] The hardness values of Si-HA compositions are lower than those of HA for low sintering temperatures as a result of the low sintered densities achieved for Si-HA at these temperatures (1000°–1100°C). As the sintered density of Si-HA increases, the corresponding hardness values become greater than those obtained for HA, and at 1200°C all of the Si-HA compositions have hardness values greater than HA. As the sintered densities of the Si-HA compositions are all slightly less that that of HA at 1200°C (Fig. 3), the improved hardness can be attributed to the smaller grain sizes obtained for Si-HA ceramics compared with HA ceramics at this temperature, as observed by SEM analysis (Figs. 4(a–d)). At 1300°C, when all of the density values are comparable, the hardness values of all compositions, except the composition with the highest silicon content (HA-1.6Si), are similar. The composition HA-1.6Si still has a high hardness value at this temperature, again as a result of the enhanced microstructure.

These effects can be visualized diagrammatically by plotting the hardness values as a function of sintered density for all compositions (Fig. 6). In general, there is a fairly linear relationship between hardness and density, but with some data points that lie outside of this trend. These points can be attributed to (a) HA-0.8Si and HA-1.6Si compositions with very low densities of 60 and 53%, respectively, (b) the HA-1.6Si values with the highest density (92%–94%) and the smaller grain size, and (c) the higher density values of HA and HA-0.4Si (94%–96%) with corresponding large grain sizes.

As for carbonate-substituted HA ceramics that show enhanced mechanical properties[23,37] compared with stoichiometric HA, there is no clear evidence that suggests that the improved hardness values obtained for the Si-HA materials in this study are a result of anything more than the ionic substitution having an effect of reducing the grain size of the final ceramic, relative to stoichiometric HA. To confirm this, a model would have to be devised that allowed comparison of the mechanical properties of substituted HA ceramics with stoichiometric HA ceramics that all had identical grain sizes and sintered densities.

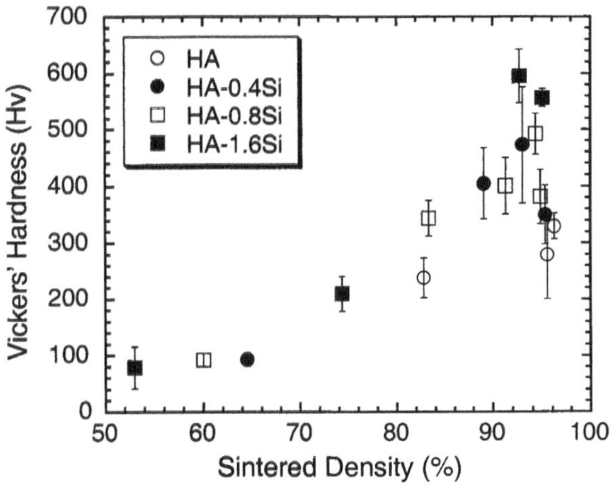

Fig. 6. Relationship between Vickers hardness (H_v) and sintered density of silicon substitution hydroxyapatite ceramics.

V. Conclusions

A range of silicon-substituted HA compositions were prepared that had the same phase composition and physical powder characteristics as stoichiometric HA; the only difference between the materials was the chemical composition. The silicon substitution had the effect of retarding the sintering of HA, with a higher temperature required to begin the onset of sintering. This effect was related to the amount of silicon substituted into the HA. As a result, the Si-HA samples achieved near-full densities at significantly higher temperatures than stoichiometric HA; temperatures of 1150° and 1300°C were required for HA and HA-1.6Si to achieve 95% of the theoretical density, respectively. The positive effect that silicon substitution did have was that it reduced grain growth, so that for a given sintering temperature, e.g., 1200°C, the Si-HA ceramics had significantly smaller grain sizes than stoichiometric HA ceramics. This was reflected in the hardness values of the ceramics, with Si-HA compositions having higher Vickers hardness values than stoichiometric HA.

Acknowledgments

We thank Dr. John Merry for his assistance with the Vickers hardness measurements, and Mr. Bob Whitenstall for his technical assistance with the scanning electron microscopy.

References

[1]G. de With, H. J. A. van Dijk, N. Hattu, and K. Prijs, "Preparation Microstructure and Mechanical Properties of Dense Polycrystalline Hydroxyapatite," *J. Mater. Sci.*, **16** [6] 1592–98 (1981).

[2]C. P. A. T. Klein, A. A. Driessen, K. de Groot, and A. van den Hooff, "Biodegradation Behaviour of Various Calcium Phosphate Materials in Bone Tissue," *J. Biomed. Mater. Res.*, **17** [5] 769–84 (1983).

[3]N. Ikeda, K. Kawanabe, and T. Nakamura, "Quantitative Comparison of Osteoconduction of Porous, Dense A-W Glass-Ceramic and Hydroxyapatite Granules (Effects of Granule and Pore Size)," *Biomaterials*, **20** [12] 1087–95 (1999).

[4]W. Bonfield, M. D. Grynpas, A. E. Tully, J. Bowman, and J. Abram, "Hydroxyapatite Reinforced Polyethylene—A Mechanically Compatible Implant Material for Bone Replacement," *Biomaterials*, **2** [3] 185–86 (1981).

[5]K. Ioku, M. Yoshimura, and S. Somiya, "Microstructure and Mechanical Properties of Hydroxyapatite Ceramics with Zirconia Dispersion Prepared by Post-Sintering," *Biomaterials*, **11** [1] 57–61 (1990).

[6]J. D. Santos, R. L. Reis, F. J. Monteiro, J. C. Knowles, and W. Bonfield, "Liquid Phase Sintering of Hydroxyapatite by Phosphate and Silicate Glass Additions: Structure and Properties of the Composites," *J. Mater. Sci.: Mater. Med.*, **6** [6] 348–52 (1995).

[7]C. Schwartz, P. Liss, B. Jacquemaire, P. Lecestre, and P. Frayssinet, "Biphasic Synthetic Bone Substitute Use in Orthopaedic and Trauma Surgery: Clinical, Radiological and Histological Results," *J. Mater. Sci.: Mater. Med.*, **10** [12] 821–25 (1999).

[8]K. Anselme, B. Noël, B. Flautre, M. C. Blary, C. Delecourt, M. Descamps, and P. Hardouin, "Association of Porous Hydroxyapatite and Bone Marrow Cells for Bone Regeneration," *Bone*, 25 [2] 51S–54S (1999).

[9]R. Z. LeGeros, "Effect of Carbonate on the Lattice Parameters of Apatite," *Nature (London)*, **205**, 403–404 (1965).

[10]D. G. A. Nelson and J. D. B. Featherstone, "Preparation, Analysis and Characterisation of Carbonated Apatites," *Calcif. Tissue Int.*, **34** [2] S69–81 (1982).

[11]F. C. M. Driessens, "The Mineral in Bone, Dentin and Tooth Enamel," *Bull. Soc. Chim. Belg.*, **89**, 663 (1980).

[12]Y. Doi, T. Shibutani, Y. Moriwaki, T. Kajimoto, and Y. Iwayam, "Sintered Carbonate as Resorbable Bone Substitutes," *J. Biomed. Mater. Res.*, **39** [4] 603–10 (1998).

[13]J. Barralet, M. Akao, H. Aoki, and H. Aoki, "Dissolution of Dense Carbonate Apatite Subcutaneously Implanted in Wistar Rats," *J. Biomed. Mater. Res.*, **49** [2] 176–82 (2000).

[14]K. A. Hing, J. C. Merry, I. R. Gibson, L. Di Silvio, S. M. Best, and W. Bonfield, "Effect of Carbonate Content on the Response of Human Osteoblast-like Cells to Carbonate-Substituted Hydroxyapatite"; pp. 195–98 in *Bioceramics*, Vol. 12, Proceedings of the 12th International Symposium on Ceramics in Medicine (Nara, Japan, November 1999). Edited by H. Ohgushi, G. W. Hastings, and T. Yoshikawa. World Scientific Publishing Co. Ltd., London, U.K., 1999

[15]A. Yasukawa, S. Ouchi, K. Kandori, and T. Ishikawa, "Preparation and Characterization of Magnesium-Calcium Hydroxyapatites," *J. Mater. Chem.*, **6** [8] 1401–405 (1996).

[16]L. J. Jha, S. M. Best, J. C. Knowles, I. Rehman, J. D. Santos, and W. Bonfield, "Preparation and Characterisation of Fluoride-Substituted Apatites," *J. Mater. Sci.: Mater. Med.*, **8** [4] 185–91 (1997).

[17]E. A. P. DeMaeyer and R. M. H. Verbeeck, "Possible Substitution Mechanism for Sodium and Carbonate in Calcium Hydroxyapatite," *Bull. Soc. Chim. Belg.*, **102** [9] 601–609 (1993).

[18]S. M. Best, W. Bonfield, I. R. Gibson, L. J. Jha, and J. D. Santos, "Silicon-Substituted Apatites and Process for the Preparation Thereof," U.S. Pat. No. 6 312 468.

[19]I. R. Gibson, S. M. Best ,and W. Bonfield, "Chemical Characterisation of Silicon-Substituted Hydroxyapatite," *J. Biomed. Mater. Res.*, **44** [4] 422–28 (1999).

[20]I. R. Gibson, J. Huang, S. M. Best, and W. Bonfield, "Enhanced *In Vitro* Cell Activity and Surface Apatite Layer Formation on Novel Silicon-Substituted Hydroxyapatites"; pp. 191–94 in *Bioceramics*, Vol. 12, Proceedings of the 12th International Symposium on Ceramics in Medicine (Nara, Japan, November 1999). Edited by H. Ohgushi, G. W. Hastings, and T. Yoshikawa. World Scientific Publishing Co. Ltd., London, U.K., 1999.

[21]Y. Doi, T. Koda, N. Wakamatsu, T. Goto, H. Kamemizu, Y. Morinaki, M. Adachi, and Y. Suma, "Influence of Carbonate on Sintering of Apatites," *J. Dent. Res.*, **72** [9] 1279–84 (1993).

[22]J. E. Barralet, S. M. Best, and W. Bonfield, "Grain Growth Behaviour of Carbonate Hydroxyapatite," *Rep. Inst. Med. Dent. Eng.*, **29**, 39–43 (1995).

[23]J. C. Merry, I. R. Gibson, S. M. Best, and W. Bonfield, "Synthesis and Characterisation of Carbonate Hydroxyapatite," *J. Mater. Sci.: Mater. Med.*, **9** [12] 779–83 (1998).

[24]Powder Diffraction File, Card No. 9-432. International Centre for Diffraction Data, Newton Square, PA.

[25]M. I. Mendelson, "Average grain Size in Polycrystalline Ceramics," *J. Am. Ceram. Soc.*, **52** [8] 443–46 (1967).

[26]ASTM E 384-84, Standard Test Method for Microhardness Of Materials. ASTM Committee on Standards, Philadelphia, PA, 1984.

[27]S. Best and W. Bonfield, "Processing Behaviour of Hydroxyapatite Powders with Contrasting Morphology," *J. Mater. Sci.: Mater. Med.*, **5** [8] 516–21 (1994).

[28]A. Royer, J. C. Viguie, M. Heughebaert, and J. C. Heughebaert, "Stoichiometry of Hydroxyapatite: Influence on the Flexural Strength," *J. Mater. Sci.: Mater. Med.*, **4** [1] 76–82 (1993).

[29]I. R. Gibson, S. Ke, S. M. Best, and W. Bonfield, "Effect of Powder Characteristics on the Sinterability of Hydroxyapatite Powders," *J. Mater. Sci.: Mater. Med.*, **12** [2] 163–71 (2001).

[30]N. Patel, I. R. Gibson, S. Ke, S. M. Best, and W. Bonfield, "Calcining Influence on the Powder Properties of Hydroxyapatite," *J. Mater. Sci.: Mater. Med.*, **12** [2] 181–88 (2001).

[31]J. Cihlar and M. Trunec, "Injection Moulded Hydroxyapatite Ceramics," *Biomaterials*, **17** [19] 1905–11 (1996).

[32]W. Suchanek, M. Yashima, M. Kakihana, and M. Yoshimura, "Hydroxyapatite Ceramics with Selected Sintering Additives," *Biomaterials*, **18** [13] 923–33 (1997).

[33]T. Kanazawa, T. Umegaki, K. Yamashita, H. Monma, and T. Hiramatsu, "Effects of Additives on Sintering and Some Properties of Calcium Phosphates with Various Ca/P Ratios," *J. Mater. Sci.*, **26** [2] 417–22 (1991).

[34]N. Senamaud, D. Bernache-Assollant, E. Champion, M. Heughebaert, and C. Rey, "Calcination and Sintering of Hydroxyfluorapatite Powders," *Solid State Ionics*, **101–103** [2] 1357–62 (1997).

[35]Y. Doi, T. Koda, M. Adachi, N. Wakamatsu, T. Goto, H. Kamemizu, Y. Moriwaki, and Y. Suwa, "Pyrolysis-Gas Chromatography of Carbonate Apatites Used for Sintering," *J. Biomed. Mater. Res.*, **29** [11] 1451–57 (1995).

[36]P. van Landuyt, F. Li, J. P. Keustermans, J. M. Streydio, F. Delannay, and E. Munting, "The Influence of High Sintering Temperatures on the Mechanical Properties of Hydroxyapatite," *J. Mater. Sci.: Mater. Med.*, **6** [1] 8–13 (1995).

[37]I. R. Gibson and W. Bonfield, "Novel Synthesis and Characterisation of an AB-Type Carbonate-Substituted Hydroxyapatite," *J. Biomed. Mater. Res.*, **59** [4] 697–708 (2001). □

journal

J. Am. Ceram. Soc., **85** [11] 2785–91 (2002)

Wear Simulation of Alumina-on-Alumina Prosthetic Hip Joints Using a Multidirectional Motion Pin-on-Disk Device

Vesa Saikko

Department of Mechanical Engineering, Helsinki University of Technology, FIN-02015 HUT, Finland

Jaakko Keränen

Department of Materials Engineering, Tampere University of Technology, FIN-33101 Tampere, Finland

The wear of a state-of-the-art implant alumina against itself was studied with a circularly translating pin-on-disk (CTPOD) device, a wear simulator for prosthetic hip joint materials. The direction of sliding changed continually relative to the pin, preventing erroneous uniaxial grooving typical of ordinary pin-on-disk devices. The dominating wear mechanism was mild abrasion manifested as a relieflike surface, which agreed with clinical findings. The wear factor ranged from 1×10^{-8} to 6×10^{-8} $mm^3/(N \cdot m)$. The CTPOD device, validated earlier for ultrahigh molecular weight polyethylene, was shown to be the first simple wear test device to produce wear similar to that known to occur clinically in alumina-on-alumina total hip prostheses.

I. Introduction

For the past two decades, alumina-on-alumina articulation has constituted a low-wear alternative to metal-on-polyethylene in total hip arthroplasty. The wear particles removed from acetabular cups made of conventional ultrahigh molecular weight polyethylene have caused a large-scale clinical problem of osteolysis and implant loosening. Recent advances both in the material properties of alumina and in the implant design have reduced the risk of fracture in alumina femoral heads, and of catastrophic wear in alumina-on-alumina articulations, which have often been under discussion, to a very low level.[1,2] The wear behavior of alumina-on-alumina has been studied in laboratory conditions using hip joint simulators.[3–7] The wear rate of alumina-on-alumina in simulators is typically so low that the amount of material removed from the spherical surfaces is difficult to measure accurately. Gravimetric and dimensional methods have been used. The principal outcome of these studies is qualitative, that is, the evaluation of the prevailing wear mechanisms. The typical wear process is grain loosening → multidirectional scratching → production of smaller abrasive wear particles → mild abrasion manifested as a relieflike surface.[6] On the relief surface, individual grains are readily distinguished because of the differences in wear resistance between adjacent grains. The wear resistance of each grain is determined by the crystal orientation relative to the surface. These phenomena agree with observations from retrieved components.[4,8] Under some abnormal circumstances however, such as with malposition of the acetabular cup, the wear may be much higher than that predicted by a "benign" wear simulation.

The difficulty of the quantification of wear can be overcome with a circularly translating pin-on-disk (CTPOD) test arrangement with a spherical-ended pin against a flat disk. This is because the calotte-shaped piece worn from the pin has a distinct edge. As the wear surface thus produced is flat, the volume of missing material is easily calculated with precision, despite the fact that the volume is of the order of 1×10^{-3} mm^3 only. The weight loss corresponding to a volumetric wear of 1×10^{-3} mm^3 of alumina is 4 μg, which is difficult to quantify accurately using gravimetric methods. In the CTPOD device,[9] the direction of sliding changes continually relative to the pin. Hence, unidirectional grooving does not occur, which is in agreement with clinical retrieval studies of total hip prostheses.[4,8] A biomechanical study of the hip joint showed that in walking, the direction of sliding changes continually.[10] In ordinary reciprocating and unidirectionally rotating pin-on-disk devices, unidirectional grooving does occur.[9,11] The CTPOD device has produced a realistic hip wear simulation for ultrahigh molecular weight polyethylene.[9] The present study was done to evaluate the applicability of the CTPOD principle to the hip wear simulation of alumina-on-alumina, using specimens made of Biolox® forte alumina. Although the wear of state-of-the-art alumina-on-alumina articulations, such as Biolox forte against itself, is generally low, it has not been shown that the wear is clinically insignificant. Therefore, to improve the knowledge of the wear not only of Biolox forte against itself, but also of other ceramic-on-ceramic combinations in the human body environment, a validated method of wear simulation is valuable, particularly if the accurate quantification of wear is easy.

II. Experimental Procedure

The pins and disks were manufactured by CeramTec AG (Plochingen, Germany), from Biolox forte alumina. For Biolox forte the elastic modulus is 380 GPa, the hardness 2000 HV, the fracture toughness 4 $MPa \cdot m^{1/2}$, the four-point bending strength 580 MPa, the density 3.98 mg/mm^3, and the average grain size below 1.8 μm. The material was hot isostatically pressed, and MgO was used as a sintering additive. The pins were spherical-ended cylinders with a diameter of 6.5 mm and a length of 12 mm, cut from 54 mm nominal diameter femoral heads of a hip endoprosthesis. The true radius r of the polished spherical wear end of the pin was 26.83 mm, obtained with a three-dimensional coordinate measuring machine (Model C-700, Carl Zeiss, Oberkochen, Germany), and the surface roughness R_a below 0.01 μm. The disks were of 25 mm diameter and 6 mm thickness. As the wear surface of the disks was flat, exceptional polishing methods, not previously needed in the manufacture of prosthetic components, were required. The outcome was inferior to that of the spherical surface, the disk being more pitted (Fig. 1(a)), and the R_a value 0.06 ± 0.01 μm. Half of the disks received were sent back to the manufacturer for repolishing, after which the surface was clearly less pitted (Fig. 1(b)), albeit more scratched, and the R_a value dropped to 0.03 ± 0.01 μm. The surface roughness was

R. O. Scattergood—contributing editor

Manuscript No. 187062. Received March 28, 2002; approved August 6, 2002.
Supported by the Academy of Finland, under Grant No. 43328, and Dr. Saikko's Senior Research Fellowship.

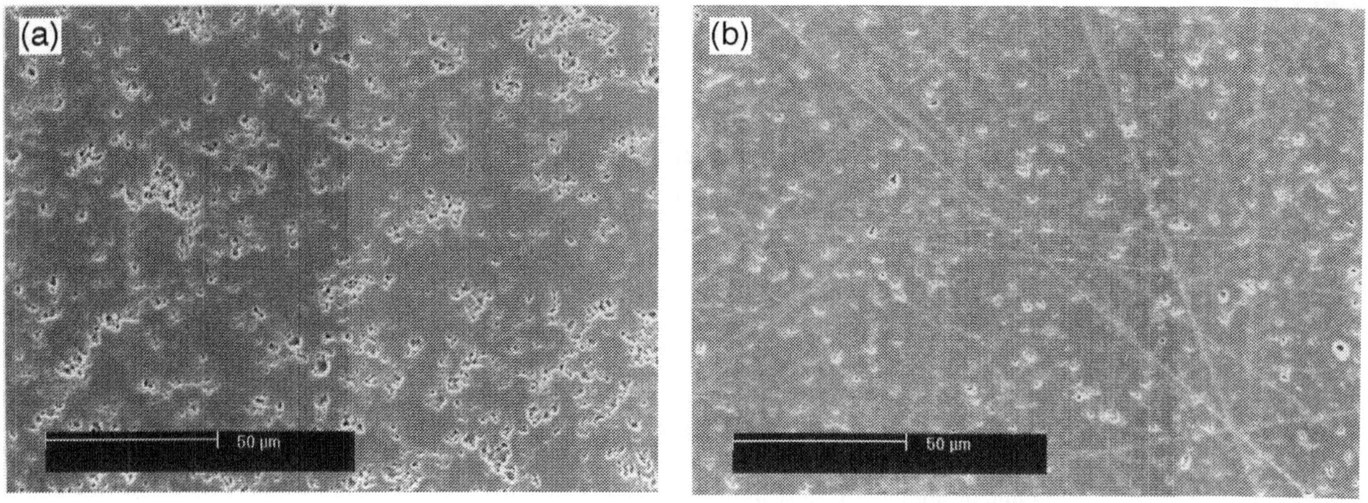

Fig. 1. Scanning electron micrographs of alumina disk before test: (a) original, (b) repolished.

measured with a diamond stylus instrument (Model Surtronic 3+, Taylor Hobson, Leicester, U.K.) using 0.8 mm cut-off and 4 mm evaluation length.

The tests were done with a CTPOD device described in detail elsewhere.[9] The principal original characteristic of the device was that the pin translated, without rotation, along a circular track of 10 mm diameter on the disk, which made the direction of sliding change continually relative to the pin. This was shown to be a key issue in producing a realistic hip wear simulation for ultrahigh molecular weight polyethylene.[9] One lap is called a cycle, in conformity with hip simulator tests. The sliding distance was 31.4 mm/cycle. The cycle frequency was 1.02 Hz, resulting in a constant sliding speed of 32 mm/s, which is between the mean and the maximum sliding speeds during a walking cycle at the point of resultant load in a total hip prosthesis with 28 mm diameter.[10] The disk was horizontal and the pin vertical. The disk made the circular translation in a horizontal plane. The pin was located above the disk, and vertically loaded against it. As the contact was nonconforming, ball-on-flat, and the elastic modulus of Biolox forte very high, the load L used in the tests was 1 N only. With r = 26.83 mm, the initial maximum Hertzian contact pressure was 220 MPa. In alumina-on-alumina total hip joints, such a contact pressure value is a result of a load of several kilonewtons, depending on the diameter and clearance.[12] In level walking, hip joint peak load may be up to 5 times body weight.[13]

In the tests, two lubricants were compared: Milli-Q-grade distilled water and HyClone Alpha Calf Fraction serum (HyClone Laboratories, Inc., Logan, UT), Cat. No. SH30076.03, diluted 1:1 with Milli-Q-grade distilled water. The former has been found to be a suitable lubricant in hip wear tests for alumina-on-alumina,[5,6] and the latter for polyethylene against various counterfaces.[14,15] Moreover, two types of disks were compared, original and repolished. The tests were done at room temperature. The volume of lubricant in the test chamber was 12 mL. The test lengths n were 0.37×10^6, 1.06×10^6, and 1.84×10^6 cycles, which took 100, 290, and 500 h to run. In the wear testing of prosthetic joint materials, 1×10^6 cycles is assumed to correspond to 1 year *in vivo*. The wear was evaluated only after the completion of each test. No intermediate wear measurements were done, because it is likely that in the reassembly, the relative position of the specimens could not be restored as accurately as needed, considering the high elastic modulus of the material, so that the contact conditions would remain unchanged.

The wear surfaces were examined with a scanning electron microscope (SEM, Model XL 30, Philips, the Netherlands) equipped with an energy dispersive spectrometer (EDS, Model DX-4, EDAX International, USA), and with a contact atomic force microscope (AFM, Model Nanoscope II, Digital Instruments, USA) in the constant force mode using a 200 µm long triangular silicon nitride cantilever and a pyramidal probe with a spring constant of 0.12 N/m. Wear particles were obtained for SEM so that a droplet of distilled water lubricant was placed on a silicon substrate and was allowed to evaporate. The chemical composition of the particles remaining on the substrate was identified by EDS.

III. Results

Wear proved to be too low to be quantified with a balance having a resolution of 0.01 mg (Model AT261 DeltaRange, Mettler-Toledo AG, Greifensee, Switzerland). The microscopy of the pins showed that a calotte-shaped piece was worn away. The wear surface thus formed was flat (Fig. 2), indicating that after the start of the test, the contact changed from ball-on-flat into flat-on-flat, and the nominal contact pressure decreased. The edge of this circular wear surface was easily distinguished (Fig. 3), and

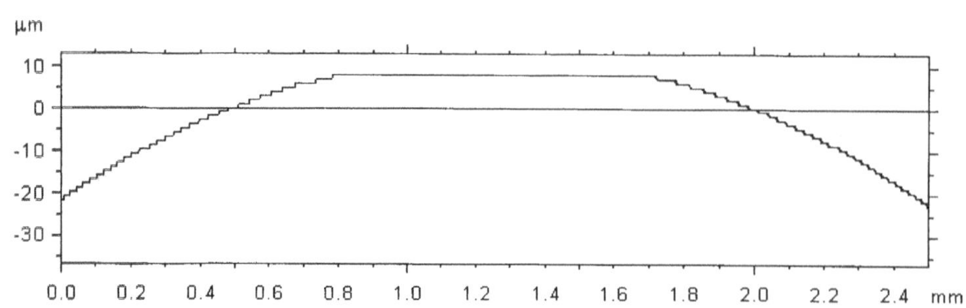

Fig. 2. Profile of alumina pin wear end after 1.06×10^6 cycle test against original disk in serum, obtained with diamond stylus instrument Surtronic 3+. Note flat wear surface created by sliding against flat disk.

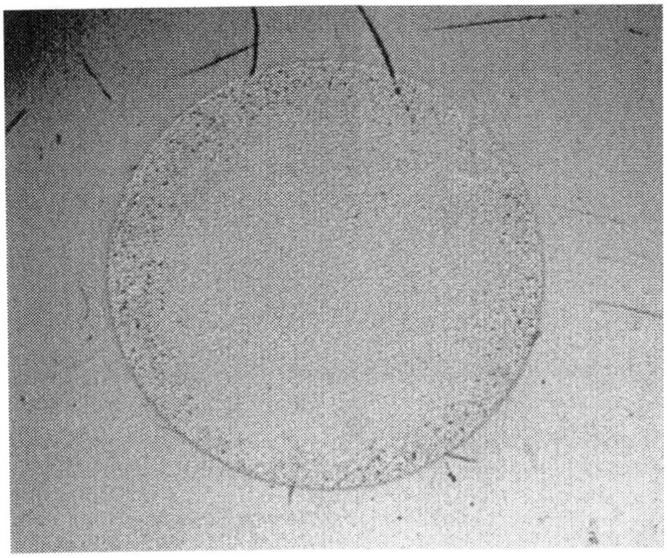

Fig. 3. Low-magnification optical micrograph of pin wear end after 1.84×10^6 cycle test against original disk in distilled water showing wear surface with a diameter $d = 0.81$ mm.

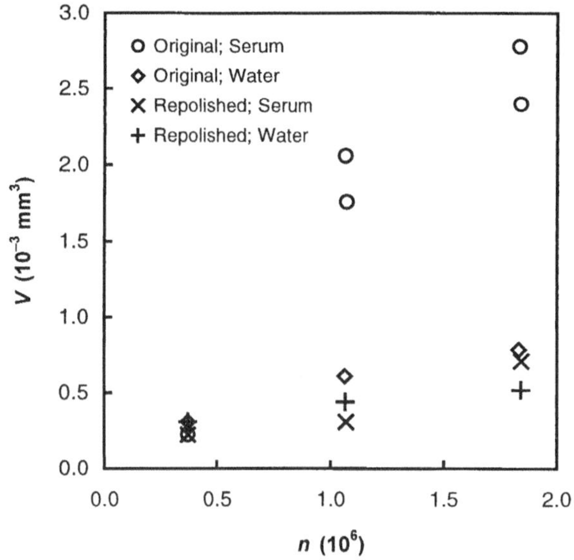

Fig. 4. Volumetric wear V of pins with different test lengths (number of cycles n) against original and repolished disks in serum and water lubricants. Each marker point represents a separate test.

so its diameter d was readily measured with a microscope, the error being ± 0.005 mm at the most. Using the measured d values, which ranged from 0.59 to 1.11 mm, the height h and the volume V of the missing calotte, the wear factor k, and the nominal contact pressure p at the end of the test were computed (see Nomenclature, Table I, Figs. 4 and 5). The ranges for V and k were 0.2×10^{-3}–2.8×10^{-3} mm^3 and 0.9×10^{-8}–6.2×10^{-8} mm^3/(N·m), respectively. The pin wear rate was of similar magnitude in the water-lubricated tests against both original and repolished disks, and in the serum-lubricated tests against repolished disks. However, in serum-lubricated 1.06×10^6 and 1.84×10^6 cycle tests against original disks, the pin wear rate was clearly higher than in all other tests. Therefore, these two tests were repeated, which confirmed the difference (Fig. 4).

On the wear surface of all pins, occasional pits with a diameter in the micrometer range, and relieflike surface revealing the grain boundaries, were observed (Fig. 6 and 7). A sectional profile analysis of AFM data showed that the average height difference between adjacent grains was 15 nm (Fig. 7(b)). Scratches were subtle compared with the original spherical, polished surface. Grooving did not occur.

On the disks, an annular wear track of 10 mm diameter could be seen with the naked eye. Microscopy revealed that on the track, the surface was smoother than elsewhere on the disk. The pits and the original polishing scratches had been partly smoothed away, the polishing scratches sometimes even entirely (Fig. 8). However, the wear was too low to be quantified by weighing or by the Surtronic 3+. Grooving did not occur.

The majority of the wear particles were below 0.4 μm in size (Fig. 9). The particles were identified as alumina by EDS.

IV. Discussion

The CTPOD tests for Biolox forte alumina against itself reproduced the dominating clinical wear mechanism of alumina-on-alumina total hip joints, that is, mild abrasion resulting in a relieflike surface (Figs. 6, 7, and 10). Moreover, the CTPOD test arrangement with a ball-on-flat contact proved to be suitable for easy and accurate quantification of extremely low volumetric wear. Clinically retrieved Biolox forte components were not available for examination, because of their recent introduction. Hence, the microscopy was done for retrieved Biolox components representing the older, conventional sintered material with larger grain size. Nevertheless, the relief surface observed on them was similar to that of the test pins. The results clearly indicated that in the simulation of the wear of total hip prostheses, the importance of constantly changing direction of sliding is not limited to

Table I. Summary of Wear Test Results for Biolox Forte Pins

Disk	Lubricant	n† (×10^6 cycles)	d‡ (mm)	h§ (μm)	V¶ (×10^{-3} mm^3)	k†† (×10^{-8} mm^3/(N·m))	p‡‡ (MPa)
Original	Serum	0.37	0.59	1.6	0.22	1.9	3.7
Original	Serum	1.06	1.03	4.9	2.06	6.2	1.2
Original	Serum	1.06	0.99	4.6	1.76	5.2	1.3
Original	Serum	1.84	1.11	5.7	2.78	4.8	1.0
Original	Serum	1.84	1.07	5.3	2.40	4.1	1.1
Original	Water	0.37	0.64	1.9	0.31	2.7	3.1
Original	Water	1.06	0.76	2.7	0.61	1.8	2.2
Original	Water	1.84	0.81	3.1	0.79	1.4	1.9
Repolished	Serum	0.37	0.59	1.6	0.22	1.9	3.7
Repolished	Serum	1.06	0.64	1.9	0.31	0.9	3.1
Repolished	Serum	1.84	0.79	2.9	0.71	1.2	2.0
Repolished	Water	0.37	0.64	1.9	0.31	2.7	3.1
Repolished	Water	1.06	0.70	2.3	0.44	1.3	2.6
Repolished	Water	1.84	0.73	2.5	0.52	0.9	2.4

†Test length. ‡Diameter of worn calotte. §Height of worn calotte. ¶Volume of worn calotte. ††Wear factor. ‡‡Nominal contact pressure at the end of the test.

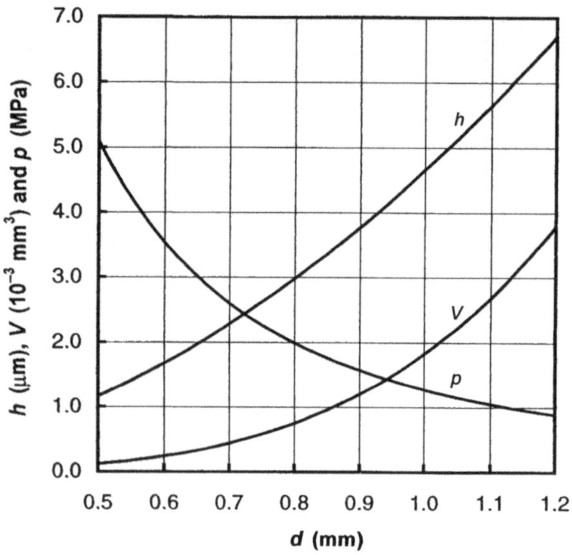

Fig. 5. Computed variation of worn calotte height h, calotte volume V, and nominal contact pressure p with calotte diameter d.

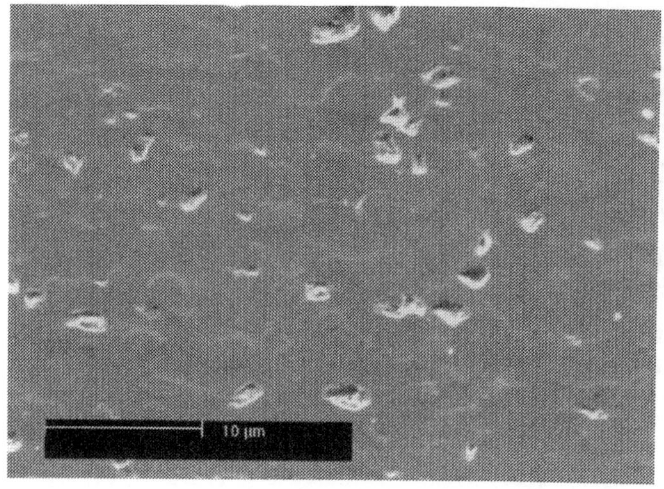

Fig. 6. Scanning electron micrograph from wear surface of pin after 1.06×10^6 cycle test against original disk in distilled water showing pits from which grains have loosened, and relief topography.

polyethylene. It is equally important in the case of alumina-on-alumina. The constantly changing direction of sliding prevents the uniaxial grooving which occurs in the widely used rotating and reciprocating pin-on-disk devices, but not in prosthetic hip joints *in vivo*. The ring-on-disk device specified in the ISO 6474 standard[16] is also uniaxial, and is clearly an obsolete test method for prosthetic hips.

The wear particles produced in the present tests agreed with those isolated from periprosthetic tissues of patients with alumina-on-alumina prostheses.[17] In both studies, the majority of particles had a diameter below 0.4 µm. The particles were clearly smaller than the average grain diameter, apparently being secondary particles resulting from the crushing of loosened grains. Multidirectional scratching did not occur in the way it did in hip simulator studies.[5,6] Possibly, the loosened grain could not leave its place, because the flat sliding surfaces were in such close contact all the time.[3] Instead, the grain was crushed *in situ*, and the secondary particles started to move only when they were small enough to fit between the sliding surfaces. Finally, just the pit remained. This was supported by scanning electron microscopy, which showed some subtle scratches originating from the pits. In the simulator tests,[6] there was no load during the swing phase, and so the surfaces were slightly separated due to the structure of the simulators. This made it possible for the whole loosened grain to leave its place, and consequently cause more severe scratching.[3]

The avalanche-like severe abrasive wear observed in retrieved early alumina-on-alumina designs,[18] and successfully simulated in hip simulator tests,[3] is nowadays so rare that it was not considered necessary to simulate it with the CTPOD device. In early alumina materials, the grain size was considerably higher and the strength lower compared with contemporary alumina, such as Biolox forte. Therefore, the loosened grains could cause an avalanche-like loosening of more grains, resulting in a total destruction of the bearing surface, and the linear wear could be in the millimeter range.[3,18] This problem has been solved by the development of materials and implant designs, the key being the prevention of rim contact. Only in the case of a defective operation leaving the joint lax, due to, for example, an insufficient neck length, is it possible that the wear rate is increased substantially. This could be attributable to a rim contact resulting from a head–cup separation during the swing phase, which was deliberately caused in one set of tests.[19]

In the present test arrangement, the increase of contact area and consequent decrease of contact pressure was rapid in the beginning of the test. Such a change, although in a less pronounced way, takes place also in alumina-on-alumina total hips during the running-in period. In addition to the tests summarized in Table I, numerous shorter tests of 100, 1000, 10 000, and 100 000 cycles duration were done against original disks in distilled water, to see whether the running-in wear mechanism differed from the steady-state one. In these tests, the average calotte diameters were 0.17, 0.24, 0.31, and 0.48 mm, respectively, and the wear factor distinctly decreased with increasing test length (Fig. 11). Irrespective of the test length, the wear surface always showed similar relief topography. Interestingly, this was the case even in the longest tests which showed a wear depth (calotte thickness h) of several micrometers, i.e., clearly in excess of grain diameter, and final contact pressure of approximately 1 MPa only (Table I). Obviously, mild abrasion was the dominating wear mechanism from the very beginning, and continued to be that in the long term. The mild abrasion wear mechanism resembles polishing, and the resulting smoothness was striking. Only the original spherical surface was smoother (Fig. 7). The difference in the smoothness between the original and the worn surface was caused by the fact that in the manufacture of the spherical surface, the polishing was done with diamond particles, whereas in the alumina-on-alumina sliding, the third bodies were of softer material, alumina, and probably also of smaller size. On the wear track of the disks, original polishing scratches were even partly or entirely smoothed away by the further polishing done by the pin and alumina third bodies rolling and sliding between the surfaces (Fig. 8). After water-lubricated tests, elongated debris, several micrometers long, was seen outside the track, similar to that seen in dry reciprocating ball-on-flat tests, and identified as aluminum hydroxide.[20] This indicates that a tribochemical wear mechanism was also acting.

In ceramic-on-ceramic sliding, substantial vibrations are inevitable because of the high elastic modulus.[21] The pin did not slide along the disk as smoothly as a polyethylene pin, and this could be heard as a creaky sound. The sound was loudest in the beginning of the tests. The vibrations caused contact stress peaks that were likely to be much above the calculated nominal values (Table I). Consequently, the pin *kept wearing* even though the nominal contact pressure had decreased to a "comfortable" level of a few megapascals (see Figs. 4 and 5). The modes, frequencies, and amplitudes of the vibrations are highly machine-dependent, the method of loading and pin guiding being important.[21] In the present device, loading was done with a weight, and pin guiding by a double-cantilever beam made from two thin strips of spring steel.[9] Presumably, the vibrations contributed to the crushing of the loosened grains. Vibrations are an essential,[21] but so far mostly neglected, issue in wear testing.

Microscopy and diamond stylus measurements showed that the wear surface of the pin was flat (Figs. 2, 3, 6, and 7). The amount of tilting caused by frictional force depends on the realization of

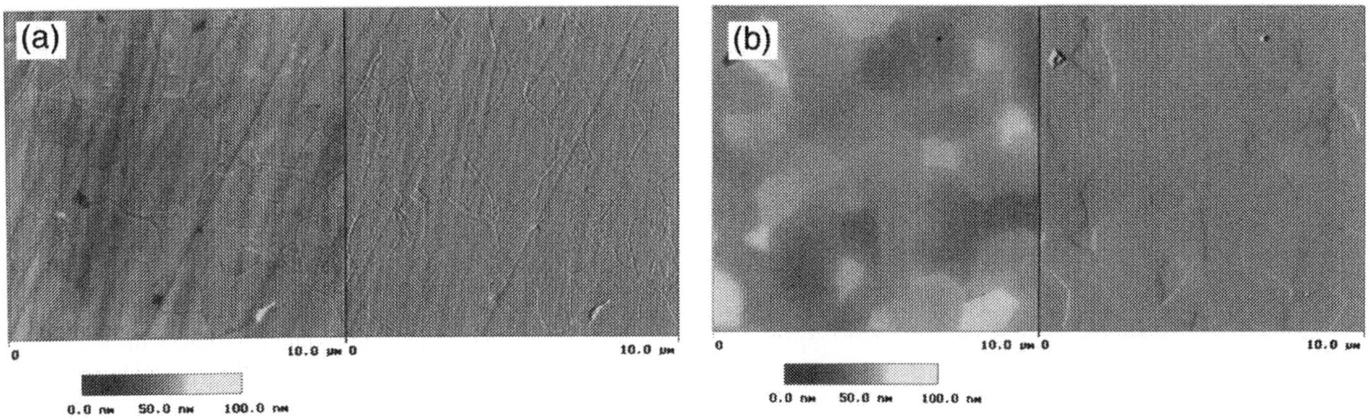

Fig. 7. Atomic force micrograph from (a) original spherical surface of pin, and (b) flat wear surface of pin showing relief topography. Same pin as in Fig. 6. Note original polishing scratches in (a), and subtle scratches on the heights in (b). If heights appear to be valleys and vice versa, rotate the picture. Scan size 10 μm × 10 μm. Left-hand image taken in topographic mode, right-hand image in deflection mode.

pin guiding. It is unlikely that the size and shape of the present wear surfaces were affected by tilting of the pin caused by frictional force. If tilting was significant in the CTPOD device, the wear surface would be convex. The observed flatness proves that the calotte computations were on a sound basis. The calotte height was small compared with the diameter (Fig. 5), and so the calculations would severely overestimate the volumetric wear if the wear surface was clearly convex, with, say, the center being more than 1 μm above the edge. The measurements showed that the deviations from flatness were below 0.1 μm. In an ordinary pin-on-disk test arrangement with a flat-ended cylinder against a flat disk, the high elastic modulus of alumina (380 GPa) would lead to edge contact problems. Even the slightest initial misalignment of the specimens would make the contact pressure distribution skew, strongly affecting the wear behavior. Such problems were not encountered in the present study, because the wear surface of the pin *ensued from* the test.

The present tests confirmed that water is a suitable lubricant in the hip wear simulation of alumina-on-alumina.[5,6] Nevertheless, it was interesting that with the more pitted original disks, serum resulted in a clearly higher pin wear rate compared with water (Fig. 4). This may have been due to adverse vibration conditions, as lubricant pockets (pits) and viscosity affect the modes, frequencies, and amplitudes. It does not seem likely, however, that there would be a difference between the two lubricants if the disk surface finish was of prosthesis-quality, because against the repolished disks, there was no difference in the pin wear rate between the two lubricants. Regarding the pin wear mechanisms, the R_a value of the disks was unimportant, apparently because the deviations from the nominal surface were pits, harmful abrasive asperities being absent.

In hip simulator tests, the wear of Biolox forte against itself is typically so low that its accurate measurement is difficult.[6] In one set of water-lubricated hip simulator tests, the average wear rate of presumably 28 mm diameter Biolox forte alumina-on-alumina joints was measured to be 0.23 mm^3 per 10^6 cycles.[5] With the help of a biomechanical study,[10] this value can be calculated to correspond to a wear factor of 1×10^{-8} $mm^3/(N{\cdot}m)$, which is in agreement with the present results. In the simulator study, however, both the head and the cup were found to lose material, and the above wear rate was a sum of the wear rate of the two components. In the present study, wear could be measured in the pin only. This is easy to understand by noting that the ratio of the area of the annular wear track on the disk to the area of the circular wear surface on the pin was $4D/d$. With the present d values (Table I), the ratio ranged from 36 to 68. Naturally, the pin was therefore the principal object of investigation.

The present wear factors were 2 orders of magnitude lower than typical wear factors measured for acetabular cups made from conventional ultrahigh molecular weight polyethylene, which are

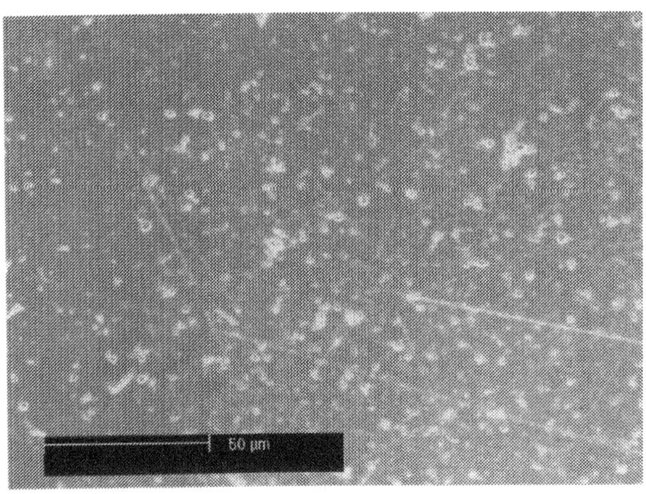

Fig. 8. Scanning electron micrograph from edge of wear track of repolished disk after 1.84×10^6 cycle test in serum. Unworn surface in lower right corner. Note how original polishing scratches have been partly smoothed away on wear track.

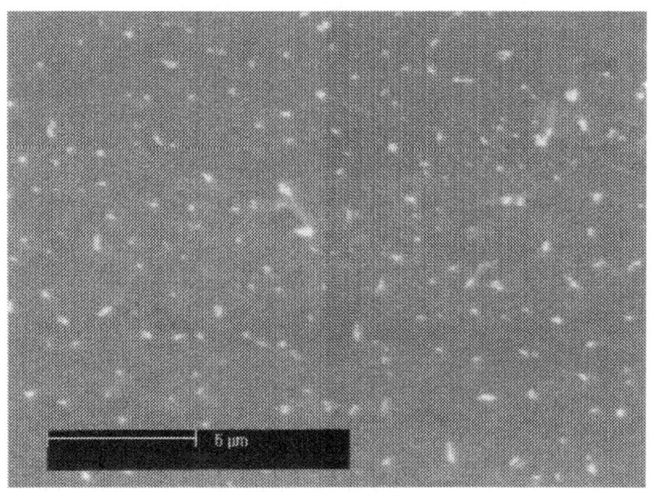

Fig. 9. Scanning electron micrograph of wear particles, identified as alumina by EDS.

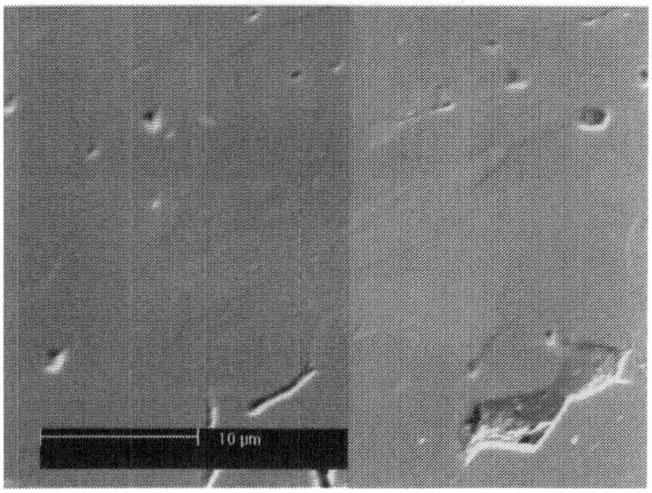

Fig. 10. Scanning electron micrograph from center of contact zone of retrieved Biolox alumina femoral head, worn *in vivo* against alumina cup. Note similarity to Fig. 6.

approximately 2×10^{-6} $mm^3/(N{\cdot}m)$.[14,22] This value was produced also by the CTPOD device for conventional polyethylene pins against polished CoCr disks.[15] The majority of polyethylene wear particles are, unfortunately, in the biologically most active 0.1–1 μm size range.[14,15,23,24] Hence, it appears likely that in total hip arthroplasty employing a state-of-the-art alumina-on-alumina articulation instead of a conventional polyethylene cup against a metallic or ceramic head, the risk of osteolysis and implant loosening caused by wear particle production is reduced.

V. Conclusions

The CTPOD device validated earlier for hip wear simulation of ultrahigh molecular weight polyethylene was shown to be the first simple wear test device to produce wear similar to that known to occur clinically in alumina-on-alumina total hip prostheses. The principal original characteristics of the device, the constantly changing direction of sliding, proved again crucial, preventing erroneous uniaxial grooving occurring in ordinary pin-on-disk devices. Against two different counterface roughnesses, and both in water and in serum lubricants, the dominating wear mechanism was mild abrasion manifested as a relieflike surface, which is in agreement with clinical observations. The test configuration, being initially ball-on-flat, made it possible to accurately quantify extremely low volumetric wear through the detection of the edge of the calotte missing from the spherical-ended pin. The wear factor was of the order of 10^{-8} $mm^3/(N{\cdot}m)$, 2 orders of magnitude lower than that shown by acetabular cups made from conventional ultrahigh molecular weight polyethylene. The low wear of alumina-on-alumina is likely to contribute to the durability of total hip arthroplasty. In the Biolox forte alumina studied, the loosening of grains did not lead to an avalanche-like loosening of more grains, which sometimes occurred in early alumina-on-alumina designs. In general, the effects of vibrations of a wear test device on the results appears to be an important subject of study in the future.

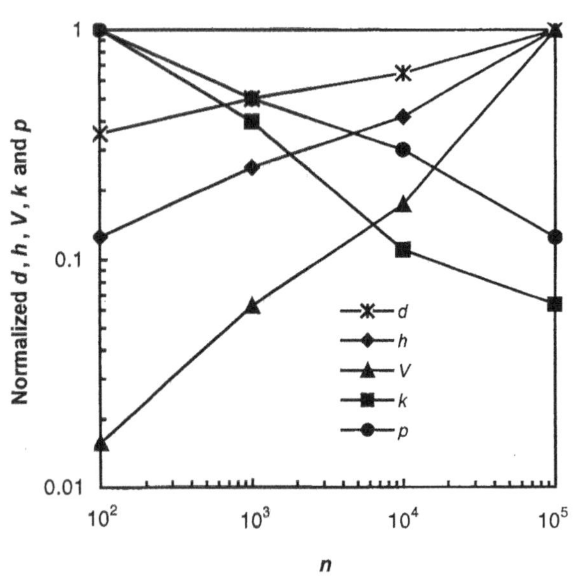

Fig. 11. Normalized calotte diameter d, calotte height h, calotte volume V, wear factor k, and final nominal contact pressure p with different test lengths (number of cycles n) in short tests against repolished disks in distilled water. Unity corresponds to d = 0.48 mm, h = 1.1 μm, $V = 9.7 \times 10^{-5}$ mm^3, $k = 4.9 \times 10^{-7}$ $mm^3/(N{\cdot}m)$, and p = 44 MPa.

Nomenclature

CTPOD	Circularly translating pin-on-disk
d	Diameter of calotte worn from the pin
D	Diameter of wear track on disk (=10 mm)
h	Height of calotte $(=r\{1 - \cos[\arcsin(d/2r)]\})$
k	Wear factor $(=V/(nL\pi D))$
L	Load (=1 N)
n	Number of cycles
p	Nominal contact pressure $(=L/(\pi(d/2)^2))$
r	Radius of spherical wear end of pin (=26.83 mm)
R_a	Arithmetical mean surface roughness
V	Volume of calotte $(=\pi h[3(d/2)^2 + h^2]/6)$

Acknowledgments

The specimens were donated by CeramTec AG (Plochingen, Germany).

References

[1]G. Willmann and W. von Chamier, "The Improvements of the Material Properties of Biolox Offers Benefits for THR"; pp. 19–24 in *Bioceramics in Orthopaedics—New Applications*. Edited by W. Puhl. Ferdinand Enke Verlag, Stuttgart, Germany, 1998.

[2]C. Piconi, M. Labanti, G. Magnani, M. Caporale, G. Maccauro, and G. Magliocchetti, "Analysis of Failed Alumina THR Ball Head," *Biomaterials*, **20** [18] 1637–46 (1999).

[3]A. Walter and W. Plitz, "Wear Mechanism of Alumina-Ceramic Bearing Surfaces of Hip-Joint Prostheses"; pp. 55–60 in *Biomaterials and Biomechanics 1983*. Edited by P. Ducheyne, G. Van der Perre, and A. E. Aubert. Elsevier Science Publishers B.V., Amsterdam, Netherlands, 1984.

[4]A. Walter, "On the Material and the Tribology of Alumina–Alumina Couplings for Hip Joint Prostheses," *Clin. Orthop. Relat. Res.*, **282**, 31–46 (1992).

[5]A. Walter, "Investigations on the Wear Couple Biolox Forte/Biolox Forte and Earlier Alumina Materials"; pp. 123–35 in *Performance of the Wear Couple Biolox Forte in Hip Arthroplasty*. Edited by W. Puhl. Ferdinand Enke Verlag, Stuttgart, Germany, 1997.

[6]V. Saikko and H.-G. Pfaff, "Low Wear and Friction in Alumina/Alumina Total Hip Joints: A Hip Simulator Study," *Acta Orthop. Scand.*, **69** [5] 443–48 (1998).

[7]S. Affatato, B. Bordini, A. Sudanese, and A. Toni, "Wear Behaviour of Ceramic-on-Ceramic System: *In Vitro* Studies on Hip Joint Simulator"; pp. 305–307 in *World Tribology Forum in Arthroplasty*. Edited by C. Rieker, S. Oberholzer, and U. Wyss. Hans Huber, Bern, Switzerland, 2001.

[8]J.-M. Dorlot, "Long-Term Effects of Alumina Components in Total Hip Prostheses," *Clin. Orthop. Relat. Res.*, **282**, 47–52 (1992).

[9]V. Saikko, "A Multidirectional Motion Pin-on-Disk Wear Test Method for Prosthetic Joint Materials," *J. Biomed. Mater. Res.*, **41** [1] 58–64 (1998).

[10]O. Calonius and V. Saikko, "Force Track Analysis of Contemporary Hip Simulators," *J. Biomech.*, submitted for publication.

[11]E. Serra, A. Tucci, L. Esposito, and C. Piconi, "Volumetric Determination of the Wear of Ceramics for Hip Joints," *Biomaterials*, **23** [4] 1131–37 (2002).

[12]M. Ungethüm, "Tribological–Biomechanical Study of the Total Prosthesis of the Human Hip" (in German); Doctoral Dissertation. Aachen University of Technology, Aachen, Germany, 1976.

[13]R. D. Crowninshield, R. C. Johnston, J. G. Andrews, and R. A. Brand, "A Biomechanical Investigation of the Human Hip," *J. Biomech.*, **11** [2] 75–85 (1978).

[14]V. Saikko, T. Ahlroos, O. Calonius, and J. Keränen, "Wear Simulation of Total Hip Prostheses with Polyethylene against CoCr, Alumina and Diamond-like Carbon," *Biomaterials*, **22** [12] 1507–14 (2001).

[15]V. Saikko, O. Calonius, and J. Keränen, "Effect of Counterface Roughness on the Wear of Conventional and Cross-Linked Ultrahigh Molecular Weight Polyethylene

Studied with a Multidirectional Motion Pin-on-Disk Device," *J. Biomed. Mater. Res.*, **57** [4] 506–12 (2001).

[16]International Standard ISO 6474, "Implants for Surgery—Ceramic Materials Based on Alumina," 1st Ed., International Organization for Standardization, Geneva, Switzerland, 1981.

[17]S. Lerouge, O. Huk, L'H. Yahia, and L. Sedel, "Characterization of *In Vivo* Wear Debris from Ceramic–Ceramic Total Hip Arthroplasties," *J. Biomed. Mater. Res.*, **32** [4] 627–33 (1996).

[18]W. Plitz and H. U. Hoss, "Wear of Alumina–Ceramic Hip Joints: Some Clinical and Tribological Aspects"; pp. 187–96 in *Biomaterials 1980.* Edited by G. D. Winter, D. F. Gibbons, and H. Plenk Jr. Wiley, Chichester, U.K., 1982.

[19]T. Stewart, J. Tipper, R. Streicher, E. Ingham, and J. Fisher, "Long-Term Wear of HIPed Alumina on Alumina Bearings for THR under Microseparation Conditions," *J. Mater. Sci.: Mater. Med.*, **12** [10–12] 1053–56 (2001).

[20]S. Jahanmir and X. Dong, "Wear Mechanisms of Aluminum Oxide Ceramics"; pp. 15–49 in *Friction and Wear of Ceramics.* Edited by S. Jahanmir. Marcel Dekker, New York, 1994.

[21]M. G. Gee, "Effect of Test Machine Dynamics on the Sliding Wear of Alumina"; pp. 24–44 in ASTM Special Technical Publication, Vol. 1167, *Testing of Advanced Materials.* Edited by R. Divakar and P. J. Blau. American Society for Testing and Materials, Philadelphia, PA, 1992.

[22]R. M. Hall, A. Unsworth, P. Siney, and B. M. Wroblewski, "Wear in Retrieved Charnley Acetabular Sockets," *J. Eng. Med.*, **210** [H3] 197–207 (1996).

[23]P. A. Revell, N. AL-Saffar, and A. Kobayashi, "Biological Reaction to Debris in Relation to Joint Prostheses," *J. Eng. Med.*, **211** [H2] 187–97 (1997).

[24]J. D. Mabrey, A. Afsar-Keshmiri, G. A. McClung II, M. A. Pember II, T. M. Wooldridge, and C. M. Agrawal, "Comparison of UHMWPE Particles in Synovial Fluid and Tissues from Failed THA," *J. Biomed. Mater. Res. Appl. Biomater.*, **58** [2] 196–202 (2001). □

journal

J. Am. Ceram. Soc., **85** [12] 3129–31 (2002)

Calcium Phosphate Bioceramics with Various Porosities and Dissolution Rates

Soon-Ho Kwon, Youn-Ki Jun, Seong-Hyeon Hong,* In-Seop Lee, and Hyoun-Ee Kim*

School of Materials Science and Engineering, Seoul National University, Seoul 151-742, Korea

Ye Yeon Won*

Department of Orthopaedic Surgery, Ajou University, Suwon 442-721, Korea

Porous bioceramics, such as hydroxyapatite (HA), tricalcium phosphate (TCP), and biphasic HA/TCP, were fabricated using the polyurethane sponge technique. The porosity of the ceramics was controlled by a multiple coating of the porous body. When a porous body was produced by a single coating, the porosity was ~90%, and the pores were completely interconnected. When the sintered body was coated five times after the porous network had been made, the porosity decreased to 65%. As the porosity decreased, the strength increased exponentially. The TCP exhibited the highest dissolution rate in a Ringer's solution, and the HA had the lowest rate. The biphasic HA/TCP showed an intermediate dissolution rate.

I. Introduction

CALCIUM-PHOSPHATE-BASED bioceramics have received considerable attention as bone-graft substitutes, primarily because of their excellent biocompatibility, bioactivity, and osteoconduction characteristics.[1,2] These ceramics are used in porous, granular, and dense forms. Porous calcium phosphate ceramics are quite effective in substituting for and regenerating damaged bones. The appropriate porosity, coupled with the bioactivity of the material, allow in-growth of bone tissue to achieve full integration with the living bones.

The most widely used calcium-phosphate-based bioceramics are hydroxyapatite (HA, $Ca_{10}(PO_4)_6(OH)_2$) and β-tricalcium phosphate (β-TCP, $Ca_3(PO_4)_2$). HA is stable in a body fluid, whereas TCP is rather soluble in the fluid.[2] Many studies have indicated that the dissolution of well-crystallized HA in the human body after implantation is too low to achieve optimum results. On the other hand, the dissolution rate of β-TCP ceramics is too fast for bone bonding. To achieve an optimum dissolution rate of bone-graft materials, research has focused mainly on biphasic calcium phosphate ceramics composed of HA and TCP.[3–7]

For bone in-growth and attachment to the body tissue, pore characteristics are essential features for the bone-graft materials. These materials should have the proper pore size, morphology, and interconnectivity.[8–11] Even though there is wide disagreement about the optimal pore size, it is generally agreed that the pores should be interconnected for actual clinical applications.

To reproduce the pore structure of natural bone, various processing methods have been used.[12–17] To a reasonable extent, these techniques have successfully produced a pore structure similar to that of natural bone, but further improvements are still required. In particular, for load-bearing applications, the mechanical strength should be enhanced while the high porosity of the body is maintained. Consequently, several attempts have been made to correlate mechanical strength with pore size and porosity.[13,18]

In this study, HA, TCP, and HA/TCP composite powders were synthesized by a coprecipitation method. Porous bioceramics with various porosities and biocompatibilities were fabricated using polyurethane foams. The mechanical properties and *in vitro* dissolution behavior of those bioceramics were investigated.

II. Experimental Procedure

HA, TCP, and HA/TCP composite powders were synthesized by the coprecipitation method, using $Ca(NO_3)_2{\cdot}4H_2O$ and $(NH_4)_2HPO_4$. The details of the powder synthesis have been described elsewhere,[7] and the processing parameters for each powder are shown in Table I. All precipitates were calcined at 800°C for the fabrication of porous bodies.

Porous bodies were fabricated by impregnating the struts of polyurethane foam with a ceramic slurry composed of ceramic powders, triethylphosphate (dispersant), polyvinyl butyral (binder), and ethanol (solvent). A 45 ppi (pore/inch) polyurethane sponge was used as a rectangular shape. After the sponge had been impregnated and dried, it was heated at the rate of 1°C/min to 600°C, to remove the polymeric struts, and then sintered. To control the porosity, the sintered bodies were impregnated with the slurry and densified repeatedly. This multiple-coating technique resulted in ceramic bodies with a porosity of 65%–90%. HA ceramics were sintered at 1250°C, and TCP and HA/TCP composites were sintered at 1150°C, to avoid the β- to α-TCP phase transformation.

The total porosity of an as-sintered body was determined by its weight and dimensions and had a variation of 1%–2%. The actual pore size of the porous ceramics was estimated from scanning electron micrographs. An X-ray microscope-microtomograph (Model 1072, SkyScan, Aartselaar, Belgium) was used to produce cross-sectional and three-dimensional (3D) images of the porous body. The porosity was also obtained from the reconstructed 3D images. For the mechanical test, a sample was machined into a rectangular bar shape with dimensions of 5 mm × 5 mm × 10 mm, and the top and bottom surfaces of the bars were infiltrated with paraffin to minimize the edge effects. The compressive strength was measured using a universal testing machine (Model 5565, Instron Corp., Danvers, MA) at a crosshead speed of 0.5 mm/min. For the dissolution experiments, porous bodies were immersed in a commercially available Ringer's solution (Hartmann solution, Cheil Jedang, Seoul, Korea) for up to 30 d. After the porous bodies had

P. Greil—contributing editor

Manuscript No. 187708. Received April 9, 2002; approved August 23, 2002.
This research was sponsored by the Ministry of Science and Technology of Korea, through the 21C Frontier R and D Program and the National Research Laboratory (NRL) Program of the Ministry of Science and Technology of Korea.
*Member, American Ceramic Society.

Table I. Processing Parameters for Powder Synthesis under the Coprecipitation Method

Powder	Initial Ca/P ratio	pH of solution	Aging temperature (°C)
HA	2.0	11	80
HA/TCP	1.55	8.0	40
TCP	1.0	7.4	40

been immersed for a predetermined period of time, the composition of the solution was analyzed by inductively coupled plasma atomic-emission spectroscopy (ICP-AES).

III. Results and Discussion

The X-ray diffraction (XRD) patterns shown in Fig. 1 confirmed that the powders synthesized were pure HA, pure TCP, and a biphasic HA/TCP under the given sintering conditions. The HA/TCP composite powder consisted of ~50% HA and ~50% TCP and had a Ca/P molar value of 1.58.

Scanning electron microscopy (SEM) and cross-sectional microtomographic images of a typical porous HA ceramic (80% total porosity) are shown in Fig. 2. In the microtomographic image (Fig. 2(B)), the pores are displayed as white and the solid walls as black, because of X-ray absorption differences between the pores and walls. The sample sintered immediately after removal of the sponge had a total porosity of 90%, an average pore size of ~600 μm, and a wall thickness of ~100 μm. Macropores in this sample were spherical, almost identical in size, and completely interconnected. The pore interconnections were in the range of 400–500 μm. With multiple coatings, the wall thickness increased and the total porosity decreased (Fig. 2(A)). The pores were interconnected until the sample had been coated five times. However, further coatings resulted in pore isolation. This sample had a total porosity of 65%, an average pore size of ~500 μm, and a wall thickness of ~250 μm, characteristics similar to those of the porous HA derived from the genus *Goniopora* coral skeleton.[2] The pore size and the wall thickness measured by X-ray microtomographic images were consistent with the previous SEM results (Fig. 2(B)). However, the macroporosity calculated from the 3D reconstruction differed from the total porosity determined from the weight and dimensions of the samples. The estimated macroporosity was 12%–15% lower than the total porosity. This discrepancy was attributed to the microporosity of the solid wall, shown in Fig. 2(C). TCP and biphasic HA/TCP composite ceramics also exhibited similar microstructures and porosities.

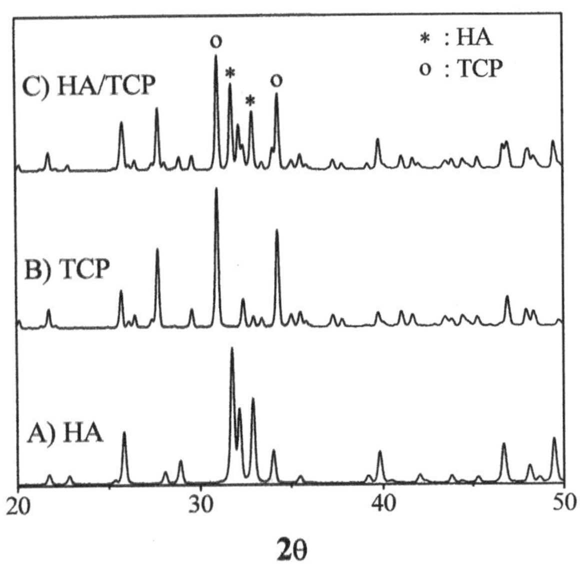

Fig. 1. XRD patterns of (A) HA powder, (B) TCP powder, and (C) HA/TCP composite powder calcined at 1000°C.

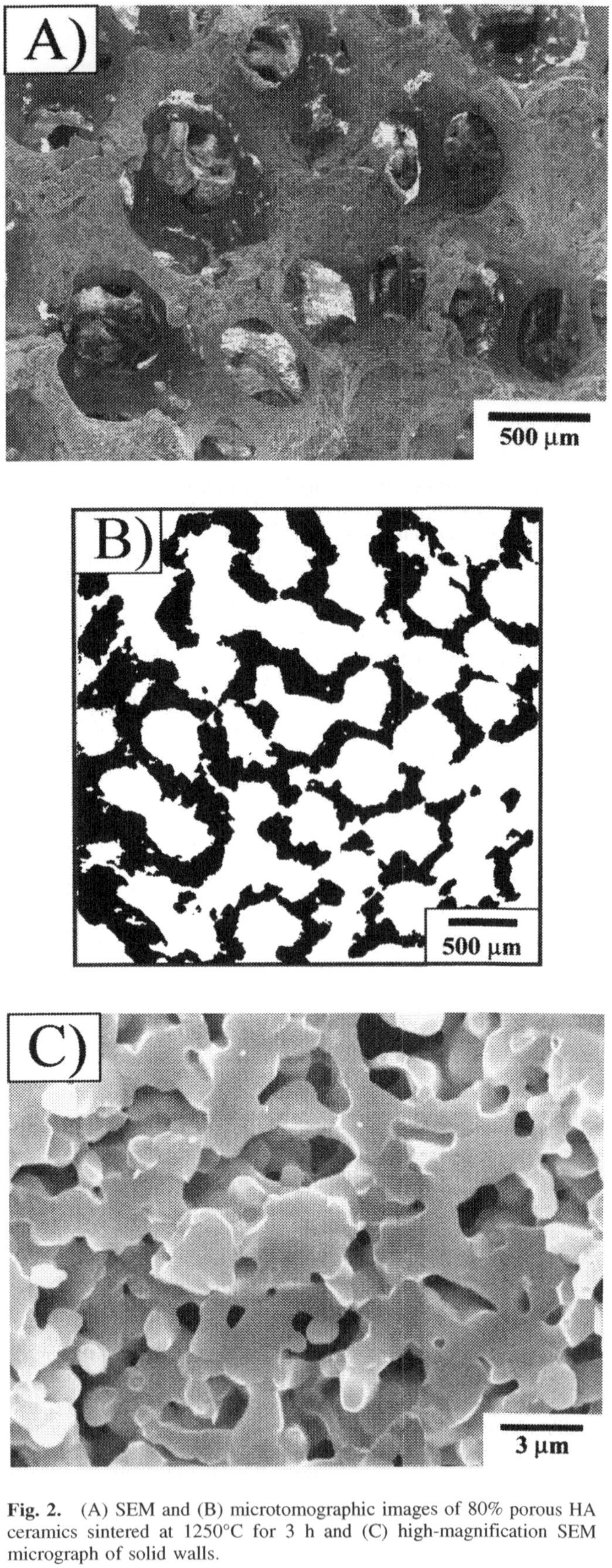

Fig. 2. (A) SEM and (B) microtomographic images of 80% porous HA ceramics sintered at 1250°C for 3 h and (C) high-magnification SEM micrograph of solid walls.

The compressive strengths of the porous bodies are shown in Fig. 3. The strength increased exponentially as the porosity decreased in all sample types. A similar exponential dependency

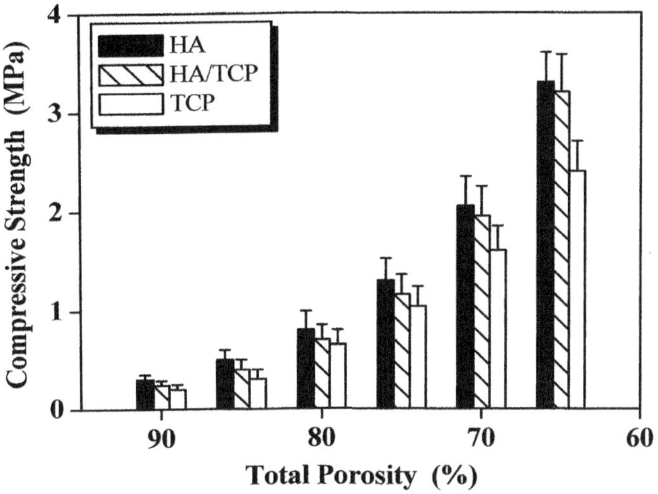

Fig. 3. Compressive strength of porous HA, TCP, and HA/TCP composite ceramics as a function of total porosity.

between strength and porosity has been reported previously.[19] The present work extends this relationship up to 90% porosity. HA had a higher compressive strength than TCP, and HA/TCP composites exhibited an intermediate value. In addition to the inherent weakness of TCP, compared with HA, the low sintering temperature of TCP used to avoid the β- to α-phase transformation is believed to have further decreased the strength of the TCP. At 65% total porosity, the compressive strength of the HA ceramics was >3 MPa, which is comparable to that of the commercial coral-derived porous HA.[20]

The Ca^{2+} concentrations, as released from the porous bodies immersed into Ringer's solution, are represented in Fig. 4. The Ca^{2+} concentration in the HA immersed solution increased initially but stabilized after 1 d. The PO_4^{3-} concentration also remained at a very low level, suggesting that HA was rather stable in the solution. On the other hand, the dissolution rate of TCP was significantly higher than that of HA. The concentrations of Ca^{2+} and PO_4^{3-} released from the TCP samples increased continuously up to 30 d. Like the other properties examined, the biphasic HA/TCP composites exhibited an intermediate dissolution behavior between that of HA and TCP ceramics. The dissolution rate is affected by both macroporosity and microporosity in the wall. Similar dissolution results were obtained from the HA, TCP, and HA/TCP powders used in these experiments. However, further studies are required to address comprehensively the relationships among microstructure, compressive strength, and dissolution rate.

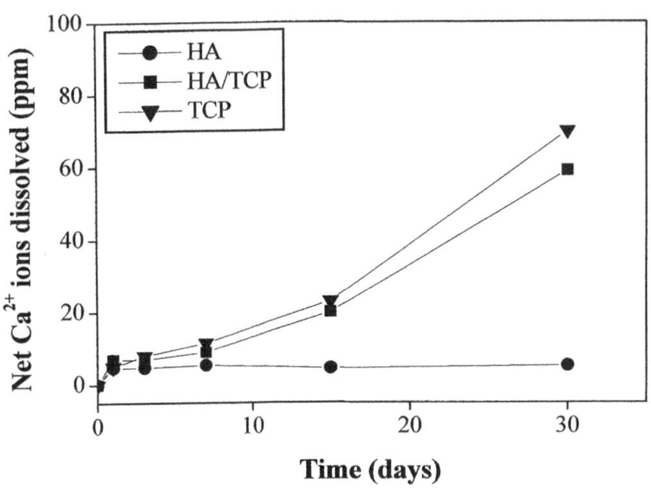

Fig. 4. Net Ca^{2+} concentrations released from HA, TCP, and HA/TCP porous bodies immersed in the Ringer's solution.

IV. Summary

Porous bioceramics with variable porosity were successfully fabricated using the polyurethane sponge technique. Porosity was controlled by the number of coatings on the sponge struts and ranged from 90%–65%. The compressive strength was strongly dependent on the porosity and weakly dependent on the type of ceramics, HA, TCP, or HA/TCP composite. At the 65% porosity level, the strength was ~3 MPa, comparable to that of the commercially available porous ceramics. The dissolution results confirmed that the biodegradation of calcium phosphate ceramics could be controlled by simply adjusting the amount of HA or TCP in the ceramics.

References

[1]K. de Groot, *Bioceramics of Calcium Phosphate*. CRC Press, Boca Raton, FL, 1983.

[2]L. L. Hench and J. Wilson, *An Introduction to Bioceramics*. World Scientific, London, U.K., 1993.

[3]M. Kohri, K. Miki, D. E. Waite, H. Nakajima, and T. Okabe, "*In Vitro* Stability of Biphasic Calcium Phosphate Ceramics," *Biomaterials*, **14** [4] 299–304 (1993).

[4]E. B. Nery, R. Z. LeGeros, K. L. Lynch, and K. Lee, "Tissue Response to Biphasic Calcium Phosphate Ceramics with Different Ratios of HA/β TCP in Periodontal Osseous Defects," *J. Periodontol.*, **63** [9] 729–35 (1992).

[5]P. Frayssinet, J. L. Trouillet, N. Rouquet, E. Azimus, and A. Autefage, "Osseointegration of Macroporous Calcium Phosphate Ceramics Having a Different Chemical Composition," *Biomaterials*, **14** [6] 423–29 (1993).

[6]X. Yang and Z. Wang, "Synthesis of Biphasic Ceramics of Hydroxyapatite and β-Tricalcium Phosphate with Controlled Phase Content and Porosity," *J. Mater. Chem.*, **8** [10] 2233–37 (1998).

[7]N. Kivrak and A. C. Tas, "Synthesis of Calcium Hydroxyapatite–Tricalcium Phosphate (HA–TCP) Composite Bioceramic Powders and Their Sintering Behavior," *J. Am. Ceram. Soc.*, **81** [9] 2245–52 (1998).

[8]J. J. Klawitter and S. F. Hulbert, "Application of Porous Ceramics for the Attachment of Load-Bearing Internal Orthopedic Applications," *J. Biomed. Mater. Res. Symp.*, **2** [1] 161–229 (1971).

[9]T. Flatley, K. L. Lynch, and M. Benson, "Tissue Response to Implants of Calcium Phosphate Ceramics in the Rabbit Spine," *Clin. Orthop.*, **179**, 246–52 (1983).

[10]O. Gauthier, J.-M. Bouler, E. Aguado, P. Pilet, and G. Daculsi, "Macroporous Biphasic Calcium Phosphate Ceramics: Influence of Macropore Diameter and Macroporosity Percentage on Bone Ingrowth," *Biomaterials*, **19**, 133–39 (1998).

[11]B. S. Chang, C.-K. Lee, K.-S. Hong, H.-J. Youn, H.-S. Ryu, S.-S. Chung, and K.-W. Park, "Osteoconduction at Porous Hydroxyapatite with Various Pore Configurations," *Biomaterials*, **21,** 1291–98 (2000).

[12]D. M. Roy and S. K. Linnehan, "Hydroxyapatite Formed from Coral Skeletal Carbonated by Hydrothermal Exchange," *Nature (London)*, **247**, 220–22 (1974).

[13]D.-M. Liu, "Control of Pore Geometry on Influencing the Mechanical Property of Porous Hydroxyapatite Bioceramic," *J. Mater. Sci. Lett.*, **15**, 419–21 (1996).

[14]P. Sepulveda, F. S. Ortega, M. D. M. Innocentini, and V. C. Pandolfelli, "Properties of Highly Porous Hydroxyapatite Obtained by the Gelcasting of Foams," *J. Am. Ceram. Soc.*, **83** [12] 3021–24 (2000).

[15]A. Slosarczyk, "Highly Porous Hydroxyapatite Material," *Powder Metall. Int.*, **21** [4] 24–25 (1989).

[16]M. Milosevski, J. Bossert, D. Milosevski, and N. Gruevska, "Preparation and Properties of Dense and Porous Calcium Phosphate," *Ceram. Int.*, **25**, 693–96 (1999).

[17]A. Curodeau, E. Sachs, and S. Caldarise, "Design and Fabrication of Cast Orthopedic Implants with Freeform Surface Textures from 3-D Printed Ceramic Shell," *J. Biomed. Mater. Res.*, **53** [5] 525–35 (2000).

[18]J. C. Le Huec, T. Schaeverbeke, D. Clement, J. Faber, and A. Le Rebeller, "Influence of Porosity on the Mechanical Resistance of Hydroxyapatite Ceramics under Compressive Stress," *Biomaterials*, **16**, 113–118 (1995).

[19]D.-M. Liu, "Influence of Porosity and Pore Size on the Compressive Strength of Porous Hydroxyapatite Ceramic," *Ceram. Int.*, **23**, 135–39 (1997).

[20]M. Sous, R. Bareille, F. Rouais, D. Clement, J. Amedee, B. Dupuy, and Ch. Baquey, "Cellular Biocompatibility and Resistance to Compression of Macroporous β-tricalcium Phosphate Ceramics," *Biomaterials*, **19**, 2147–53 (1998). □

J. Am. Ceram. Soc., 84 [2] 295–300 (2001)

Molten Salt Synthesis of Calcium Hydroxyapatite Whiskers

A. Cüneyt Taş*,†

Department of Metallurgical and Materials Engineering, Middle East Technical University, Ankara 06531, Turkey

Calcium hydroxyapatite (HA) whiskers and crystals were produced by the route of molten salt synthesis. The effects on whisker morphology of chosen flux, flux-to-HA ratio, synthesis temperature, and reaction time were investigated. The thermal stabilities of the produced whiskers were tested at 1300°C in an air atmosphere. A tentative X-ray diffraction pattern was proposed for the HA whiskers. Molten salt synthesis with a K_2SO_4 flux was found to be a simple and sturdy technique for manufacturing short (≤60 μm) HA whiskers in the temperature range from 1080° to ~1200°C. The alternative use of fluxes such as KCl, KBr, $CaCl_2$, or Na_2SO_4, rather than K_2SO_4, over the temperature range 850°–1000°C resulted in the formation of large (~25 μm) single crystals of HA.

I. Introduction

Calcium hydroxyapatite ($Ca_{10}(PO_4)_6(OH)_2$) is one of the most biocompatible ceramics, because of its significant chemical and physical resemblance to the mineral constituents of human bones and teeth. For load-bearing orthopedic and dental applications, densified HA ceramics are needed. However, dense HA ceramics manufactured by using synthetic HA powders have always exhibited a low fracture toughness, of ~1 MPa·m$^{1/2}$, in contrast to the values observed for human bones, in the range 2–12 MPa·m$^{1/2}$.[1]

Reinforcement by whiskers has been considered as a way of improving the fracture toughness of pure HA bioceramics; thus, whiskerlike or needlelike crystals of HA have been synthesized in recent years, mainly by the hydrothermal method or precipitation routes.[2–9] However, the whiskers synthesized by these methods[4–6] suffer from nonstoichiometry (i.e., calcium deficiency) and have low thermal stability, i.e., they partially decompose into a β-TCP phase (5–35 vol% TCP), even after 1 h of heating at 1100°C. Moreover, Suchanek *et al.*[5] have reported that, for HA composite ceramics reinforced with hydrothermally synthesized HA whiskers (~30 vol% whiskers), the whiskers disappear within the HA matrixes at sintering temperatures ≥1000°C and turn themselves into large, equiaxed grains.[6] The fracture toughness values of these samples have been reported[5] to remain only in the modest range of 1.4–2.0 MPa·m$^{1/2}$.

Molten salt synthesis (MSS) is reported to be one of the simplest techniques for preparing ceramic powder bodies with whiskerlike, needlelike, or platelike morphology and, as well, complex stoichiometry.[10] The MSS technique is based on the use of low-melting solvents, such as alkali chlorides, sulfates, carbonates, or hydroxides, as the medium of reaction for the ceramics. The literature on molten salt synthesis is quite extensive and, to name just a few cases, this technique has been used (with different alkali salts) to prepare ferrites,[10] titanates,[11–13] niobates,[14–17] mullite,[18] aluminum borate,[19,20] wollastonite,[21] and carbonated apatite ($Ca_{9.8}((PO_4)_{5.6}(CO_3)_{0.4})(CO_3)$, by using a high-melting flux of $CaCO_3$).[22] The selection of the salt in MSS is critical for obtaining desirable powder morphology and characteristics. There are two major requirements for the selection of a salt:[16] First, the melting point of the salt should be low and appropriate for the synthesis of the required phase; second, the salt should have sufficient aqueous solubility that it will be eliminated easily by simple washing, after synthesis.

In the present study, we used submicrometer-sized HA powders synthesized by a previous method[23–25] as the starting material for the MSS method. The effects on whisker morphology of the alkali salt chosen, the temperatures/times of synthesis, and the salt-to-HA powder ratio used were studied. To our knowledge, this report is the first describing the successful preparation of monodisperse HA whiskers, using K_2SO_4 salt, by the simple technique of MSS.

II. Experimental Procedure

(1) Preparation of HA Powders

The single-phase calcium hydroxyapatite powders used as the starting material for the MSS of the HA whiskers were synthesized as follows.[23–25] (The following procedure is the derivative of a route described earlier by Hayek and Newesely,[26] Moreno *et al.*,[27] and Jarcho *et al.*[28]) A 3 mL aliquot of 0.1 g/L methyl cellulose solution (99% purity, Sigma–Aldrich Corp., St. Louis, MO) was mixed (to act as a dispersant) with 1440 mL of deionized water. Next, 0.152 mol of $Ca(NO_3)_2{\cdot}0.4H_2O$ (99.8% purity, Merck, Darmstadt, Germany) was dissolved in the above-described solution. Then, 0.090 mol of $(NH_4)_2HPO_4$ (99.8% purity, Merck) was dissolved in that solution. Following that step, 115 mL of 24 vol% NH_4OH was added, in its entirety, to the above-described opaque solution. The solution was heated and vigorously stirred at 60°–70°C for 3 h, on a hot plate. The precipitates that formed were recovered from the supernatant, by filtering, and washed five times with deionized water. The filtrates were dried at 100°C overnight. Finally, the HA precursors were calcined in an air atmosphere at 1000°C for 6 h and then lightly ground by hand, with an agate mortar and pestle.

(2) Synthesis of HA Whiskers

HA powders calcined at 1000°C were dry-mixed in an agate mortar with potassium sulfate (K_2SO_4, 99.9% purity, Merck) at K_2SO_4-to-HA weight ratios in the range 1.2–3.0, for a total sample weight of 2 g. In several experiments, the K_2SO_4 (melting point (MP) = 1069°C) flux was replaced by sodium sulfate (Na_2SO_4, MP = 884°C), calcium chloride ($CaCl_2$, MP = 782°C), potassium chloride (KCl, MP = 771°C), or potassium bromide (KBr, MP = 734°C). The mixtures, as loose powder compacts, were then placed into clean alumina boats with a volume of 7.5 cm^3 and set inside a box furnace. The samples were heated from the ambient to the peak temperature of whisker synthesis at a rate of 5°C/min. Following soaking times ranging from 0.5 to 3.5 h at the peak temperatures (850°–1190°C), the samples were cooled naturally to room temperature within the shut-off furnace. The single-crystal whiskers or particles were separated from the solidified mass by washing the mass several times with hot (~90°C) deionized water.

P. W. Brown—contributing editor

Manuscript No. 188607. Received April 24, 2000; approved September 19, 2000.
*Member, American Ceramic Society.
†Present address: Max-Planck-Institut für Metallforschung, Heisenbergstrasse 5, Stuttgart D-70569, Germany.

Washing was repeated until the specific conductance of the decanted liquid fell to <2.4 μS, measured[11] using a conductance meter (Model No. Digi610, WTW, Weilheim, Germany), knowing that the conductance of deionized water was 1.4 μS. Finally, the washed whiskers were dried in an oven, at 100°C, overnight.

(3) *Investigation of Thermal Stability of Whiskers*

The morphology and phase stability of the HA whiskers after heating (with heating/cooling rates of 5°C/min) at 1300°C for 9 h, as a loose powder compact, in an air atmosphere, were evaluated by scanning electron microscopy (SEM), X-ray diffractometry (XRD), and Fourier transform infrared spectrometry (FT-IR).

(4) *Sample Characterization*

The phase constitution of the whiskers was analyzed by XRD (Model No. D-5000, Siemens Aktiengesellschaft, Karlsruhe, Germany) and CuK_α radiation (40 kV, 30 mA). For lattice-parameter determinations, a scan rate of 0.2° 2θ/min (over the range 10°–70° 2θ), using a silicon external standard to correct for systematic errors, was used, along with the Appleman Least-Squares Refinement Program.[29] The morphologic and semiquantitative elemental distribution information on the samples were obtained by SEM (Model No. DSM 982-Gemini, Karl Zeiss, Inc., Oberkochen, Germany), and by energy dispersive X-ray spectroscopy (EDS), respectively. Quantitative chemical analyses were performed by inductively coupled plasma atomic-emission spectroscopy (ICP-AES; Model No. JY-70Plus, Jobin Yvon S.A., Longjuveau, France). An FT-IR spectrophotometer (Model No. IFS66, Bruker, Karlsruhe, Germany) was used to measure the infrared transmission spectra of the whiskers, after the whiskers had been mixed with dry KBr (1 wt%), to form pellets.

III. Results and Discussion

The SEM micrographs given in Fig. 1 show the morphology of the starting HA powders used in this study in molten salt whisker synthesis. The chemically precipitated HA precursors, following filtration from the mother liquor and 100°C drying, consisted of nanosized, but aggregated, particles, as depicted in Fig. 1(a). These precursors were poorly crystalline, but not completely amorphous. Their crystallization behavior, as a function of calcination temperature, has been published elsewhere.[25] Figure 1(b) shows the microstructure of the same powders after calcination (as a loose powder compact) in air at 1000°C for 6 h. The average particle size was ~100 nm. Calcined HA powders were determined, by XRD, to be "single-phase" HA (with only a small amount of CaO, not readily detectable by rapid XRD scans) with a Ca/P atomic ratio (measured by ICP-AES) of 1.68 ± 0.01.[24,25] This Ca/P ratio in the calcined powders was intentionally adjusted to that value by the specific Ca/P ratio used in the chemical precipitation of precursors. The XRD pattern of the calcined (1000°C, 6 h) HA powders is shown as the bottom trace of Fig. 2.

HA powders precalcined at 1000°C (to ensure that the starting materials consisted of single-phase hydroxyapatite) were then mixed with the alkali salts listed in Table I for MSS. K_2SO_4 was first[20] tested as the fluxing agent in MSS runs at four different salt-to-HA weight ratios and four different temperatures. The samples, labeled W1–W12 (see Table I), all produced single-phase HA whiskers. The XRD pattern of the W4 sample is shown by the middle trace of Fig. 2. The same XRD trace was observed for all of the samples, labeled as W*xx* in Table I. That trace represents the characteristic XRD pattern for calcium hydroxyapatite, although the intensities of the 211 and 300 planes are changed, because of whisker orientation. This result was also the case for previously reported[3–6] hydrothermally synthesized HA whiskers, and the whiskers were apparently elongated along the *c* axis. Moreover, all of the HA whiskers of samples W1–W12 were totally transparent, according to examination by optical microscopy.

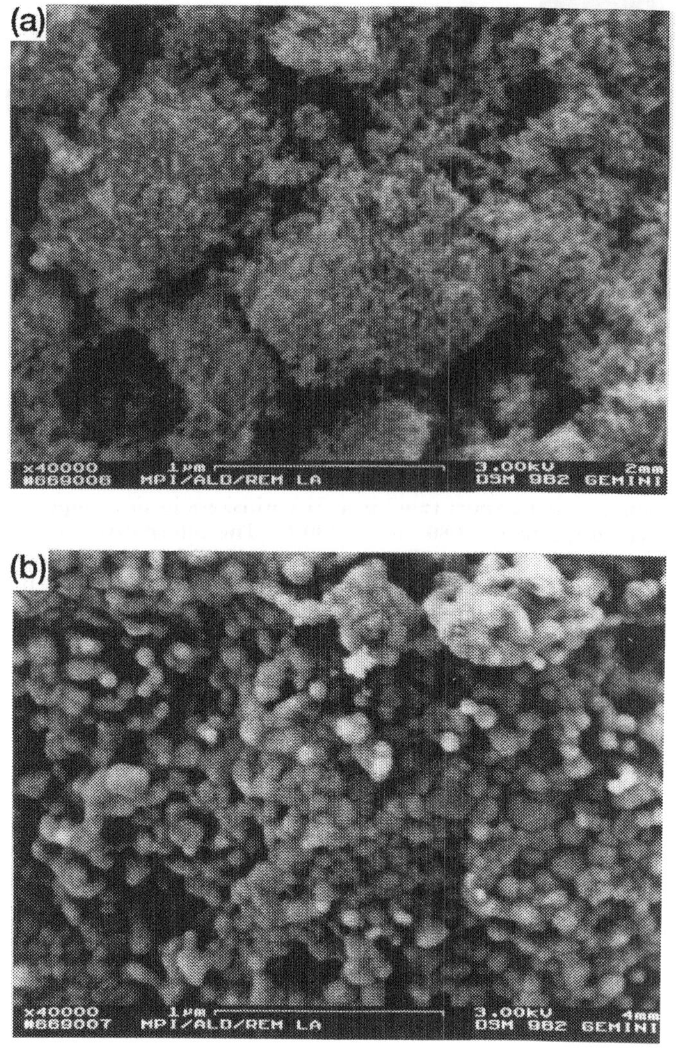

Fig. 1. SEM micrographs of HA powders at (a) 100° and (b) 1000°C.

ICP-AES analyses performed on the W*xx* samples showed the presence of 0.55–0.60 wt% potassium in the whiskers, regardless of the salt-to-HA ratios and synthesis temperatures/times used in this study. Potassium was expected to substitute the calcium sites of the HA lattice. No sulfur was detected in the whiskers by the ICP-AES analyses. Thus, the crystals produced in the present study could not be regarded as "pure" calcium hydroxyapatite whiskers, and they had the typical formula of $Ca_{1-x}K_x(PO_4)_6(OH)_{2-x}$, where x varied between 0.140 (i.e., 0.55 wt%) and 0.155 (i.e., 0.60 wt%).

However, human bones and tooth enamel are also known[30] to contain significant quantities of alkali and alkali earth cations, such as Na^+, K^+, and Mg^{2+}. The sum of these three ions in human bones reaches ~1.3 wt%, whereas, in enamels, the same figure has been reported[30] to be ~1 wt%. On the other hand, the Ca/P molar ratio of the present MSS whiskers was found, by ICP-AES analyses, to be 1.64 ± 0.01. These whiskers may also be regarded as calcium-deficient, in comparison with stoichiometric HA, which has a Ca/P molar ratio of 1.667. However, the Ca/P ratios of dental enamel and human bones are known[30] to be 1.62 and 1.65, respectively.

The lattice parameters of the W4 whiskers (middle XRD trace in Fig. 2) were determined, by least-squares analysis,[29] to be a = 9.4189 and c = 6.8827 Å. The hexagonal unit cell (of the space group of $P6_3/m$) had a cell volume of 528.79 Å^3. The lattice parameters of these whiskers resembled those reported previously[30] for the apatite of human bones, although these whiskers and human bones do not have the same chemical constitution. The

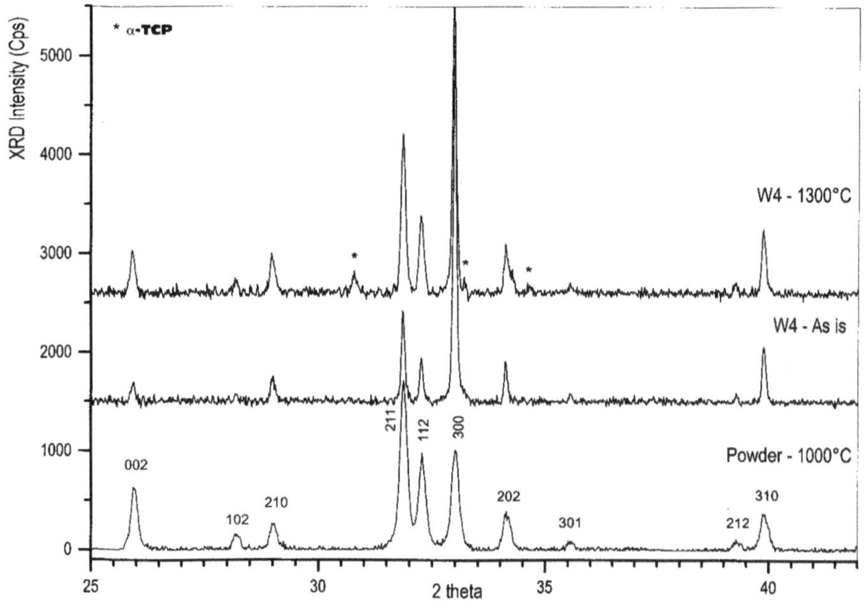

Fig. 2. XRD patterns of HA powders and whiskers.

Table I. Molten-Salt-Synthesized Samples

Sample	Salt	Salt/HA (by weight)	Reaction temperature (°C)	Reaction time (h)
W1	K_2SO_4	1.2	1190	3.5
W2	K_2SO_4	1.2	1150	2.0
W3	K_2SO_4	1.2	1100	1.0
W4	K_2SO_4	1.6	1190	3.5
W5	K_2SO_4	1.6	1150	2.0
W6	K_2SO_4	1.6	1100	1.0
W7	K_2SO_4	2.4	1190	3.5
W8	K_2SO_4	3.0	1190	3.5
W9	K_2SO_4	3.0	1150	2.0
W10	K_2SO_4	3.0	1100	2.0
W11	K_2SO_4	3.0	1100	1.0
W12	K_2SO_4	3.0	1080	0.5
P1	KCl	1.6	880	3.0
P2	KCl	1.6	1000	3.0
P3	KBr	1.6	850	3.0
P4	KBr	1.6	1000	3.0
P5	Na_2SO_4	3.0	1000	3.0
P6	$CaCl_2$	3.0	850	3.0
P7	$CaCl_2$	3.0	1000	3.0

presence of K^+ in the lattice also has been reported previously[30] to have no influence on the lattice parameters of hydroxyapatite. Therefore, a tentative XRD pattern for the HA whiskers (with the strongest XRD peak assigned to the 300, rather than the 211, plane) was created and is given in Table II.

Figures 3(a) and (b) show the SEM micrographs of molten-salt-synthesized HA whiskers of samples W1 and W4, respectively. The aspect ratios (i.e., length/diameter) varied in the range 2–18, with the median whisker diameter and length 9 μm and 55 μm, respectively. Whiskers were monodisperse and were not fused to one another. Interestingly, samples W2, W3, and W5–W11 produced almost the same microstructures and whisker morphologies. Thus, the K_2SO_4-to-HA weight ratio (in the range 1.2–3.0), the reaction temperature (in the range 1100°–1190°C), and the reaction time (in the range 1–3.5 h) were almost unable to influence the resultant HA whisker morphology. On the other hand, Fig. 3(c) shows that sample W12 (i.e., 1080°C, 0.5 h, K_2SO_4-to-HA weight ratio = 3.0) exhibited the formation of monodisperse, but much thinner, HA whiskers, with an aspect ratio >30 and a typical diameter and length of 2 μm and 65 μm, respectively. The XRD

Table II. Experimental XRD Pattern of HA Whiskers[†]

2θ	*d* (Å)	*hkl*	I/I_0
10.8335	8.1600	100	8
16.8416	5.2601	101	4
18.8287	4.7092	110	3
21.7654	4.0800	200	9
22.8615	3.8868	111	8
25.8647	3.4419	002	7
28.1278	3.1699	102	2
28.9355	3.0832	210	8
31.7870	2.8128	211	26
32.1873	2.7788	112	13
32.9093	2.7194	300	100
34.0553	2.6305	202	12
35.4751	2.5284	301	3
39.1983	2.2964	212	3
39.8151	2.2622	310	18
42.0046	2.1492	311	2
42.3272	2.1336	302	3
43.8628	2.0624	113	6
44.3859	2.0393	400	3
45.3132	1.9997	203	2
46.7025	1.9434	222	9
48.0899	1.8905	312	4
48.6156	1.8713	320	3
49.4793	1.8406	213	9
50.5031	1.8057	321	6
51.2834	1.7800	410	9
52.0951	1.7542	402	4
53.1910	1.7206	004	3
54.4593	1.6835	104	2
55.8807	1.6440	322	7
57.1331	1.6109	313	5
58.0628	1.5873	501	2
59.9570	1.5416	420	3
60.4326	1.5306	331	3
61.6848	1.5025	214	7
63.0029	1.4742	502	8
63.4444	1.4650	510	2
64.1687	1.4502	323	9
65.0382	1.4329	511	6
66.3987	1.4068	422	2
69.7071	1.3479	512	1

[†]For W4 at 1190°C.

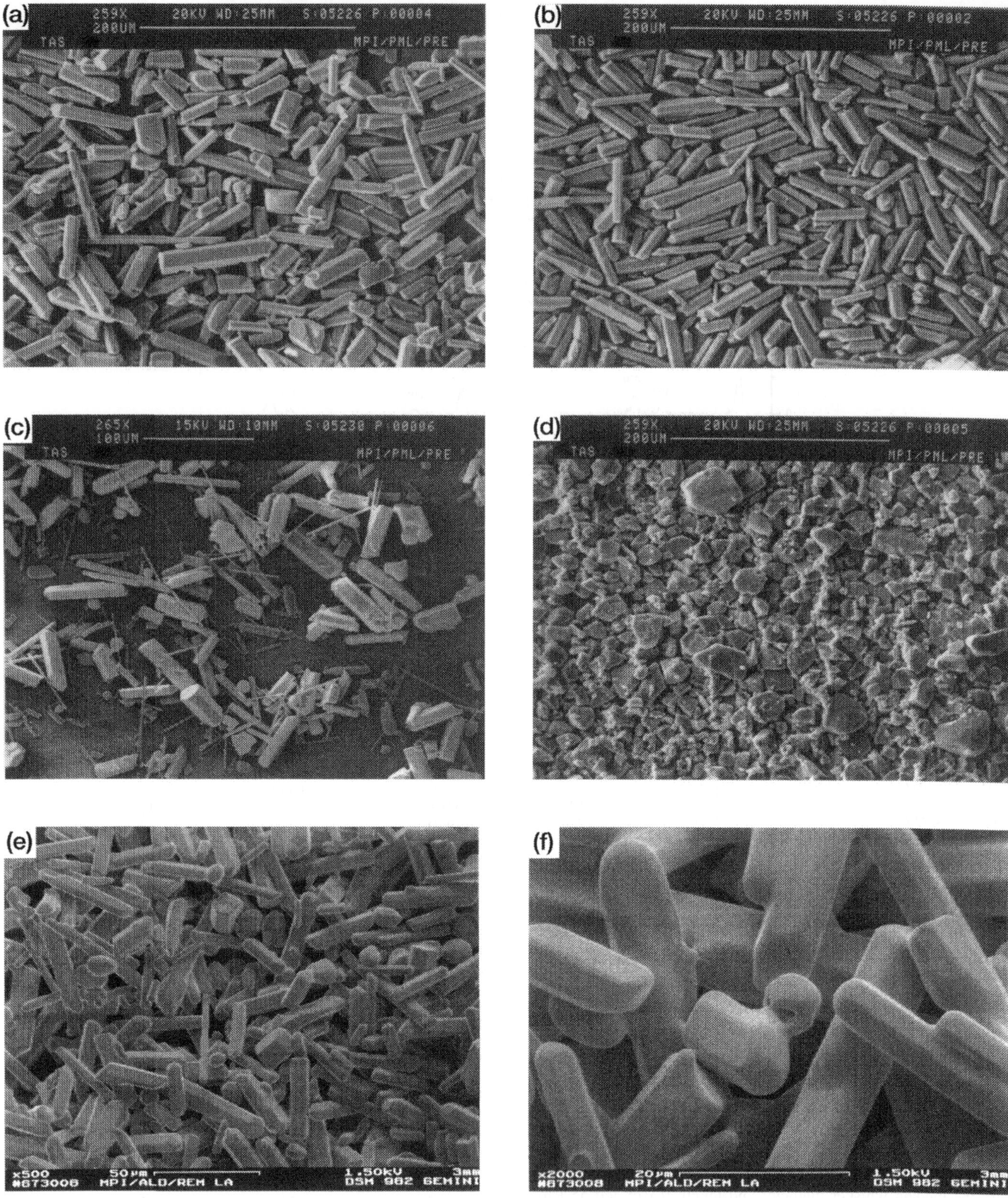

Fig. 3. SEM micrographs of HA whiskers and crystals: (a) W1, (b) W4, (c) W12, (d) P1, (e) and (f) W4 at 1300°C (see Table I for sample designations).

pattern of this sample again showed the presence of calcium hydroxyapatite only.

The above set of experimental data, obtained using K_2SO_4 as the fluxing agent, implies the following process:

(1) The liquid phase formed during the MSS process by the molten K_2SO_4 (i.e., the flux) first dissolves all of the initial ceramic raw material.

(2) With further heating, particles of the apatite phase are formed through the nucleation and growth processes.[16]

(3) As the molten ionic bath cools, while passing through its melting point down to room temperature, rapid crystallization occurs along the preferred growth axes of the ceramic phase.

(4) HA whisker growth occurs during MSS, by a sequential "dissolution–crystallization–whisker-growth" process.

(5) Solubility of the ceramic raw material in the molten flux (which is a function of temperature) must have a significant role in the crystallization process to follow.

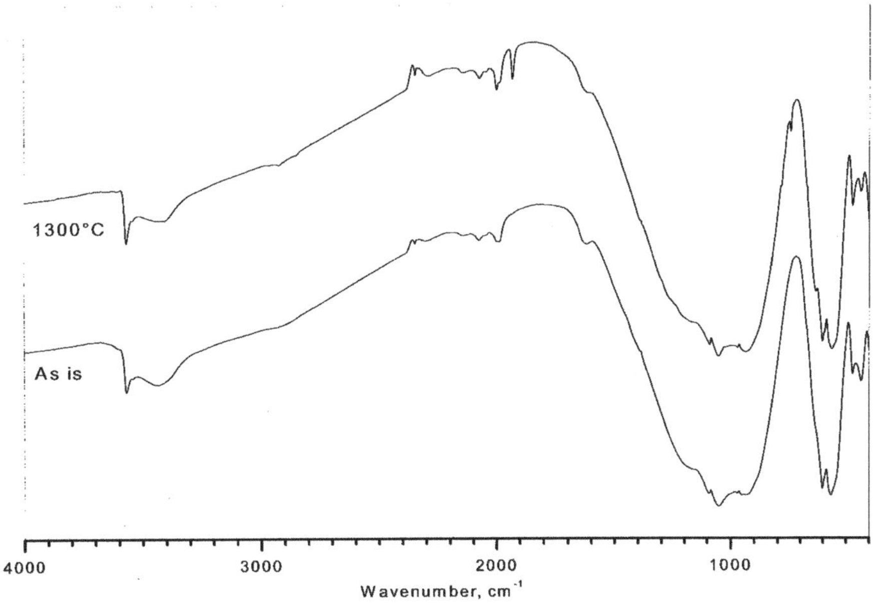

Fig. 4. FT-IR spectra (transmittance) of HA whiskers.

(6) The extent of superheating of the molten flux must also have a rather strong effect on the resultant aspect ratio of the formed whiskers (as evidenced by the case of sample W12).

(7) The morphology of the whiskers growing out of the cooling molten salt bath must be strongly dependent on soaking time at the peak temperature.

Whiskers with the highest aspect ratio were obtained at the lowest temperature and time combination, i.e., sample W12 of Table I, a result suggesting that time and temperature are the most significant variables in altering the whisker morphology, along with the use of an appropriate fluxing agent, in which the ceramic raw material has sufficient solubility.

To test the feasibility of decreasing the MSS temperature, we also tried using KCl, KBr, Na_2SO_4, and $CaCl_2$, rather than K_2SO_4, with the MSS parameters given in Table I. These samples were labeled P1–P7. Interestingly, none of the samples were able to produce HA whiskers, and the reason(s) for this failure may also be found in the above paragraph. Figure 3(d) shows the SEM micrograph of the P1 powders, and this morphology was also encountered with the other samples, P2–P7. The product phase in all of these P*x* samples was, again, calcium hydroxyapatite, with an average particle size of 25 μm. The finer portion of the powder body (of Fig. 3(d)) is believed to have been the undissolved, initial HA powder, and the larger portion consisted of single crystals of HA. Such hydroxyapatite powders, with a large average particle size, may be useful for applications such as plasma-spraying. However, ICP-AES analyses performed on the P1 and P2 samples indicated the presence of chlorine (in the range 1.5%–1.7%) in the final powders. It can be inferred that using KCl as the molten salt facilitates at least the partial transformation of hydroxyapatite into chloroapatite.

Figures 3(e) and (f) show the microstructures of W4 whiskers at two different magnifications, after heating as loose powder compacts in alumina boats, at 1300°C, for 9 h in a stagnant air atmosphere. For the molten-salt-synthesized HA whiskers of the present study, the previously mentioned problem (for the whiskers synthesized by the hydrothermal method)[3–6] of morphologic degradation apparently was not present. The W4 whiskers retained their shapes perfectly, formed a skeleton of HA, and just fused together at the points of mutual contact. However, the XRD pattern of the whiskers heated at 1300°C (see Fig. 2) showed the presence of a second phase of α-TCP (ICDD No. PDF 9–348[‡]), the high-temperature orthorhombic polymorph of tricalcium phosphate, $Ca_3(PO_4)_2$. The formation of TCP, as a decomposition product of HA, in samples heated at 1300°C in an air atmosphere, is well-known and normal.[1,30] Previous reports[31] have also noted that, for synthetic hydroxyapatites cooled rapidly (as in the present study) from temperatures >1250°C, the crystallographic form of TCP observed will always be the high-temperature polymorph.

The FT-IR spectrum of the as-synthesized W4 whiskers shown in the bottom trace of Fig. 4 is characteristic for calcium hydroxyapatite. All bands originating from PO_4 and OH groups are clearly visible. The absence of any distinct bands in the range 1500–1400 cm^{-1} means that the HA whiskers do not contain significant quantities of carbonate ions.[32] Bands in the region 1190–975 cm^{-1} result from the ν_3 vibrational mode of the phosphate group. A phosphate ν_1 band is present at ~962 cm^{-1}. A phosphate ν_4 band is present in the region 605–560 cm^{-1}, and two sites are observed for these whiskers at 602 and 569 cm^{-1}. A phosphate vibration, ν_2, is observed in the form of two discrete peaks at 471 and 433 cm^{-1}. The OH vibrations at 3571 cm^{-1} (stretching) and 634 cm^{-1} (bending) are well-defined, and the band in the region 1638–1600 cm^{-1} is a result of H–O–H deformation. Atmospheric CO_2 is indicated by the band at 2349 cm^{-1}.

The infrared spectrum of the W4 whiskers calcined in air at 1300°C for 9 h (depicted by the top trace in Fig. 4) shows, as well as all of the above-mentioned bands, a unique band at 743 cm^{-1}, which is characteristic of the P–O–P vibrational mode of pyrophosphates,[32] although their XRD patterns did not indicate the presence of $Ca_2P_2O_7$ as a decomposition product. The band at 1933 cm^{-1} could not be identified.

Biocompatible HA whiskers prepared by the MSS technique could be useful for numerous applications involving the reinforcement of hydroxyapatite-based bioceramics. As shown in this report, the MSS process for calcium hydroxyapatite whisker manufacture is quite robust, because it does not require the achievement of precise, up-to-the-last-digit control over many of the processing parameters, such as the flux-to-HA ratio, reaction temperature, and time.

IV. Summary

Molten salt synthesis (MSS) of monodisperse calcium hydroxyapatite whiskers was accomplished using a K_2SO_4 flux. Single-phase, potassium-doped HA whiskers proved possible to synthesize over the temperature range 1080°–1190°C, and the K_2SO_4-to-HA ratios in the initial mixtures could be varied between 1.2 and 3.0 without significantly affecting the whisker morphology.

[‡]Powder Diffraction File, No. PDF 9–348. International Centre for Diffraction Data, Newtown Square, PA.

HA whiskers produced by the K_2SO_4 flux retained their initial shapes and aspect ratios, even after heating in air at 1300°C for 9 h, although they started to decompose into TCP. Fluxing agents such as KCl, KBr, $CaCl_2$, and Na_2SO_4, when used in place of K_2SO_4, produced large single crystals of HA, with an average particle size of 25 μm, rather than whiskers, over the MSS temperature range 850°–1000°C.

Acknowledgments

The author gratefully acknowledges the Max-Planck-Institut für Metallforschung, Stuttgart, Germany, for the award of Visiting Professorship, from February 1999 to February 2001. The author also expresses his personal appreciation to H. Labitzke (SEM), F. Predel (SEM/EDS), G. Kaiser (ICP-AES), M. Thomas (XRD), and W. König (FT-IR) of MPI for their help with sample characterization.

References

[1]L. L. Hench, "Bioceramics: From Concept to Clinic," *J. Am. Ceram. Soc.*, **74**, 1487–510 (1991).

[2]L. Yubao, K. De Groot, J. De Wijn, C. P. A. T. Klein, and S. V. D. Meer, "Morphology and Composition of Nanograde Calcium Phosphate Needle-like Crystals Formed by Simple Hydrothermal Method," *J. Mater. Sci.: Mater. Med.*, **5**, 326–31 (1994).

[3]M. Yoshimura, H. Suda, K. Okamoto, and K. Ioku, "Hydrothermal Synthesis of Biocompatible Whiskers," *J. Mater. Sci.*, **29**, 3399–402 (1994).

[4]W. Suchanek, H. Suda, M. Yashima, M. Kakihana, and M. Yoshimura, "Biocompatible Whiskers with Controlled Morphology and Stoichiometry," *J. Mater. Res.*, **10**, 521–29 (1995).

[5]W. Suchanek, M. Yashima, M. Kakihana, and M. Yoshimura, "Hydroxyapatite/Hydroxyapatite-Whisker Composites without Sintering Additives: Mechanical Properties and Microstructural Evolution," *J. Am. Ceram. Soc.*, **80**, 2805–13 (1997).

[6]W. L. Suchanek and M. Yoshimura, "Preparation of Fibrous, Porous Hydroxyapatite Ceramics from Hydroxyapatite Whiskers," *J. Am. Ceram. Soc.*, **81**, 765–67 (1998).

[7]T. Iizuka and A. Nozuma, "Effects of pH of the Aqueous Solutions on the Growth of Hydroxyapatite Whiskers," *J. Ceram. Soc. Jpn.*, **106**, 820–23 (1998).

[8]T. Iizuka and A. Nozuma, "Effects of the Buffer Solutions on the Growth of Hydroxyapatite Whiskers," *J. Ceram. Soc. Jpn.*, **107**, 442–48 (1999).

[9]A. Nakahira, K. Sakamoto, S. Yamaguchi, M. Kaneno, S. Takeda, and M. Okazaki, "Novel Synthesis Method of Hydroxyapatite Whiskers by Hydrolysis of α-Tricalcium Phosphate in Mixtures of Water and Organic Solvent," *J. Am. Ceram. Soc.*, **82**, 2029–32 (1999).

[10]R. H. Arendt, "The Molten Salt Synthesis of Single Magnetic Domain $BaFe_{12}O_{19}$ and $SrFe_{12}O_{19}$ Crystals," *J. Solid State Chem.*, **8**, 339–47 (1973).

[11]P. A. Fuierer and R. E. Newnham, "$La_2Ti_2O_7$ Ceramics," *J. Am. Ceram. Soc.*, **74**, 2876–81 (1991).

[12]A. Aboujalil, J. P. Deloume, F. Chassagneux, J. P. Scharff, and B. Durand, "Molten Salt Synthesis of the Lead Titanate $PbTiO_3$, Investigation of the Reactivity of Various Titanium and Lead Salts with Molten Alkali-Metal Nitrites," *J. Mater. Chem.*, **8**, 1601–606 (1998).

[13]K. Katayama, Y. Azuma, and Y. Takahashi, "Molten Salt Synthesis of Single-Phase $BaNd_2Ti_4O_{12}$ Powder," *J. Mater. Sci.*, **34**, 301–305 (1999).

[14]C. C. Li, C. C. Chiu, and S. B. Desu, "Formation of Lead Niobates in Molten Salt Systems," *J. Am. Ceram. Soc.*, **74**, 42–47 (1991).

[15]D. M. Wan, J. Wang, S. C. Ng, and L. M. Gan, "Formation and Characterization of Lead Magnesium Niobate Synthesized from the Molten Salt of Potassium Chlorate," *J. Alloys Compd.*, **274**, 110–17 (1998).

[16]K. H. Yoon, Y. S. Cho, and D. H. Kang, "Review: Molten Salt Synthesis of Lead-based Relaxors," *J. Mater. Sci.*, **33**, 2977–84 (1998).

[17]B. Brahmaroutu, G. L. Messing, and S. Trolier-McKinstry, "Molten Salt Synthesis of Anisotropic $Sr_2Nb_2O_7$ Particles," *J. Am. Ceram. Soc.*, **82**, 1565–68 (1999).

[18]S. Hashimoto and A. Yamaguchi, "Synthesis of Needlelike Mullite Particles Using Potassium Sulfate Flux," *J. Eur. Ceram. Soc.*, **20**, 397–402 (2000).

[19]H. Wada, K. Sakane, T. Kitamura, and H. Hata, "The Reaction Sequence in the Synthesis of Aluminum Borate Whiskers," *J. Mater. Sci.*, **31**, 537–44 (1996).

[20]I. E. Gonenli and A. C. Tas, "Chemical Preparation of Aluminum Borate Whiskers," *Powder Diffr.*, **15**, 104–107 (2000).

[21]S. Hayashi, M. Sugai, Z. Nakagawa, T. Takei, K. Kawasaki, T. Katsuyama, A. Yasumori, and K. Okada, "Preparation of $CaSiO_3$ Whiskers from Alkali Halide Fluxes," *J. Eur. Ceram. Soc.*, **20**, 1099–103 (2000).

[22]Y. Suetsugu and J. Tanaka, "Crystal Growth of Carbonate Apatite Using a $CaCO_3$ Flux," *J. Mater. Sci.: Mater. Med.*, **10**, 561–66 (1999).

[23]A. C. Tas, "Production of the Two Inorganic Phases [$(Ca_{10}(PO_4)_6(OH)_2$: Calcium Hydroxyapatite and $Ca_3(PO_4)_2$: Tri-Calcium Phosphate] of Synthetic Bones by Using a Chemical Precipitation Technique," Turk. Pat. No. TR 1995 01422 B, Turkish Patent Institute, Ankara, Turkey.

[24]A. C. Tas, F. Korkusuz, M. Timucin, and N. Akkas, "An Investigation of the Chemical Synthesis and High-Temperature Sintering Behaviour of Calcium Hydroxyapatite (HA) and Tricalcium Phosphate (TCP) Bioceramics," *J. Mater. Sci.: Mater. Med.*, **8**, 91–96 (1997).

[25]B. Mavis and A. C. Tas, "Dip-Coating of Calcium Hydroxyapatite on Ti-6Al-4V Substrates," *J. Am. Ceram. Soc.*, **83**, 989–91 (2000).

[26]E. Hayek and H. Newesely, "Pentacalcium Monohydroxyorthophosphate," *Inorg. Syn.*, **7**, 63–65 (1963).

[27]E. C. Moreno, T. M. Gregory, and W. E. Brown, "Preparation and Solubility of Hydroxyapatite," *J. Res. Natl. Bur. Stand. (U.S.)*, **72A**, 773–82 (1968).

[28]M. Jarcho, C. H. Bolen, M. B. Thomas, J. Bobick, J. P. Kay, and R. H. Doremus, "Hydroxyapatite Synthesis and Characterization in Dense Polycrystalline Form," *J. Mater. Sci.*, **11**, 2027–35 (1976).

[29]D. E. Appleman and H. T. Evans, "Indexing and Least-Squares Refinement of Powder Diffraction Data," U.S. Geol. Survey Rept. No. GD-73–003, 1973.

[30]R. Z. LeGeros and J. P. LeGeros, "Dense Hydroxyapatite"; pp. 139–80 in *An Introduction to Bioceramics*. Edited by L. L. Hench and J. Wilson. World Scientific, Singapore, Republic of Singapore, 1993.

[31]N. Kivrak and A. C. Tas, "Synthesis of Calcium Hydroxyapatite-Tricalcium Phosphate (HA-TCP) Composite Bioceramic Powders and Their Sintering Behavior," *J. Am. Ceram. Soc.*, **81**, 2245–52 (1998).

[32]A. C. Tas, "Synthesis of Biomimetic Ca-Hydroxyapatite Powders at 37°C in Synthetic Body Fluids," *Biomaterials*, **21**, 1429–38 (2000). □

J. Am. Ceram. Soc., **84** [9] 2123–25 (2001)

Gel-to-Ceramic Conversion during Hydroxyapatite Synthesis

Ming-Fa Hsieh and Tsung-Shune Chin

Department of Materials Science and Engineering, National Tsing Hua University, Hsinchu, Taiwan 30043, Republic of China

Li-Hsiang Perng and Huann-Guang Perng

Department of Chemical Engineering, Ta-Hwa Institute of Technology, Chiunglin, Hsinchu, Taiwan 30703, Republic of China

Conversion of hydroxyapatite (HA, $Ca_{10}(PO_4)_6(OH)_2$) synthesis from gel to ceramic using solid-state nuclear magnetic resonance (NMR) spectroscopy and X-ray diffraction was studied. The sol was prepared by dissolving calcium nitrate tetrahydrate and triethyl phosphate in 2-methoxyethanol. In solid-state ^{31}P magic-angle spinning nuclear magnetic resonance (MAS NMR) spectra, gel calcined at 250°, 350°, and 600°C showed a conversion from gel to glassy phosphate, then HA ceramic. Spin-lattice relaxation experiments of samples calcined at 600°C indicated that the existence of a CaO impurity might affect $OH\cdots O{=}PO_3$ linkages in a HA unit cell and result in longer ^{31}P spin-lattice time.

I. Introduction

Hydroxyapatite (HA, $Ca_{10}(PO_4)_6(OH)_2$) is known for its biocompatibility with mammalian calcified tissues,[1,2] and has been prepared for use in orthopedic and dental applications. The evolution of phosphorus bonding state in material processing can be mostly resolved by spectroscopy methods, such as infrared or nuclear magnetic resonance spectroscopy (NMR). For example, chemical reaction analysis using liquid-state NMR is especially helpful for the analysis of the sol-to-gel conversion.[3,4] However, in the past, the conversions from gel-to-ceramic were mostly studied by infrared method and X-ray diffractometry (XRD).[5] This study utilizes solid-state NMR spectroscopy to explore this conversion.

Solid-state NMR spectroscopy is used to investigate structural roles of different phosphates.[6–7] For instance, ^{1}H magic-angle spinning nuclear magnetic resonance (MAS NMR) spectra of HA indicate that there are four structural sites: acid phosphate (8.7 ppm), surface-adsorbed water (5.5 ppm), octacalcium phosphate defect (1.5 ppm), and structural OH (0.2 ppm).[7] In addition, local chemical structure and bonding of glassy phosphates are explored[8] by analyzing deconvoluted NMR spectra. Therefore, physical and chemical properties of phosphate glasses could be deduced from NMR analysis in collaboration with other instrumentations, such as infrared spectroscopy.

Spin-lattice relaxation of ^{31}P nuclei, in nature, depends on fluctuations near the nuclear spins of observation.[9,10] Allcock *et al.*[10] studied interactions of synthetic polymers and metal ions; the complexation behaviors were characterized by chemical shift variation and T_1 times of associated spins. They proposed that atoms in a flexible side chain would have longer relaxation time because of increased mobility. However, in contrast to the solid state, nuclear spins in the liquid state have more opportunities to return to the equilibrium state, i.e., spins are all aligned with external magnetic field. Therefore, T_1 times of spins are generally smaller (larger relaxation rates) than those in the solid-state samples. Therefore, spin-lattice relaxation experiments can be used to study local bonding nature (few bond lengths) of materials, whether they are amorphous or crystalline. In the clinical applications, enhancement of magnetic resonance imaging (MRI) availability to access human bone mineral density *ex vivo* was achieved. Recently, a feasibility study for applying solid-state ^{31}P NMR projection imaging to discriminate synthetic HA and natural bones indicated ~70% ^{31}P T_1 contrast.[11]

This paper presents a detailed investigation on the nature of the chemical bonding during the gel-to-ceramic conversion process using ^{31}P MAS NMR in conjugation with XRD. Moreover, the relation between chemical composition and spin-lattice relaxation of HA ceramic was exploited by measuring ^{31}P T_1 times.

II. Experimental Procedure

The preparation of the sol solution, described in detail elsewhere,[12] was done by mixing $Ca(NO_3)_2{\cdot}4H_2O$ (98%; Ferak Laborate, Berlin, Germany) and triethyl phosphate (99%; $(C_2H_5O)_3PO$, Janssen Chemicals, Geel, Belgium) in 2-methoxy ethanol (ACS grade, TEDIA Chemicals, Fairfield, OH). The route includes aging of the sol solution followed by a gelation. On aging, the sol-contained vessel was tightly capped and placed in an oil bath of 80°–90°C for 16 h. On gelation (drying), the solvent was evaporated in the same oil bath for 48 h.

The dried gels (xerogels) were then calcined in an air atmosphere from 25°–600°C using a ramp of 100°C/h. For the study of gel-to-ceramic conversion, calcined samples collected at 250°, 350°, and 600°C were analyzed by the solid-state ^{31}P NMR method. To understand the relationship between chemical composition and ^{31}P spin-lattice relaxation of HA ceramic, a HA and CaO sample was prepared as a control using a method described elsewhere.[5] Solid-state ^{31}P NMR was performed using MAS mode. A NMR spectrometer (Model DSX400WB, Bruker Analytic GmbH, Karlsruhe, Germany) was operated under a field strength 9.4 T. The sample rotation rate was 7 kHz. The chemical shift is referenced to external H_3PO_4. A high-power proton decoupling technique was applied in the experiments, except in the ^{31}P T_1 time measurements. The measurement of spin-lattice relaxation times, ^{31}P T_1, was made for the calcined sample (calcined at 600°C) and the control. A typical inversion recovery method[9] (d-180°-t-90°-acquire pulse sequences) was applied. The

P. W. Brown—contributing editor

Manuscript No. 188397. Received July 17, 2000; approved April 25, 2001.
Supported by the National Science Council of the Republic of China under Grant Nos. NSC87-2216-E-233-001 and NSC90-2815-C-233-005-E.
Presented at the 102nd Annual Meeting of The American Ceramic Society, St. Louis, MO, May 1, 2000 (Paper No. B1-004-00).

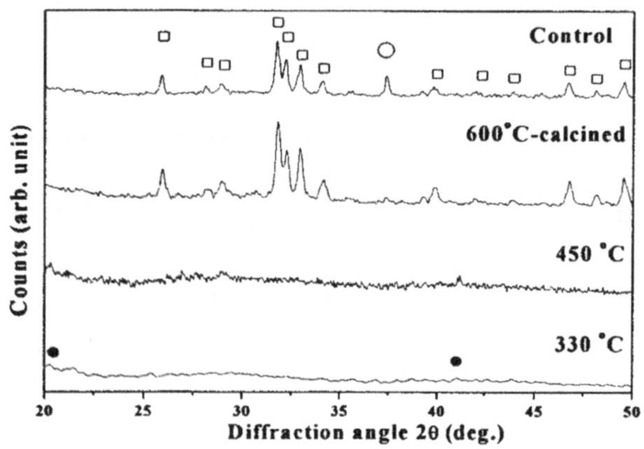

Fig. 1. XRD patterns of powders derived from calcined precursors of Ca/P = 1.67 and calcined at temperatures shown ((●) $Ca(NO_3)_2$ and (○) CaO; other peaks denote the HA control containing XRD-observable CaO, as prepared elsewhere[5]).

experiment used at least twelve sequences with a different delay time (*t*) between the 180° pulse and the 90° pulse to observe the recovery of the *z*-magnetization. The decay time (*d*) between the pulse sequences was >5 times the spin-lattice relaxation time, which ensured equilibrium of magnetic moments. ^{31}P T_1 times were then determined by the data processing system equipped with the spectrometer.

III. Results and Discussion

Figure 1 presents crystalline phase evolution during calcining at 330°, 450°, and 600°C. The XRD patterns of the gel calcined below 600°C are mainly amorphous state and show faint peaks corresponding to $Ca(NO_3)_2$ anhydride. From the XRD pattern of the powder calcined at 600°C, the HA phase and minor calcium oxide (CaO) phase were observed.

^{31}P NMR spectra of samples calcined at different temperatures are shown in Fig. 2 and the chemical shifts of assigned peaks are summarized in Table I. The spectrum of the sample calcined at 250°C shows a single chemical shift that peaked at −2.55 ppm with a set of spinning sidebands and corresponds to the gel state. For the 350°C-calcined sample, two peaks located at −7.72 ppm and 0.57 ppm are assigned to Q^1-species (0.57 ppm) and $_1Q^2$-species (−7.72 ppm), respectively. Q^1 represents P atoms in chain-end-type phosphate glasses and $_1Q^2$ represents P–O–Ca linkages in PO_4 tetrahedron.[13] The sidebands became more intense. The XRD pattern of the gel calcined at 330°C shows an amorphous phase, and the $_1Q^2$ peaks in the ^{31}P NMR spectrum are characteristic of the glassy phosphate.[13] After calcining at 600°C,

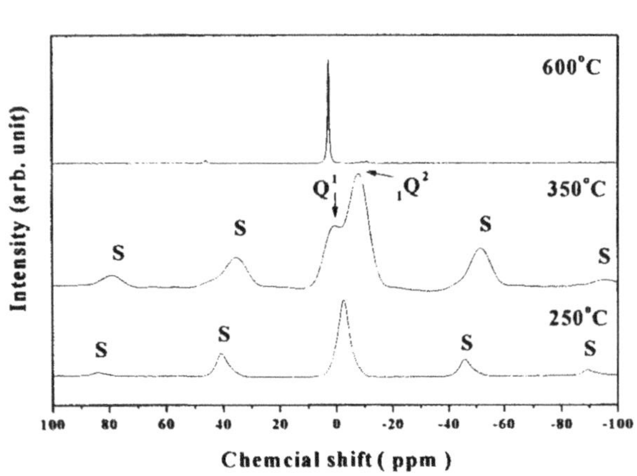

Fig. 2. Solid-state ^{31}P MAS NMR spectra of sample calcined at different temperatures. "S" represents spinning sidebands.

Table I. Isotropic Chemical Shifts (δ) of Samples Calcined at Different Temperatures†

Calcining temperature (°)	Chemical shift (ppm) δ_1	δ_2
250	−2.55	
350	−7.72	0.57
600	2.73	

†Spectra were recorded in high-power proton decoupling (HPPD) mode of MAS ^{31}P NMR.

sidebands of the spectrum disappeared and a sharp peak at 2.73 ppm appeared. These spectroscopic features are related to the HA phase formation at 600°C, as confirmed by the XRD pattern. The spinning sideband patterns are diagnostic of the particular symmetries.[14] A protonated phosphate group (HPO_4^{2-}) in brushite, for instance, has a very strong sideband pattern, which corresponds to a more random structure, but the nonprotonated one (PO_4^{3-}) in HA shows a weak pattern. Therefore, sideband patterns in these samples clearly indicate that from the gel-to-ceramic process, phosphate groups in samples undergo a pathway from a random bonding state to an ordered crystalline state. However, a spinning sideband is only qualitative by nature in the interpretation of NMR spectra, and may be diminishing by the line broadening as a result of chemical shift anisotropy and dipolar interactions.

The most powerful parameter in NMR spectra interpretation is the chemical shift anisotropy variation caused by the shielding or deshielding of the electron clouds from the neighbors. The presence of electronegative atoms in the neighborhood withdraws the electron cloud from P atoms, thereby resulting in deshielding of the P nucleus. In general, a positive chemical shift represents deshielding. Thus, a chemical shift represents local bonding structures in atoms within a few single bonds. The relationship between isotropic chemical shifts and the crystalline structure of calcium phosphate was reported by Miquel *et al.*[6] and is summarized in Table II. It is well-known that the apatite content in the hard tissues of humans is not always 100% by weight, and only synthetic materials can have pure apatite structure. From Table II, rabbit bones have a polycrystalline structure and larger positive chemical shifts. As the crystallininty of the calcined gel increases, the peak shifts toward downfield. Recently, Sahai *et al.*[15] theoreotically calculated ^{31}P isotropic and anisotropic chemcial shifts of orthophosphate minerals (DCPD, OCP, HA, ACP). The results gave the ^{31}P isotropic chemical shift a value of 2.8 ppm (with reference to 85% H_3PO_4), with a distinguishable tenfold scale for anisotropic ones. In addition, the halfwidth of the peak can be used to verify the crystallinity of the HA ceramics, such as the apparently different halfwidths of glassy state and crystalline state, as shown in Fig. 2.

In the spin-lattice relaxation experiments for ^{31}P T_1 values, the HA peak intensity at ~2.73 ppm was recorded as a function of delay time (*t*). A best-fit by the spectrometer yields ^{31}P T_1 times of the control and 600°C-calcined sample of 201.4 and 161.6 s, respectively (Table II). There is a large difference in ^{31}P T_1 samples in the present study. Wu *et al.*[11] found that the T_1 of natural bones, such as bovine bones, are 60–80 times longer than that of the stoichiometric HA. It is well-recognized that calcium-to-phosphorus ratios of natural bones generally deviate from that

Table II. Relation between Isotropic Chemical Shifts, Relaxation Time (T_1), and Crystalline Structure of HA Ceramics

Sample	δ (ppm)	T_1 value (s)
HA†	2.9	
Poorly crystallized HA†	3.3	
Rabbit bones†	3.1	
Control	2.79	201.4
600°C-calcined HA	2.73	161.6

†Data adopted from Miquel *et al.*[6]

of the stoichiometric HA, i.e., Ca:P = 1.67. So, T_1 times could be correlated to the stoichiometry of the calcium phosphate materials.

In general, there are two pathways for relaxation: chemical shift anisotropy and dipolar interaction. In this study, the former was partially avoided because MAS mode was used. Thus, the latter pathway, because of hydrogen bonding in HA ceramic, might be highly efficient. The high gyromagnetic ratio of protons and the short bond length lead to this efficient relaxation. The relaxation rate is related to $\gamma_H^2\gamma_P^2R^{-6}$, where γ denotes the gyromagnetic ratios of the unlike nuclei and R the internuclear distance.[9] In inorganic materials, it is believed that the interaction between the protons and phosphorus contribute less to the relaxation pathways because of the absence of protons. However, the hydrogen bond in an HA unit cell is in the form of $OH\cdots O{=}PO_3$ linkages. In addition, hydrogen bond length of $OH\cdots O{=}PO_3$ linkages found in the literature is in a range of 0.24–0.31 nm.[13,16] So, the dipolar interaction (^1H–^{31}P) relaxation facilitated through the hydrogen bond would be the main contribution. In this study, the presence of CaO might influence the linkages, because the ionic bond nature of CaO might insert into the linkages to form locally stable charged pairs. As a result, the hydrogen bond length is extended and the relaxation rate is longer than that of pure HA ceramic calcined at 600°C.

IV. Conclusions

We have successfully elucidated phase and chemical structures during gel-to-ceramic conversion of HA synthesized by a sol–gel method using solid-state NMR and XRD. XRD shows that during calcinations, dried gel calcined at 330°C remains amorphous and, finally, the HA phase emerges at 600°C. The solid-state ^{31}P MAS NMR spectra show the same evolution. The gel converts to a glassy phosphate at 350°C, then HA ceramic at 600°C. In the glassy phosphate, most of the calcium ions are incorporated into the glassy structure, as indicated by the $_1Q^2$ peak. The ^{31}P T_1 time measurement for HA containing CaO has a larger T_1 value, indicating elongated $OH\cdots O{=}PO_3$ linkages in a HA unit cell, as compared with normal linkages in pure HA ceramic.

Acknowledgments

The authors thank Ms. Mei-Yueh Chien and Ms. Suh-Yun Fang for the help in taking the NMR spectra, and Dr. Rabi Narayan Panda for fruitful discussion and proofreading.

References

[1] H. Plenk, "Biocompatibility of Ceramics in Joint Prostheses"; pp. 269–95 in *Biocompatibility of Orthopedic Implants*, Vol. 1. CRC Press, Boca Raton, FL, 1982.

[2] L. L. Hench, "Bioceramics—From Concept to Clinic," *J. Am. Ceram. Soc.*, **74** [7] 1487–510 (1991).

[3] W. Weng, L. Huang, and G. Han, "The Alkoxide Sol–Gel Process in the Calcium Phosphate System and its Applications," *Appl. Organomet. Chem.*, **13** [8] 555–64 (1999).

[4] L. Wang, W. D. Samuels, G. J. Exarhos, B. I. Lee, and Z. Cao, "^{31}P and ^{29}Si NMR Study of Sol–Gel-Synthesized Phosphate Ceramics," *J. Mater. Chem.*, **8** [1] 165–69 (1998).

[5] G. Kordas and C. C. Trapalis, "Fourier Transform and Multi Dimensional EPR Spectroscopy for the Characterization of Hydroxyapatite Gels," *J. Sol–Gel Sci. Technol.*, **8** [1–3] 305–309 (1997).

[6] J. L. Miquel, L. Facchini, A. P. Legrand, C. Rey, and J. Lemaitre, "Solid State NMR to Study Calcium Phosphate Ceramics," *Colloids Surf.*, **45**, 427–33 (1990).

[7] J. P. Yesinowski and H. Eckert, "Hydrogen Environments in Calcium Phosphates: ^1H MAS NMR at High Spinning Speeds," *J. Am. Chem. Soc.*, **109** [21] 6274–82 (1987).

[8] R. J. Kirkpatrick and R. K. Brow, "Nuclear Magnetic Resonance Investigation of the Structures of Phosphate and Phosphate-Containing Glasses: A Review," *Solid State Nucl. Magn. Reson.*, **5** [1] 9–21 (1995).

[9] R. Jaeger, G. J. Vancso, D. Gates, Y. Ni, and I. Manners, "Chain Flexibility and ^{31}P NMR Spin-Lattice Relaxation Measurements on Melts of Halogenated Poly(thionylphosphaxenes)," *Macromolecules*, **30** [24] 6869–72 (1997).

[10] H. R. Allcock, M. E. Napierala, D. L. Olmeijer, S. A. Best, and K. M. Merz Jr., "Ionic Conduction in Polyphosphazen Solids and Gels: ^{13}C, ^{31}P, and ^{15}N NMR Spectroscopy and Molecular Dynamics Simulations," *Macromolecules*, **32** [3] 732–41 (1999).

[11] Y. Wu, J. L. Ackerman, D. A. Chesler, J. Li, R. M. Neer, J. Wang, and M. J. Glimcher, "Evaluation of Bone Mineral Density Using Three-Dimensional Solid State Phosphorus-31 NMR Projection Imaging," *Calcif. Tissue Int.*, **62** [6] 512–18 (1998).

[12] M. F. Hsieh, L. H. Perng, T. S. Chin, and H. G. Perng, "Phase Purity of Sol–Gel Derived Hydroxyapatite Ceramic," *Biomaterials*, **22** [19] 2601–607 (2001).

[13] H. S. Liu and T. S. Chin, "Low Melting PbO–ZnO–P_2O_5 Glasses, Part 2. A Structural Study by Raman Spectroscopy and MAS-NMR," *Phys. Chem. Glasses*, **38** [3] 123–31 (1997).

[14] P. S. Belton, R. K. Harris, and P. J. Wilkes, "Solid-State Phosphorus-31 NMR Studies of Synthetic Inorganic Calcium Phosphates," *J. Phys. Chem. Solids*, **49** [1] 21–27 (1988).

[15] N. Sahai and J. A. Tossel, "Molecular Orbital Study of Apatite ($Ca_5(PO_4)_3(OH)$) Nucleation at Silica Bioceramic Surfaces," *J. Phys. Chem. B*, **104** [18] 4322–41 (2000).

[16] T. Kanazawa, "Hydroxyapatite"; pp. 27–30 in *Inorganic Phosphate Materials*. Elsevier Science Publications, New York, 1989. □

J. Am. Ceram. Soc., **84** [9] 2135–37 (2001)

journal

Hydroxyapatite Coating on Thermally Oxidized Titanium Substrates

Minkmas Vatanatham and Shoichi Kimura*

Department of Chemical Engineering, Oregon State University, Corvallis, Oregon 97331

Titanium substrates were oxidized in oxygen or air at temperatures of 600°–800°C, then immersed in solutions of 2.0m*M*–20.7m*M* $CaCl_2$ and 1.2m*M*–12.4m*M* KH_2PO_4 for aging periods of 0.5–10 d. The titanium surface was successfully coated with hydroxyapatite (HAP) when the substrates were oxidized in oxygen gas at 610°C for 1 h and then aged in a solution of 2.00m*M* Ca^{2+} and 1.20m*M* PO_4^{3-}. The Ca/P ratio of the surface coating increased toward its stoichiometric HAP value ($^{10}/_{6}$) as the aging time increased; the Ca/P ratio attained a value of 1.66 after 10 d.

I. Introduction

Hydroxyapatite ($Ca_{10}(PO_4)_6(OH)_2$, or HAP) has been used in the medical field in various forms because of its presence as bone apatite or the mineral calcium phosphate that is present in biological hard tissue. Although these features cause HAP to have excellent bioactivity (or capability to bind with living tissue), HAP has some disadvantages, such as brittleness, when applied to implantation processes.

To compensate for the disadvantages of HAP, several methods have been developed for applying a HAP coating on titanium that is intended for use as a load-bearing material. Recently, Soten and Ozin[1] developed a method to grow HAP that was a few micrometers thick on titanium substrates. Before the HAP coating was applied, TiO_2 was sputter-deposited onto the titanium surface. Soten and Ozin[1] implied that both the rutile and anatase phases of TiO_2 are important in the surface nucleation of HAP.

This research examines the possibility of using thermal oxidation to prepare a mixture of rutile and anatase on the titanium surface. Thermal oxidation can easily accommodate any shape of implant material, in contrast to the limitations that result from the use of sputtering. After thermal oxidation at different conditions, HAP surface nucleation in solutions of calcium and phosphate (at different concentrations) was tested. Two oxidation sources were compared: oxygen and air.

II. Experimental Procedure

In this study, $CaCl_2$ and KH_2PO_4 were chosen as the respective sources of calcium and phosphate ions[1,2] to crystallize HAP via the reaction

$$10Ca^{2+} + 6PO_4^{3-} + 2OH^- \rightarrow Ca_{10}(PO_4)_6(OH)_2$$

In an aqueous system of calcium and phosphate, many forms of calcium phosphate can crystallize. Solubility isotherms of several calcium phosphates by Gregory *et al.*[3] suggest that β-tricalcium phosphate (TCP) is second only to HAP in stability at pH >6.36. HAP is increasingly more stable than other calcium phosphates at higher pH. However, $Ca(OH)_2$ has a tendency to form at pH >8.0. In this study, the pH was maintained in the range of 6.5–7.5 throughout the aging periods to sustain the domination of HAP among all the calcium phosphates.

Titanium foil (99.7% purity) and potassium phosphate (monobasic anhydrous, 99%) (each supplied by Sigma, St. Louis, MO) and commercial-grade $CaCl_2$ (Mallinckrodt, Phillipsburg, NJ) was used. A suspension of HAP (Lot 97H5236, Sigma) in a 0.001*M* phosphate buffer solution (pH 6.8) was used as a reference to index the X-ray diffraction (XRD) patterns of HAP.

Titanium samples (cross-sectional area of 10 mm × 10 mm, 2 mm thick) were first polished, degreased, and then acid-treated to remove an oxide layer that had formed naturally. Samples were oxidized in an alumina tube (38 mm inside diameter, 1.5 m long) for different periods of time (1–6 h). Oxidation temperatures were in the range of 600°–800°C. Two systems were studied: oxygen and simulated air (79% nitrogen and 21% oxygen).

The tube was purged with argon during the temperature ramp. When the temperature reached the set point, oxygen or air was fed into the tube at a rate of 1.75 L/min. The oxidation was terminated by switching the oxygen or air to argon immediately after the oxidation period ended.

Preliminary runs indicated that the oxidation of titanium substrates in oxygen at temperatures of >800°C yielded a thick oxide layer that had a high tendency to flake off, whereas titanium was hardly oxidized at temperatures of <600°C. The phase diagram for the titanium–TiO_2 system presented by Hauff[4] also suggests that a temperature of <800°C is appropriate to form both the anatase and rutile phases. Thus, the oxidation temperature was set at 600°–800°C.

Solutions of calcium and phosphate were prepared through the slow mixing of a phosphate solution into a calcium solution while maintaining a pH of 6.5–7.5 with a 0.01*M* KOH solution to prevent the formation of any calcium-deficient HAP.[5] The calcium and phosphate concentrations were adjusted at three levels: low concentration (2.00m*M* Ca^{2+} and 1.20m*M* PO_4^{3-}), intermediate concentration (9.10m*M* Ca^{2+} and 5.45m*M* PO_4^{3-}), and high concentration (20.73m*M* Ca^{2+} and 12.43m*M* PO_4^{3-}), while maintaining a Ca/P ratio of $^{10}/_{6}$ (~1.67). Oxidized substrates were immersed in 200 mL of one of these solutions in a stirred container for 0.5–10 d with its pH adjusted in the 6.5–7.5 range, using a 0.01*M* KOH solution.

X-ray photoelectron spectroscopy (XPS) (Model SSX-100, ESCA) and scanning electron microscopy (SEM) (Model 4700, Hitachi, Tokyo, Japan) were used to examine the prepared surfaces. A monochromatized Al*K*α X-ray source was used (20 mA, 10 kV) in the XPS apparatus. The corresponding precipitate obtained in the bulk solution was examined via XRD (Model D5000, Siemens, Karlsruhe, Germany) with Cu*K*α radiation and a step size of 2θ = 0.02°.

D. S. Wilkinson—contributing editor

Manuscript No. 187969. Received February 5, 2001; approved May 7, 2001.
Based in part on the thesis for a M.S. degree in Chemical Engineering submitted by author MV at Oregon State University.
*Member, American Ceramic Society.

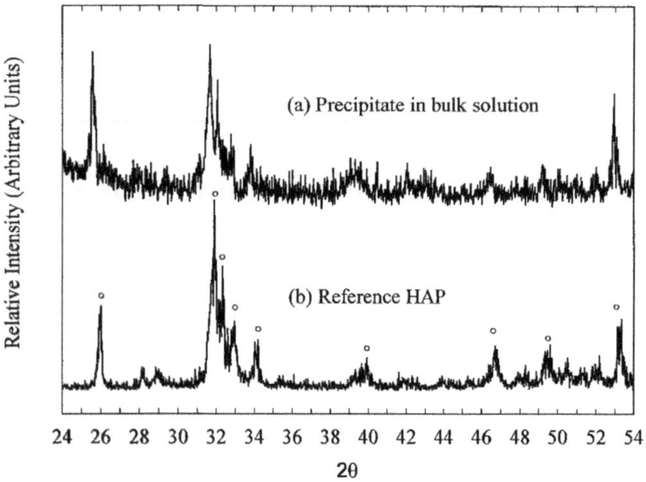

Fig. 1. XRD pattern of precipitate formed in the low-concentration bulk solution, compared with that of reference HAP.

III. Results

When the $CaCl_2$ and KH_2PO_4 solutions were mixed, HAP crystals could precipitate on the titanium substrates and in the bulk solution, when their concentrations were appropriate. The first visible precipitate was formed in the bulk solution after 2 h of mixing the two solutions at the low concentration; precipitation was immediate at the intermediate and high concentrations.

The XRD spectrum of the precipitate that was obtained at the low concentration only demonstrated good matching with the reference HAP at all main peaks: 26.0°, 31.9°, 32.3°, 33.0°, 34.2°, 39.9°, 46.7°, 49.6°, and 53.3°,[6,7] as shown in Fig. 1. The XRD patterns of the precipitates that were obtained at the high and intermediate concentrations[8] exhibited the biggest peaks that corresponded to a main characteristic peak of TCP[6,7] and some minor peaks that were characteristic of HAP. A mixture of TCP and HAP is suggested to crystallize at the intermediate and high concentrations, as demonstrated by other investigators.[9,10] However, only HAP precipitated at the low concentration.

The atomic concentrations and binding energies, as obtained from XPS analysis, of selected substrates that were obtained in different solutions are displayed in Table I. The oxidation of these substrates was conducted at 610°C for 1 h. Based on the equation that was proposed by Unnam *et al.*[11] for the oxidation of titanium with oxygen gas, an oxide layer thickness of 130 nm was estimated after oxidation for 1 h in oxygen gas at 610°C.

A positive energy shift, calibrated with the C 1*s* peak, indicates that an insulating layer is present on top of the metal substrate. A higher energy shift can be attributed to a thicker insulating layer that is either oxide or calcium phosphate. Samples A, B, and C are plain surfaces without being aged in any solution. Sample A is the starting plain titanium substrate (after polish and cleaning steps).

Samples D, E, and F have been oxidized in oxygen gas but aged in different solutions. At the high concentration, a calcium phosphate coating with a Ca/P ratio of only 1.07 is present on the surface; this Ca/P ratio is much less than the Ca/P ratio of HAP (1.67). The titanium concentration is still high, which indicates an incomplete surface coating. At the intermediate concentration, no phosphorus is observed, with a minor amount of calcium and much titanium still remaining on the surface. At the low concentration, the titanium concentration has decreased to zero while the calcium and phosphorus concentrations are high (Ca/P ratio of 1.66), which is very close to that for HAP.

Comparison of the Ca/P ratios of the coated surface for samples G, H, I, and D, which have been oxidized in oxygen gas and aged in the low-concentration solution for 0.5–10 d, reveals the growth of HAP on the titanium substrate. After aging for 0.5 d, the entire oxide surface is already completely covered with calcium phosphate, as evidenced by the zero titanium concentration (sample G). However, its Ca/P ratio is still 1.41. After aging for 2 d (sample H), the Ca/P ratio drastically increases to 1.62 and gradually increases as the aging time increases (sample I). The Ca/P ratio of 1.66 after aging for 10 d (sample D) is almost the same as that of HAP.

Figure 2 is an SEM image (15 000× magnification) of sample D. This image shows that the morphology of the coated surface consists of roselike structures similar to the HAP structures that have been reported by Soten and Ozin;[1] this morphology is unlike the round white clumps comprising the TiO_2 structures that have been shown by Narayana *et al.*,[12] which indicates the formation of HAP on the oxidized surface.

XRD patterns of the precipitate that formed simultaneously in the low-concentration solution used to obtain sample D were essentially identical to those shown in pattern "(a)" in Fig. 1[8] and demonstrated good matching with the reference HAP. Thus, one may conclude that HAP is formed, covering the entire surface of the titanium substrate that has been oxidized in oxygen gas, during a 10-d aging process in the low-concentration solution.

XPS analyses of plain titanium and titanium that was oxidized in simulated air (and aged in the low-concentration solution) are also shown in Table I, as samples J and K, respectively. Results of the plain titanium obviously indicate incomplete coverage with very low calcium and phosphorus concentrations at a low Ca/P ratio. The scanning XPS spectrum of sample J was not much different from that of unaged titanium and showed only very small Ca 2*p* and P 2*p* peaks, at 347.0 and 132.9 eV, respectively.[8]

For sample K, which was oxidized in air, the surface was also completely covered after aging for 10 d but had a Ca/P ratio of 1.29. No phosphorus or calcium was detected on the surface when substrates were oxidized in air at any other temperatures, although they were also immersed in the low-concentration solution.[8] All this evidence confirms that the oxide layer that formed in oxygen gas at low temperature is indispensable for enhancing the nucleation of HAP on the titanium surface.

Table I. XPS Analysis of Different Substrates in Different Solutions

Sample	Oxidation†	Solution	Aging (d)	Concentration (at.%) P	Ca	O	Ti	Ca/P ratio	C 1*s* binding energy shift (eV)	Corrected binding energy (eV) P	Ca	O	Ti
A	Plain titanium	No		0	0	45.7	13.1		+0.7			529.9	457.6
B	O_2	No		0	0	55.3	11.4		+0.9			529.4	458.4
C	Air	No		0	0	53.6	11.7		+0.8			529.7	458.5
D	O_2	Low	10	12.7	21.1	54.5	0	1.66	+5.9	132.9	346.8	530.6	
E	O_2	Intermediate	10	0	3.7	59.9	16.1		+0.8		347.6	529.6	458.3
F	O_2	High	10	2.9	3.1	55.8	23.1	1.07	+2.9	131.6	345.7	527.6	456.6
G	O_2	Low	0.5	13.0	18.2	54.7	0	1.41	+3.7	132.8	346.7	530.6	
H	O_2	Low	2	10.9	17.8	57.7	0	1.62	+4.1	132.7	346.6	530.5	
I	O_2	Low	5	12.2	19.9	56.1	0	1.63	+5.3	132.8	246.7	530.5	
J	Plain titanium	Low	10	2.3	2.1	40.5	17.7	0.92	+1.0	132.9	347.0	532.4	458.2
K	Air	Low	10	14.4	18.5	51.1	0	1.29	+4.7	133.0	346.8	530.7	

†The oxidation was performed in the gas indicated at 610°C for 1 h; "plain" denotes no oxidation.

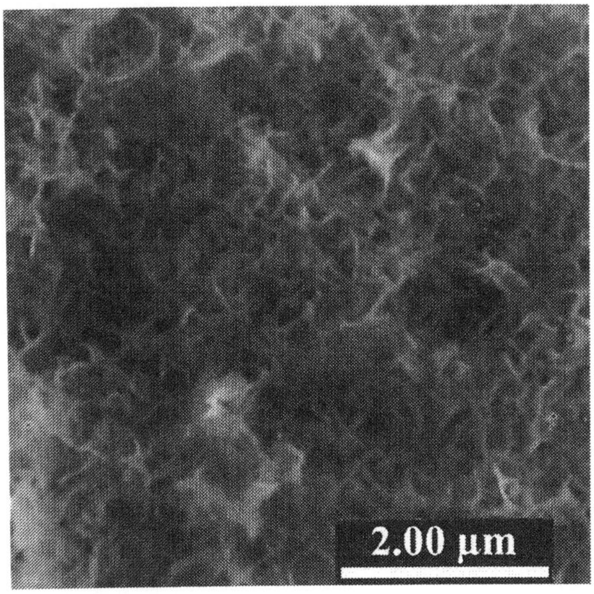

Fig. 2. SEM image showing the morphology of HAP formed on the titanium substrate immersed in the low-concentration solution for 10 d.

Rutile-phase TiO_2 is known to be hydroxylated, and Brønsted acid and base hydroxyl sites exist at the surface. The O 1*s* spectrum of a titanium substrate after 1 h of oxidation in oxygen gas at 610°C has three main peaks (not shown):[8] the largest, at 530.3 eV, corresponds to the bulk H_2O overlayer; the medium peak, at 532.6 eV, is ascribed to Ti—OH, or basic sites; and the smallest peak, at 531.8 eV, is assigned to OH(s), or acidic sites.[13] The acidic and basic sites are both formed from the chemisorption of H_2O; the former attracts PO_4^{3-} ions, whereas the latter attracts Ca^{2+} ions.

The lattice matching between the OH groups of the anatase-TiO_2 layer and HAP plane,[14] and the existence of both the acidic and basic sites on rutile-phase TiO_2,[8,13] provides convincing evidence that a mixture of rutile and anatase TiO_2 (from an oxidation in oxygen gas) on titanium substrates is necessary for HAP surface nucleation.

IV. Conclusions

The surface of titanium was successfully coated with hydroxyapatite (HAP) when the titanium substrates were oxidized in oxygen gas at 610°C for 1 h and then aged in a solution of 2.00m*M* $CaCl_2$ and 1.20m*M* KH_2PO_4 (with a starting Ca/P ratio of 1.67). After aging for 0.5 d, the surface was completely covered with calcium phosphate that had a Ca/P ratio of 1.41. After aging for 10 d, the surface concentration of calcium increased to 21.1% and that of phosphorus increased to 12.7%, with a Ca/P ratio of 1.66, forming HAP structures with a roselike morphology. X-ray diffraction patterns of the precipitate that formed simultaneously in the bulk solution matched that of the reference HAP very well.

References

[1] I. Soten and G. A. Ozin, "Porous Hydroxyapatite–Dodecylphosphate Composite Film on Titania–Titanium Substrate," *J. Mater. Chem.*, **9**, 703–10 (1999).

[2] A. A. Campbell, G. L. Graff, L. Song, and K. R. Sump, "Bioactive Void Metal Composites for Orthopedic Implant Devices," *Mater. Res. Soc. Symp. Proc.*, **414**, 177–82 (1996).

[3] T. M. Gregory, E. C. Moreno, J. M. Patel, and W. E. Brown, "Solubility of β-$Ca_3(PO_4)_2$ in the System $Ca(OH)_2$–H_3PO_4–H_2O at 5, 15, 25, and 37°C," *J. Res. Natl. Bur. Stand. (U.S.)*, **78A** [6] 667–75 (1974).

[4] K. Hauff, *Oxidation of Metal*. Premium Press, New York, 1965.

[5] A. L. Boskey and A. S. Posner, "Formation of Hydroxyapatite at Low Supersaturation," *J. Phys. Chem.*, **80**, 40–46 (1976).

[6] D.-M. Liu, "Fabrication of Hydroxyapatite Ceramic with Controlled Porosity," *J. Mater. Sci.: Mater. Med.*, **8**, 227–32 (1997).

[7] W. F. Jayne, P. A. Moor Jr., and D. M. Miller, "Solubility and Ion Activity Products of Calcium Phosphate Minerals," *J. Environ. Qual.*, **28**, 530–36 (1999).

[8] M. Vatanatham, "Surface Nucleation of Hydroxyapatite onto Titanium Substrates Thermally Treated with Oxygen"; M.S. Dissertation. Oregon State University, Corvallis, OR, 2000.

[9] M. A. Fanovich and J. M. P. Lopez, "Influence of Temperature and Additives on the Microstructure and Sintering Behavior of Hydroxyapatite with Different Ca/P Ratios," *J. Mater. Sci.: Mater. Med.*, **9**, 53–60 (1998).

[10] S. Zhang and K. E. Gonsalves, "Preparation and Characterization of Thermally Stable Nanohydroxyapatite," *J. Mater. Sci.: Mater. Med.*, **8**, 25–28 (1997).

[11] J. Unnam, R. N. Shenoy, and R. K. Clark, "Oxidation of Commercial Purity Titanium," *Oxid. Met.*, **23**, 231–52 (1986).

[12] K. V. Narayana, A. Venugopal, K. S. Rama Rao, K. Masthan, V. V. Rao, and P. K. Rao, "Ammoxidation of 3-picoline over V_2O_5/TiO_2 (Anatase) System. II. Characterisation of the Catalysts by DTA, SEM, FTIR, ESR and Oxygen and Ammonia Chemisorption," *Appl. Catal. A.*, **167**, 11–22 (1997).

[13] T. K. Sham and M. S. Lazarus, "X-ray Photoelectron Spectroscopy (XPS) Studies of Clean and Hydrated TiO_2 (Rutile) Surface," *Chem. Phys. Lett.*, **68**, 426–32 (1979).

[14] C. Mao, H. Li, F. Cui, Q. Feng, H. Wang, and C. Ma, "Oriented Growth of Hydroxyapatite on (001) Textured Titanium with Functionalized Self-Assembled Silane Monolayer as Template," *J. Mater. Chem.*, **8** [12] 2795–801 (1998). □

IV. Conclusion

The surface of titanium was successfully [illegible] hydroxy-apatite (HAP) when the titanium substrates were [illegible] [illegible]

References

AMERICAN CERAMIC SOCIETY BULLETIN

NANOPHASE CERAMICS AS

Improved Bone Tissue Engineering Materials

Altering the particulate size of existing materials to the nanometer regime might be a solution to improving current orthopedic implants.

Thomas J. Webster
Dept. of Biomedical Engineering, Purdue University, West Lafayette, Ind.

Nanotechnology can be broadly defined as the use of materials and systems whose structures and components exhibit novel and significantly changed properties when control is gained at the atomic, molecular and supramolecular levels. Advances in several critical research fields (such as processing, catalytic, optical, actuation, electrical and mechanical) have begun to benefit from new technological advancements in the area of nanotechnology. Specifically, such advances have been found for materials when particulate or grain size is decreased to <100 nm.

However, to date, relatively few advantages have been elucidated for biological applications (specifically, for implants and/or tissue-engineering applications). This article seeks to demonstrate the promise that nanophase ceramics have to improve biological applications, such as tissue regeneration. In this manner, this article adds another novel property of ceramics with grain sizes <100 nm: improved cytocompatibility. Although works are currently focused on the use of nanophase materials in dental, bladder, neurological, vascular and cardiovascular graft applications, this article specifically concentrates on the use of nanophase ceramics as better orthopedic implants.

Fibrous Encapsulation of Implanted Orthopedic Materials

In 1990, the total medical device sales for orthopedic implants totaled ~2.2 trillion dollars.[1] Since 1990, this number has been steadily growing. In fact, the 152 000 total hip replacements in 2000 is a 33% increase from the number performed in 1990 and a little over half of the projected number of total hip replacements (272 000) by the year 2030 in the United States alone.[1] Unfortunately, however, in 1997, 12.8% of the total hip arthroplasties were revisions of previously failed hip replacements.[1]

The fact that such a high percentage of hip replacements performed every year are revision surgeries is not surprising when considering the life expectancy of the implant versus that

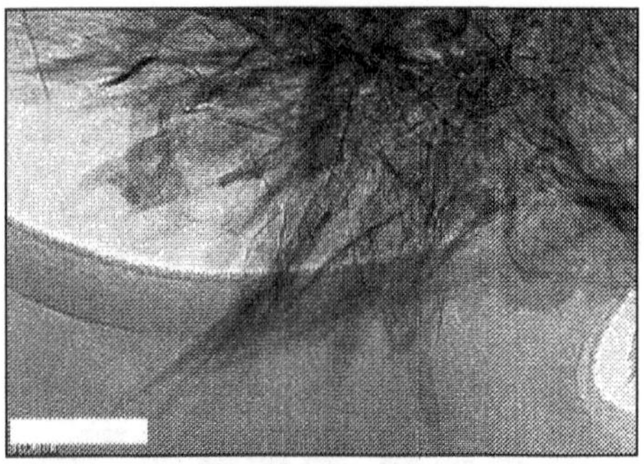

Representative TEM of individual alumina nanodimensional fibers (bar = 100 nm). Bone cell function is enhanced on nanofibrous compared with nanosperical alumina. Photograph courtesy of Argonide Corp.

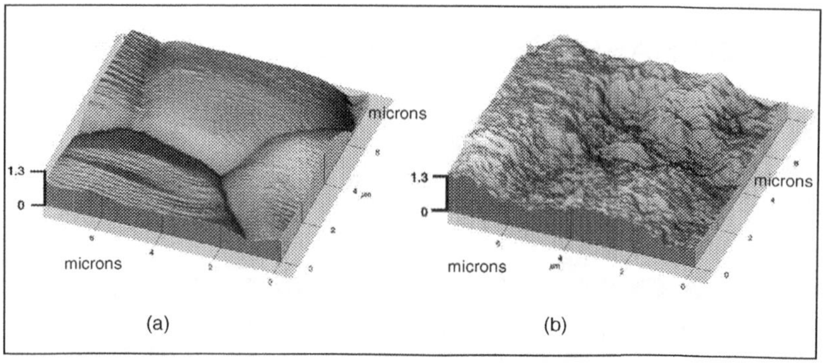

Representative atomic force images of (a) conventional and (b) nanophase titania ceramics. Bone cell function is enhanced on nanophase compared with conventional ceramics.

of the patient receiving the implant. Consistently, over 30% of those requiring total hip replacements have been below the age of 65. However, the longevity of orthopedic implants ranges only ~12–15 years. Therefore, the majority of those who receive an implant at age 65 or younger will require at least one revision surgery. This suggests that the life expectancy of orthopedic prostheses is a recurring problem that has to be dealt with because current approaches fail.

The characteristics vital for the effective functioning of orthopedic implants in the host tissue include lack of toxicity tendencies, resistance to corrosion by surrounding tissue fluids, sufficient strength to support normal physical motion or loading, resistance to bodily fatigue forces and ability to promote cellular adhesion, which leads to juxtaposed bone tissue regeneration.[2] The healing response immediately following biomaterial implantation determines the long-term functionality of the device. The healing process involves recruitment of a variety of body fluids, proteins and unwanted cell types to the tissue–implant interface.

Healing characteristics common of unsuccessful bone prosthetic wound-healing include fibrous encapsulation and chronic inflammation. Fibrous encapsulation (or callus formation) at the interface or at the implant–body tissue site decreases the bonding effectiveness and often results in clinical failures. This slows down rapid attainment of the physical strength in the region that would be juxtaposed to that of normal tissue.

Most importantly, to date, these failures (common to conventional orthopedic implant materials) often lead to insufficient bonding with juxtaposed bone. This event is necessary to stabilize the implant for subsequent physiological loading. That is, select, timely and desirable responses from surrounding bone cells are required to enhance deposition of the mineralized matrix at the tissue–implant interface, which provides crucial mechanical stability to implants. Therefore, modulating the healing response may improve biomaterial efforts to increase new bone regeneration and decrease unwanted fibrous tissue formation. This is the role envisaged of the next generation of materials for orthopedic applications.

Nanophase Ceramics

Many definitions are attached to the term "nanophase materials" by various experts. The commonly accepted concept defines nanomaterials as those materials with basic structural units in the range of 1–100 nm (nanostructured), crystalline solids with grain sizes of 1–100 nm (nanocrystals), individual layer or multilayer surface coatings in the range of 1–100 nm (nanocoatings), extremely fine powders with an average particle size in the range of 1–100 nm (nanopowders) and fibers with a diameter in the range of 1–100 nm (nanofibers).[3]

Nanostructure science and technology create materials and products that potentially outperform, at several boundaries, existing advanced materials (such as advanced/fine ceramics, advanced polymers and composites).[3,4] Assisted by these developments, there has emerged, concurrently, nanotechnology (an endeavor able to work at the molecular level, atom by atom to create large structures) and fundamentally new molecular organization (with at least one characteristic dimension measured in nanometers).

There are many bulk-material advantages of nanophase materials (such as mechanical properties in nanophase ceramics closer to bonelike increased toughness because of greater grain-boundary sliding) that clearly make these novel materials attractive for bone implant applications.[3] Mechanical properties of the next generation of orthopedic implants must match those of surrounding bone to decrease stress and strain imbalances that often lead to bone implant failure.[2]

However, numerous less obvious advantages exist as well. For example, living systems are governed by molecular behavior at nanometer scales. The molecular building blocks of life—proteins, nucleic acids, lipids and carbohydrates—are examples of materials that possess unique properties determined by the size, folding and patterns at the nanoscale.[5]

More importantly, for the present article, bone is a nanophase material. It is composed of proteins (for example, collagen) that possess nanometer features. In addition, other inorganic constituents in natural bone (such as hydroxyapatite fibers) possess dimensions 2–5 nm in width and ~50 nm in length.[2] For this reason, cells in the body are accustomed to interacting with nanostructured surfaces on a daily basis. However, conventional materials used for orthopedic implants are composed of micron grain sizes and resulting nonbiologically inspired topographies.[2]

Nanophase ceramics can be formulated to simulate the nanometer surface roughness of bone.[6] In this manner, nanophase ceramic implants seek to mimic the nanotopography that proteins and inorganic hydroxyapatite crystals create in natural bone tissue.

Increased Bone Regeneration on Nanophase Ceramics

The first reports correlating increased bone cell function with decreased ceramic grain sizes into the nanometer regime date back to 1998.[7] Specifically, compared with conventional (micron-sized) ceramic formulations, nanophase ceramic compacts made separately from nanometer spherical particles of alumina, titania and hydroxyapatite provided evidence of enhanced adhesion of osteoblasts (bone-forming cells), while, at the same time, decreased adhesion of fibroblasts (cells that contribute to fibrous encapsulation and callus formation events that may lead to implant loosening and failure).

Equally as interesting, a step-function increase in osteoblast adhesion appeared specifically at ceramic spherical grain sizes <60 nm. Thus, direct proof was provided to show for the first time that the ability of nanophase ceramics to increase bone cell function is indeed limited to grain sizes <100 nm. Ceramics below this same grain size have been noted by others to possess special mechanical, catalytic and other properties.[3,4] These studies further reported enhanced calcium deposition (calcium deposition is an index of mineralization of the bone matrix) by osteoblasts as well as increased functions of osteoclasts (bone-resorbing cells) on nanospherical over larger grain-size ceramics.[8–11]

Specifically, deposition of calcium by osteoblasts on nanospherical alumina and titania was over four and three times greater than on respective conventional ceramic formulations.[8] Coordinated functions of osteoblasts and osteoclasts are imperative for the formation and maintenance of healthy new bone juxtaposed to an orthopedic implant. Frequently, newly formed bone juxtaposed to implants is not remodeled by osteoclasts and, thus, becomes unhealthy or necrotic.[2]

Researchers have further modified nanophase ceramics to simulate the nanometer dimension and the aspect ratio of proteins and hydroxyapatite found in bone.[12] For example, consolidated substrates formulated from nanofibrous alumina (diameter of 2 nm, length of >50 nm) increased osteoblast functions in comparison with similar alumina substrates formulated from the aforementioned nanospherical particles.[12] Thus, perhaps not only is the nanometer grain size of components of bone important to mimic in ceramics, but the aspect ratio also may be important to simulate in synthetic materials.

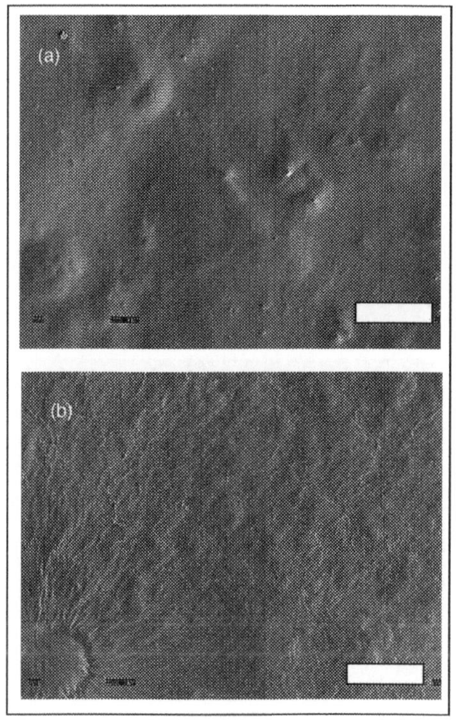

SEM images depicting poly(lactic-co-glycolic acid) (PLGA) composites containing (a) conventional titania (4.120 μm in grain size) compared with (b) nanophase titania (32 nm in grain size) (bar = 10 μm). Composite is 70/30 wt% PLGA/titania. Bone cell function is enhanced on polymer composites containing nanophase compared with conventional ceramics.

Recent evidence has been provided that the special cytocompatibility properties as pertaining to bone implants are not specific only to alumina, titania and hydroxyapatite bulk ceramics.[13–15] For example, studies in the literature show similar increases in bone cell function when nanophase (compared with conventional) ceramic particles are incorporated into polymer composites.[14] Specifically, up to three times more osteoblasts adhered to poly(lactic-co-glycolic acid) when it contained nanophase compared with conventional titania particles.

Moreover, Elias et al.[13] showed significantly greater osteoblast

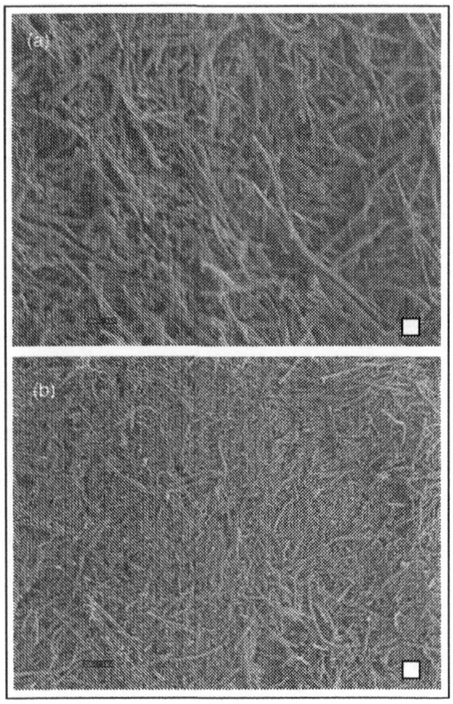

SEM images depicting (a) conventional carbon fibers (0.125 μm in diameter) compared with (b) nanophase carbon fibers (60 nm in diameter) (bar = 10 μm). Bone cell function is enhanced on nanophase compared with conventional carbon fibers.

function leading to new bone synthesis on bulk compacts containing carbon fibers with nanometer compared with conventional dimensions. Such novel cytocompatibility properties have been seen when carbon nanofibers were incorporated into polymer composites. Specifically, increased osteoblast adhesion was observed in polyurethane with increased weight percentages of nanometer, not conventional, dimension carbon fibers. In fact, there was even preferred alignment of osteoblasts along the carbon nanofibers present on the surfaces of the polymer composites.

Osteoblasts have been observed to align on the surfaces of bone in the body.[2] Thus, this may be another important consequence of using nanophase fibers in orthopedic design. These positive cellular behaviors, combined with the high specific strength of carbon nanofibers/nanotubes, can readily

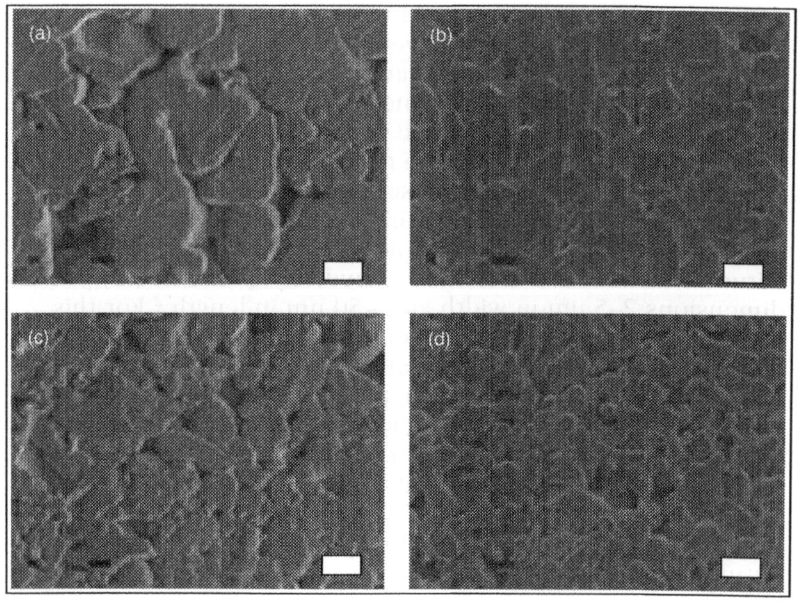

SEM images depicting (a) conventional titanium compared with (b) nanophase titanium and (c) conventional Ti–6Al–4V compared with (d) nanophase Ti–6Al–4V (bar = 10 μm). Bone cell function is enhanced on nanophase compared with conventional metals.

be exploited as a reinforcing component for composite orthopedic implant materials. Lastly, Ejiofor and Webster[15] have recently provided evidence that such novel properties for enhanced bone cell functions observed on all of the prior nanophase materials also are present for nanophase compared with conventional metals (specifically, titanium and Ti–6Al–4V).[15]

Although nanophase ceramics may have increased wear fatigue properties,[3] debris may form from articulating components of orthopedic implants composed of nanophase ceramics when subjected to physiological loading properties. Conventionally sized wear debris particles induce bone loss, which leads to implant loosening and sometimes results in clinical failure of bone prostheses.[3] In a recent report, however, results of a more well-spread morphology and increased cell proliferation in the presence of nanophase wear debris demonstrated less adverse influences on bone and cartilage cell function in comparison with larger conventional ceramic wear particles.[11] For this reason, nanophase wear debris may not be as harmful as its conventional counterparts.

Although much more testing must be conducted on this new classification of materials, collectively, these findings consistently testify to unprecedented and excellent cytocompatibility properties of nanophase materials with regard to regenerating bone. This condition is critical for the fixation of orthopedic implants so that patients can resume and continue a normal active lifestyle for the remainder of their lives.

Following these significant discoveries, extremely fine bioceramic powders can be used as components in a wide range of biomedical implants, from hard sintered ceramic disk implants to porous bone grafts (bone replacement), coatings, controllable setting calcium phosphate-based bone cements (for implant fixation) and nanocomposites that have superior biological properties. At this point, although the opportunities seem widespread, little is known about how bone cells recognize and respond favorably to nanophase materials.

Bone Cell Recognition of Nanophase Ceramics

Surface properties (such as area, charge and morphology) depend on the particulate (such as grain) or fiber size of a material. As mentioned, the increased surface defects (such as at the edge/corner sites) and the high number of grain boundaries in nanophase materials have special advantageous properties that are being exploited in the development of biocompatible implants. To date, the increased surface reactivity of nanomaterials has been utilized for catalytic applications almost exclusively.[4]

For example, compared with conventional magnesia, nanophase magnesia possesses an increased number of atoms at the surface, higher surface area, less acidic OH^- groups (because of a much higher proportion of edge sites for the nanophase magnesia to cause delocalization of electrons) and a subsequent increased adsorption of acidic ions as well as destructive adsorption of organophosphorous/chlorocarbons. Are these properties of nanophase materials important for catalytic applications also influencing bone cell function? Right now, the answer seems to be yes.

Recent reports demonstrated that similar special interactions observed in catalytic applications exist between nanophase ceramics and proteins contained in body fluids to mediate bone cell function.[6,9] Proteins initially adsorb to a biomaterial surface within milliseconds of implantation from surrounding body fluid.[5] The type of protein and the manner in which that protein adsorbs (that is, its conformation) determines whether a bone cell will adhere.

Specifically, osteoblasts adhere to select amino acid sequences (such as arginine-glycine-aspartic acid (RGD)) in adsorbed proteins.[5] Surface properties of an implant determine whether this and/or other important amino acids are available for osteoblast adhesion. Because bone cell adhesion on newly implanted orthopedic surfaces is necessary for those cells to synthesize bone, initial optimal protein adsorption events are important to implant success.

To be more specific, biomaterial surface features (such as roughness, charge, chemistry and wettability) and the select properties of each protein influence protein adsorption and, ultimately, affect implant biocompatibility with host tissue. For nanophase ceramics, it has been found that smaller surface grain sizes increase the number of grain boundaries at the surface to enhance material surface wettability for optimal protein adsorption, which, subsequently, promotes select cell function.[6, 9]

Nanophase ceramics have special surface properties because of an increased number of atoms at the surface than in the bulk, when compared with conventional ceramics. In addition, because the

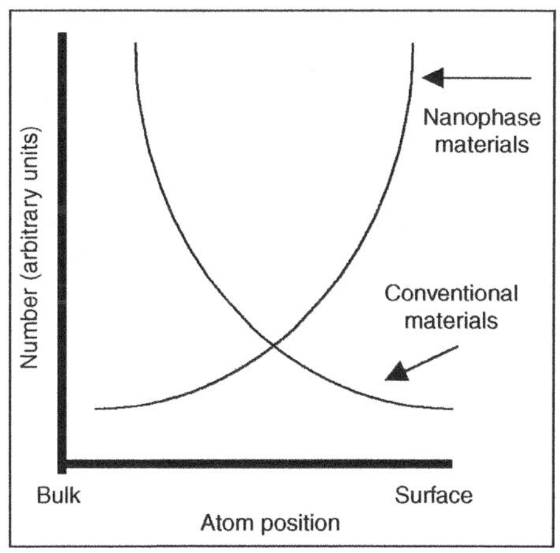

Higher number of atoms at the surface for nanophase compared with conventional materials. Increased number of atoms at the surface gives nanophase ceramics special properties to regenerate bone.

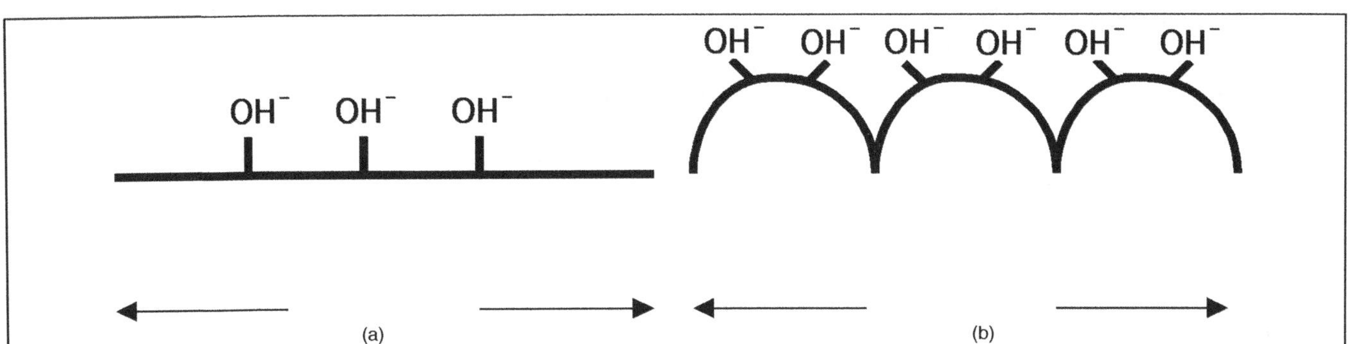

Special surface properties of nanophase ceramics pertinent for protein interactions and subsequent cell interactions. Compared with (a) conventional materials, (b) nanophase materials possess higher surface area and less acidic OH^- groups (because of an increase in electron delocalization) in the hydroxide layer. Adapted and redrawn from Ref. 4. Special surface properties of nanophase ceramics for catalytic applications also can be used in bone tissue regeneration.

dimensions of proteins that mediate cell adhesion are at the nanometer level, a surface with a nanometer topography can influence the availability of amino acids for cell adhesion to a greater extent than conventional surfaces that are smooth at the nanoscale.

Indeed, literature reports demonstrate that the cumulative adsorption of proteins contained in body fluids is significantly higher on smaller, nanometer, grain-sized ceramics.[6,9] In particular, the interaction of four proteins—fibronectin, vitronectin, laminin and collagen—known to enhance osteoblast function, increased greatly on nanophase compared with conventional (micron-sized grains) ceramics.[6,9]

Furthermore, a novel adaptation of the standard surface-enhanced Raman scattering (SERS) technique has provided evidence of increased unfolding of the aforementioned proteins adsorbed on nanophase versus conventional ceramics.[9] This is important, because unfolding of these proteins, once they are adsorbed, promotes availability of specific cell-adhesive epitopes (collections of amino acids in proteins) to increase bone–cell adhesion and function.

It is now believed that the novel surface properties (nanometer topography, increased number of grain boundaries at the surface, wettability, charge, etc.) of nanophase ceramics influence initial interactions with proteins to subsequently increase osteoblast response and new bone formation.

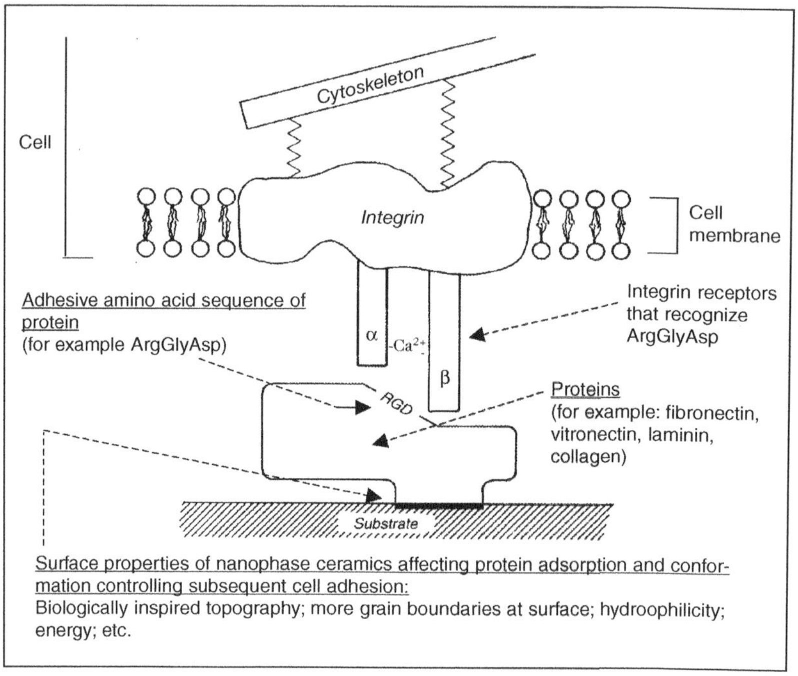

Surface properties of nanophase ceramics that manipulate protein interactions for altered cell functions. Redrawn and adapted from Ref. 5. Nanophase ceramics alter initial interactions with proteins to promote bone cell function.

Potential Risks

Because the research on and the use of nanophase ceramics remains in its infancy, risks to human health and environment must not be overlooked. Many issues relating to safe and healthy fabrication of nanophase ceramics need to be addressed. For example, the health effects of small nanoparticles entering the human body through pores and accumulating in the cells of the respiratory or other organ systems (for example, when also becoming dislodged through wear debris) are practically unknown.

These effects would happen during commercial-scale processing of the nanoparticles as well as through the use of these materials as implants. There should be a need for continuous monitoring of potential effects of newly designed and fabricated nanomaterials, especially under in vivo situations

The scientific developments reported above do not exhaust the current global research efforts on the biological potentials of nanophase ceramic particulates as implants. It is believed, however, that following the trends of these impressive application properties of nanomaterials in bone applications, there exists a bright future for therapies and treatments.

Recent developments in modifying existing conventional materials to possess nanoscale dimensions may increase new bone synthesis to offer exciting promising alternatives to bone tissue engineering. This is a much easier route to exploiting the beneficial properties of nanostructured materials as biomedical implants than by creating new chemistries that have not been recommended for inside-the-body use. By simply altering particulate size of existing materials into the nanometer regime, a solution to improving current orthopedic implants may be obtained. ■

Editor's Note

The list of references to this article is available on the Internet, www.ceramicbulletin.org; by E-mail, references@acers.org; or by fax, 614-794-5822. Request Data Depository File No. 397.

3-D CT IMAGES FOR

Biomimetic Artificial Bone Design and Manufacture

The combination of simplified computed tomography images and modern rapid-prototyping processes produces biomimetic artificial bone similar in microstructure to natural bone.

Jiemo Tian, Xiangang Wang, Chaozong Zhang and Zhiping Guo
State Key Laboratory of New Ceramics and Fine Processing, Institute of Nuclear Energy Technology, Tsinghua University, Beijing, Peoples Republic of China

During recent years, biomimetic artificial materials have become widely used in clinics. These materials are mainly fabricated as the substitution of human hard tissue, such as artificial bones and false teeth. As medical implants, the artificial bones that have a structure similar to human bone have better biocompatibility and osteoinductional property.

A new method for designing and manufacturing artificial bone, computed tomography- (CT-) assisted artificial bone design and manufacturing, has been proposed to overcome the shortcomings of traditional computer-assisted design (CAD) methods, such as drawing a graph after manually measuring an actual bone. The essence of CT-assisted artificial bone manufacturing and engineering is to design, evaluate, process and control quality using CT. The essence of CT-assisted artificial bone design is a generated bone model, using CT-provided data.

First, a 3-D image of a natural bone is acquired using CT. Second, a model of the bone is generated using a simplified CT image. Third, a biomimetic artificial bone (BMAB) is manufactured using 3-D rapid-prototyping technology.[1] Comparison between the BMAB CT image and the bone model shows the success of the 3-D rapid-prototyping manufacturing process. To evaluate onsteogenesis, the CT image of an implant sample can be compared with the BMAB model. The quantity of new bone is compared with osteoinduction performance.

CT Measuring and Evaluation

X-ray CT is an important and powerful tool in industrial imaging for obtaining shape and dimension information of an industrial part.[2] A 3-D image of the microstructure can be obtained using X-ray CT, which also greatly enhances our knowledge of bone. CT yields images having superior resolution and dimensional accuracy to traditional manual-measuring methods, especially in accuracy of boundaries and interior dimensions.

CT is a convenient way to study the interior microstructure of materials. Therefore, CT is an ideal tool to describe the exterior and interior complex structures and dimensions of a bone. An important feature of CT is its nondestructive measuring capability.[3]

A CT image is composed of points and point values. CT maps

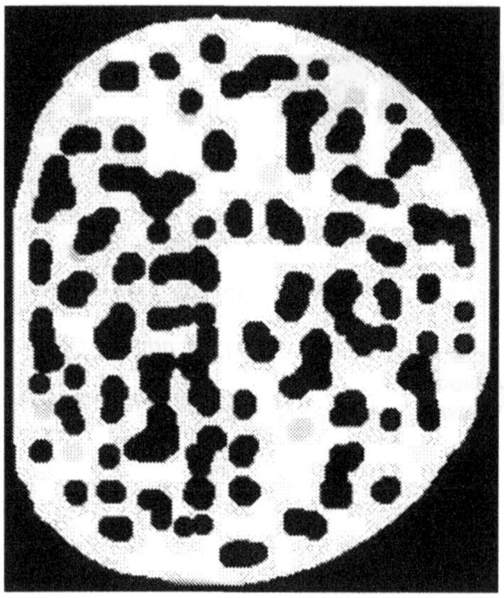

Lattice model of bone (bright regions are higher density and dark regions are lower density).

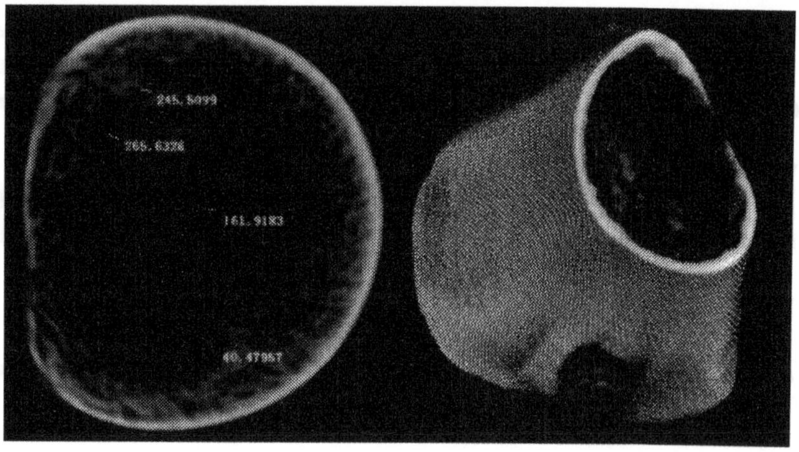

Typical CT slice and 3-D shape of natural bone.

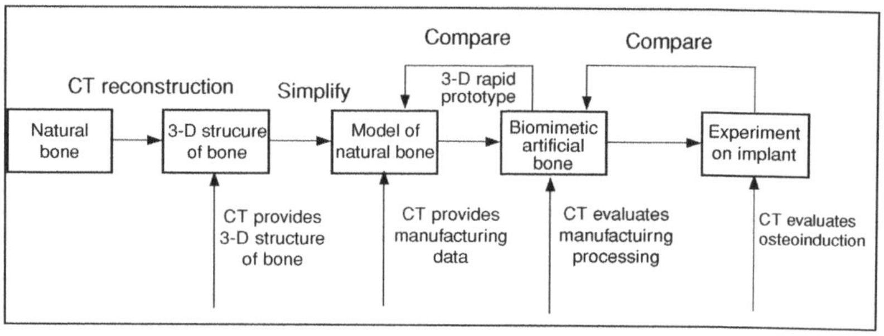

Process diagram of CT-assisted artificial bone design, manufacturing and evaluation.

the density of actual bone. The brighter the signal, the higher the density—the darker the signal, the lower the density. A CT image-derived model is called a lattice model in this article.

CT-Assisted Artificial Bone Design

Artificial bone design is the first step of producing a bone. In many factories, industrial parts are designed and manufactured using a CAD model; i.e., industrial parts are described using lines, arcs and planes. However, a CAD model cannot fully express the complex shape and dimensional information of a bone, especially its 3-D spatial structure.

On the other hand, a lattice model is composed of pixels (points). Pixel values represent density information located in a 3-D space. A graph with 1000 lines is complex, but a typical CT slice contains 512 × 512 pixels, and 512 × 512 × 100 if a 3-D structure is expected.

Generally, a bone model designed for one person is not perfectly suitable for another person, because particular bones from different people are not exactly the same. A traditional bone model is generated on the basis of human anatomy.

The dimensions of a bone must be measured manually or by machine, such as a coordinate-measuring machine (CMM), before design can begin. Then, a CAD model is generated by the designer using the information contained in the measured data. Therefore, automated designing is important.

Measuring the interior structure of bone is difficult. Moreover, the precision of manual measuring is poor because it is difficult for traditional methods to generate a large data set. This often produces ambiguity in continuity and connectivity. For example, porosity in a specified region is difficult to determine using traditional methods. Therefore, exactly describing the complex curve of a human bone using a sparse data set is not exact and results in poor biocompatibility.

CT overcomes the difficulty of manual measuring. CT can be used to nondestructively inspect the interior structure and density of human bone, providing complete dimensional and structural information for the inaccessible region of the bone. Another problem of the CAD model is that design is performed manually and, possibly, destructibly. On the other hand, a CT-image-derived lattice model can be generated automatically using a computer, making automation of design and manufacturing possible.

The true 3-D structure must be simplified before manufacturing, because a CT slice is too complex for direct implementation in factories.[4] Few machines can manufacture a part having high resolution and high complexity at the same time. Another reason for simplifying is that pores whose diameters are <200 μm provide little contribution for osteogenesis, according to Klawitter.[5] Therefore, it is not necessary to manufacture such

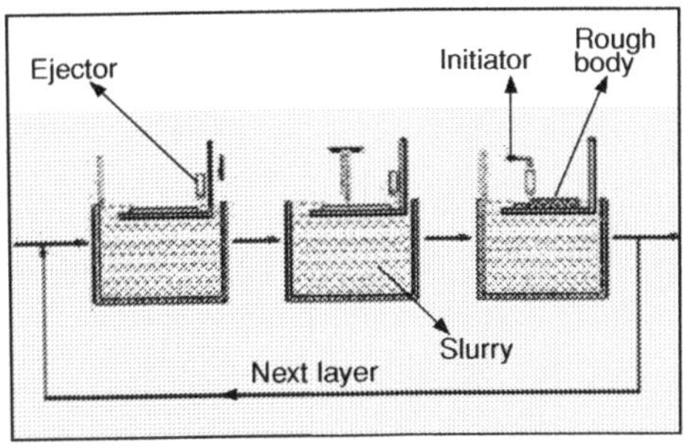

Principle of 3-D gel casting.

complex parts, which reduces costs. Small pores are reduced from the CT image by digital image-processing methods, e.g., noise elimination to smooth the image edge.

Usually, the CT slice is converted to a binary system, using point values of zero or one, because it is more convenient to form using a single material. Zero (darker) represents voids and one (bright) represents solids. For those bodies that are made from several types of materials, the cross section is quantified to several values according to density, such as 0, 0.4, 0.8 and 1. Various material densities are mapped to various gray values. Therefore, the lattice model can be defined as a quantified slice whose shape and density are represented using pixel position and gray values, respectively.

Some small pores are <1 mm in diameter. More small pores can be generated using a foaming agent.

Manufacturing

Some modern rapid-prototyping processes can be combined with the simplified CT image (lattice model), such as laser selection sintering methods, 3-D printing and 3-D gel-casting. All the processes have the feature that the body is built up point-by-point and layer-by-layer.

For example, 3-D gel-casting is used to form the hydroxyapatite skeletal framework in our laboratory.[6] A computer-controlled nozzle moves and ejects material based on the information provided by a simplified CT image. When the nozzle moves to a position where its corresponding position in the CT image is not zero, it ejects initiator into a slurry. If the position is zero, it ejects nothing.

The initiator then solidifies the piece of slurry. After one layer is completed, the platform moves down one layer thickness (~100 μm) and repeats the process on the basis of the neighboring CT slice. A new layer then is formed. In this way, a rough body is built up, layer by layer.

Therefore, artificial bone is manufactured using 3-D rapid prototyping on the basis of a simplified bone model. Further implant experiments can be performed to study the oeteogenesis factor. In this process, CT provides 3-D true structure and design data, evaluates the manufacturing process and controls quality using a comparison between a simplified bone model and the product slice. The osteogenesis factor is evaluated using a study on new bone implant experiments. ■

Acknowledgments

This work is supported by the National Major Fundamental Research Program about biomaterials (National 973 program, P.R. China) under Contract No. G19990647-02 and National Natural Science Foundation of China under Contract No. 69972023.

References

[1] J.M. Tian and S.F. Yang, "Freeform Fabrication of Bone Hydroxyapatite Artificial Bone"; 5th IUMRS-ICAM '99, Beijing, China, July 13–19, 1999.

[2] X.G. Wang, Z.P. Guo, Y.H. Peng, et al., "Fast 3-D Reconstruction CT Image by Using Geometric Parameter Table," *Journal of Tsinghua University (Scientific and Technology)*, **42** [5] 655–58 (2002).

[3] C.Z. Zhang, Z.P. Guo, Y.F. Dong, H.P. Zhang and J.M. Tian, "Testing Advanced Structural Ceramics," *Am. Ceram. Soc. Bull.*, **75** [1] 64–66 (1996).

[4] G.T. Herman and A. Kuba, *Discrete Tomography: Foundations, Algorithms and Applications,* 346–61, Birkhser Press, Boston, Mass., 1999.

[5] J. Klawitter, "A Basic Investigation of Bone Growth into a Porous Ceramic Material"; Ph.D. Thesis. Clemson University, Clemson, S.C., 1970.

[6] L. Zhang, "Study on the Preparation of Biomimetic Artificial Bone Using 3-D Gel-Lamination Method"; Ph.D. Thesis. Tsinghua University, Beijing, China, 2000.

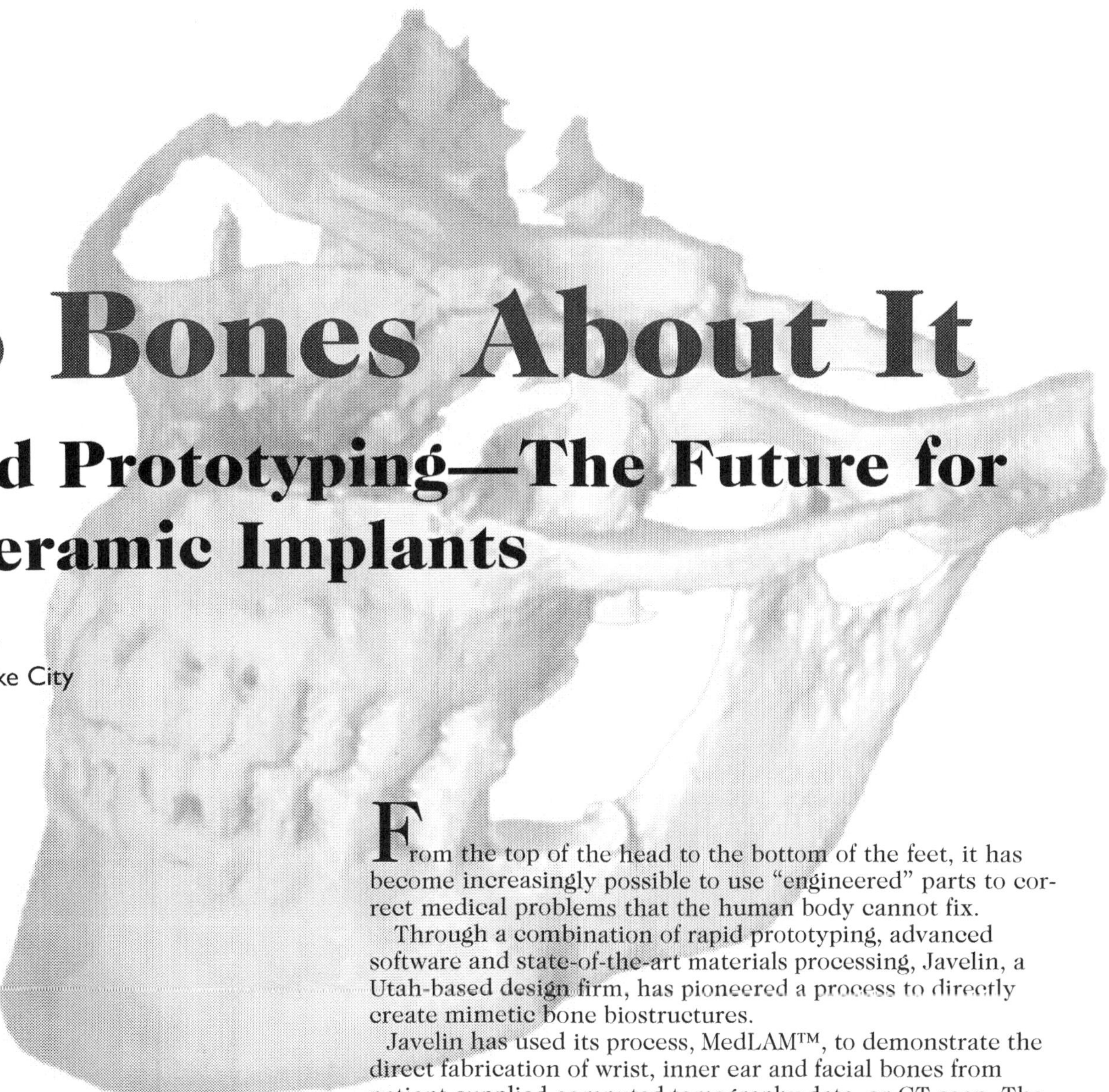

No Bones About It

Rapid Prototyping—The Future for Bioceramic Implants

Alair Emory
Javelin, Salt Lake City

From the top of the head to the bottom of the feet, it has become increasingly possible to use "engineered" parts to correct medical problems that the human body cannot fix.

Through a combination of rapid prototyping, advanced software and state-of-the-art materials processing, Javelin, a Utah-based design firm, has pioneered a process to directly create mimetic bone biostructures.

Javelin has used its process, MedLAM™, to demonstrate the direct fabrication of wrist, inner ear and facial bones from patient-supplied computed tomography data, or CT scan. The process has been used to demonstrate bone biostructures out of alumina, zirconia and phosphate-based bioceramic materials.

Reconstruction Background

The CT scan uses X-ray technology to create images of internal organs. Unlike a traditional X-ray, CT scans are able to distinguish between obscured and overlapping parts of the body. They also are capable of producing images of several different internal components, including soft tissue, blood vessels and bones.

The CT scan creates detailed images by using X-ray beams that pass through sections of the patient. The scanner, invented by Hounsfield, is basically an X-ray tube that rotates in a circle around the patient, making many pictures as it rotates.

While lying down on a flat, moving table, the patient enters a circular CT machine where the images are created by the X-ray beams. The beams are aimed at the body at different angles in order to show various "slices" or smaller areas of concentration. A computer analyzes the data received by the detector, and transforms the information into a digital image. Each slice can be examined separately.

Although each image may be examined separately, for bio-

Javelin is a registered DBA name for Lone Peak Engineering Inc., Salt Lake City
MedLAM is a Javelin, Salt Lake City, trademark
Velocity^2 Pro is an Image3 LLC, Salt Lake City, trademark
Laminated Object Manufacturing is a Helisys Inc., Torrance, Calif., trademark
SteamRoller is a Javelin, Salt Lake City, trademark

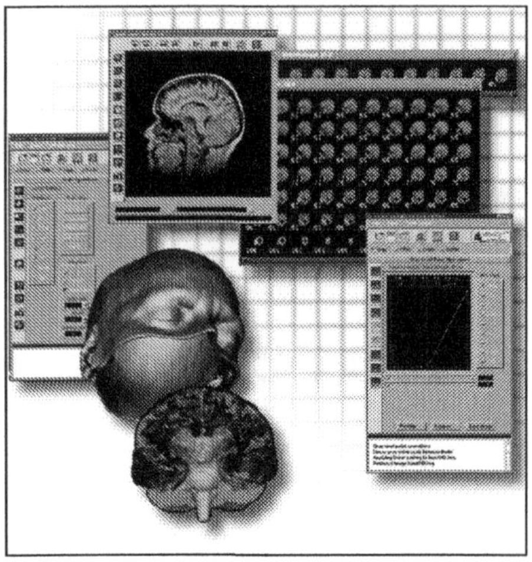

Velocity² Pro for NT interface supports direct import of CT and MR images and export of smooth 3-D reconstructions.

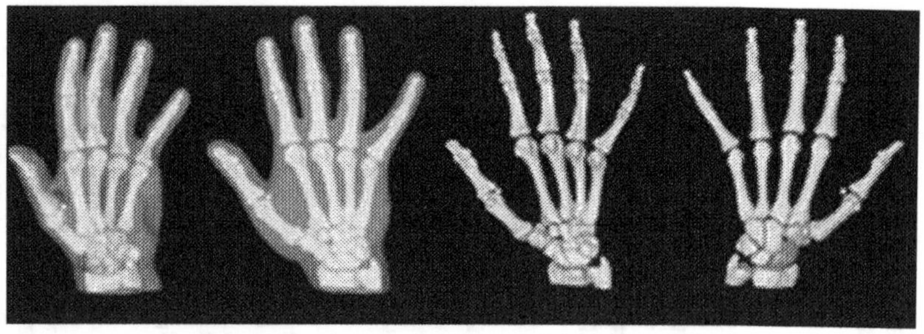

Using Javelin's MedLAM, approach it may be possible one day to produce custom bioceramic implants directly from patient-specific data.

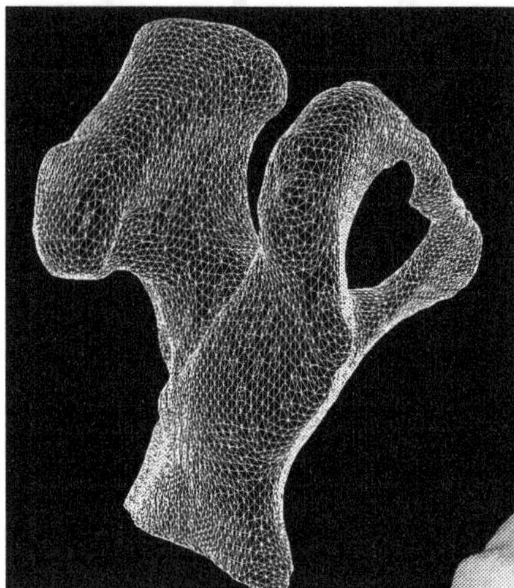

Patient-supplied CT data are imported into Velocity². Once the image reconstruction is completed, a triangulated iso-surface can be viewed.

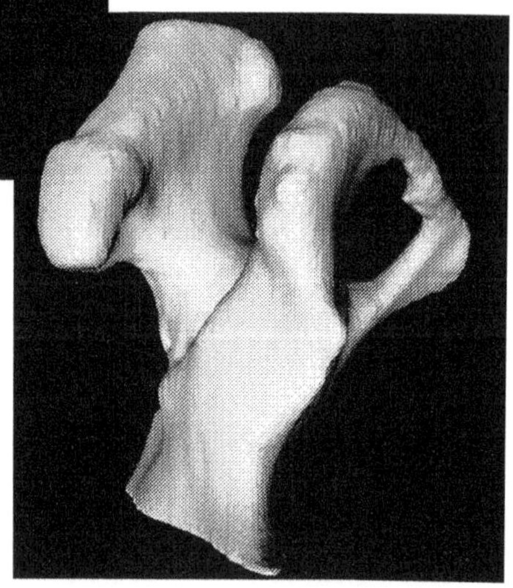

After defining the surface characteristics—with respect to color, material choice and lighting effects—the same model can be examined in a 3-D mode.

model building purposes, it is necessary to reconstruct the object from individual slice data. Reconstruction is the "rebuilding" of an item that has been "torn" apart. 3-D reconstruction also requires the ability to view or visualize all of the data once it has been put back together.

Software for Medical Models

Javelin considers Velocity² Pro™ for NT as the first step in the MedLAM process. In order to build accurate bioceramic models for implant evaluation, a complete software solution for creating 3-D computer models from CT data sets is necessary. Velocity's advanced segmentation tools and 3-D viewing allows Javelin professionals to undertake medical image reconstruction from patient-supplied data.

Velocity² Pro combines gray level, algebraic, geometric, morphological and masking operations to accomplish image reconstruction. 3-D geometry models are created through high-resolution surface triangulation. The resulting geometry models are then exported in the rapid prototyping STL file format.

Rapid Prototyping

Javelin's MedLAM process incorporates a modified Laminated Object Manufacturing™ (LOM) technique to produce green (unfired) bioceramic models based on the reconstructed patient data.

LOM systems normally use rolls of paper to build up a wood-like component. Javelin has modified the LOM rapid prototyping technique to allow sheets of bioceramic materials to be used. In order to adapt the system to work with bioceramic materials, Javelin has developed strong and flexible tape-cast ceramic sheet materials suitable for lamination.

Javelin also has designed an add-on sheet-feed system that bypasses the LOM roller mechanism and automatically feeds single sheets. This system, called the SteamRoller™, interfaces directly with the LOM operating software and significantly expands materials options for LOM rapid prototyping.

During the LOM build process, a laser, controlled by the machine's software, cuts the part cross-section onto the paper

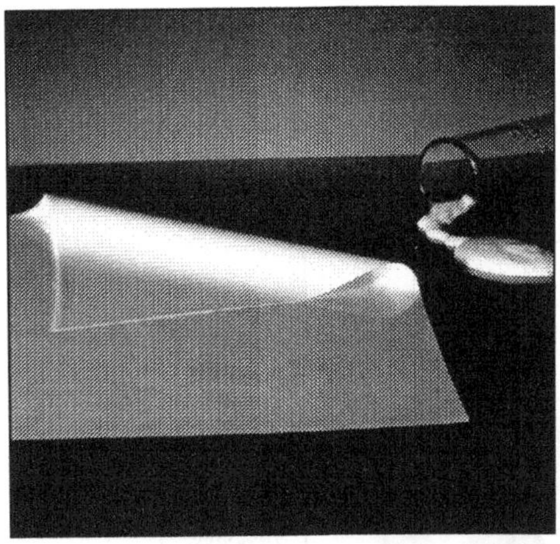

Alumina tape-cast sheet material used in the MedLAM process and produced by Javelin.

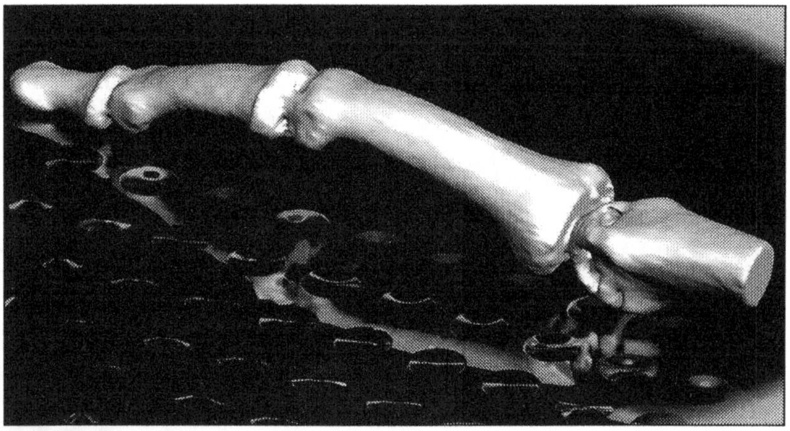

Reconstruction of human finger bone from CT data. Courtesy of Image3. Reconstructed computer model can be exported in the STL file format to a rapid-prototyping machine.

(or flexible ceramic tape). A new layer of material is laminated to the previously cut layer. The computer-directed laser then cuts the next layer, and the process is repeated until the part is finished.

The excess material around the part area remains with the part to support it as it is built. The laser cuts tile into the support material to facilitate the removal of the part at the end of the build cycle.

Prior to firing, Javelin's MedLAM parts have strength and appearance similar to green parts formed using more conventional ceramic injection molding techniques. In the MedLAM process, bioceramic parts undergo tape-cast binder removal and sintering in a conventional furnace. This process has been used by Javelin to produce alumina, zirconia, and phosphate-based mimetic bone biostructures for research purposes.

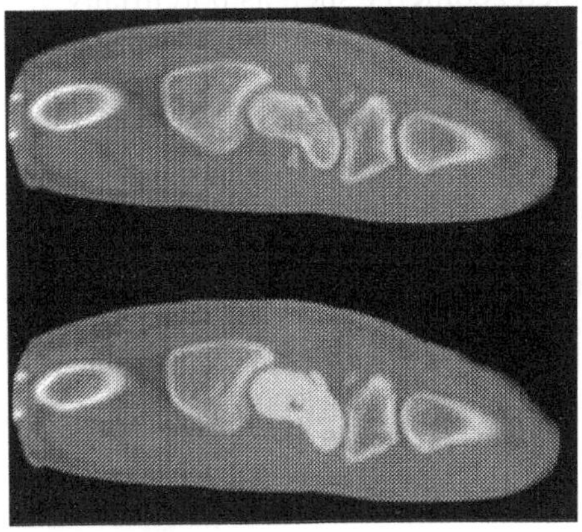

CT slice data with the bone of interest selected for reconstruction.

Alumina

High-density, high-purity (>99.5%) alumina was basically the first bioceramic widely used clinically. It was used in load-bearing hip prostheses and dental implants because of its combination of excellent corrosion resistance, good biocompatibility, wear resistance and high strength. This material was the first ceramic developed by Javelin for the MedLAM process.

Alumina has been used in orthopedic surgery for nearly 20 years, largely because of its acceptance by the body and minimal scar formation (which permits cementless fixation of prostheses) and its exceptionally low coefficients of friction and wear rates. Using the MedLAM process, Javelin has produced alumina ceramic duplicates of every bone in an adult male hand CT data set.

Densities of 95–98% theoretical are achievable for alumina MedLAM prototypes. Design factors have been developed by Javelin to account for shrinkage encountered during sintering to obtain tolerances of ±0.010 in.

Javelin produces the green tape, typically in thicknesses of 0.002, 0.005 and 0.010 in., although thicker tapes can be used in the MedLAM process.

Better surface definition of the finished prototype is obtained by using a thinner tape. However, thinner tape increases the time to build the part, resulting in a more expensive prototype.

Zirconia

The higher toughness and the lower modulus of elasticity of zirconia, in stabilized and transformation-toughened forms, provides some advantages over alumina and metals for use in orthopedics.

Javelin produces a partially-stabilized zirconia tape for the MedLAM process. The tape is available in two thicknesses, 0.005 and 0.010 in.

MedLAM prototypes produced from this composition have

theoretical densities of 96%. Zirconia prototypes rapidly produced by Javelin have strengths and fracture toughness properties similar to zirconia ceramics produced by conventional methods. Biomimetic structures prototyped by Javelin in zirconia include inner ear bones and bone anchors.

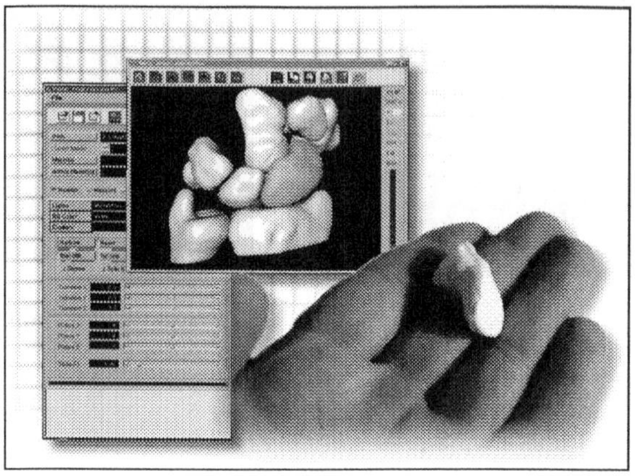

Alumina ceramic scaphoid medical prototype produced from patient data via the MedLAM process.

Phosphate-Based Bioceramics

Calcium phosphate-based bioceramics have been in use in medicine and dentistry for nearly 20 years. Applications include dental implants, skin treatment, gum treatment, jaw bone reconstruction, orthopedics, facial surgery, ear, nose and throat repair, and spinal surgery.

Different phases of calcium phosphate ceramics are used depending upon whether a resorbable or bioactive material is desired. These include dicalcium phosphate (C_2P) and hydroxyapatite ($Ca_{10}(PO_4)_6(OH)_2$(HA)).

Tape casting of phosphate-based ceramics is not as prevalent as the more common alumina and zirconia ceramics. However, using the methods and procedures established for alumina and zirconia, Javelin has produced flexible bioceramic tapes in both calcium phosphate and hydroxyapatite compositions. Currently, these tapes are only available in the 0.010-in. thickness.

Lamination characteristics are similar to those of alumina and zirconia. Additionally, these tapes have been used to build prototypes with complex-shaped geometry such as potentially implantable facial reconstruction sections.

Into the Future

Javelin has demonstrated the ability to take medical scan data and rapidly prototype models in a variety of bioceramic materials. The ability to rapidly produce bioceramic prototypes efficiently and consistently should allow the medical design community to tailor composition, microstructure and chemistry of various types of ceramics to match the specific biological and metabolic requirements of tissues and/or disease states.

Using Javelin's MedLAM approach, it may be possible one day to produce custom bioceramic implants directly from patient-specific data. ■

Ceramic Transactions

THE ROLE OF CERAMICS IN AN AGE OF BIOLOGY

Larry L. Hench
Department of Materials
Imperial College London
Room B403 Bessemer Building
South Kensington Campus
Exhibition Road
London SW7 2AZ
United Kingdom

ABSTRACT

Meeting the healthcare needs of an ageing population is one of the great challenges of this century. This lecture explores the use of ceramics to stimulate the regeneration and repair of human tissues at a genetic level. Approximately 3.5 billion years ago life emerged on earth. This transformation from disorder to order has been passed on by countless generations of descendants in the form of genes, microscopic bundles of DNA. The cells of many present day life forms, including humans, contain as many as 60,000 genes that direct the growth, maintenance and replication of our cells. The genes encode proteins that control all phases of the bone cell cycle; including growth, replication of DNA, repair of DNA, cell division (mitosis), programmed cell death (apoptosis) and differentiation of the cells to form bone matrix and control bone mineralization. Special compositions of silicate based glasses act as gene-activating ceramics. Analysis of the reaction kinetics of the bioactive glass surfaces reveals that it is release of soluble silica and calcia ions in very specific concentrations that activates the genes. Gene activation occurs only when the temporal sequence of the cell cycle is matched by the temporal sequences of the glass surface reactions. When the two are synchronised the bone cells quickly form new bone, even when the cells are obtained from old humans. The implications of this discovery extend from understanding the origin of species that contain mineralised bones to the loss of bone mass in space travel. It also establishes a scientific foundation for designing a personalised, genetic basis for repair and regeneration of tissues in patients and offers hope for eventual inhibition of the deterioration of bones and joints as we age.

It also provides direction for molecular design of ceramics for tissue engineering scaffolds and living cell bio-optical sensor systems for monitoring chemical and biological warfare agents and testing the toxicity of industrial materials and wastes. New types of bioceramics provide an innovative approach to controlling human biology and maintaining a high quality of life for ageing people. First generation biomaterials were developed to be as bioinert as possible to minimise rejection by host tissues. Second-generation biomaterials were designed to be either resorbable or bioactive, achieving positive interactions with the body. The next generation of biomaterials is combining these two properties, with the aim of developing materials that, once implanted, will help the body heal itself. The function of first and second generation biomaterials is to replace diseased or damaged parts of the body. Third generation biomaterials are designed to regenerate tissues.

INTRODUCTION

Several billion years ago life evolved form the seas. An irreversible transformation occurred that resulted in order coming from disorder[1]. This transformation created a world of organic chemistry from a world that was originally composed of only inorganic compounds. The dissolution of rocks into the water of the seas, along with changes in the atmosphere, provided the ingredients for the first biological organisms to appear. In the aeons since, the world of biology has become immensely diverse. This diversity has culminated in the evolution of beings; i.e. humans, that are also capable of producing irreversible transformations of nature. The field of ceramics results from the irreversible transformations of naturally occurring inorganic minerals into man made materials. Discovery of the ability to transform naturally occurring clays through control of fire into ceramics was a seminal event in the cultural development of mankind. Throughout the millennia ceramics have provided innovative approaches to harnessing the forces of nature for the good of mankind. As shown in Figure 1 ceramics first appeared as a science and technology by understanding the transformation of the earth into man made products through use of earth sciences, chemistry and physics. Ceramics have evolved as one of the primary driving forces for achieving and maintaining a high quality of human life. During the last several decades a new challenge has emerged for the field of ceramics. This challenge is to harness the science and technology of inorganic materials to enhance the understanding and control of biological organisms, including ourselves (Figure 1). This challenge requires us to return to our beginnings, to the origins of life and biology, which evolved from the inorganic world.

CHALLENGE OF THE 21ST CENTURY: THE AGE OF BIOLOGY

In this new century we face the consequences of several revolutions that are heralded as the "age of biology". The first revolution is the control over life and death. The technology now exists to be able to determine when children are born.

The understanding of the human genome and the manipulation of DNA also make it possible to influence the nature of a child that is born. The age of biology gives rise to many moral and ethical questions and dilemmas. Many of these ethical uncertainties are addressed in my recent book, "Science, Faith & Ethics"[1]. Among the most important of these questions that now face every reader is the ultimate balance between our length of life and our quality of life.

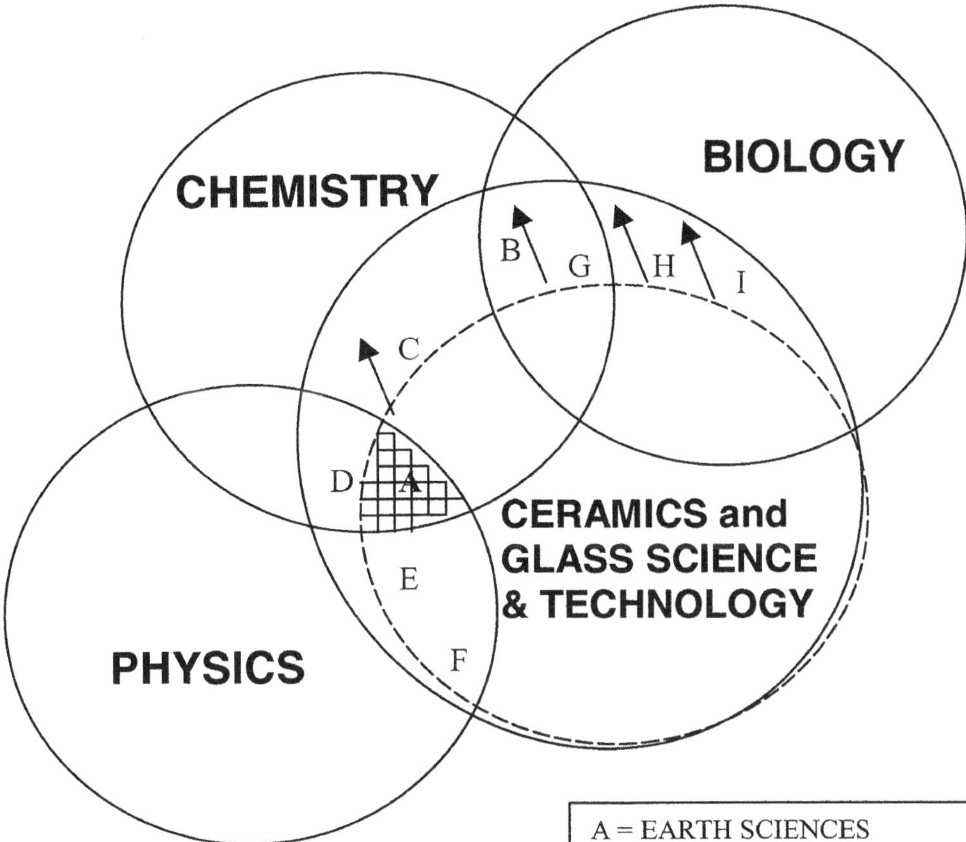

A = EARTH SCIENCES
- GEOLOGY
- MINERALOGY
- MINING

B = ORGANIC CHEMISTRY
C = INORGANIC CHEMISTRY
D = SURFACE CHEMISTRY
E = SURFACE PHYSICS
F = MICROMECHANICS
G = BIOMATERIALS
H = CELL BIOLOGY
I = MOLECULAR BIOLOGY

Figure 1. Growth of ceramics field to incorporate physics, chemistry and biology.

During the last 100 years the average age of the population in the developed world has increased by 30 years. This trend will continue. The problem that faces us is that the percentage of the population that generate the resources to maintain life are now less than the percentage of the population which depends on others for their quality of life. The number of individuals from infant-hood until twenty years of age combined with the number of individuals from the age of 65 to 100 is greater than the number of productive individuals from 20 to 65 years of age. Thus the resources to maintain quality of life for all individuals are shrinking. This important shift in the average age and distribution of age has occurred simultaneously with the ability of the medical community to maintain life for long periods of time using life support systems. Living a long life is good. However, living a long life with deteriorating quality of life is bad. It is now well established that the quality of tissues, including skeletal tissues, cardiovascular tissues and nervous tissues, all deteriorate with age. As described in references 1-4 it is well known that by the time people reach the age of 60 years or more that the quality of their tissues has degraded by 20% to 50% compared to their tissues when they were 20 to 30 years of age. The medical community supported by the biomaterials community, including bioceramics, have responded to this need[1-5].

During the last 50 years more than 40 different parts of the body have become routinely replaced by prostheses and implants. It is now commonplace to replace tissues with spare parts: more than 3 million people receive implants each year. The use of man made implants to replace living parts of the body was an excellent solution for millions of people. However, people are now outliving their implants. Survivability of replacement parts are typically in the range of 10 to 15 years[6], whereas the life expectancy of the individuals receiving the implants is increasing from 10, to 20, to 30 years. The consequences of patients outliving their implants is a growing incidence of revision surgery which drains the resources of hospitals, medical staff, private or national insurances and greatly deteriorates the quality of life of the patients. The use of transplants, parts from other patients or animals, does not provide a viable alternative for the problem of survivability of implants[1]. The incidence of viral infections and/or prions combined with the deterioration of transplants over a period of time and the requirement for a lifetime use of immuno-suppressant drugs combined with the difficulty and ethical problems of obtaining sufficient donors limits the use of transplants. Another solution is required. Without another alternative we will, as a society, be faced with a growing in-balance between our infinite desires for a long, healthy, high quality of life versus the finite resources to achieve those aims.

EXPANDING ROLE OF CERAMICS IN HEALTHCARE

Numerous reviews and books[1-6] have documented that ceramics have played an important part in the maintenance of high quality of life. Medical grade alumina and zirconia are excellent examples. Bioactive glasses heralded the development of a new generation of biomaterials, as did resorbable calcium phosphate ceramics[7]. Recent results, which will follow, show that a third generation of biomaterials, materials that serve to activate the genes of the tissues in contact with the materials, are now feasible[8]. In the remaining sections of this presentation we will review the first, second and third generation of bioceramics and discuss the potential use of ceramics to control biology.

First Generation Biomaterials: The goal of all early biomaterials was to "*achieve a suitable combination of physical properties to match those of the replaced tissue with a minimal toxic response in the host*"[2]. These materials resulted in a revolution in healthcare; i.e., the reliable replacement of diseased or damaged parts of the body. In 1980 there were more than 50 implanted devices (prostheses) in clinical use made from 40 different materials[2], approximately 3 million prosthetic parts were implanted in patients in the United States and Europe annually. A common feature of most of the materials was their "bioinertness." Tens of millions of individuals have had their quality of life enhanced for 5 to 25 years by use of implants made from first generation, bioinert biomaterials.

Second-Generation Biomaterials: During the 1970s the field of biomaterials began to produce bioactive components that could elicit a controlled action and reaction with tissues[3]. Bioactive glasses (composed of Na_2O-CaO-P_2O_5-SiO_2) were developed to bond to living tissue[7]. Interfacial bonding involved a sequence of 11 reaction steps[4]. The first five steps occurred on the surface of the material due to rapid ion exchange of Na^+ with H^+ and H_3O^+ followed by a polycondensation reaction of surface silanols to create a high-surface area silica gel. These surface reactions provided a large number of sites for heterogeneous nucleation and crystallisation of a biologically reactive hydroxy-carbonate apatite (HCA) layer equivalent to the inorganic mineral phase of bone. The growing HCA layer on the surface of the material is synergistic with six cellular reaction steps that include colonization by osteoblasts, followed by proliferation and differentiation of the cells to form new bone that produces a mechanically strong bond to the implant surface.

By the mid-1980s bioactive materials reached clinical use in many orthopaedic and dental applications[4-5]. Synthetic hydroxyapatite (HA) ceramics were used as porous implants, powders, and coatings on metallic prostheses to provide bioactive fixation[4-6]. The HA coatings led to a tissue response (termed osteoconduction) in which bone grew along the coating and formed a mechanically strong interface. Bioactive glasses and glass-ceramics were used as middle-ear prostheses to restore the ossicular chain and treat conductive hearing loss[6]. They were also used as dental implants to preserve the alveolar ridge from the bone resorption that follows tooth extraction[6]. A strong and tough bioactive glass-ceramic, A-W glass-ceramic, was used for replacement of vertebrae in patients with spinal tumors[5]. By the 1990s bioactive composites, composed of HA particles in a polyethylene matrix, became important in the repair and replacement of bones in the middle ear[9]. Another advance achieved in second generation biomaterials was the development of resorbable biomaterials that exhibited controlled chemical breakdown and resorption when implanted in the body. The implant material is ultimately replaced by regenerating tissues, and ultimately there is no discernible difference between the implant site and the host tissue[2]. An example of this is the biodegradable suture, in which the polymer composed of polylactic (PLA) and polyglycolic (PGA) acids hydrolytically decomposes into CO_2 and H_2O. By 1984 clinical use of resorbable polymers as sutures was routine[3]. Resorbable fracture fixation plates and screws in orthopaedics and controlled-release drug-delivery systems were in their infancy[10]. An important characteristic of this second generation of biomaterials is their design especially for medical applications, in contrast to first generation biomaterials which were selected from "off the shelf" compositions[2-5].

THE CLINICAL CHALLENGE FOR THE FUTURE

The clinical success of first and second generation biomaterials has been excellent. However, survival analyses of skeletal prostheses[6-11] and artificial heart valves[12] show that a third to half of prostheses fail within 10 to 20 years. Years of research have had only small effects on failure rates[6]. Improvements of first- and second-generation biomaterials are limited in part because all man-made biomaterials used for repair or restoration of the body represent a compromise[1]. Living tissues can respond to changing physiological loads and biochemical stimuli, but synthetic materials cannot. This limits the lifetime of artificial body parts. Continuing this path of trial-and-error experiments that require the use of many animals and human clinical trials is prohibitively expensive. We have reached a limit to our current medical paradigm that emphasises replacement of tissues. It is time to emphasize a more biologically based method for the repair and regeneration of tissues. The biological response of cells to bioactive ceramics provides an insight towards creating a third generation of biomaterials[8].

Third Generation Biomaterials: Third-generation biomaterials are being designed to stimulate specific cellular responses at the molecular level[8]. The separate concepts of bioactive materials and resorbable materials have converged. Bioactive materials are now made resorbable. Resorbable polymers are being made bioactive. Molecular modifications of resorbable polymers and bioactive composite systems elicit specific interactions with cell integrins. Consequently third generation biomaterials can enhance cell proliferation, differentiation, and extracellular matrix production and organization. Recent findings show that third generation bioactive glasses and macroporous foams can be used to activate genes that stimulate regeneration of living tissues. Two alternative routes of repair are now available with the use of these third generation molecularly tailored biomaterials.

Tissue engineering: The engineering of tissues starts with the seeding of progenitor cells onto biologically active resorbable scaffolds. The cells grow outside the body and become differentiated and mimic naturally occurring tissues. These tissue-engineered constructs are then implanted into the patients to replace diseased or damaged tissues. With time the scaffolds are resorbed and replaced by host tissues that include a viable blood supply and nerves. The living tissue-engineered constructs adapt to the physiological environment and should provide long-lasting repair.

In situ tissue regeneration: The concept of tissue regeneration involves the use of biomaterials in the form of powders, solutions, or doped microparticles to stimulate local, *in situ*, tissue repair. Bioactive materials release chemicals in the form of ionic dissolution products, or growth factors such as bone morphogenic protein (BMP), at controlled rates, by diffusion or network breakdown, that activate the cells in contact with the stimuli. The cells produce additional growth factors that in turn stimulate multiple generations of growing cells to self-assemble into the tissues *in situ* along the biochemical and biomechanical gradients that are present. For example, when a particulate of bioactive glass is used to fill a bone defect there is rapid regeneration of bone that matches the architecture and mechanical properties of bone at the site of repair. Both *osteoconduction* and *osteoproduction*[13] occur as a consequence of rapid reactions on a bioactive glass surface[3-4]. The surface reactions release critical concentrations of soluble Si, Ca, P, and Na ions that give rise to both intracellular and extracellular responses at the interface of the glass with its cellular environment.

CELL CYCLE CONTROL AND GENE ACTIVATION

Rapid repair of bone requires differentiation as well as proliferation of osteoblasts. A synchronised sequence of genes must be activated in the osteoblasts so that they undergo cell division called mitosis. The bone cells then synthesize an extracellular matrix that is capable of mineralizing to become bone. We now know that there is genetic control of the cellular response of osteoblasts to bioactive glasses. Seven families of genes are up regulated within 48 hours of the exposure of primary human osteoblasts to the ionic dissolution products of bioactive glasses[14]. The activated genes express numerous proteins that influence all aspects of differentiation and proliferation of osteoblasts:

Transcription factors and cell-cycle regulators;
Signal transduction molecules;
Proteins involved in DNA synthesis, repair, and recombination;
Growth factors and cytokines that influence the inflammatory response to the material;
Cell-surface antigens and receptors;
Extracellular-matrix components
Apoptosis regulators.

Use of the dissolution products of resorbable bioactive gel-glasses to stimulate cellular repair at a molecular level offers promise for creating scaffolds for bone tissue engineering as well as *in situ* regeneration of tissues. Under appropriate culture conditions, differentiating embryonic stem (ES) cells can be induced to form bone nodules[15]; Bone nodules are multi-layers of bone cells embedded in a mineralised extracellular matrix that contains type I collagen and osteocalcin. When a standard osteoblast differentiation medium is conditioned by exposure to resorbable bioactive gel-glasses for 24 hours and then applied to differentiating ES cells, a dose-dependent increase in the numbers of bone nodules is formed. This is a unique response to the activation of genes by the ionic dissolution products of the bioactive glasses[16]. Bioactive scaffolds have been made that release optimal concentrations of the ionic dissolution products as they resorb in the presence of adherent human osteoblasts[17]. Molecular modifications of the three-dimensional resorbable inorganic scaffolds by chemisorption of surfactant proteins have been made to enhance attachment and proliferation of lung cells[18]. Clinical trials of these third generation biomaterials will soon be underway.

Regeneration of Soft Connective Tissues

Obtaining and maintaining a blood supply in tissue engineered constructs is necessary for their long-term stability following implantation. Recent studies by the author, and colleagues at Imperial College London, have used third generation bioactive, resorbable composites to enhance vascularization of a regenerated soft tissue construct in rats. A novel composites processing method was developed to impregnate polyglycolic acid (PGA) meshes and foams with controlled concentrations of sub 5-micron particles of 45S5 Bioglass®[19-21]. An optimal concentration of bioactive particles was established by using a rat fibroblast model with monitoring of cell proliferation and production of vascular endothelial growth factor (VEGF) [22-23]. Samples of the bioactive, resorbable composite mesh were implanted subcutaneously in adult rats. The composite meshes were infiltrated by fibroblasts and blood vessels. There were significantly greater numbers of blood vessels at 28 and 42 days post implantation within the composite meshes compared with control PGA polymer meshes without the bioactive phase[23]. The results indicate that the increased neo-vascularization occurring with meshes coated with 45S5 Bioglass® particles may be due to the bioactive phase stimulating release of VEGF, a highly pro-angiogenic factor that acts solely on endothelial cells[24].

IMPLICATIONS FOR THE FUTURE

We now know that bioactive glasses can be used to activate genes. Control of genes by ceramics offers a vision for the role of ceramics in the age of biology. A cellular and molecular basis for development of third-generation biomaterials provides the scientific foundation for molecular design of scaffolds for tissue engineering and for *in situ* tissue regeneration and repair, with minimally invasive surgery. The economic advantages of these new approaches may aid in solving the problems of caring for an ageing population. It should be feasible to design a new generation of gene-activating biomaterials tailored for genetic activation of specific patients and disease states. Tissue-engineered constructs based on a patient's own cells may be produced. Bioactive stimuli may be used to activate genes in a preventive treatment to maintain the health of tissues as they age. Only a few years ago this concept would have seemed unimaginable. But we need to remember that only 34 years ago the concept of a material that would not be rejected by living tissues also seemed unimaginable. Biology evolved from an inanimate, inorganic world. Our goal should be to use the science of ceramics to maintain harmony between the physical and biological worlds.

Acknowledgements

The author acknowledges the U.K. Engineering and Physics Research Council, the Medical Research Council.

REFERENCES

[1]L.L. Hench, *Science, Faith & Ethics*, Imperial College Press and World Scientific, London and Singapore, 2001.

[2]L. L. Hench, *Science* **208**, 826 (1980).

[3]L.L. Hench and J. W. Wilson, *Science*, **226** 630 (1984).

[4]L. L. Hench, *J. Am. Ceram. Soc.* **81**, 1705 (1998).

[5]T. Yamamuro, L. L. Hench, J. Wilson, Eds., *CRC Handbook of Bioactive Ceramics*, Vol. 1, "Bioactive Glasses and Glass-Ceramics", Vol. 2, "Calcium Phosphate and Hydroxylapatite Ceramics" (CRC Press, Boca Raton, FL, 1990).

[6]L. L. Hench, J. Wilson, Eds., *Clinical Performance of Skeletal Prostheses* (Chapman & Hall, London, 1996), chaps. 13 and 15.

[7]L. L. Hench, R. J. Splinter, W. C. Allen, T. K. Greenlee Jr., *J. Biomed. Mater. Res.* **2**, 117 (1971).

[8]L. L. Hench and J. M. Polak, "Third-Generation Biomedical Materials", *Science* **295**:1014-1017 (2002).

[9]W. Bonfield, in *CRC Handbook of Bioactive Ceramics*, T. Yamamuro, L.L. Hench, J. Wilson, Eds., vol. 2, *Calcium Phosphate and Hydroxylapatite Ceramics* (CRC Press, Boca Raton, FL, 1990), chap. 16.

[10]G. Hastings, P. Ducheyne, *Eds. Macromolcular Biomaterials* (CRC Press, Boca Raton, FL, 1984).

[11]B. M. Wrobelewski, P. A. Fleming, P. D. Siney, *J. Bone Jt. Surg. Br.* Vol. 81, 427 (1999).

[12]F. J. Schoen, R. J. Levy, H. R. Piehler, *J. Soc. Cardiovasc. Pathol.* **1**, 29 (1992).

[13]J. Wilson and S. B. Low, *J. Appl. Biomater.* **3**, 123 (1992).

[14]D. Xynos, A. J. Edgar, L. D. K. Buttery, L. L. Hench, J. M. Polak, *J. Biomed. Mater. Res.* **55**, 151 (2001).

[15]L. D. K. Buttery, et al., *Tissue Eng.* **7**, 89 (2001).

[16]R. Bielby, R. Pryce, L. L. Hench, J. M. Polak, *Tissue Eng.* **6**, 693 (2000).

[17]P. Sepulveda, J.R. Jones and L.L. Hench, "Bioactive Sol-Gel Foams for Tissue Repair", *J. Biomed. Mater. Res.* **59** (2), 340-348 (2002).

[18]R.F. S. Lenza, J. R. Jones, W. Vasconcelos, L. L. Hench, *J. Mater Sci. Mater. Med.*, (2003) in press.

[19]J. A. Roether, A. R. Boccaccini, L. L. Hench, V. Maquet, S. Gautier, R. Jérôme, "Development and in-vitro characterisation of novel bioresorbable and bioactive composite materials based on polylactide foams and Bioglass® for tissue engineering applications", *Biomaterials* **23**, 3871-3878 (2002).

[20]R. Boccaccini, J. A. Roether, L. L. Hench, V. Maquet, R. Jérôme, "A Composites Approach to Tissue Engineering", *Ceram. Eng. Sci. Proc.* **23**, 805-816 (2002).

[21]A. G. Stamboulis, A. R. Boccaccini, L. L. Hench, "Novel Biodegradable Polymer/Bioactive Glass Composites for Tissue Engineering Applications", *Adv. Eng. Mat.* **4**, 105-109 (2002).

[22]R. Day, A. R. Boccaccini, J.A. Roether, S. Surey, A. Forbes, L. L. Hench, S. Gabe, "The effect of Bioglass® on epithelial cell and fibroblast proliferation and incorporation into a PGA matrix", *Gastroenterology* **122** (4): Suppl. 1, T875 (2002).

[23]R. Day, S. Surey, A. R. Boccaccini, J. A. Roether, A. Forbes, L. L. Hench, S. Gabe, "Assessment of polyglycolic acid mesh and bioactive glass for soft tissue engineering scaffolds", *Biomaterials 2002*: submitted.

[24]P. J. Polverini, "The Pathophysiology of Angiogenesis", *Crit Rev Oral Biol Med.* **6**, 230-247 (1995).

A REVIEW OF BONE SUBSTITUTES IN BONE REMODELING: INFLUENCE OF MATERIALS CHEMISTRY AND POROSITY

A. Cuneyt Tas
Turkish Academy of Sciences, Ataturk Bulvari No. 221, 06100 Ankara, Turkey

Abstract. Given the bone tissue's superb ability to adapt its mass and morphology to *in vivo* functional necessities, its aptitude to repair itself without leaving a scar, and its capacity to rapidly mobilize mineral supplies on metabolic demand, it is in fact the ultimate "smart" material in biological systems.

Scientific efforts which may eventually lead to the synthesis of materials that mimic the *natural bones* have started about four decades ago [1, 2], and it should be open-heartedly confessed now that the calcium phosphate-based synthetic bone substitute materials are still too far away from taking over the *golden standard* status of autologous bone chips/grafts which are harvested from the patient, in real time, during the surgery together with the bone marrow and living cells. The current paper tries to concisely bring together what perspectives are needed to develop new synthetic bone substitute materials exhibiting higher levels of participation in the bone remodeling process.

Requirements. Considering the ever-growing number of patients who suffer from devastating disorders of the skeleton, it becomes more critical for the material scientists to be able to design bone substitutes, which can:

1) readily take part in bone remodeling (i.e., *osteoconduction*: the direct anchorage of an implant by bony tissue surrounding it, without the onset and growth of fibrous tissue at the bone-implant interface),
2) itself cause the formation of bone tissues (i.e., *osteoinduction*), even if it is not in interfacial contact with natural bones,
3) maintain their mechanical strength even during the intermediate stages (3-4 months) of cellular (i.e., osteoclasts) or active resorption, and
4) be gradually but fully replaced, within the 48 to 52 weeks following the surgery, by new bone (i.e., *osseointegration* via osteoblastic activity) at the implantation site.

Unfortunately, until now, there are no synthetic biomaterials which simultaneously satisfy all of the above criteria required by the clinicians.

Bone Mineral. Bone mineral has commonly been referred to the perfectly stoichiometric compound *calcium hydroxyapatite* [$Ca_{10}(PO_4)_6(OH)_2$], but this can be a dangerously misleading oversimplification of this "smart material." Actually, it is a rather defective and complex substance (whose Ca sites were simultaneously doped (to a total percentage of about 1.5%) by several mono- or divalent cations (Na, K, Mg, Zn, Fe, Sr, Pb, Ba, Cu, etc.) and the hydroxyl and phosphate groups being doped with carbonate ions of around 5% by weight) with a generic formula of $Ca_{8.3}(PO_4)_{4.3}(HPO_4, CO_3)_{1.7}(OH, CO_3)_{0.3}$ [3-5]. The determination of the influence of collagen (and the organic molecules it supplies) on the formation (and dissolution and reprecipitation) of nanocrystals of bone mineral must be regarded as a task of colossal importance still needing the joint efforts of clinicians and the materials specialists. To summarize, bone mineral is not simply a hydroxyapatite ceramic, and it should be named as *biological, calcium-deficient carbonate apatite.*

Bone Remodeling. Bones contain three distinct types of cells: the matrix-forming *osteoblast*, the tissue-resorbing *osteoclast*, and the *osteocyte* [6]. Osteoblasts are the cells present in bones which actually build the extracellular matrix and regulate its mineralization. The lifespan of an osteoblast ranges up to 8 weeks in humans, during which time it lays down 0.5 to 1.5 µm osteoid per day [6, 7]. Cells named as osteoclasts, on the other hand, are able to resorb fully mineralized bone as they are equipped with a variety of enzymes which lower the local pH to values between 3 and 4 (i.e., cell-mediated acidification). Osteocytes are the principal (they account for about 90% of all cells in the adult skeleton) cells present in adult bones, and their special construction may actually orchestrate the spatial and temporal recruitment of the cells that form and resorb bone. Modeling is the processes whereby bone is laid down onto available surfaces, and in the case of *remodeling*, osteoclastic resorption of bone leaves pockets that are then filled by osteoblast activity [6]. When the bones no longer have any osteoblasts or osteoclasts, all the modeling/remodeling processes would cease.

Bone Substitutes. Calcium phosphate-based bone substitute materials should ideally be implanted with the design consideration that the osteoclastic resorption will be able to slowly and gradually degrade the implanted material, and in such pockets or crevices created by the osteclasts, new bone will simultaneously be deposited by the osteoblasts [6]. If a material is not resorbed by the osteoclasts (such as, crystalline alumina (mostly used as caps on metallic implants used for hip arthroplasty) or zirconia), then such bioinert materials may not be used as a successful bone substitute bioceramic, which can take part in bone turnover. On the other hand, if an implant material is rapidly eroded away in physiological fluids (such as, $CaSO_4 \cdot ½H_2O$ or $Ca_4(PO_4)_2O$) by passive dissolution, then it also can not help much in the bone remodeling processes, due to the lack of that precise interaction and crosstalk which must be present between the *resorbing* osteoclasts and *depositing* osteoblasts. Such a crosstalk is strictly essential for the successful replacement of the synthetic material by natural bone at the defect site.

Resorbability. It is known that perfectly stoichiometric (Ca/P=1.67), sintered synthetic hydroxyapatite ceramics do not actively participate in bone remodeling, but they can only display *osteoconductive* behavior [8]. In other words, bone can grow in apposition or in close contact with the hydroxyapatite implant interfaces, but hydroxyapatite ceramics can not be fully resorbed *in vivo* by the osteoclasts even after five years. On the other hand, in the course of natural biomineralization/calcification processes, the bone mineral forms (within a continuum of precipitation-dissolution sequences) petal- or needle-like calcium-deficient hydroxyapatite crystals 100-150 nm in length and 10-20 nm thick (Fig. 1), and since these are less perfect (as compared to stoichiometric apatite) in chemical and crystallographic structure, and since they are more reactive and soluble; these non-stoichiometric apatitic calcium phosphate nanocrystals facilitate chemical turnover or bone remodeling. Proteins and other organic macromolecules present in collagen of the bone tissues govern the dissolution/precipitation mechanisms for these nanocrystals.

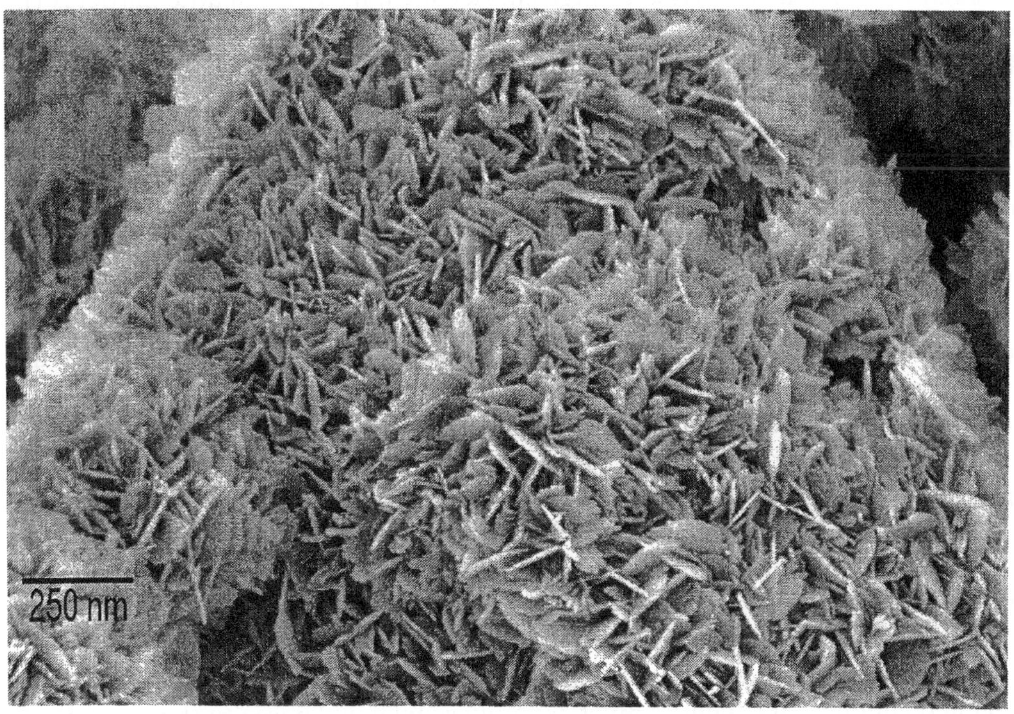

Fig.1 Calcium-deficient hydroxyapatite nanoplates grown on a calcium phosphate ceramic (with a Ca/P ratio of 1.30) immersed in synthetic body fluid

Active resorption of the bioceramic implant, by the osteoclastic action, is a crucial starting condition if the *in vivo* biological participation of the material in bone remodeling is desired. Therefore, any biomaterial left (without being resorbed) in the human body must be considered as a potential focus for infection or further clinical complications [9], especially if it is known to be a bioinert material (such as, bioinert ceramics or PMMA-polymers).

Material Form. Another important question which needs to be addressed in the design of calcium phosphate-based biomaterials is the form of the implant material. Nowadays, commercially available bioceramics (including the bioglasses) do typically come to the perusal of the clinician in the form of powders, granules, porous blocks (as either fully synthetic or of bovine-origin), pre-coated metallic implants or injectables. Powders may not find much of a widespread use in clinical practice, mainly because of the fact that defects which need to be filled are constantly wetted by blood, and the powders (especially if they are nanosize or submicron-particulated) to be applied to such a dynamic defect site would easily migrate and get washed away within a short time, and thus they would not function well. Injectable apatitic putties [10], which do not harden *in vivo*, do have the ability to readily penetrate the macropores of trabecular bones, and comprised of high surface area, nanosize apatite particles (in water) as a viscous paste, categorically fall in between the loose powders and hard calcium phosphates in terms of their applied forms. Such putties would, of course, have no applicability in load-bearing defect sites. Pre-shaped prismatic blocks, which are designed for use in load-bearing areas [11], do also have certain limitations, and they may require a certain extent of "machining/sizing-by-the-surgeon" on the operation table to fit those into the actual defects. However, granules within the size range of 1 to 5 mm, which can be *on site* impregnated with bone marrow cells harvested from the patient and packed into a gelated porous compact with the help of blood clotting, or granules which have previously been impregnated with certain antibiotics or growth factors (depending on the clinical application), can remedy some of the geometrical limitations associated with the use of dense or porous blocks. Injectable calcium phosphates (either in the form of a putty or self-setting cement), by quickly reaching quite high compressive strength values ($\geq$ 55 MPa) upon hardening *in vivo*, obviously present an attractive alternative [12-15] to the above-mentioned preshaped bone substitutes. On the other hand, the main concern for the injectable self-hardening cements still remains as their lack of macroporosity.

Porosity. For the osteoclasts to simultaneously attack even the bulk of the implanted ceramic, the material must have *interconnected* porosity (between 55 to 70%), and the pore sizes must be over the range of 150 to 700 μm [16], just like the natural bones. The presence of such a high porosity in the bone substitute materials facilitates the complete (i.e,, both bulk and the surface) invasion of the implant by the osteoclasts and osteoblasts from the very beginning, leading to *osseointegration* and further *vascularization*. If the material does not have the stated porosity, osteoclasts can only degrade the external surface of the implant, and this initial surface attack lasts for a relatively short period of time and then it may totally stop, if the osteoblasts regard the material as a foreign body. By using the ceramic manufacturing technology it is not difficult at all to produce calcium phosphate-based bone subsitute materials as shown in Fig. 2 below. Ca/P molar ratio (over the range of 1.05 to 1.67), phase assemblage, as well as the percentages of the monovalent or divalent dopant elements (as mentioned previously), can again be easily adjusted or tailored in such porous bioceramics to control the *in vivo* response (cytotoxicity, resorption rate, the rate of bone ingrowth, mechanical strength following the first few weeks of implantation, etc.) to these implants.

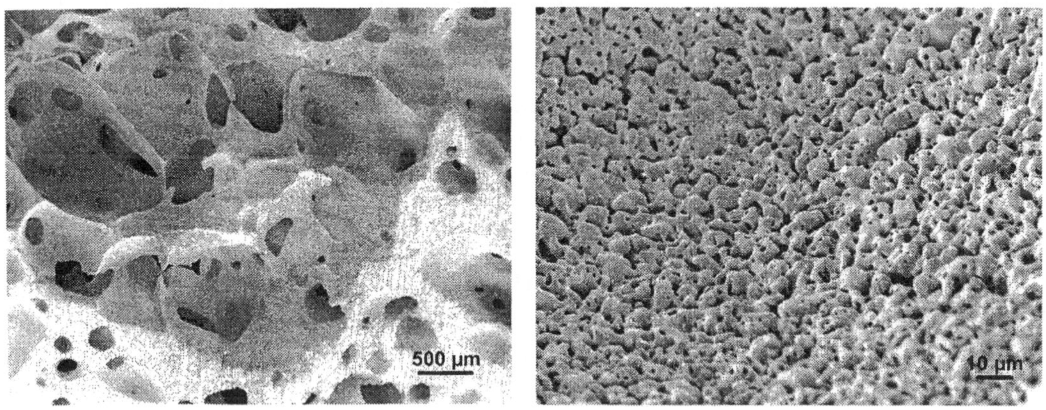

Fig. 2 Porous calcium phosphate scaffold material (Ca/P=1.45), after calcination at 1000°C; 35±2 MPa compressive strength: (*left*) interconnected macropores, (*right*) magnified view of the same sample, which thus reveals the microporous nature of those dense-looking struts/walls

Material Chemistry. However, physical factors like porosity and material form alone are not enough to allow a bone substitute implant to show the ability of full resorbability and participating in bone remodeling. A good example to this situation can be seen in the case of commercially available porous blocks or granules, which were manufactured from the trabecular bones of animal (bovine) origin [17, 18]. These materials are able to perfectly retain the magnificent porosity present in bovine bones, but since they are sintered at temperatures above 1200°C (to safely burn out the organic residues), they simply lose the material chemistry aspects of the original bones, and they convert into well-crystallized calcium hydroxyapatite, contaminated with only trace amounts of phases like CaO, $Ca_3(PO_4)_2$, and $Ca_4(PO_4)_2O$. Since the material after sintering is the *ceramic* and crystalline phase of hydroxyapatite with a Ca/P ratio slightly greater than 1.67, these samples were shown to be non-resorbable even after several years of implantation. With these kinds of blocks used in defect-filling applications, it was seen that the bone ingrowth is perfect but the implant stayed as an almost inert material. Moreover, a ceramic bone substitute which sits in the bone for long years without being absorbed, could be a potential spot for the development of an inflammatory response. On the other hand, when the same porous bovine hydroxyapatite ceramic blocks were first blended with human bone marrow cells and then implanted *in vivo*, it was observed that the material showed positive and strong signs of participating in *osteogenesis* and remodeling processes [19].

As a different facet of the impact of material chemistry on the *in vivo* behavior of a calcium phosphate-based bone substitute, the surface chemistry of the implanted material becomes of extreme importance. In case of bone substitute materials with an acidic pH value at their interface they would form with the natural bone (for instance, when α–TCP powders are mixed with citric acid to form a cement for implantation [20]), the fibrous tissue formation and the onset of foreign body reactions are well-known. In contrast, in case of using implants with excessively alkaline surfaces, cell necrosis [21] may be the initial undesired *in vivo* response. Cytotoxicity of the bone substitute candidate materials must be carefully addressed and evaluated before their clinical use.

A delicate control to be achieved in the surface chemistry (for instance by the use of an acid phosphatase [22]) of the calcium phosphate-based bone substitute implants may in turn be used to adjust and monitor the extent of crosstalk between the osteoclasts and osteoblasts. As described by Lee, *et al.* [22], "the acid phosphatase coatings on porous hydroxyapatite bone substitutes serves to attract osteoclast progenitor cells from the bone marrow or bloodstream to the surface of the prosthetic device. The recruited osteoclast population then etches the bone mineral or hydroxyapatite surface of the implant and thereby provides the natural signals to recruit osteoblasts to lay down new bone that will abut and integrate with the graft or prosthetic surface mimicking the natural process of bone deposition on an osteoclast resorbed bone surface [22]. The acid phosphatase-induced stimulation of osteoclast recruitment results in osteointegration and enhanced bonding of the graft or prosthesis to the patient's bone. This, as claimed by Lee, *et al.*, reduces recovery time from the operation and lengthens the life of implants by reducing their tendency to loosen over several years [22]."

Challenges. The bone mineral which embrace about 70 wt% [23] of human bones

(1) is not a crystalline, simply stoichiometric ceramic,
(2) is a complex and rather defective material,
(3) is not soluble in physiological fluids, but can only be degraded, when necessary, by the osteoclastic environment,
(4) contains trace elements in differing but small percentages,
(5) resembles to *hydroxyapatite*, but both the A- and B-sites of the bone mineral are partially doped with carbonate ions,

(6) has its Ca-sites minimally doped with the above-mentioned cations,
(7) has a unique crystal structure [24] which places the hydroxyl and carbonate ions on its cell edges for easier chemical interaction with the surrounding cells and tissues, and
(8) the unit cell parameters of human bone mineral, as well as its overall Ca/P atomic ratio, display fluctuations as a function of bone maturation [25-27].

Predictions and Speculations. Hydroxyapatite-like bioceramics designed to mimic the bone mineral and intended for use in *in vivo* implantations should not possess steps of *heating/firing/calcination* at or above 650°C in any phase of their processing, manufacturing and shaping operations. The reason for this is clear that at or above 650°C carbonate ions which may be present in the apatitic structure are opt to readily leave the material [28]. The same also applies to the case of HPO_4^{2-} ions present in the bone mineral, and the materials chemist must face this challenge in preparing bioceramics which should resemble *the bone mineral* to the most possible extent. Sophisticated chemical techniques which involve the loading of several proteins, organic molecules, biopolymers or inorganic salts into the aqueous media of the synthesis reactors would become increasingly important in the manufacture of *next-generation macroporous* bioceramics. The total weight percentage of Na, K, and Mg, which altogether amount to a value greater than 1.25 wt% in the bone mineral, must be considered in preparing synthetic bioceramic bone substitute materials [4, 29]. Low-temperature (<100°C) chemical processing of Ca, Na, K, Mg and Sr phosphates and carbonates, to be selected from a tentative list of chemicals, such as α- or β-$Ca_3(PO_4)_2$, $Ca_4(PO_4)_2O$, $Ca_8(PO_4)_4(HPO_4)_2{\cdot}5H_2O$, $Ca_2P_2O_7$, $CaHPO_4$, $CaHPO_4{\cdot}2H_2O$, $Ca(H_2PO_4)_2{\cdot}H_2O$, $MgHPO_4{\cdot}3H_2O$, $Na_4P_2O_7$, Na_2HPO_4, NaH_2PO_4, KH_2PO_4, K_2HPO_4, $NaHCO_3$, Na_2CO_3, $CaCO_3$, $SrCO_3$, K_2CO_3, and to be later processed in synthetic body fluids [28], which contain trace amounts of Zn, Sr, Fe, and Cu ions [30], might yield bioceramics of higher resemblance to the bone mineral. Ca/P atomic ratio in the ideal synthetic bioceramic, as a tool of controlling resorbability, must be easily adjustable within the range of 1.05 to 1.67 by controlling the synthesis parameters. If the bioceramic undergoes *in vivo* osteoclastic resorption and osteoblastic deposition without a difficulty [31], then the Ca- and P-rich environment needed for *in situ* bone formation (i.e., *osteoinduction*) would have been provided even in cases of intramuscular implantation.

Summary. Stoichiometric calcium hydroxyapatite ceramic, especially if it is heated, prior to its clinical use, at elevated temperatures, does not take part in the bone remodeling process. Calcium-deficient hydroxyapatite (with a Ca/P ratio ranging from 1.3 to 1.6) doped with alkali and alkali-earth elements, such as Na, K, and Mg, resorb much faster and allow the natural bone to proceed with its remodeling process. Porosity (i.e., highly interconnected macropores) in bone substitute implant materials should be regarded as the bare necessity.

References

[1] W. Neumann and M. Neumann, *The Chemical Dynamics of Bone Mineral*, p. 34, University of Chicago Press, Chicago, 1958.

[2] E. Hayek and H. Newesely, "Pentacalciummonohydroxyorthophosphate," *Inorganic Syntheses*, 7, 63 (1963).

[3] L.L. Hench, "Bioceramics: From Concept to Clinic,"*J. Am. Ceram. Soc.*, **74**, 1487-1510 (1991).

[4] R.Z. LeGeros and J.P. LeGeros, "Dense Hydroxyapatite"; pp. 139-180 in *An Introduction to Bioceramics*. Edited by L.L. Hench and J. Wilson. World Scientific Publishing, Singapore 1993.

[5] D.D. Lee, C. Rey, M. Aiolova, and A. Tofighi, "Methods and Products Related to the Physical Conversion of Reactive Amorphous Calcium Phosphate," U.S. Pat. No. 6 117 456, Sep. 12, 2000.

[6] R. Gunzburg, M. Szpalski, N. Passuti and M. Aebi, *The Use of Bone Substitutes in Spine Surgery*, pp. 2-11, Springer-Verlag, Berlin, 2002.

[7] G. Bourne, *The Biochemistry and Physiology of Bone*, Academic Press, New York, 1972.

[8] F. Korkusuz, K. Karamete, B. Irfanoglu, H. Yetkin, G. W. Hastings, and N. Akkas, "Do Porous Calcium Hydroxyapatite Ceramics Cause Porosis in Bone? A Bone Densitometry and Biomechanical Study on Cortical Bones of Rabbits," *Biomaterials*, .**16**, 537-543 (1995).

[9] A.G. Gristina, "Biomaterial-centered Infection: Microbial Adhesion versus Tissue Integration," *Science*, **237**, 1588-1595 (1987).

[10] Ostim® Paste, Osartis GmbH & Co. KG, Obernburg, Germany (http://www.osartis.de/start.htm)

[11] P. Frayssinet, J.L. Trouillet, N. Rouquet, E. Azimus, and A. Autefage, "Osseointegration of Macroporous Calcium Phosphate Ceramics Having a Different Chemical Composition," *Biomaterials*, **14**, 423-429 (1993).

[12] K. Kurashina, H. Kurita, M. Hirano, A. Kotani, C.P.A.T. Klein, and K. de Groot, "In Vivo Study of Calcium Phosphate Cements: Implantation of an α-Tricalcium Phosphate/Dicalcium Phosphate Dibasic/Tetracalcium Phosphate Monoxide Cement Paste," *Biomaterials*, **18**, 539-543 (1997).

[13] B.R. Constantz, B.M. Barr, I.C. Ison, M.T. Fulmer, D.C. Delaney, J. Ross, and R.D. Poser, "Histological, Chemical and Crystallographic Analysis of Four Calcium Phosphate Cements in Different Rabbit Osseous Sites," *J. Biomed. Mater. Res (Appl. Biomater.)*, **43**, 451-461 (1998).

[14] D. Knaack, M.E.P. Goad, M. Aiolova, C. Rey, A. Tofighi, P. Chakravarthy, and D.D. Lee, "Resorbable Calcium Phosphate Bone Substitute," *J. Biomed. Mater. Res.(Appl. Biomater.)*,**43**, 399-409 (1998).

[15] E.M. Ooms, J.G.C. Wolke, J.P.C.M. van der Waerden, and J.A. Jansen, "Trabecular Bone Response to Injectable Calcium Phosphate (Ca-P) Cement," *J. Biomed. Mater. Res.*, **61**, 9-18 (2002).

[16] M. Milosevski, J. Bossert, D. Milosevski, and N. Gruevska, "Preparation and Properties of Dense and Porous Calcium Phosphate," *Ceram. Int.*, **25**, 693-696 (1999).

[17] S. Joschek, B. Nies, R. Krotz, A. Gopferich, "Chemical and Physicochemical Characterization of Porous Hydroxyapatite Ceramics Made of Natural Bone," *Biomaterials*, **21**, 1645-1658 (2000).

[18] F.H. Lin, C.J. Liao, K.S. Chen, and J.S. Sun, "Preparation of a Biphasic Porous Bioceramic by Heating Bovine Cancellous Bone with $Na_4P_2O_7 \cdot 10H_2O$ Addition," *Biomaterials*, **20**, 475-484 (1999).

[19] R. Bareille, M.H. Lafage-Proust, C. Faucheux, N. Laroche, R. Wenz, M. Dard, and J. Amedee, "Various Evaluation Techniques of Newly Formed Bone in Porous Hydroxyapatite Loaded with Human Bone Marrow Cells Implanted in na Extra-Osseous Site," *Biomaterials*, **21**, 1345-1352 (2000).

[20] S. Minagawa, A. Uchida, M. Takei, and S. Ishiyama, "Biocompatibility of α–TCP Cement," *Orthop. Ceram. Implants*, **7**, 199-202 (1987)

[21] A. Lebugle, A. Rodrigues, P. Bonnevialle, J.J. Voigt, P. Canal, and F. Rodriguez, "Study of Implantable Calcium Phosphate Systems for the Slow Release of Methotrexate," *Biomaterials*, **23**, 3517-3522 (2002).

[22] M.Y. Lee, D.R. Eyre, and M.A.E. Weis, "Compositions for Medical Implantation," U.S. Pat. No. 6 508 838, Jan. 21, 2003.

[23] P. Ducheyne, "Bioceramics: Material Characteristics versus In Vivo Behavior," *J. Biomed. Mater. Res:. Appl. Biomater.*, **21**, 219-236 (1987).

[24] T.I. Ivanova, O.V. Frank-Kamenetskaya, A.B. Koltsov, and V.L. Ugolkov, "Crystal Structure of Calcium-Deficient Carbonated Hydroxyapatite," *J. Solid State. Chem.*, **160**, 340-349 (2001).

[25] J.M. Burnell, E.J. Teubner, and A.G. Miller, "Normal Maturational Changes in Bone Matrix, Mineral and Crystal Size in the Rat," *Calcified Tissue Int.*, **31**, 13-19 (1980).

[26] A.C. Oyedepo and D.L. Henshaw, "Calcification of the Lumbar Vertebrae During Human Fetal Development," *Calcified Tissue Int.*, **61**, 179-182 (1997).

[27] M.C. Dalconi, C. Meneghini, S. Nuzzo, R. Wenk, and S. Mobilio, "Structure of Bioapatite in Human Foetal Bones," *Nucl. Instrum. Meth. B.*, **200**, 406-410 (2003).

[28] A.C. Tas, "Synthesis of Biomimetic Ca-Hydroxyapatite Powders at 37°C in Synthetic Body Fluids," *Biomaterials*, **21**, 1429-1438 (2000).

[29] F.C.M. Driessens, M.G. Boltong, E.A.P. de Maeyer, R. Wenz, B. Nies, and J.A. Planell, "The Ca/P Range of Nanoapatitic Calcium Phosphate Cements," *Biomaterials*, **23**, 4011-4017 (2002).

[30] A.C. Tas, "Combustion Synthesis of Calcium Phosphate Bioceramic Powders," *J. Eur. Ceram. Soc.*, **20**, 2389-2394 (2000).

[31] K. Kurashina, H. Kurita, Q. Wu, A. Ohtsuka, and H. Kobayashi, "Ectopic Osteogenesis with Biphasic Ceramics of Hydroxyapatite and Tricalcium Phosphate in Rabbits," *Biomaterials*, **23**, 407-412 (2002).

MANUFACTURING OF THERMALLY SPRAYED TRICALCIUM PHOSPHATE (TCP) COATINGS FOR BIOMEDICAL APPLICATIONS

M. Baccalaro, R.Gadow and K. von Niessen
Institute for Manufacturing Technologies of Ceramic Components and Composites, University of Stuttgart,
Allmandring 7b, D-70569, Germany

ABSTRACT

Resorbable calcium phosphates for biomedical applications play an important role in a growing number of surgical disciplines. In contrast to bioactive materials like hydroxyapatite (HAP), which are intended to remain stable and chemically unchanged as long as possible in the human body, resorbable bioceramics are applied to dissolve gradually in body environment and new bone will replace the absorbed material. Tricalcium phosphate (TCP) appears to be the most suitable bioceramic of this type. It is known in its two polymorphs, the high temperature α-TCP and the more stable β-TCP phase. A promising application of these bioceramics is the coating of bioinert metal alloys, bioresorbable polymeric substrates or composite structures made thereof. The use of a TCP coating for a structural composite implant makes it possible to realize surfaces which dissolve gradually in the body and lead to bone formation. The spray-granulation technique was applied to produce new β-TCP powders suitable for Atmospheric Plasma Spraying (APS) with different grain size and grain size distributions. The powders were sprayed onto commercially available titan rods and onto aramide fabrics, in order to investigate the possibility to apply these bioceramics coating also to thermally sensitive substrates. The phase change from β to α and therefore the presence and amount of β-phase in the coatings after plasma spraying is strongly influenced by the powder mean grain size and by the heat content of the plasma during plasma spray deposition. XRD qualitative and quantitative analysis revealed that the obtained coatings are made of pure α-TCP, mixtures of α– and β– phase and, after a post heat treatment, pure β-TCP. The porosity of the coatings was determined by electronic image processing.

INTRODUCTION

In the last years there is an increasing interest in ceramics consisting of physiological minerals, among these calcium phosphates, has been increasing and many efforts have been made to develop clinical applications. Among the large number of calcium phosphates which have been studied, HAP [$Ca_{10}(PO_4)_6(OH)_2$] and TCP [$Ca_3(PO_4)_2$] are considered the most promising for this kind of applications. In particular HAP is well known for being a bioactive ceramic material which remains stable in the physiological environment and is able to create an interfacial bond with the surrounding tissue, reproducing the type of interface that is formed when natural tissues repair themselves. On the other hand TCP is a resorbable ceramic material, degrading gradually with time when surrounded by the physiological environment of the human body. The resorbed material is replaced by new bone. TCP is known in two polymorphs, α and β phase. The biodegradation of HAP and TCP has been found to be roughly related to their solubility. In previous studies [1], various solubilities of powdered calcium phosphates in aqueous environment were investigated, and the results showed an increasing solubility from HAP to α-TCP (HAP$\ll$ β-TCP $\ll$ α-TCP). Both β- and α-TCP are bioresorbable materials, but the α phase has a much higher resorption rate than the β phase and therefore it is of great importance to distinguish between the two. Due to their poor mechanical properties, it is not possible to produce massive prostheses components made of HAP or TCP. These ceramic materials are therefore applied only as bone fillers (TCP) or as coatings on light metal substrates and steel alloys (HAP). The thermal spraying of HAP is a state-of-the-art process. On the other hand, so far specific experiments to develop thermally sprayed TCP coatings on different substrates such as light metals, polymers and composites have not been yet carried out or reported.

POWDER MANUFACTURING PROCESS FOR THERMAL SPRAYING

One of the main parameters influencing the properties of the APS coating is the powder quality, particularly its grain size, grain size distribution, phase composition and morphology. The raw β- TCP powder is a commercially available powder for food industry, and due to its splintery grain morphology it is not suitable for thermal spraying. The grain size distribution is too broad and the mean grain size is too small for APS (D_{10} = 1 µm, D_{50} = 3 µm, D_{90} = 10 µm). Therefore it was necessary to prepare granulates suitable for APS by spray drying of β-TCP slurries. The powder obtained consists of spherical granules with the appropriate grain size distribution and good flowability for thermal spray processing. Four different slurries containing deionized water, surfactants and binders were produced. The elements of the mixtures and their quantities are summarized in Table I. The effect of a surfactant is to avoid untimely agglomeration of the particles, leading to higher slurry's stability (Fig. 1). The surfactant molecules have a non polar tail and a polar head which is bonded to the polar particles in the suspension. The non polar tails lead to repulsion between the particles, avoiding thereby their agglomeration.

Table I: Composition of the slurries

Powder (wt. %)	50 ÷ 65
H_2O content (wt. %)	35 ÷ 50
Surfactant type	Trusan 450
Surfactant (wt %)	0.01 ÷ 0.2
Binder	PVA 22000, PEG 2000
Binder soluted in H_2O (wt. %)	1 ÷ 1.6

Fig. 1: Effect of the surfactant in the suspension

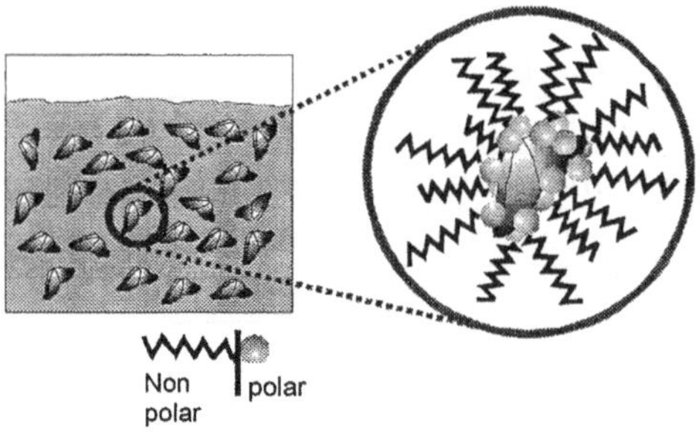

The binder ensures good mechanical stability of the granules during bagging and conveying. The binders frequently employed in spray granulation are low- to high- molecular weight polymer molecules which adsorb on the surfaces of particles in the suspension and bridge them together or form a polymer-polymer bonded network among the particles [2].

The suspensions were investigated and characterized by means of Z potential measurements to determine their stability (Fig. 2) and by means of oscillation rheometry (Fig. 3,4).

Fig.2: Zeta potential of a β-TCP slurry

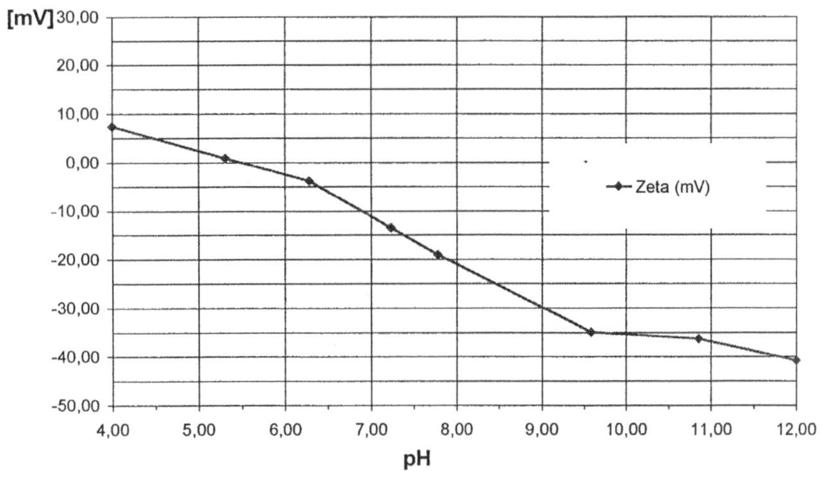

The particles in the suspension possess a pH value dependent charge, which may be indicated as Z potential. Applying an electric field to the slurry the particles are forced to move and therefore is it possible to determine their surface's charge [3]. By means of this measure the repulsion between the particles and therefore the stability of the slurry can be estimated. The stability of a suspension depending from the Z potential is classified in Table II [4].

Tab.II: Levels of stability of a suspension depending from the Z potential

Level of stability	Zeta potential (mV)
Good stability	+60 ÷ +80
Maximum agglomeration	+3 ÷ 0
Pronounced agglomeration and sedimentation	-1 ÷ -4
Small agglomeration and sedimentation	-5 ÷ -10
Threshold for sedimentation	-11 ÷ -20
Slight agglomeration	-21 ÷ -30
No agglomeration	-31 ÷ -40
Good stability	-41 ÷ -60
Maximum stability	-80 ÷ -100

As the pH value of the slurry was too low (pH = 7.65) it was necessary to adjust it to a value of 9.82 by adding NH_3 in order to obtain maximum slurry stability. The rheological properties of the suspension were also investigated, since a good flowability is required to obtain a continuous and constant feeding of the spray-drying tower. Changes in the microstructure of the system produced during flow may affect the pumping proficiency in the spray-drying process. The measurements were carried out before and after the adding of the bonding agent, in order to determine its influence on the rheological properties of the suspension (Figures 3 and 4). The measurements were carried out at the IMTCCC with a viscometer (Physica Universal Dynamic Spectrometer 200).

Fig. 3: Rheological properties of a TCP suspension without bonding agent

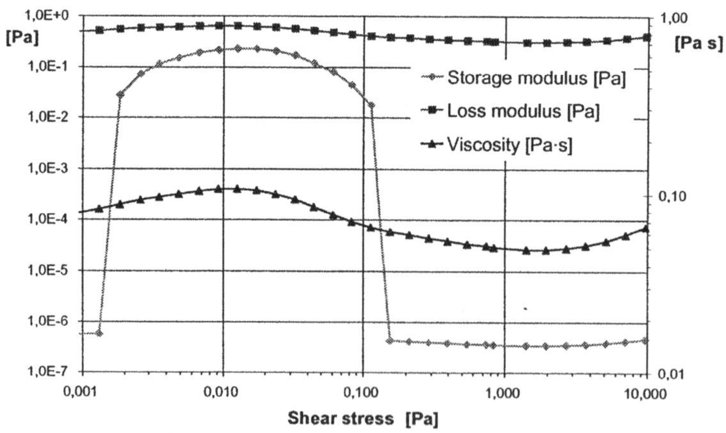

The required rheological slurry properties are low viscosity and low storage modulus. Low viscosity allow for good pumpability. Low storage modulus means that the slurry does not tend to thicken if the shear rate is increased (e.g. at the nozzle of the spray-drier). Figures 3 and 4 show a discontinuity in the storage modulus at low shear rates. The increase of the storage modulus is caused by formation of structures of particles and surfactants which are broken up at higher shear rates. Addition of the binder has caused a narrowing of the critical shear stress range. The viscosity is at a low value, ensuring good pumpability.

Fig. 4: Rheological properties of a TCP suspension with bonding agent PEG 2000

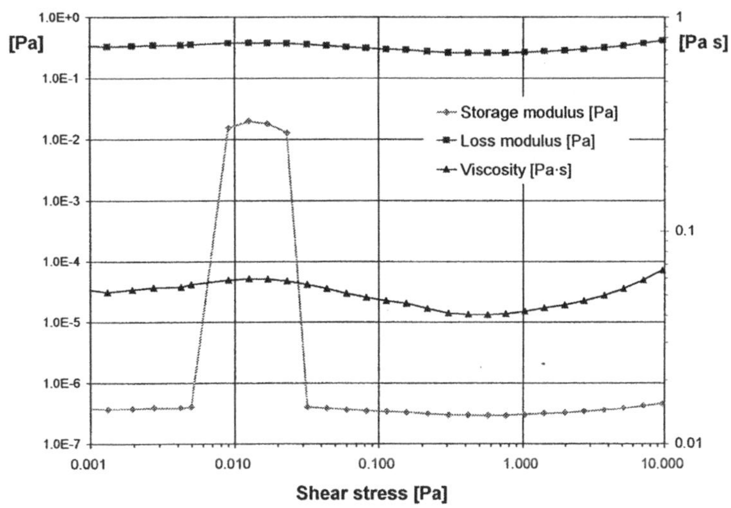

The agglomeration of the suspensions was carried out by means of a top down co-current flow spray-drying tower of the IMTCCC. It is equipped with a Laval nozzle, which uses a pressurized air jet to break up and atomize the slurry into droplets. A pump feeds the suspension into the two-fluid centrifugal atomizer at the top of the tower. The atomized slurry is dried in the stream of heated gas (air) and the moisture contained in the droplets evaporates during flight in the drying chamber. The solid particles are collected in the powder collector at the bottom of the tower. The droplet-air mixing process determines properties of the resulting powder such as the degree of moisture content in the particles, the mean grain size and the grain size distribution. By tuning the processing parameters of the tower (in particular slurry flow rate and amount of compressed air introduced through the nozzle) is it possible to control the final mean grain size of granulates.

Fig.5: P4 morphology (SEM analysis)

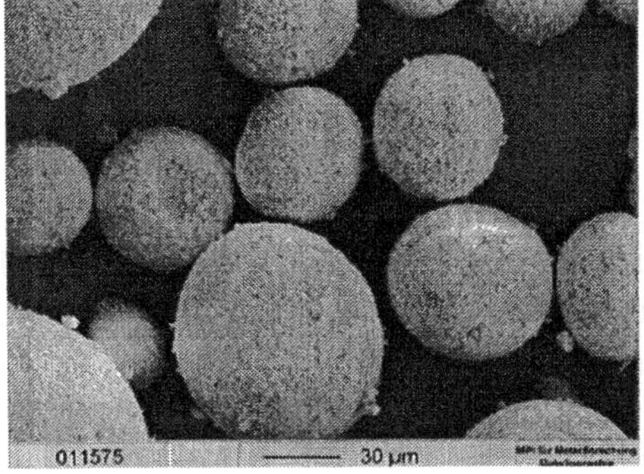

Fig.6: Particle size distribution (P4)

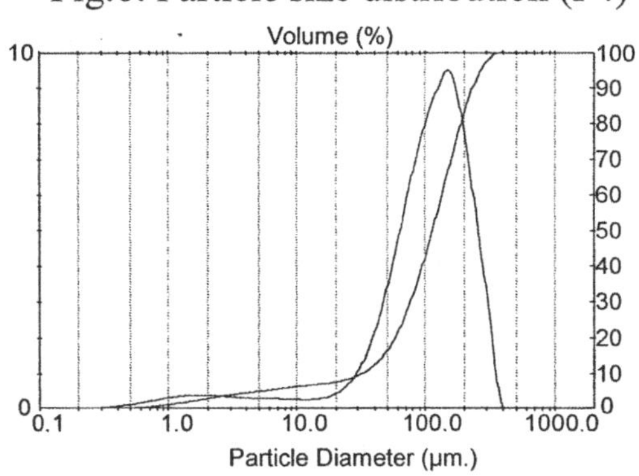

The agglomerated powders were investigated to determine their morphology, mean particle size and particle size distribution by means of SEM analyses (fig. 5) and optical measurement devices (fig. 6). The spray-dried particles present mostly a well defined round shaped morphology (fig. 5) and narrow particle size distribution (fig.6). Only P1 has a too high mean particle size and particle size distribution and therefore it was not used in the thermal spraying experiments. The particle size dimensions D_{10}, D_{50} and D_{90} of the four manufactured β-TCP powders are showed in table III.

Tab. III: Particle size dimensions of the manufactured powders

Powder	P1	P2	P3	P4
D_{10} [µm]	134	33	32	12
D_{50} [µm]	300	119	115	82
D_{90} [µm]	597	340	234	194

ATMOSPHERIC PLASMA SPRAYING (APS)

Among the various appropriate coating techniques (CVD, PVD, sol-gel, sputtering), thermal spraying is a cost effective and well established process for deposition of ceramic, metallic and composite coatings up to the mm thickness range. The principal energy source in APS is an electrical arc discharge with high frequency high voltage current. The powders are injected into the plasma and accelerated toward the substrate, where they cool down and form the coating with the typical lamellar structure [5]. A plasma torch is schematically represented in fig. 7.

Fig. 7: Sketch of a modern APS torch [6]

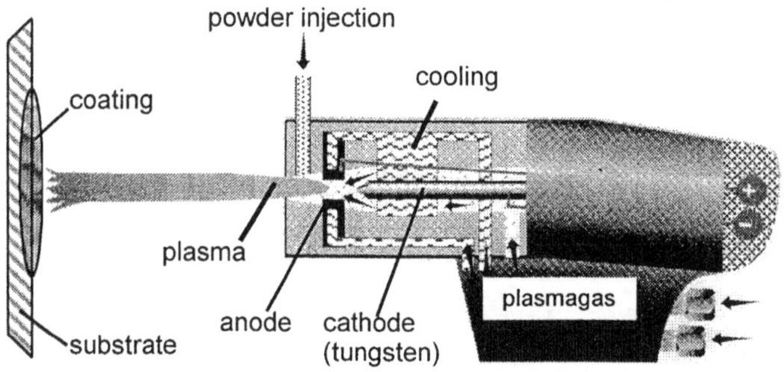

Courtesy Linde AG

An outstanding advantage of APS is the relatively low thermal load on the substrate during the coating process, so that it is possible to coat thermally sensitive substrates in an appropriate mechanical assembly with robot controlled plasma torches. Due to advanced cooling and APS parameters is it possible to control the thermal load on the substrate and it has been possible to coat temperature sensitive polymer fabrics.

EXPERIMENTAL PROCEDURES - XRD ANALYSIS OF THE COATINGS

The Ti rods were prepared by means of sand-blasting in order to achieve an adequate roughening for the mechanical adhesion of the powder particles. In APS the powder particles are completely or partially melted and accelerated against the substrate, determining this way a change in their phase composition. The following extremely quick cooling of the coating does not permit the restoring of the initial conditions.

Fig. 8: XRD of pure α-TCP coating

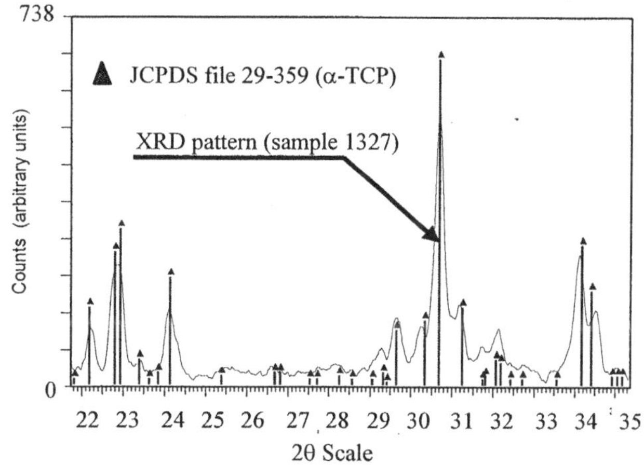

Fig. 9: XRD of thermally sprayed coating made of α/β phase mixtures

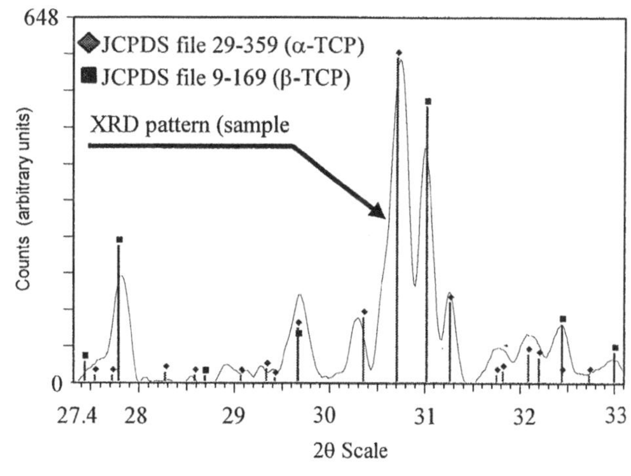

In particular regarding to TCP coatings is it of crucial importance to know whether α- or β-phase is present, or eventually a combination of the two, because of their different solubilities in the human body. Our experiments evidenced that is it possible to obtain thermally sprayed coatings made of pure α- TCP (fig. 8) but also coatings made of a mixture of the two phases (fig. 9). This is possible by means of a very accurate tuning of the processing parameters, achieving this way the melting only of the powder external surface, whereas the core is not subjected to phase transformations. In particular the heat content of the plasma plays an important role, and it can be controlled by the H_2 mass flow and by the electric arc current. The coatings phase composition is also strongly influenced by the mean grain size of the powders. Powders with a lower mean grain size (P4) were completely molten in the plasma, whereas the powders P2 and P3 were only partially fused. The β- phase content was determined considering the external standard method for quantitative XRD analyses [7]. In case of a two-phase mixture the following equation (1) permits to calculate the weight fraction w_α for the amount of α-TCP and w_β for the amount of β-TCP [8]. If the mass absorption coefficients of the two phases ($\mu_{m\alpha}$ and $\mu_{m\beta}$) are known the ratio $I_\beta/I_{\beta p}$ between the integrated intensity of the β phase main peak in the coating's XRD pattern (I_β, located at 2θ = 31.027°) and the same peak in the XRD pattern of the original powder ($I_{\beta p}$) can be calculated (fig. 10):

$$\frac{I_\beta}{I_{\beta p}} = \frac{w_\beta \cdot \mu_{m\beta}}{w_\beta \cdot \left(\mu_{m\beta} - \mu_{m\alpha}\right) + \mu_{m\alpha}}. \qquad (1)$$

Fig. 10: Main peak to be integrated for XRD quantitative analysis

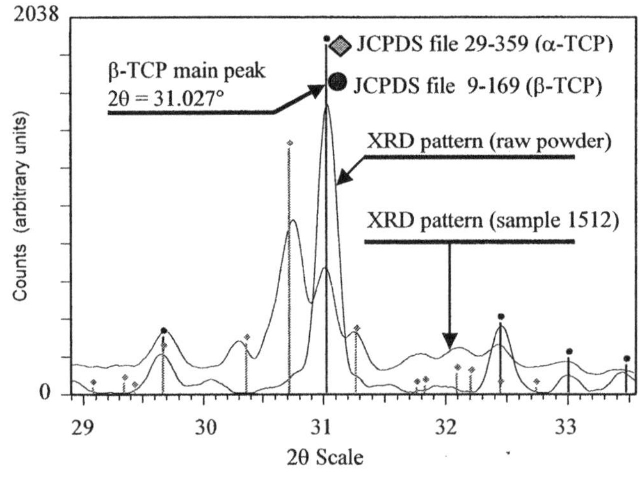

If we consider that α-TCP and β-TCP are two allotropic forms and therefore the mass absorption coefficients are equal it is possible to simplify the equation (1) in the form (2):

$$\frac{I_\beta}{I_{\beta p}} = W_\beta. \qquad (2)$$

The results of the measurements indicate a β-phase weight percentage in the coatings comprised between 11 wt. % and 26 wt. %. A heat treatment of the coatings sprayed on Ti was carried out. The results are promising concerning the desired phase formation, because after a 2 hours heat treatment at 900 °C the diffraction patterns of the samples show that the only phase in the coatings is pure β -TCP (fig. 11).

Fig. 11: Phase composition before and afterwards heat-treatment at 900 °C

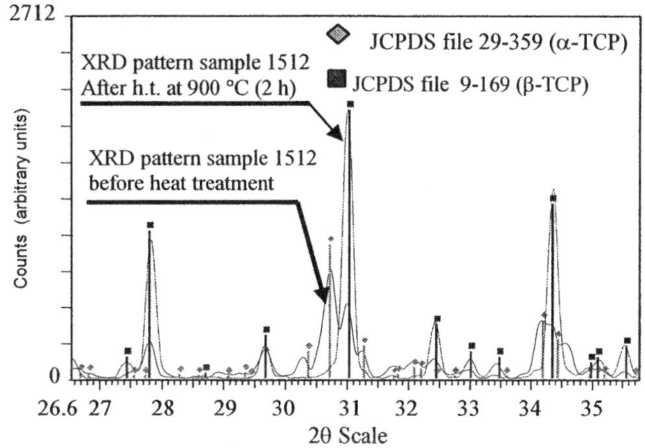

POROSITY OF THE COATINGS

In biomedical applications the porosity of the coatings is a remarkable property. A porous implant serves as a structural bridge and model or scaffold for bone formation. The measurements carried out with a light microscope (point analysis) showed very high porosity content comprised between 11% and 14% (vol.) for powder P4 and between 25% and 48% (vol.) for powders P2 and P3. The light microscope shots (figures 12, 13) evidence the presence of micro and macropores.

Fig. 12: macropores in a TCP coating

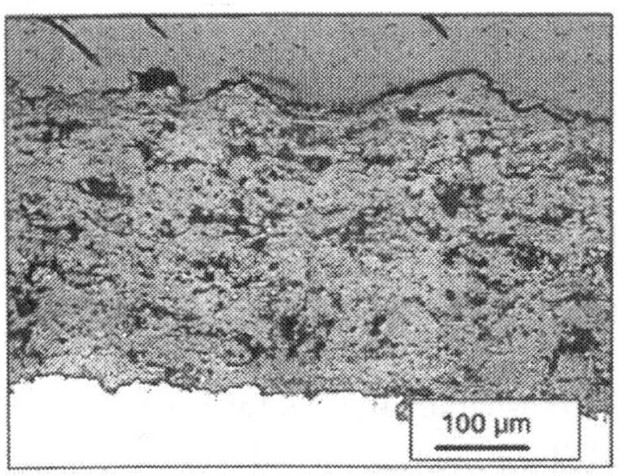

Fig. 13: micropores in a TCP coating

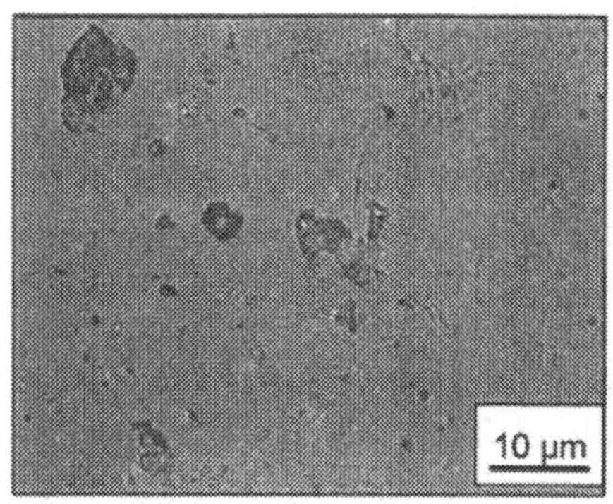

The amount of porosity in the coating is influenced by the amount of unmolten particles, i.e. from the combined effect of spraying parameters, powders grain size and grain size distribution. P4 actually is the powder with the lower mean grain size and besides it was sprayed with higher plasma heat content, in order to obtain pure α-TCP coatings. P2 and P3 have a higher mean grain size and they were sprayed with lower plasma heat content, in order to get only partially molten particles and therefore coatings made of a mixture of the two TCP phases.

SUMMARY AND CONCLUSIONS

The spray-granulation process of aqueous ceramic slurries made from commercially available β-TCP raw powders developed in this work permits the manufacturing of suitable APS spray powders. It is possible to influence the mean grain size of the final powders, and to produce spherical aggregates. The different powder types were successfully sprayed by means of the APS process onto aramide fabrics and Ti substrates. By tuning the spraying parameters and in combination with the different powder characteristics (lower/higher mean grain size) it has been possible to get coatings made of pure α-TCP and also made of α/β phase mixtures. The coatings sprayed on Ti were heat-treated at 900 °C for 2 hours in order to obtain the α to β phase transformation, and after the heat treatment they resulted to be composed of pure β-TCP. The samples were analyzed via XRD both qualitatively and quantitatively. The quantitative XRD analysis revealed that in the coatings composed of α/β phase mixtures the β phase content is between 11 and 26 %. By means of image analysis the porosity was also investigated, showing that the coatings possess a very high porosity between 11 % and 48 % (vol.) mainly influenced by the spraying parameters and the powders mean grain size.

OUTLOOK

Future work includes the optimization of the mechanical properties and the developing of combined implants made of TCP and Polylactide substrates. Polylactide is a bioresorbable polymer which is employed for instance in bone repairing as fixing element. A TCP coating should ensure a better controlled resorption of the implant itself in various medical applications.

REFERENCES

[1] LeGeros J.P., LeGeros R.Z., 1993: "Dense Hydroxylapatite", in "An Introduction to Bioceramics", Advanced Series in Ceramics – Vol. 1, Editors Hench and Wilson, World Scientific

[2] Reed J.S., 1995: "Principles of Ceramic Processing – Second Edition", John Wiley & Sons Inc.

[3] Adamson A.W., 1976: "Physical Chemistry of Surfaces", Third Edition, John Wiley & Sons

[4] Riddick T.M., 1968: "Zeta-Meter Manual", Zeta-Meter Inc., New York

[5] Pawlowski L., 1995: "The Science and Engineering of Thermal Spray Coatings", John Wiley & Sons

[6] "Das Verfahrenspektrum beim thermischen Spritzen", Linde AG, Werksgruppe technische Gase, Höffrieglskreuth (1990)

[7] Alexander L., Klug H.P., 1948: "The Basic Aspects of X-ray Absorption in Quantitative Diffraction Analysis of Powder Mixtures", Anal. Chem. 20, 886-888

[8] Cullity B.D., 1978: "Elements of X-Ray Diffraction", 2nd Ed., Addison-Wesley ed., London

ELECTROCHEMICAL DEPOSITION AND PATTERNING OF CALCIUM PHOSPHATE BIOCERAMIC COATING

Ke Duan, Yuwei Fan and Rizhi Wang
Department of Metals and Materials Engineering,
University of British Columbia,
Vancouver, BC, Canada V6T 1Z4

ABSTRACT

In this study, a method based on electrochemical deposition (ECD) has been developed to deposit either continuous or patterned calcium phosphate coatings on titanium and silicon surfaces. Deposition was performed by electrolysis in calcium and phosphate containing electrolyte with metal substrate as cathode and platnum as the anode. Deposited coating is crack free and has uniform porous structure at sub-micron level. EDX and FTIR analyses have found the coating to be calcium deficient apatite with the Ca/P ratio of 1.47. Calcium phosphate coating with different patterns were made on the metallic substrates by combining photolithography technique with ECD. The patterned bio-ceramic coatings are expected to regulate cell attachment and activity and have potential applications in biomedical implants and biosensors.

INTRODUCTION

Calcium phosphate (CaP) bio-ceramics have been known to be biocompatible and widely used as coatings on metallic prostheses [1]. Although plasma spray technique [2] has been popular for making CaP coating in the past decade, the coatings usually exhibit substantial cracking due to the high temperature nature of the technique, which seriously affects the reliability and lifetime of the implants. Plasma spraying is also difficult to produce uniform CaP coatings onto implants of complex geometries, and to control the texture of the coatings with good reliability. Recent studies [3] have revealed that surface texture had synergistic effect with surface chemistry in determining cell responses and bioceramics with nano-structures could stimulate enhanced cell functions. In addition, direct control of cell localization and the following organization into higher structures is important for the success of future bio-devices, e.g. prostheses and biosensors, and has been the objective of extensive studies. One approach of realizing the above goals is to pattern bioactive materials, e.g. peptides, proteins or bioceramics, on relevant surfaces [4, 5, 6]. This is beyond the capability of current plasma spray technique.

Electrochemical deposition (ECD) is an emerging coating technique [7]. The process involves electrochemically induced crystallization on cathode. In aqueous solution with calcium and phosphate ions, the reduction reaction at cathode in an electrolytic system causes local increase in pH that reduces the solubility of CaP minerals. As a result, CaP minerals with various morphologies deposit onto the cathode surface. With modification of solution parameters it is possible to control the coating microstructure. Since ECD is usually performed at relatively low temperatures cracking may be ameliorated. In this study, we describe an ECD protocol that produced crack-free CaP coatings with controllable nano-scale texture. By combining ECD with photolithography (a mature technique in microelectronics), we demonstrated that patterned CaP deposition could also be achieved.

MATERIALS AND METHODS

Commercially pure titanium plates (20×20×3mm) were first mechanically grinded with 800 grit sand paper and then sonicated in acetone, ethanol and distilled water each for 5 min and etched in 1% HF for 5min. Plates were sonicated again in distilled water and stored in distilled water. Electrolytes were prepared by weighing proper amount of $Ca(NO_3)_2$ and $NH_4H_2PO_4$, dissolved and mixed to make 21.6mM P and 10.8mM Ca. Solution pH was controlled to 4.7 by addition of 1N NaOH stock solution. ECD was performed by electrolysis under two-electrode mode at room temperature in the prepared electrolytes. The cleaned titanium plate was used as cathode and a platinum plate as anode, separated by 5 mm. The voltage was kept constant at 2.45V and electrolysis time ranges between 15 to 30 min.

For the patterned deposition, cleaned titanium plates were spin-coated with photoresist A1410 at 200 rpm, baked at 100 °C for 10 min and exposed through a mask under 275nm UV light. The plates were then washed with developer AZ400, rinsed with distilled water, and dried with nitrogen stream. Plates with photoresist patterns on the surface were used as cathodes in the ECD process. In some experiments, smooth silicon wafers, instead of titanium, were used for patterned deposition.

After electrolysis, plates were removed and rinsed repeatedly with distilled water and followed by rinsing with absolute ethanol and dried in air. For the patterned deposition, plates were first rinsed with acetone to remove the photoresist coating, which was followed by rinsing repeatedly in distilled water and drying in air.

Samples were characterized with optical microscope (Nikon Epiphot 300) and scanning electron microscope (SEM Hitachi 3000 for low magnification and Hitachi 4700 field emission microscope for high magnification observation). The compositions of the coatings were analyzed by energy dispersive X-ray analysis

(EDX) attached to SEM (Hitachi 3000). X-ray diffraction (XRD, Siemens D5000, Cu Kα) and Fourier transformed infrared reflective spectroscopy (FTIR microscope, Bruker Equinox 55) were used to characterize the crystal structure.

RESULTS AND DISCUSSION

Figure 1 shows the SEM results of the coating prepared by ECD. It can be seen that the coating is porous (Fig. 1a) and crystal plates about 300 nm long and less than 50 nm in thickness (Fig. 1b) form the continuous skeleton. The pores size is about 200 nm and relatively uniform. At lower magnification the porous coating perfectly followed the texture of the etched titanium surface and no cracks could be observed in the whole field (Fig. 1c). SEM study (Fig. 1d) along a scratch (tilted 24°) reveals no coating debonding indicating a coherent coating-substrate interface (white arrows in Fig. 2). The coating thickness is estimated to be about 5 μm according to the tilt angle. This value should be treated as approximate as the metal and coating were both deformed during scratching. EDX analysis (Fig. 2) indicated presence of Ti (25.2%), Ca (4.15%), P (2.83) and C (13.35%) and the Ca/P ratio is determined to be 1.47, which is higher than octacalcium phosphate (1.33: $Ca_8(HPO_4)_2(PO_4)_4.5H_2O$) and close to calcium deficient apatite (1.5: $Ca_9(HPO_4)(PO_4)_5(OH)$). The high carbon content may be related to that fact that EDX quantification is less accurate for light elements. It may also be related to contamination from chemical (e.g. ethanol) residue in the coating process.

The EDX results were further supported by the structural information obtained from FTIR. The split bands at 1020, 1108 cm^{-1} (Fig. 3) correspond to the antisymmetric stretch of phosphate group and the weak band at 872 cm^{-1} corresponds to P-OH stretch. However, the bands characteristic of OCP [8] at 917 and 1295 cm^{-1} were not observed. Above 3000 cm^{-1}, a diffused peak associated with adsorbed water or ethanol was observed and the peak characteristic of apatite was not detected (not shown herein). In general, the FTIR spectrum resembles the electrochemically deposited apatite reported by Rößler [9] *et al.* Current results suggest that the coating may be calcium deficient apatite. However, XRD gave no distinct peaks between 3° and 55° besides the signal from the substrate. This may be the result of the limited amount of the minerals and the limitation of the XRD machine used. Thin film XRD is needed for further characterization of the coating crystal structure.

Besides the continuous crack-free coating, CaP minerals can also be formed into patterns on a substrate by combining ECD with photolithography. Figure 4 shows combined optical microscopy and EDX element mapping results of a deposited CaP coating with negative patterns on titanium, where arrays of circular titanium dots are surrounded by CaP coating. This is clearly confirmed by the Ti, Ca and P element mapping. Under optical microscope (Fig. 4a), the uncoated part appears bright as contrasted to the dark coating. This is because of the micro-porous morphology of the coating does not reflect light as well as the relatively smooth titanium surface. Positive patterns (arrays of CaP islands in the titanium background) of various

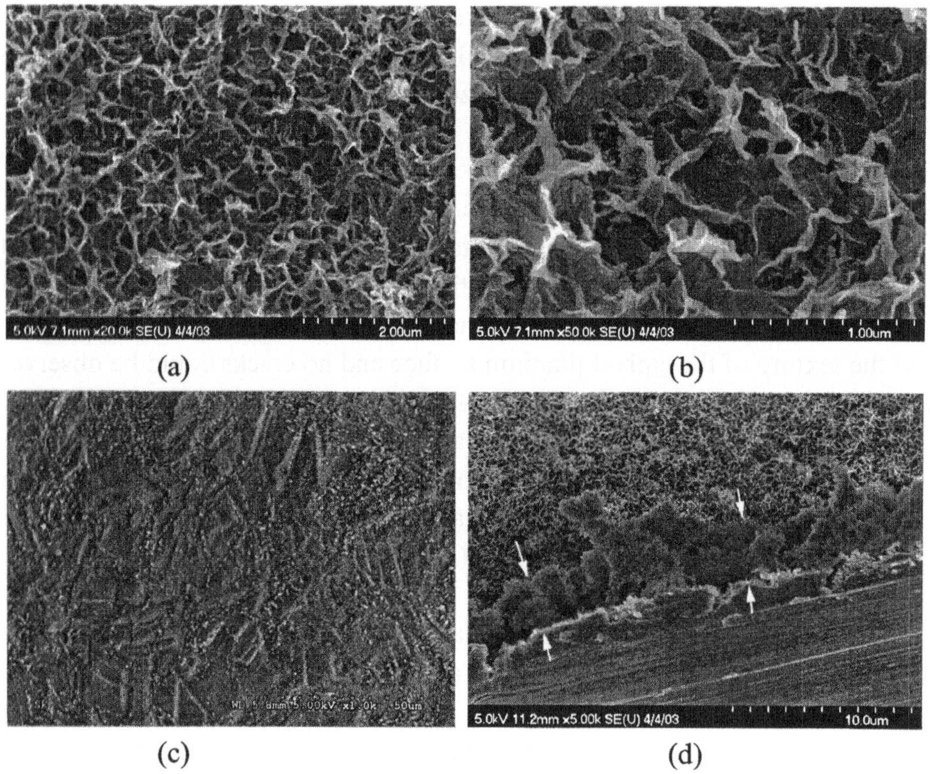

Fig. 1 Morphology of the CaP coating

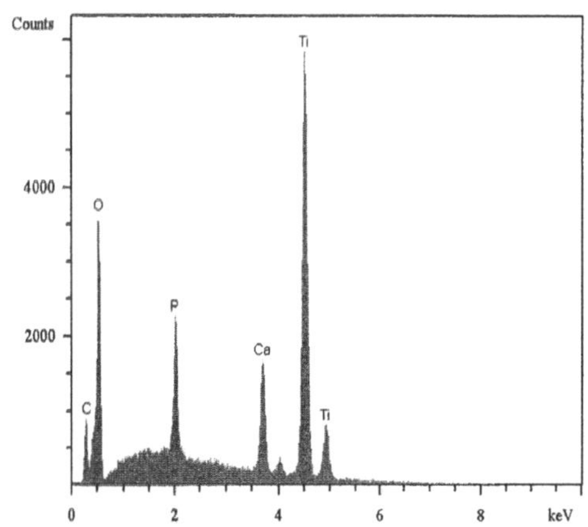

Fig. 2 EDX of the CaP coating

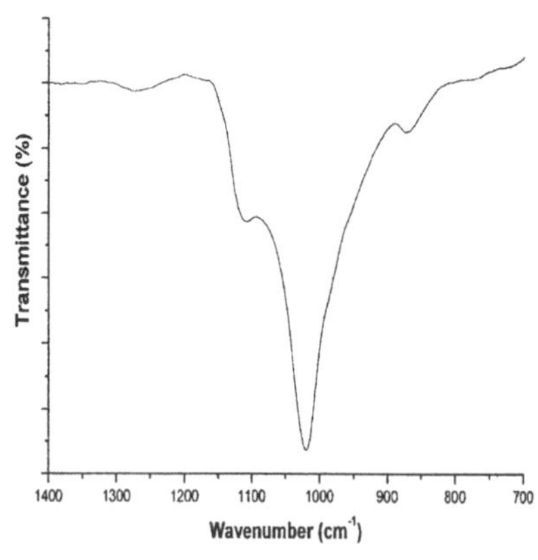

Fig. 3 FTIR of the CaP coating

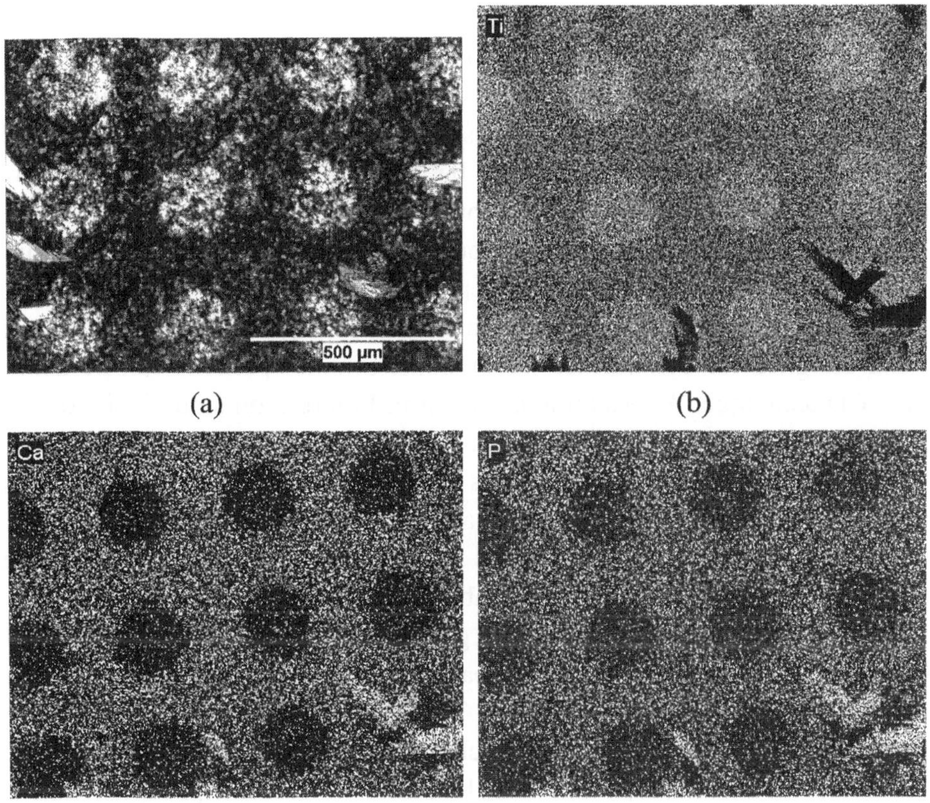

(a) (b)

(c) (d)

Fig. 4 Optical microscopy (a) and SEM/EDX mapping (b: Ti, c: Ca, d: P) of a CaP negative pattern where titanium dots are surrounded by CaP coating,

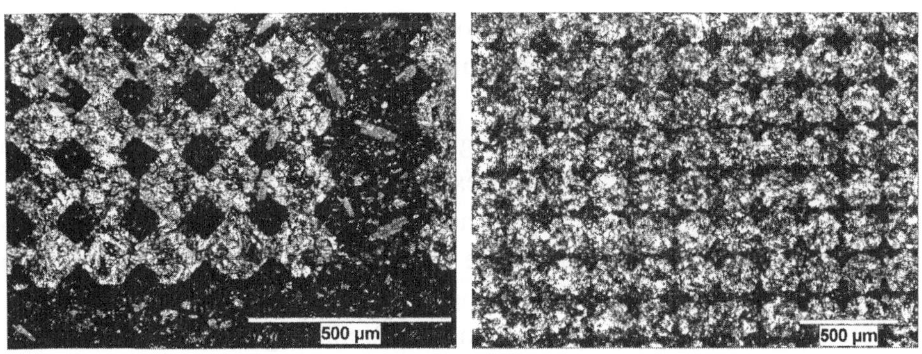

(a) (b)

Fig. 5 Optical microscopy of deposited CaP positive patterns where dark CaP arrays are surrounded by gray titanium substrate

geometries were also prepared and examples are presented in Figure 5. Figure 5a shows a cubic array of CaP rhombuses (dark areas) surrounded by regularly indented lines. Figure 5b shows a clear pattern of 8×10 array of "diamonds". It should be noted that scattered large crystals were also observed. These big crystals, identified as brushite, formed at later stages and can be avoided by reducing the electrolyte concentration or electrolysis time. Results presented in this paper represent our work at earlier stages and uniform patterns without these "impurities" have been achieved recently and will be reported in a separate report.

The patterns shown in Figures 4 and 5 are large because of the coarse photomask designed for cell surface interactions. Smaller patterns can be achieved with this ECD technique. An example is shown in Figure 6 on smooth silicon wafer. During the development of the exposed photoresist, small holes on the photoresist layer were created sometimes. CaP minerals would later form inside these small areas. The two muffin-like CaP structures were examples of such a micro-scale process. The round root about 5 μm in diameter reflects the initial crystallization confined within the photoresist patterns. The upper part is about 10 μm in diameter and shows radiant growth and may reflect the later stage of growth above the photoresist layer. It is interesting that CaP can be formed on untreated smooth silicon, which is widely used in sensors and various other micro-devices. The results demonstrate the possibility of integrating bioactive materials with silicon chip based devices.

The mechanisms of electrochemical deposition of calcium phosphate has been suggested to be as follows [10]. On pass of current, H^+ in the vicinity of cathode was consumed, i.e. $2H^+ + 2e \rightarrow H_2$, which increases the local pH near the cathode. Then calcium phosphate either formed in the solution and attracted by the electrostatic field to impinge on the cathode or heterogeneously nucleated on the titanium surface [9, 11]. It has been a challenge to deposit a porous, uniform, fine and crack free CaP coatings with ECD. Shirkhanzadeh [10] reported deposition of nano-scale apatite on titanium, but the crystal observation was performed under TEM and the coating microstructure was not described. Recently, Rőßler [9] *et al.* reported deposition of apatite under near-physiological conditions. The coating obtained was porous and consisted of crystals of similar size to this work and exhibited hierarchical pore size typical of microstructure from aggregation. With the present protocol, we demonstrated a continuous coating with uniform pore size could be formed (Fig. 1). The different microstructures reflect difference in coating formation mechanisms. In the present protocol, the current density was low ($< 1 mA/cm^2$), although the true current density was unknown as the titanium surface was etched and rough. At low current density, the local pH change was expected to be less significant and nucleation in solution to be less favorable than heterogeneous nucleation on titanium electrode. Although the detailed deposition mechanism is still not clear, the uniform microstructure at submicron scale may reflect an outward growth of CaP mineral skeletons at the later stage rather than attachment and aggregation from particles crystallized in solution.

Coating thickness is an important factor. Most electrochemically deposited

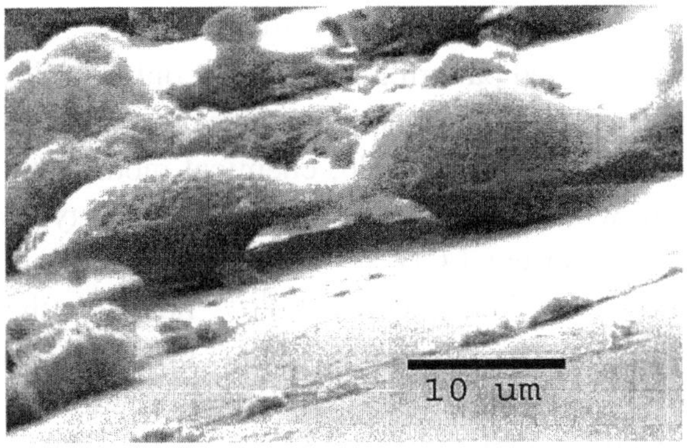

Fig. 6 SEM of muffin-like CaP structures on silicon wafer

ceramic coatings were less than 1 μm [11] since they are poorly conducting. The significantly higher thickness in this paper may be attributed to its porosity. As a comparison, Manso [12] *et al.* performed ECD at high pH conditions and obtained dense apatite coating with thickness of only 200 nm. For better mechanical integrity, thin coating is favorable. However, to survive the potential fast *in vivo* degradation caused by initial inflammation, a thick coating on bioimplant is desirable. For the present coating, with the combined porous structure and intermediate thickness, it is expected to be suitable for drug carrier coatings on biomedical devices.

In the present protocol, all procedures were performed at room temperature and therefore thermal stress was eliminated. The only possibility of cracking is capillary pressure during drying. As has been extensively discussed [13], most cracking occurs when the liquid begins receding into the pores and a curved liquid-vapor interface was formed. The capillary pressure is proportional to surface tension and inversely proportional to the curvature radii. In our experiments, water was replaced with ethanol, which has lower surface tension, and the pore size is intermediate (~200nm), the capillary pressure was reduced. As a comparison, densely packed globular CaP minerals (results not shown) of smaller crystal size were also deposited in our laboratory but was prone to substantial cracking possibly because the existence of much smaller pores which caused much higher capillary pressure. It should be noted that cracks could be initiated only when different pore sizes and consequently different drying rate and capillary pressure difference exist. As described above, the coating prepared by the present protocol exhibited relatively uniform pore size and is free of hierarchical coagulations. This may also contribute to the cracking-free nature of current coating.

Patterned surface has been extensively explored as an approach to regulate the adhesion, organization and function of living cells. Numerous studies [14, 15, 16] have been published that involved patterned immobilization of organic polymers or small molecules. Patterned calcium carbonate was also reported [17]. However patterning of bioactive inorganic materials such as CaP minerals was less studied. Ozawa [18] *et al.* reported patterning of apatite on glass substrate by a biomimetic process. We recently reported patterning of hydroxyapatite by electrophoresis [19]. Biomimetic process is flexible in coating thickness and pattern geometry but only applicable for substrate of suitable surface chemistry to induce apatite nucleation. For inert or nearly inert materials, e.g. silicon, native titanium, gold, chemical modification is required [20]. In addition, biomimetic growth is a relatively slow process and typically involves a few days, as compared to the current ECD (15~30 min.). Electrophoretic deposition is quick and independent of surface chemistry [11, 19] however the patterned coating formed through coagulation of colloidal particles is loose in microstructure and fragile in mechanical property. Post heat treatment is needed to render mechanical integrity to the electrophoretically deposited patterns. As a comparison, electrochemically deposited CaP patterns firmly attached to the substrate and can withstand rubbing with fingers. Combining these unique advantages, it is expected that electrochemically deposited bioceramic coatings and patterns have promising applications in the field of biomedical implants and biosensors.

CONCLUSIONS

An electrochemical protocol has been developed for depositing continuous calcium phosphate coating on titanium and silicon surfaces. The coating was uniform and crack free, with the mineral and pores both in sub-micron scale. By combine ECD with photolithography technique well defined patterns of CaP minerals down to micron level can be prepared onto a conducting surface.

ACKNOWLEDGEMENTS

This study was funded by the Natural Sciences and Engineering Research Council of Canada. R.W. is incumbent of the Canada Research Chair in Biomaterials.

REFERENCES

[1] K. de Groot, J.A. Jansen, J.G.C. Wolke, C.P.A.T. Klein and C.A. van Blitterswijk, "Developments in Bioactive Coatings", in *Hydroxylapatite Coatings in Orthopaedic Surgery*, Edited by R.G. T. Geesink and M. T. Manley. Raven Press, New York, 1993

[2] K. de Groot, R.G.T. Geesink, C.P.A.T. Klein and P. Serekian, "Plasma-sprayed Coatings of Hydroxyapatite", J. *Biomed. Mater. Res.*, **21,** 1375-81 (1987)

[3] T.J. Webster, C. Ergun, R.H. Doremus, R.W. Siegel and R.Biozios, "Enhanced Functions of Osteoblasts on Nanophase Ceramics", *Biomaterials*, **21,** 1803-10 (2000)

[4] Y. Ito, "Surface Micropatterning to Regulate Cell Functions", *Biomaterials*, **20,** 2333-42 (1999)

[5] R.S. Kane, S. Takayama, E. Ostuni, D.E. Ingbert and G.M. Whitesides, "Patterning Proteins and Cells Using Soft Lithography", Biomaterials, **20**, 2363-2376 (1999)

[6] S.N. Bhatia and C.S. Chen, "Tissue Engineering at the Micro-scale", *Biomedical Microdevices*, **2**, 131-44 (1999)

[7] G.H.A. Therese and V. Kamath, "Electrochemical Synthesis of Metal Oxides and Hydroxides", *Chem. Mater.*, **12**, 1195-204 (2000)

[8] B.O. Fowler, M. Marković and W.E. Brown, "Octacalcium Phosphate. 3. Infrared and Raman Vibrational Spectra", *Chem. Mater.*, **5**, 1417-23 (1993)

[9] S. Rőßler, A. Sewing, M. Stőlzer, R. Born, D. Scharnweber, M. Dard and H. Worch, "Electrochemically Assisted Deposition of Thin Calcium Phosphate Coatings at Near-physiological pH and Temperature", *J. Biomed. Mater. Res.*, **64**, 655-63 (2002)

[10] M. Shirkhanzadeh, "Direct Formation of Nanophase Hydroxyapatite on Cathodically Polarized Electrodes", *J. Mater. Sci.: Mater. Med.*, **9**, 76-72 (1998)

[11] I. Zhitomirsky, "Ceramic Films using Cathodic Electrodeposition", *JOM-e, Journal of the Minerals Metals and Materials Society*, **52**, [1] (2000) www.tms.org/pubs/journal/JOM/0001/Zhitomirsky/Zhitomirsky-0001.html

[12] M. Manso, C. Jiménez, C. Morant, P. Herrero and JM Martinez-Duart, "Electrodeposition of Hydroxyapatite in Basic Conditions", *Biomaterials*, **21**, 1755-61 (2000)

[13] C.J. Brinker and G.W. Scherer, "Drying"; pp. 453-513 in *Sol-Gel Science*, Academic Press, San Diego, 1990

[14] C.D. McFarland, C.H. Thomas, C. DeFilippis, J.G. Steele and K.E. Healy, "Protein Adsorption and Cell Attachment to Patterned Surfaces", *J. Biomed. Mater. Res.*, **49**, 200-10 (2000)

[15] Y. Ito, S. Kondo, G. Chen and Y. Imanishi, "Patterned Artificial Juxacrine Stimulation of Cells by Covalently Immobilized Insulin", *FEBS Letters*, **403**, 159-62 (1997)

[16] S.N. Bhatia, M.L. Yarmush and M. Toner, "Controlling Cell Interactions by Micropatterning in Co-cultures: Hepatocytes and 3T3 Fibroblasts", *J. Biomed. Mater. Res.*, **34**, 189-99 (1997)

[17] J. Aizenberg, "Patterned Cystallisation on Self-Assembled Monolayers with Integrated Regions of Disorder", *J. Chem. Soc., Dalton Trans.*, **21**, 3963-68 (2000)

[18] N. Ozawa and T. Yao, "Micropattern formation of apatite by combination of biomimetic process and transcription of resist pattern", *J. Biomed. Mater. Res.*, **62**, 579-86 (2002)

[19] R. Wang and Y. Hu, Patterning Hydroxyapatite Bio-coatings by Electrophoretic Deposition, *J. Biomed. Mater. Res.*, accepted for publication.

[20] T. Kokubo, "Apatite Formation on Surface of Cramics, Metals and Polymers in Body Environment", *Acta Materialia*, **46**, 2519-27 (1998)

2 AND 10 YEAR RETRIEVALS OF ZIRCONIA FEMORAL HEADS- XRD, SEM AND RAMAN SPECTROSCOPY STUDIES

D. D. Green[1], Pezzotti G[2], Sakakura S[2] M. Ries[3] and I. C. Clarke[1].

[1]Peterson Tribology Lab, Department of Orthopaedic Surgery, Loma Linda University Medical Center, Loma Linda, California, 92354, USA, ddgreen@som.llu.edu.
[2]Department of Materials, Kyoto Institute of Technology, Sakyo-ku, Matsugasaki, Kyoto, 606-8585, Japan.
[3]Deptment of Orthopaedics, University of California, San Francisco, California, USA,

ABSTRACT

Analysis of zirconia implant performance in patients is limited to one study of two Kobelco[1] implants (retrieved after 3 and 5 years use). The Japanese authors reported extensively cratered surfaces and formation of 20%-30% monoclinic phase. Here we report on two zirconia balls (Prozyr™, SGCD Inc), one retrieved at 2 years and the other at 10 years in the USA. Analysis was carried out for surface roughness, SEM, XRD and Raman Spectroscopy to determine the phases present, the residual-stress mapping and surface condition of the bearing surfaces. The bearing surfaces appeared satisfactorily preserved and XRD showed the majority of the surface was tetragonal phase with monoclinic < 8% after 10 years use. The Raman spectroscopy described close to neutral residual stresses on the surface. Thus these 2 year and 10 year Prozyr™ retrievals demonstrated satisfactory performance in the patients. This was in direct contrast to the Japanese zirconia retrieval study. Thus we may have to consider on case-by-case basis any differences in manufacturing, implant design and patient performance. In our study there was a trend for the residual compressive-stresses to decrease and the tensile-stresses to increase. This observation could imply that the tensile residual-stresses and monoclinic phase on the zirconia surface were increasing with time under the main bearing area. More detailed work is needed in this area.

INTRODUCTION

Since the introduction of zirconia balls in 1985 for orthopedic implants, the clinical outcomes and conclusions have been quite varied [1-6]. The main concern regarding the use of zirconia for total hip replacement (THR) is its metastability between two phases, tetragonal and monoclinic. Yittria-doped zirconia is a metastable material, whereby transformation toughening is induced via the transformation of tetragonal to monoclinic phase. An increase in grain volume of approximately 3-4% is produced upon transformation, thereby preventing or hindering the progression of any advancing crack(s) via this compressive dilation.

Analysis of zirconia implant performance in patients is limited to one Japanese study of two Kobelco implants retrieved after 3 and 5 years use. The authors reported much roughened, extensively cratered surfaces with evidence of 20%-30% monoclinic phase. The manufacturing literature and standards report < 2% of monoclinic phase was acceptable. Our group of collaborators had the opportunity to study two zirconia balls made by Prozyr™, SGCD Inc. One had been retrieved at 2 years and the other at 10 years, both from the Orthopedic Department of UCSF. We introduced Raman Spectroscopy for the first time in implant retrieval studies. This novel technique provided a much higher resolution of the zirconia phases as well as an understanding of the residual stresses on the surfaces.

MATERIALS AND METHODS

The University of California at San Francisco (UCSF) contributed the two zirconia balls. Both were 28mm zirconia balls manufactured by Saint-Gobain-Desmarquest (Prozyr: SGD), and were used with mating polyethylene cups for 2 years and 10 years (Table 1). Analysis was carried out for surface roughness, SEM, XRD and Raman Spectroscopy to determine the phases present, the residual-stress mapping and surface condition of the bearing surfaces.

Surfaces of the retrieved balls were imagined on a LV-SEM (Philips Electronics, model XL30-FEG) in a 30°-arc circle on the ball dome (main wear region) and at any wear scars or sites of metal-transfer. X-Ray diffraction measurements (XRD) were taken at the pole and at 30° relative to the pole (0°). Measurements were taken on a Bede D1 high-resolution X-ray Diffractometer using CuKα radiation at 40kV and 2mA. Scans were taken from 26° to 36° 2θ inclusive, with a step size 0.0175° and step time of 1.15 seconds. Surface roughness measurements were carried out on a Feinpruf Perthometer S8P analyzer using a 5um radius diamond tip stylus. Measurements were taken at 0, 15, 30, 45 60 and 90° relative to the pole (0°). The percent monoclinic phase for each ball was extrapolated from the maximum intensity 2-theta position (tetragonal = 30.167° and monoclinic = 28.190°).

Raman Spectroscopy was performed using a Raman microprobe spectrometer (ISA, T-64000, Jobin-Ivon/Horiba Group, Tokyo, Japan) at room temperature. The 488nm line of an Ar-ion laser was used as the excitation source, with a power of 400 mW. Scattered frequencies were analysed with a triple-monochromator equipped with a charge-coupled device (CCD) camera. Spectrums were collected at the pole (0°) and 90° relative to the pole in an area of 50um. It should be noted that the Raman spectroscopy is scanning an area of $50\mu m^2$ whereas the XRD takes its spectrum from an area ~$1.5mm^2$. The nature of the Raman allows for a more detailed analysis at the micro level, where XRD allows for a bulk resolution of the material properties.

Table: 1 –data for retrieved zirconia balls.

Sample	Source	Years *in vivo*	ø of ball	Manufacturer	Appearance
R62	UCSF	2	28mm	Proyzr	White and shiny
R66	UCSF	10	28mm	Proyzr	White and shiny

RESULTS AND DISCUSSION

Both balls revealed the presence of the original polishing and machine marks made at the time of manufacture. Ball R62 at 2 years revealed a greater degree of machine tracks; ball R66 showed much less as would be expected after the polishing effect of 10 years use with polyethylene cups. Both R62 and R66 showed some mild grain relief and grain pullout from the zirconia surface. This was generally visible as dark square or triangular like shapes (Figs, 1-6). There was still some evidence of a "biofilm" on the samples, i.e. not completely removed after our cleaning process. Care should be taken to discriminate between surface features of the zirconia ceramic and the biofilm.

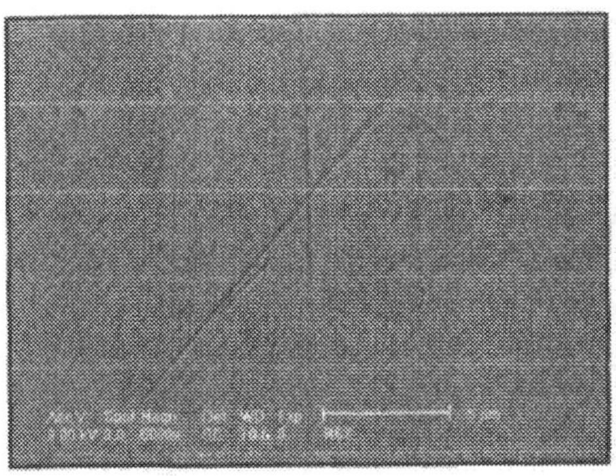

Figure: 1 – R62 micrograph showing original machine marks on 2-year retrieval.

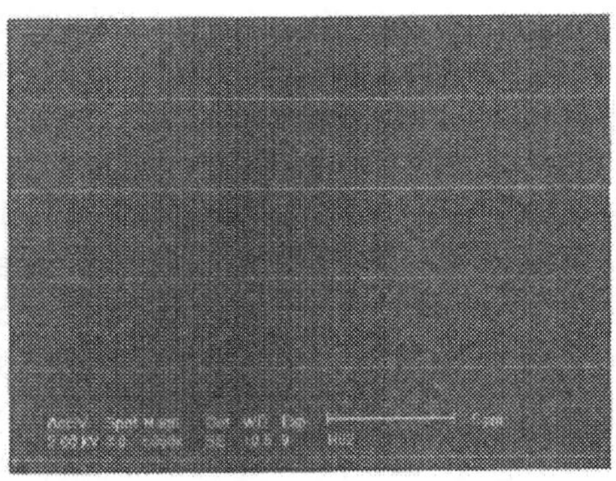

Figure: 2 – R62 micrograph showing parallel lines representing polish marks.

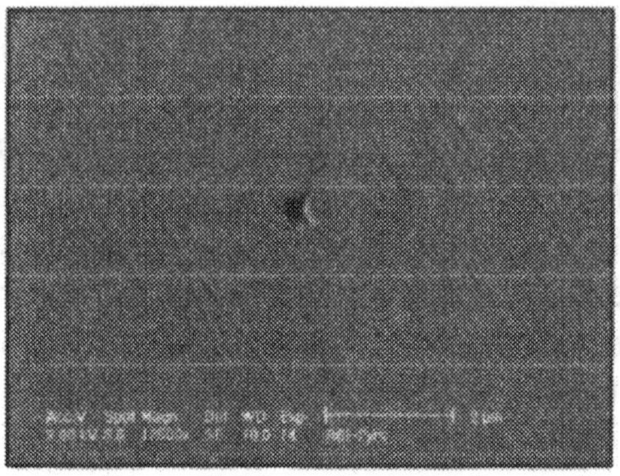

Figure: 3 – R62 micrograph grain pullout from the bearing surface.

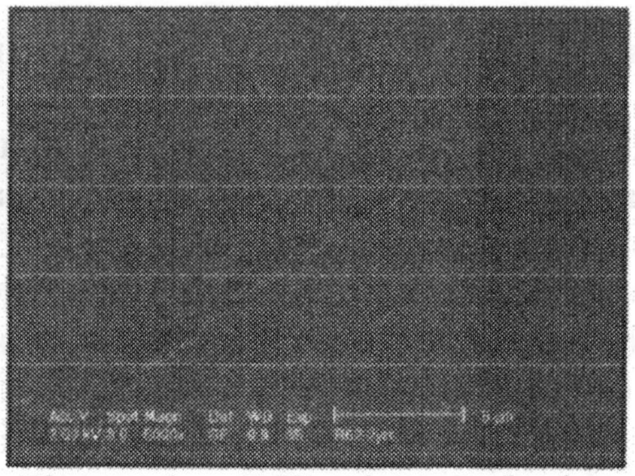

Figure: 4 – R62 micrograph showing grain relief of the bearing surface.

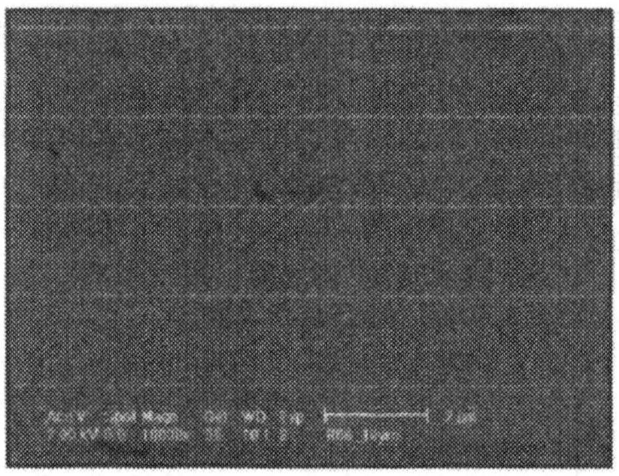

Figure: 5 – R66 micrograph showing relief of the original polish and machine marks combined with some grain relief.

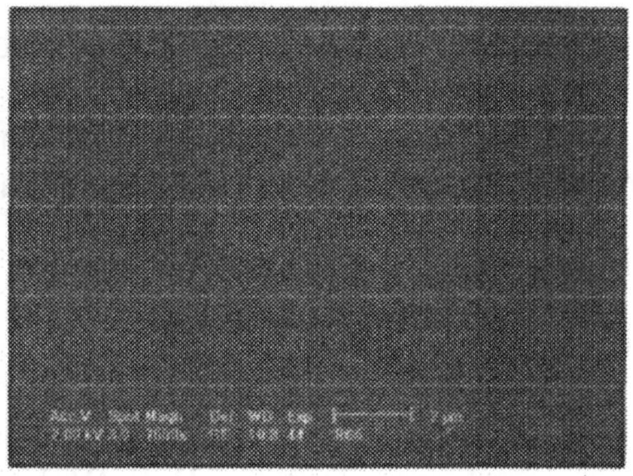

Figure: 6 – R66 micrograph showing some mild grain pullout from the bearing surface at 10 years.

XRD measurements for both balls identified the major phase for both regions (pole and 30°) on R62 and R66 as tetragonal. The monoclinic phase at the pole of R62 was ~8% and at 90°-arc was ~2%; R66 pole monoclinic was ~7% and at 90°-arc was ~2%. The XRD showed that the zirconia material has undergone mild transformation of the tetragonal phase to the monoclinic phase. Having predominant tetragonal content relays that the material is close to its original condition prior to implantation.

Raman spectroscopy was used to map the residual stresses at the bearing surface (Figs. 9 and 10). Overall the Raman data from both samples showed fairly neutral residual stresses (Figs. 9 and 10: green color). R62 showed predominantly neutral residual stresses interspersed with some islands of tension (Fig. 9: 293Mpa; yellow color, location represented by the arrows). The R62 ball with shorter follow-up had the higher compressive stresses (Table 2: 450-500 MPa) whereas R66 at 10 years showed only 60% of that magnitude at the pole and 30% at the 90°-arc. In contrast, the R66 ball showed the highest tensile residual stresses at the 90-arc (Fig. 10, location represented by arrows), 300% higher than R62. At the dome area the tensile stresses in R66 were 44% higher than R62. The Raman data illustrates that as the ball spends a longer period *in vivo* we start to see more tensile stress zones (R66). Even though the overall stress value is predominately neutral in nature, islands of monoclinic transformation were detectable where tensile stresses were present.

Table: 2 – Min and Max Stress Vales from Raman measurements.

	R62		**R66**	
	Pole (0°)	90°	Pole (0°)	90°
Min Stress (MPa)	-452	-500	-263	-162
Max Stress (MPa)	293	136	423	433

Surface roughness measurements trends were the same in both balls over the 30-90-arc (Table 3). Surface roughness measurements towards the pole of R62 appeared to show the effects of self-polishing with a lower Ra value at 2 years whereas R66 increased toward the pole, perhaps indicative of the length of time *in vivo* (10 years). These trends were confirmed in the SEM analysis where removal of the original machine marks was tracked.

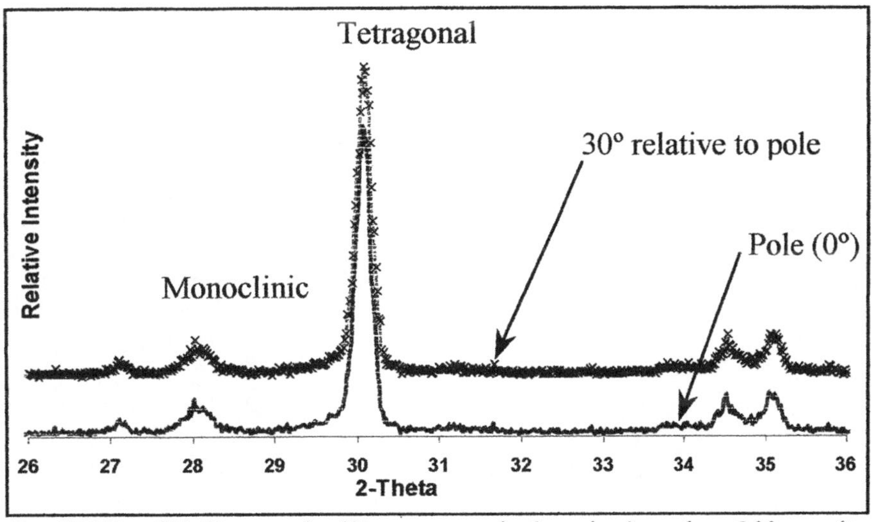

Figure: 7 – XRD of R62 at pole (2 years; main bearing) and at 30°-arc (transition from main bearing region), both regions showing same strong tetragonal signal and weak monoclinic signal

Table: 3 - Surface Roughness Data as a function of Orientation.

Orientation	Ra (nm)	
	R62	**R66**
Pole (0°)	16	24
15°	17	19
30°	19	18
45°	20	20
60°	22	22
90°	22	22

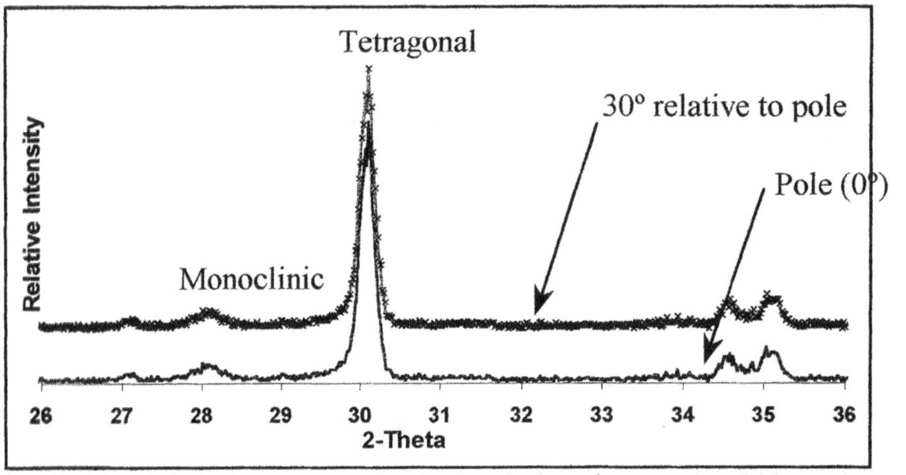

Figure: 8 – XRD of R66 (10 years) at pole (main bearing) and at 30° arc (transition from main bearing region), both showing same strong tetragonal signal and weak monoclinic signal

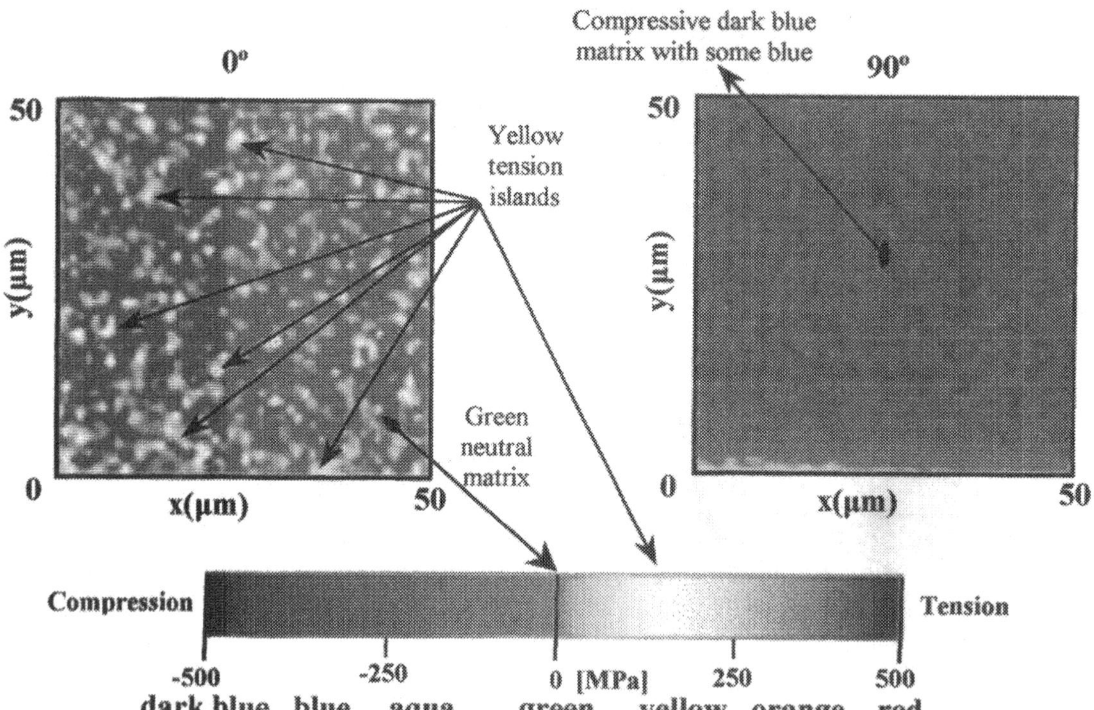

Figure: 9 - Raman Spectroscopy of R62 (2 years) at the pole and 90°, showing relatively neutral (pole) to compressive (90°) stress on the surface.

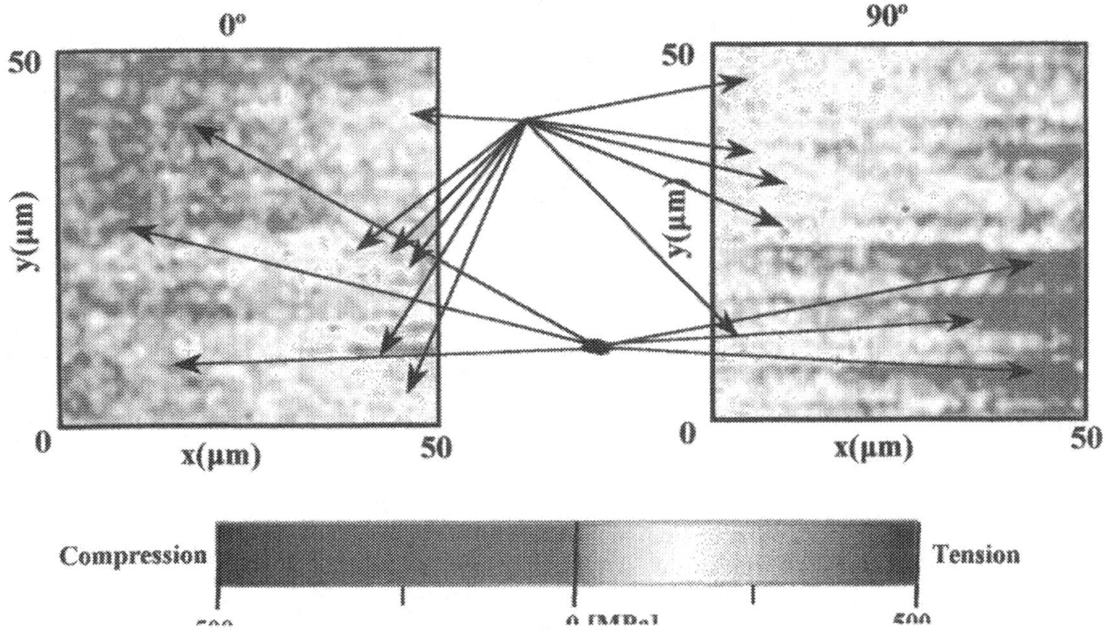

DISCUSSION AND CONCLUSIONS

Our study reports the longest follow-up for a retrieved zirconia implant. Therefore it was reassuring to see that original machine marks were still visible and the degree of monoclinic transformation was no more than 8%. This was also seen on the 2-year ball and thus there had appeared to have been no progression over 8 intervening years. Thus the Prozyr bearing had performed satisfactorily against its polyethylene cup for over a decade in our patient.

The main zirconia bearing surface is thought to be the polar region extending to 30°-arc segment. Beyond 30°-arc there will be much less habitual contact and hence less wear and transformation phenomena. Our data shows that the transformation to monoclinic was 7-8% at the pole and dropped down to <2% at the equator in both balls. This appears consistent with the hypothesis that the contact stresses and frictional heating effects in the main wear zone will be the first to contribute to higher monoclinic phase and possibly rougher surfaces.

Our 2 and 10 Year Prozyr data were in direct contrast to the Japanese study that had two cases (Kobelco Inc) complicated by implant dislocations and part-dissassociation.[1] Thus we may have to consider such zirconia retrievals on a case-by-case basis with respect to differences in manufacturing, implant design and patient performance. Our Raman data showed an interesting trend with the high compressive residual-stresses measured in the 2-year ball were greatly decreased in the 10-year ball. In contra-distinction the tensile residual stresses appeared to have greatly increased in the 10-year ball. However the observation that the tensile residual stresses and monoclinic phase could be increasing with time is somewhat troublesome. However with data from only two balls this is only an observation at this time and needs much more work to document the actual trends.

REFERENCES

[1] Haraguchi, K., Sugano, N., *et al.*, "Phase Transformation of a Zirconia Ceramic Head after Total Hip Arthroplasty". J. Bone. Jt. Surg., 83B, 996, 2001

[2] Banon F, "Experience with ceramic heads and friction with polyethylene or alumina cups in hip surgery. A new couple: ZIRCONIA-Alumina. About 163 cases", 2000 World Biomaterials Congress, April 2000, Hawaii.

[3] Dambreville A., Phillipe., Ray A., "Zirconia ceramics or 'by night, all cats are grey' ", Maitrise Orthopedique, Articles, 1999.

[4] Allain J., Le Mouel S., *et al.*, "Poor Eight Year Survival of Cemented Zirconia-Polyethylene Total Hip Replacements", J. Bone Jt. Surg., 81B,:835, 1999.

[5] Kim Y-H., Kim J-S., and Cho S-H., "A Comparison of Polyethylene Wear in Hips with Cobalt-Chrome or Zirconia Heads", J. Bone Jt Surg., 83B:742, 2001.

[6] Cales B., Stefani Y., "Mechanical properties and surface analysis of retrieved zirconia hip joints heads after an implantation time of two to three years" Biomaterials, 1994, p376-380.

3 DIMENSIONAL CT ANALYSES OF BONE FORMATION IN POROUS CERAMIC BIOMATERIALS

Y.Ikeda[1)], M.Yasutoshi[1)], M.Mizuno[1)], M.Mukaida[2)], M.Neo[2)] and T.Nakamura[2)]

1) Japan Fine Ceramics Center
2-4-1, Mutsuno, Atsuta-ku, Nagoya, 456-8587 (Japan)

2) Kyoto University, Graduate School of Medicine, Faculty of Medicine
54, Shogoin Kawaramati, Sakyou-ku, Kyoto, 606-8507 (Japan)

ABSTRACT

Bone formation on porous biomaterials implanted into living tissue has been studied quantitatively by 3-D X-ray CT. Porous apatite-wollastonite-containing glass ceramics (A-W GC) have been implanted into the thighbones of rabbits, and a few weeks after, the implantation removed from the rabbits and imaged with a 3-D X-ray CT. The 3-D structures of the materials are reconstructed from hundreds of 2-D sectional CT images obtained 100 slices at a time. The complicated 3-D structure of the A-W GC was imaged and analyzed at high resolution (4μm voxel size),. At lower resolution (14 μm voxel size), the whole volume of the implanted A-W GC specimen (6 mm dia. and 4 mm length) was imaged using volume CT. The regions where bone formed could be distinguished from the A-W GC and their volumes.

1. INTRODUCTION

In the first half of the 21th century, we will be faced with the challenge of a rapidly aging society. One of the main concerns for an aging society is the increasing incidence of osteoporosis, which causes weakening and fracture of bones. This disease is widespread already and is expected to become even more so in the future. For the elderly, recovering from bone-fracture takes a very long time as the result of the decline in bone regenerative power. One means of shortening the healing time is to introduce porous biomaterials to the damaged region to support the bone while repair and regrowth take place by marrow cells. Some bio-implantation materials, such as hydroxyapatite (HA), appear to be promising bone substitutes for medical investigation and treatment [1-3]. Porous apatite-wollastonite-containing glass ceramics (A-W GC) is a hydroxyapatite that has been studied for bone formation [4]. For clinical application, it is important to evaluate the implanted A-W GC from the point of view of its compatibility withliving tissue, its performance in vivo cell conformity and so on. These characteristics are considered to strongly depend on the porous structure of the biomaterial into which blood can permeate. Nondestructive 3-D analysis of the structure is therefore very important. In addition, a nondestructive measuring and appraisal method of bone formation for these materials in vivo may also become very important. The most powerful nondestructive method for measuring and evaluating the 3-D structures of such porous bone-like ceramics is high-resolution X-ray computed tomography (CT), which takes multiple CT slice images duringt one rotation of the sample and reconstructs a 3-D image from these [5].

2. THE 3-D HIGH-RESOLUTION X-RAY CT (HRXCT) METHOD

HRXCT begins with the imaging of a specimen using a cone-shaped beam of X-rays, so that a 2-D projection of the specimen is obtained from the transmitted x-rays with a 2-D image detector. The intensity of the X-rays transmitted through the specimen yields the projection data, as is usual in CT. By rotating the specimen and irradiating it from various angles, one set of projection data for reconstructing a CT cross-section image can be obtained. A micro-focus X-ray tube radiates a cone-shaped beam of X-rays from its small focal spot, so that when the specimen is placed in the beam, a magnified image of it is obtained at the image detector. When the ratio of the distance between the focal spot and the image detector (FID) to that between the focal spot and the specimen (FOD), we obtain a large image magnification, which makes it possible to obtain high resolution CT images with very little blurring of the image. Figure 1 shows a schematic representation of the 3-D HRXCT. From the projection

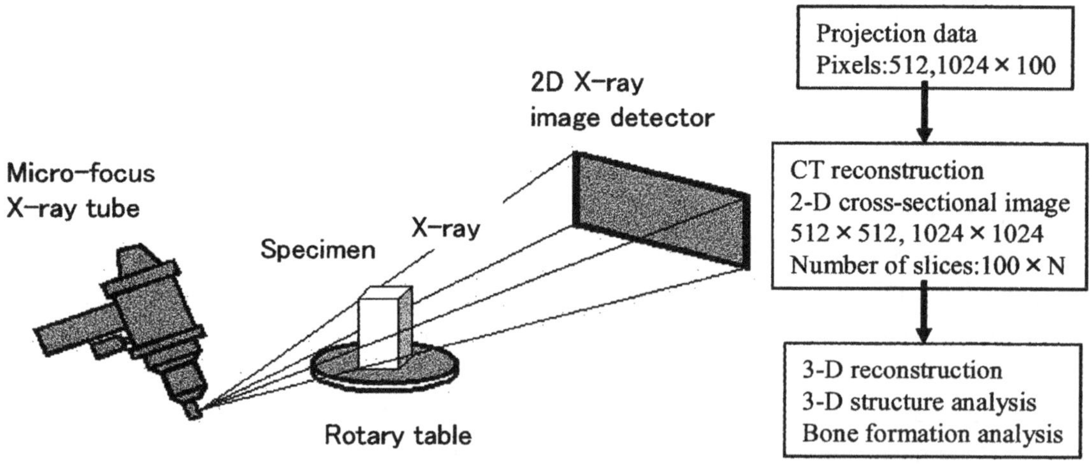

Fig.1 Schematic of the 3-D HRXCT method and computing procedure

data,2-D CT cross-sectional images are reconstructed using CT computing software. The CT reconstruction process is very similar to conventional 2-D CT, except that many cross sectional CT images are obtained at the same time. The 3-D reconstruction was carried out on computer using software with 3-D formation, 3-D analysis and 3-D viewer capabilities.

3. EXPERIMENTS

Setup for 3-D HRXCT

The HRXCT method used in this work consisted of two types of micro-focus X-ray tubes (ANDREX (now YXLON) MX-4 with a focal spot size of about 8 μ m, and HAMAMATSU PHOTONICS C8033, with a focal spot size of about 4 μ m). The 2-D image detector used was an image intensifier (TOSHIBA 9 in) with a 1.3 mega pixel digital CCD camera, which has a resolution of 7 lp/mm for X-ray images. We used two types of CT stages. The first CT stage was BIR system, controlled with the computer system PXS-ACTIS+3, developed by Bio Imaging Research Co. This system consists of Dual Pentium Ⅲ loading ACTIS+3 and VOLUME CT software. Volume CT scanning is a fast automatic 3-D scanning method, in which 100 multi-sliced CT images can be obtained in a single scan, and by going up and down the specimen automatically, allows fairly long areas to be imaged, such as 1000 cross sectional CT images for a length of 100 mm.

Another type of CT system, developed by UNIHITE SYSTEM Co can carry out tensile and compression tests for ceramic specimens during CT imaging. In future, we plan to use this system to obtain 3-D CT data during deformation of specimens under stress.

Materials and Specimens

The ceramic biomaterial used in this work was porous apatite-wollastonite-containing glass ceramic (A-W GC), which has a porosity of about 70% from Nippon Electric Glass Co. 70% porosity is considered to be the most bio-effective. First, the A-W GC specimen was imaged for structure analysis. The A-W GC specimen was cut into 2 x 2 x 5 mm^3 pieces and imaged with a high magnification of 60. By using the 3-D CT images reconstructed from 2-D CT images, the pore size distribution and the path size distributions were calculated using TRI-3D computer software, developed by RATOC SYSTEM ENGINEERING Co., Ltd.

In-vivo experiments were carried out, by implanting A-W GC rods of about 6 mm dia. and 4 mm thickness in the thighbones of rabbits. After 2 to 4 weeks, the specimens were removed from the rabbits and imaged by 3-D CT. The whole volume of each sample was imaged by the volume CT method. The volume of newly formed bone were measured and evaluated.

HEXCT Imaging And Reconstruction Conditions

The HRXCT imaging conditions are given in table 1. The imaging volumes were 2 x 2 x 0.4 mm^3 for structure analysis, and 6 x 6 x 4 mm^3 for bone formation measurement.

Table 1 CT imaging condition

X-ray tube voltage	60 kV	X-ray tube current	0.13 mA
FID	840 mm	magnification	60 (S.A.), 20(B.F.)
Number of view	800	Number of slice	100

*S.A.: Structure analysis, B.F.: Bone formation measurement

4. RESULTS AND DISCUSSION

HRXCT 3D Imaging and Analyses of an A-W GC Specimen

Figure 2 shows the 2-D CT image of the A-W GC specimen taken by HRXCT. The size of the imaged area is about 2 mm x 2 mm with a pixel size of about 4μm (number of pixels: is 512 x 512). As can be seen, the A-W GC specimen contains pores fairly round shape and almost all are connected. The connections are very important for bone formation in-vivo experiments.

By using multi-cross sectional CT images, a 3-D CT image was reconstructed using the computer software, TRI 3-D ANALYSIS. Figure 3 shows the reconstructed 3-D image of the specimen.

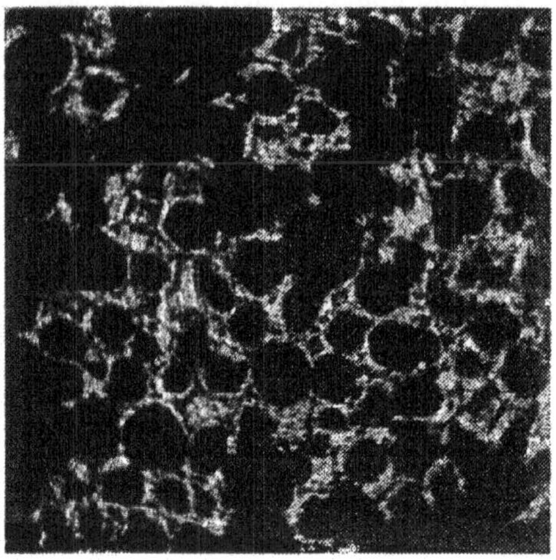

Fig.2 2-D CT image of A-W GC (porosity:70 %)

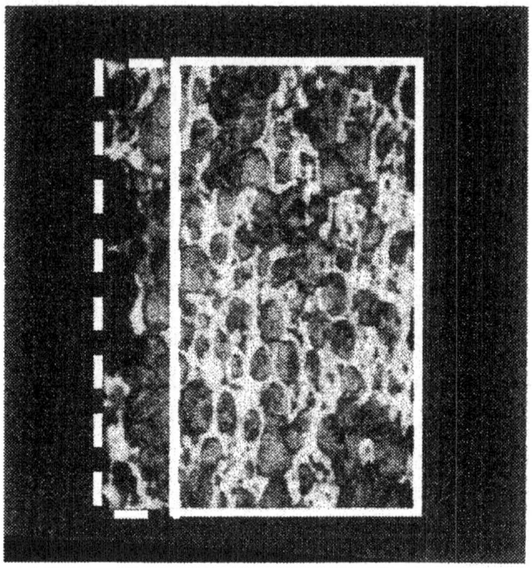

Fig.3 3-D image of A-W GC from 100 2-D images

Analysis of the 3-D CT image was carried out using TRI 3-D, which calculates both pore-size and path size distribution in the specimen. The connected pores were isolated one-by-one by an image-shrinking and dilatation process. After being isolated, each pore was labeled and the number of voxels was calculated to obtain its volume. The process was repeated for all pores. Figure 4(a) shows the pore-size distribution obtained for the porous A-W GC specimen. Using similar method, the path-size distribution in the specimen can be obtained, as shown in Fig.4(b).

This result is very interesting, because we can measure the pore-size nondestructively in stead of any mercury porosimeter and we can measure the path between pores, which may be impossible with mercury porosimeter.

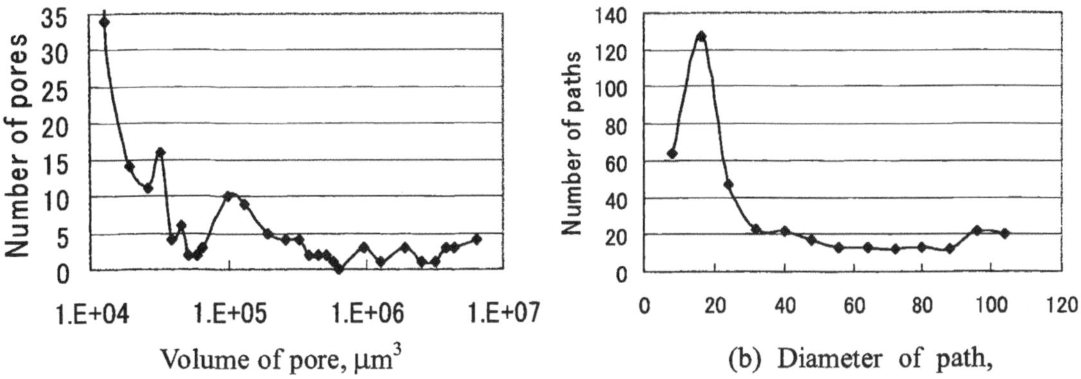

Fig.4 Histogram of pore-size and path-size in the A-W GC (porosity: 70 %)

<u>Bone-Formation Analyses of In-vivo Specimens in Rabbits</u>

A-W GC specimens were implanted in the thighbones of rabbits and removed after several weeks. The small rods of A-W GC, 6 mm dia. by 4 mm length, were imaged by HRXCT to reconstruct 3-D CT images and to measure the amount of bone-formation. Figure 5 (a) shows the 3-D CT image of an implanted specimen after a period of 4 weeks. The whole image including surrounding bone and tissue of the rabbit is shown. In the figure, the white areas correspond to A-W GC, which has the largest X-ray absorption coefficient in the specimen and indicate that the ceramic has dissolved since the shape has changed. The dark areas indicate pores or air-containing regions. The gray areas in the CT images correspond to newly formed bone since we have observed that the organic tissue areas usually are found in outer region and not inside the implanted ceramic. This result is very interesting, because we can observe and measure the effect of A-W GC in vivo experiment nondestructively and 3 dimensionally. In fact, we can study the bone formation in rats with implant periods by this method.

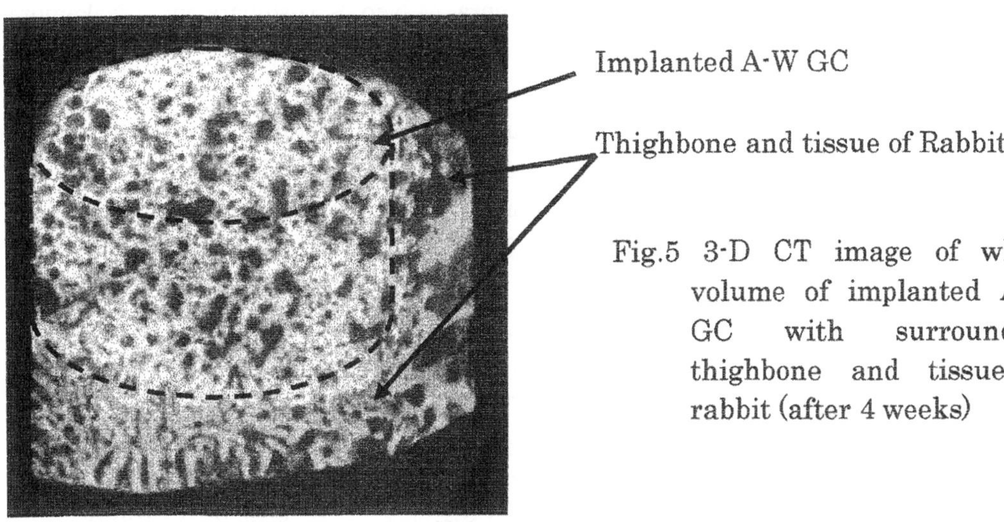

Fig.5 3-D CT image of whole volume of implanted A-W GC with surrounding thighbone and tissue of rabbit (after 4 weeks)

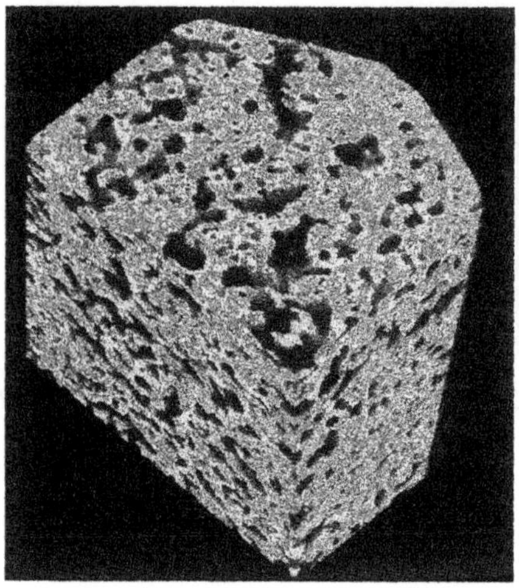

Fig.6 A section of the 3-D CT image of implanted A-W GC from Fig.5 after binary processed.

A 3-D image of the A-W GC part was cut out from the image in Fig.5, and the volume of the formed bone extracted by binary processing, shown as white parts in Fig.6. We have found that the volume of bone formed increases with longer periods of implantation. Using RATOC TRI 3D, the volumes of bone formed were calculated. For example, the volume of bone formation in the A-W GC specimen in Fig.5 and Fig.6 was calculated to be 8 mm^3 when the volume of A-W GC was 26 mm^3.

ACKNOWLEDGEMENT

This work was supported by the New Energy and Industrial Technology Development Organization (NEDO) as part of the R&D Projects in "Advanced Support System for Endoscopic and Other Minimally Invasive Surgery" entrusted to Japan Fine Ceramics Center.

REFERENCES

[1] W.Mousa, M.Kobayashi, S.Shinzato, M.Kamimura, M.Neo, S.Yoshihara and T.Nakamura, Biorogical and mechanical properties of PMMA-based bioactive bone cements, Biomaterials, 21, 2137-2146 (2000).

[2] K.Hata, N.Ozawa, T.Kokubo and T.Nakamura, Bonelike apatite formation on various kinds of ceramics and metals, J. Ceram. Soc. Japan, 109[5], 461-465 (2001).

[3] T.Miyazaki, H.Kim, T.Kokubo, C.Ohtsuka and T.Nakamura, Apatite-forming ability of niobium oxide gels in a simulated body fluid, J. Ceram.Soc. Japan, 109[11], 929-933 (2001).

[4] S.Ijiri, T.Nakamura, Y.Fujisawa, M.Hazama and S.Komatsudani, Ectopic bone induction in porous apatite-wollastonite-containing glass ceramic combined with bone morphogentic protein, J. Biomedical Mater. Res., 35, 421-432 (1997).

[5] Y.Ikeda, Y. Mizuta, M.Mizuno, K.Ohsawa, M.Neo and T.Nakamura, 3D CT analyses of porous structures of apatite ceramics and in-vivo bone formation, 26th Annual conf. on Composites, Advanced Ceram., Mater. and Structures: B, 833-838 (2002)

WEAR CHARACTERIZATION OF CLINICALLY USED HIP JOINT PROSTHESES BY A HIP SIMULATOR

Y. Takigawa, K. Jono, H. Takadama and M. Mizuno
Materials R & D Laboratory
Japan Fine Ceramics Center
2-4-1 Mutsuno, Atsuta-ku, Nagoya
456-8587, Japan

T. Nakamura

Department of Orthopaedic Surgery
Faculty of Medicine, Kyoto University
54 Kawahara-cho, Shogoin, Sakyo-ku
Kyoto 606-6507, Japan

ABSTRACT

Wear characterization of clinically used hip joint prostheses is conducted by a HIP simulator. Bovine serum solution is used for lubricant, and the tests are conducted until 5×10^6cycles. At first, the effect of testing conditions on the wear of hip joint prostheses is examined in order to determine the optimum condition of hip simulator tests. As the results, it is clarified that serum concentration in lubricant and intervals of lubricant replacement highly affect the wear of UHMWPE. Formation of protein film and increase of initial wear must be the origin, respectively. By using the determined conditions, long-term simulator tests are conducted against six types of commercial hip joint prostheses. The results clearly exhibit the difference of wear in each combination. These data are expected to be applied as the reference data on developing new type of hip joint prostheses.

INTRODUCTION

Many works have been conducted on improving wear resistance of hip joint prostheses, because the osteolysis induced by polyethylene wear particles is a key factor causing loosing failure of them [1]. For evaluating wear in these prostheses, hip joint wear simulator is very effective. However, since the result of wear is very sensitive about surroundings such as lubricant composition, it is difficult to compare the results obtained in different laboratory. Thus, it is necessary to define wear evaluation method and compare the data obtained under the same condition. In the present study, some factors to be expected to affect wear are examined for defineing wear evaluation method. Then, by using determined testing conditions, wear characterization is conducted on clinically used hip joint prostheses.

EXPERIMENTAL PROCEDURE

The combinations of hip joint prostheses examined in this study are summarized in Table 1. Three samples are examined in each combination. Wear tests are performed using 12-station hip joint simulator (MTS, USA). The tests are conducted at a rotation frequency of 1Hz, and the load is applied by Paul's walking profile [2]. Maximum load is set for 2.8kN in the profile. Bovine serum solution is used as a lubricant. The bovine serum is distiled by 7 or 25%, and 20mM EDTA and 0.1% sodium azide are added to the lubricant. Wear is evaluated by measureing the weight change of cups. The measurement is carried out every additional 250,000 or 500,000 cycles.

Table I. HIP joint prostheses examined in this study

Head and its diameter	Cup
ZrO_2 26mm	UHMWPE (A)
CoCr 26mm	UHMWPE (A)
CoCr 26mm	UHMWPE (B)
Al_2O_3 26mm	Crosslinked UHMWPE
ZrO_2 26mm	Crosslinked UHMWPE
CoCr 28mm	CoCr
Al_2O_3 28mm	Al_2O_3

RESULTS AND DISCUSSION

At first, the effect of testing conditions on the wear of hip joint prostheses is examined in order to determine the optimum condition of hip simulator tests. Figure 1 shows the results examining the effect of serum concentration in lubricant (left) and the effect of intervals of lubricant replacement (right). Both serum concentration in lubricant and intervals of lubricant replacement highly affect the wear of ZrO_2/UHMWPE. As for the effect of serum concentration in lubricant, wear in 25% serum solution is higher than that in 7% one. This result exhibits similar trend reported in metal/UHMWPE [3, 4]. It is demonstrated that the serum concentration is also important in the combination of ceramic/UHMWPE. Since the change in wear with the change in serum concentration in metal/UHMWPE is supposed to be originated from the protein film formed on joints surface, it is important to focus on protein concentration.

Since the protein concentration of fluid in the joint is in the range 20 to 35 mg/ml [5] and that of serum is about 80mg/ml, the choice of 25% serum solution seems to be reasonable. Then, the serum concentration in lubricant is determined to 25%.

In the test examining the effect of intervals of lubricant replacement (Fig.1 right), wear decreases with increasing intervals of lubricant replacement. This result seems to be corresponding with the result that degraded serum solution decreases wear [6]. However, very recent result indicates that the degree of degradation of serum solution is not so different between 3 and 6 days [7]. Another factor must be considered.

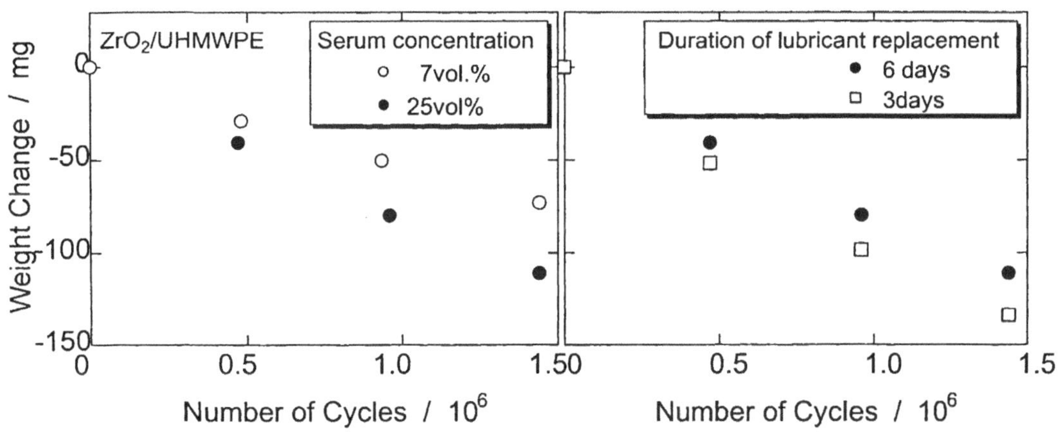

Fig. 1 Effect of serum concentration in lubricant (left) and intervals of lubricant replacement (right) on wear of ZrO_2/UHMWPE hip joint prostheses.

Figure 2 shows the comparison of relative torque change in two conditions: no replacement of lubricant (upper) and replaced twice (lower). The relative torque decreases with increasing cycles in both conditions. When the lubricant is replaced, relative torque significantly increases. Although it is difficult to explain the relationship between torque and wear quantitatively, increase in torque must lead the increase in wear in the same condition. If the amount of the change in torque is simply calculated, the change in torque in the condition replaced twice (lower) exhibits 1.5 times higher than that without replacement. This must be the origine of increasing wear in the condition replaced in 3 days. From the result, intervals of lubricant replacement are determined to be 6 days.

From these analyses together with unreported analyses, wear evaluation conditions are defined. Then, wear characterization is conducted on six types of clinically used hip joint prostheses under the conditions defined in this study.

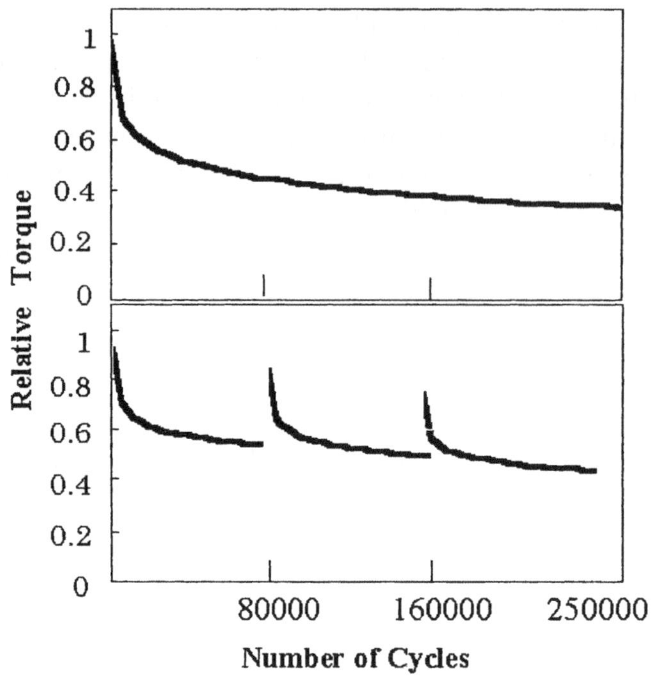

Fig. 2 Comparison of relative torque change in two conditions; no replacement of lubricant (upper) and replaced twice (lower)

Figure 3 shows the Comparison of wear in six types of commercial hip joint prostheses. The lower figure is drawn in enlarged scale. The wear characteristic is much different in each combination. In CoCr/UHMWPE, there are not so large difference in wear between two kind of joints provided from two manufacturers. The wear of UHMWPE is highly reduced by crosslinking, which is almost in the same level with that of CoCr/CoCr. Al_2O_3/Al_2O_3 exhibits extremely low wear in comparison with other combinations. From these results, the difference of wear property in each combination is clearly exhibited. These date are expected to be applied as the reference data on developing new types of hip joint prostheses or selecting combination for clinical application.

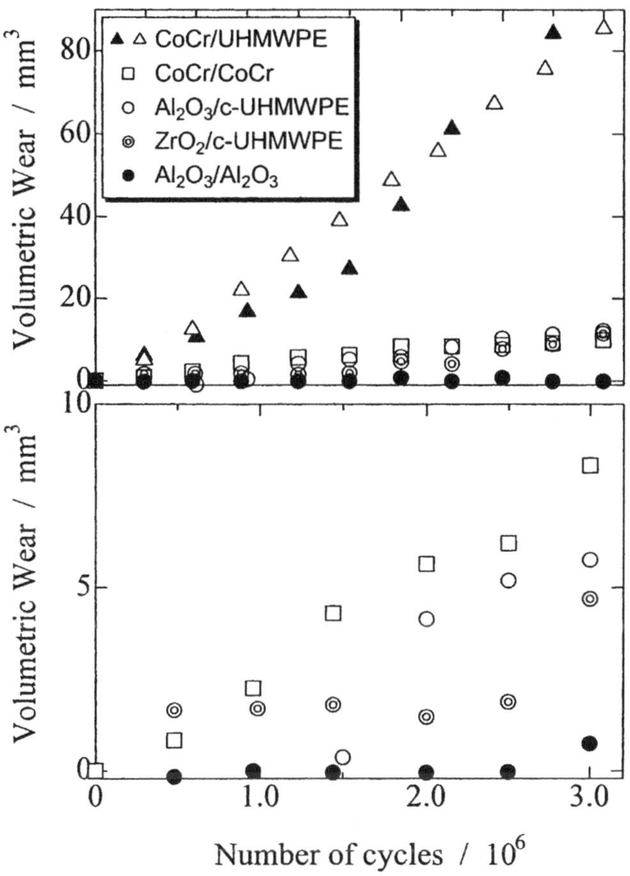

Fig. 3 Comparison of wear in six types of commercial hip joint prostheses

CONCLUSION

Wear evaluation method by a HIP simulator is examined and wear characterization of clinically used hip joint prostheses is conducted. The results are summarized as follows:

(1) It is clarified that serum concentration in lubricant and intervals of lubricant replacement highly affect the wear of ZrO_2/UHMWPE. Formation of protein film and increase of initial wear must be the origin, respectively.

(2)Wear evaluation conditions are defined from the obtained data.

(3)Wear characterization is conducted on six types of clinically used hip joint prostheses under the conditions defined in this study. The results clearly exhibit the difference of wear property in each combination.

ACKNOWLEDGEMENT

This work is in part supported by the R&D Projects in "Development of artificial hip joint prostheses and its evaluation method" entrusted from the New Energy and Industrial Technology Development Organization (NEDO) to the Japan Fine Ceramics Center.

REFERENCES

[1]P. A. Revell, N. Al Saffar and A. Kobayashi, "Biological Reaction to Debris in Relation to Joint Prostheses", *Proc. Inst. Mech. Eng.* [H], 211, 187-197 (1997).

[2]J. P. Paul, "Forces Transmitted by Joints in the Human Body", *Inst. Mech. Eng. Proc.*, 181 Part 3J, 351-68 (1966-67).

[3]V. D. Good, I. C. Clarke, G. A. Gustafson, B. Downs, L. Anissian and K. Sorensen, "Wear of Ultra-High Molecular Weight Polyethylene and Polytetrafluoroethylene in a Hip Simulator", *Acta Orthop. Scand.*, 71, 365-369 (2000).

[4]A. Wang, V. K. Polineni, A. Essner, C. Stark and J. H. Dumbleton, "The Impact of Lubricant Protein Concentration on the Outcome of Hip Joint Simulator Testing", *Proceedings of 45th Annual Meeting, Orthopaedic Research Society* 52 (1999).

[5]H. Saari, S. Santavirta, D. Nordstrom, P. Paavolainen and Y. T. Konttinen, "Hyaluronate in Total Hip Replacement", *J. Rheum.*, 20, 87-90 (1993).

[6]A. Wang, V. K. Polineni, A. Essner, C. Stark and J. H. Dumbleton, "Quantitative Analysis of Serum Degradation and its Effect on The Outcome of Hip Joint Simulator Wear Testing of UHMWPE", *Proceedings of 45th Annual Meeting, Orthopaedic Research Society* 73 (1999).

[7]E. Nishimura and Y. Okazaki, to be published.

FABRICATION OF BIOCOMPATIBLE CALCIUM PHOSPHATE CERAMICS USING EGGSHELL

S.J. Lee
Dept. of Materials Science and Eng.,
Mopko University,
Muan, 532-729
Korea

W.M. Kriven
Department of Materials Science and Engineering
University of Illinois at Urbana-Champaign
1304 W. Green St.,
Urbana, IL 61801, USA

ABSTRACT

Biocompatible β-tricalcium phosphate (β-TCP) powders have been successfully synthesized from recycled eggshells and phosphoric acid. The crystallization behavior and microstructure of the synthesized powders were dependent on the mixing ratio of eggshells and phosphoric acid, the starting condition of the eggshell and on the calcination temperature. The syntheses were achieved at about 900°C in air. Phosphoric acid-treated eggshells converted to hydroxyapatite (HA) and tricalcium phosphate (TCP). They were examined in the TEM and their chemistry determined by TEM/EDS. Ball milled β-TCP powder, having an average particle size of 0.8 μm, was sintered at 1200°C for 2 h. Fully densified β-TCP showed biocompatibility and no toxicity.

INTRODUCTION

With the increasingly widespread interest in using synthetic ceramics for bone preforms and bone repair, it is of interest to see whether it is possible to make hydroxyapatite and tricalcium phosphates from other, readily available materials apart from pure chemical sources. There are numerous phases and compositions of calcium phosphate but those currently of interest include:

(i) hydroxyapatite ($Ca_{10}(PO_4)_6(OH)_2$ or "HA"),
(ii) monoclinic, α-tricalcium phosphate ($3CaO{\bullet}P_2O_5$) or Ca_3PO_4, or "α-TCP"),
(iii) rhombohedral, β-tricalcium phosphate ($3CaO{\bullet}P_2O_5$) or Ca_3PO_4, or "β-TCP"),
(iv) orthorhombic, dicalcium phosphate α-DCP ($2CaO{\bullet}P_2O_5$ or $Ca_2P_2O_7$), also known as calcium pyrophosphate ($Ca_2P_2O_5$ or "CCP"),
(v) tetragonal, dicalcium phosphate α-DCP ($2CaO{\bullet}P_2O_5$ or $Ca_2P_2O_7$), also known as calcium pyrophosphate ($Ca_2P_2O_5$ or "CCP").

In terms of bioresorbability in simulated body fluid, the relative rates of resorption are believed to be:

HA < β-TCP < α-TCP < β-DCP < α-TCP

Lee and Ho[1] have previously reported on the synthesis of powders derived from eggshells.[1] The aim if this work is to examine by TEM/EDS, the microstructures of powders produced from eggshells and deduce whether they would be suitable ceramic starting powders for making dense ceramic bodies as bone pre-forms. Optimum sintering conditions for β-TCP were determined.

EXPERIMENTAL PROCEDURES

The methods for synthesizing the calcium phosphate starting powders are summarized in the flow chart of Fig. 1. The mixing ratios (wt %) of 900°C calcined eggshells and phosphoric acid was varied according to the ratios eggshell : acid of 1 : 1.1, 1 : 1.3, 1 : 1.5 and 1 : 1.7. A ratio of 1 : 1.3 yielded essentially HA, while higher ratios yielded β-TCP. Powders derived from a ratio of 1 : 1.5 yielded β-TCP when calcined at any temperature in the range of 700°C to 1000°C for 1 h.

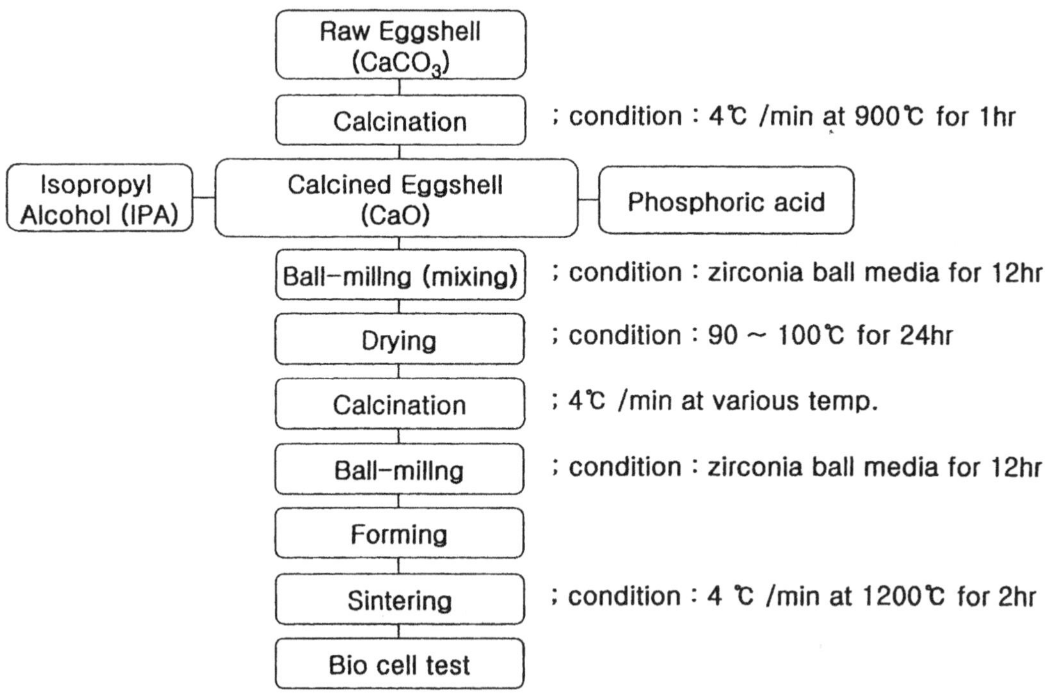

Fig. 1. Flow chart describing synthesis or calcium phosphate powders made from raw eggshells.

To break up any hard agglomerates and produce a uniform particle size, β-TCP made from a ratio of 1 : 1.5 was calcined at 900°C for 1 h, and wet ball-milled with zirconia media for 12 h, using isopropyl alcohol as the liquid phase. Dense pellets of β-TCP were prepared by heating at 4 °C in a furnace open to air and sintering at 1200°C for 2 h.

Representative powders of HA as well as of the β-TCP were prepared for TEM by crushing in an alumina mortar and pestle, suspending in isopropyl alcohol medium, and depositing onto a carbon support film mounted on a Cu TEM grid. The powders were carbon coated to provide a conducting layer following the normal practice for TEM powder preparation. The samples were examined in a Philips TEM (Philips Inc., Mawah, NJ.) operated at 120 KV and equipped with EDS capability for microchemical analysis.

RESULTS

Sedigraphy measurements of the β-TCP indicated an average particle size of 0.08 μm (Fig. 2).

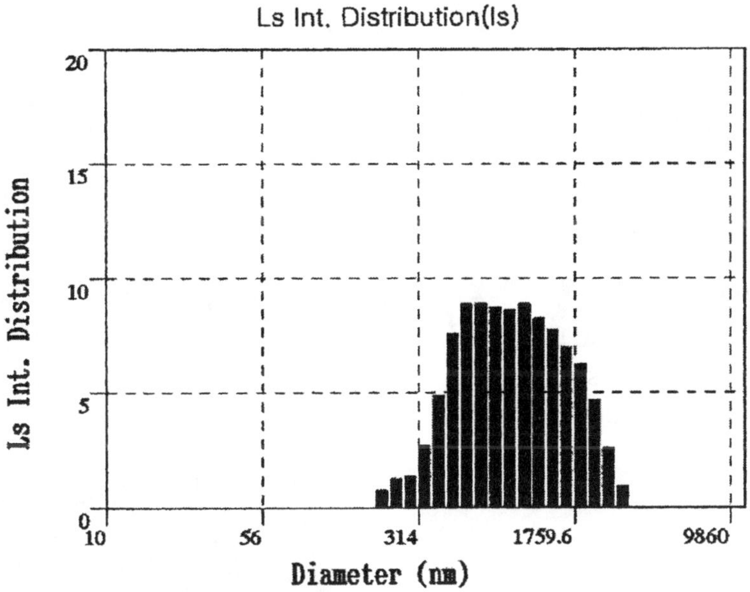

Fig. 2. Particle size distribution of β-TCP powders that had been fabricated from eggshells and wet milled in IPA using zirconia milling media, for 12 h.

SEM microstructures

The corresponding SEM microstructures of as milled and dried, phosphoric acid treated, eggshell mixture (Fig. 3) and wet milled, converted β-TCP is seen in Fig. 4. The dried mixture was widely agglomerated due to unreacted phosphoric acid. In contrast, the synthesized powder had relatively uniform particles of 2.0 μm. Relatively little grain growth had occurred.

TEM Microstructures

Hydroxyapatite Sample: TEM study of the HA sample confirmed a fine grained single crystalline powder as seen in Fig 5. Fig. 6 is the corresponding SAD pattern of a typical crystallite which was indexed as the [010] projection of the Z = 1 unit cell of hexagonal hydroxyapatite (HA). The EDS spectrum Fig. 7 indicated an atomic Ca:P ratio of 1.85, which is close to the 1.67 theoretically expected for HA.

B-TCP sample: The β-TCP sample was examined by TEM and EDS. The composition as seen in Fig. 8 had a molar ratio of $CaO:P_2O_5$ of 3.4 which is reasonably close to the expected 3.0 for tricalcium phosphate. As seen in Fig. 9, the powder consisted of submicron or micron sized single crystallites, as confirmed, for example in the selected area diffraction pattern (SADP) of Fig. 10. The pattern was indexed in the R-3c rhombohedral unit cell of $3CaO{\bullet}P_2O_5$.

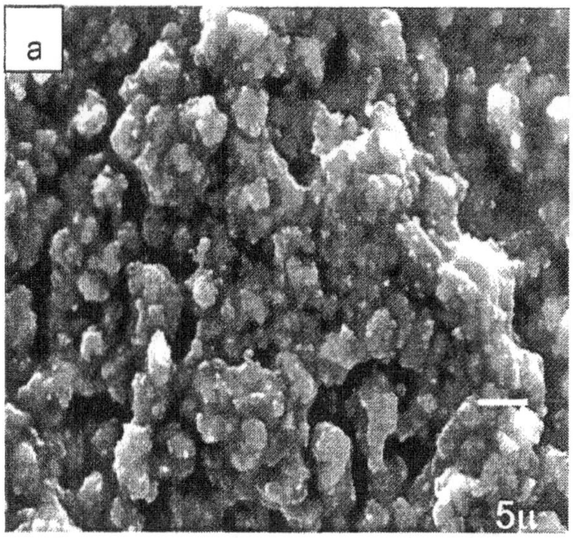

Fig. 3. SEM micrograph of as-milled, acid-treated and dried mixture.

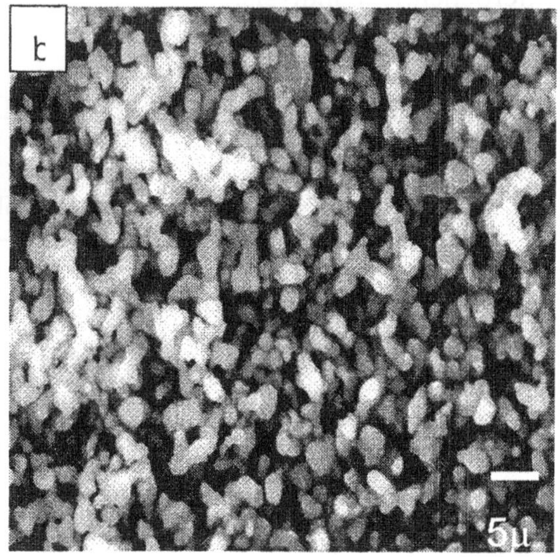

Fig. 4. SEM micrograph of calcined and converted β-TCP

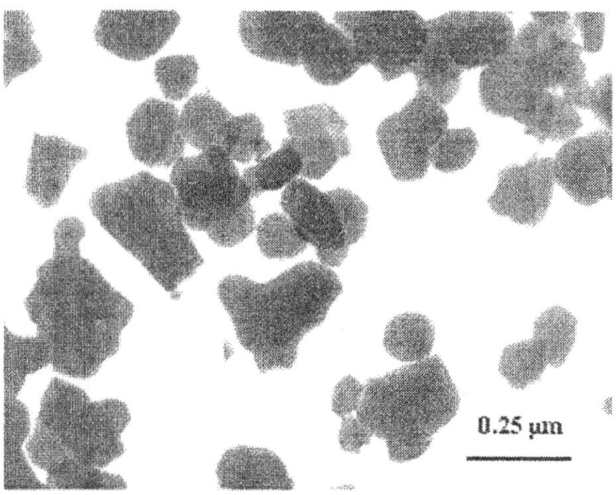

Fig. 5 BF TEM micrograph of HA powder

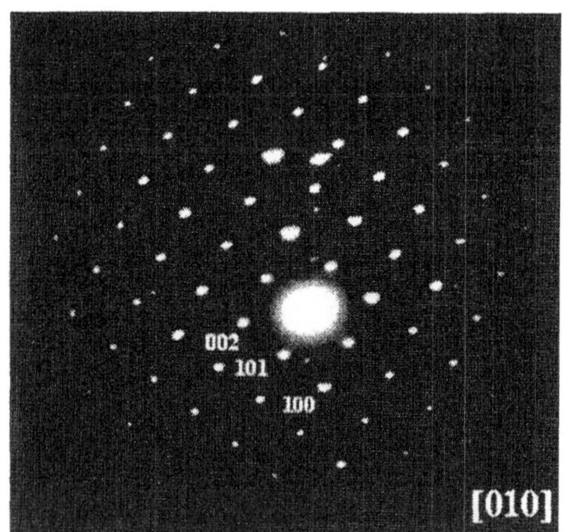

Fig. 6. TEM/SAD pattern of HA

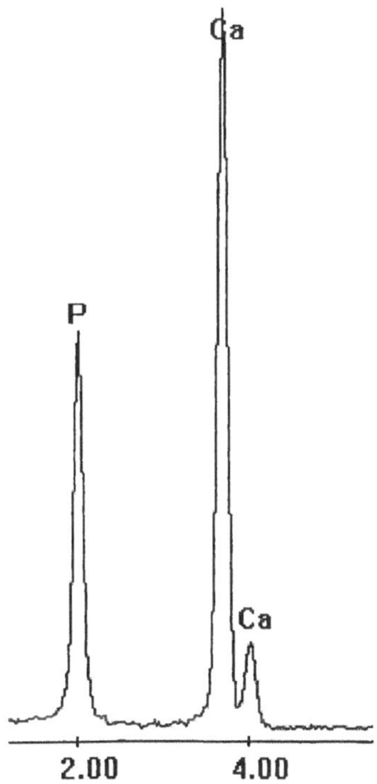

Fig. 7 EDS spectrum corresponding to a HA crystallite of Figs. 3 and 4. The Ca:P atomic ratio of 1.85 compares with1.67 for stoichiometric HA.

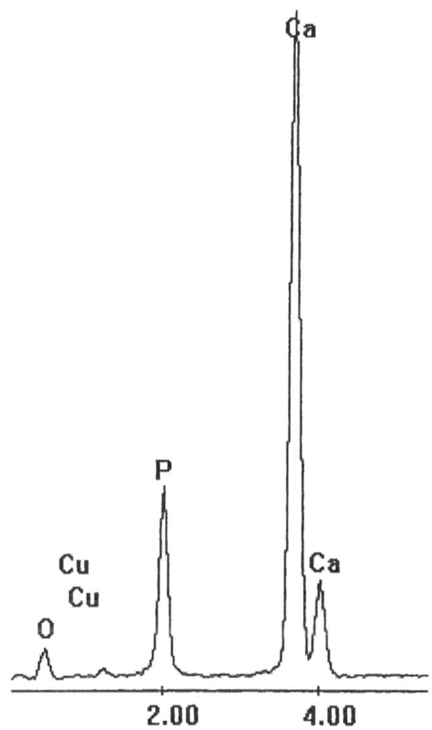

Fig. 8.EDS spectrum from a β-TCP grain containing a $CaO:P_2O_5$ ratio of 77 mol % CaO to 23 mol % P_2O_5, giving a ratio of 3.3 as compared to 3.0 for TCP.

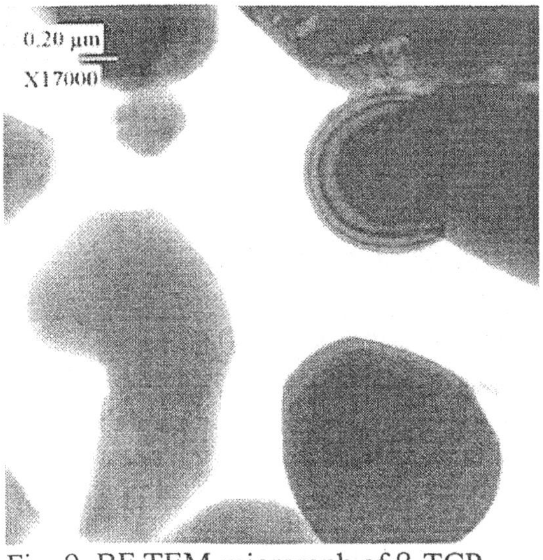

Fig. 9. BF TEM micrgraph of β-TCP

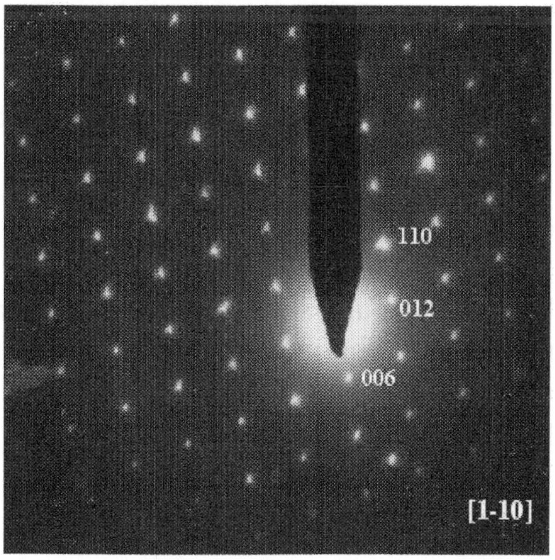

Fig. 10. TEM/SAD pattern of β-TCP

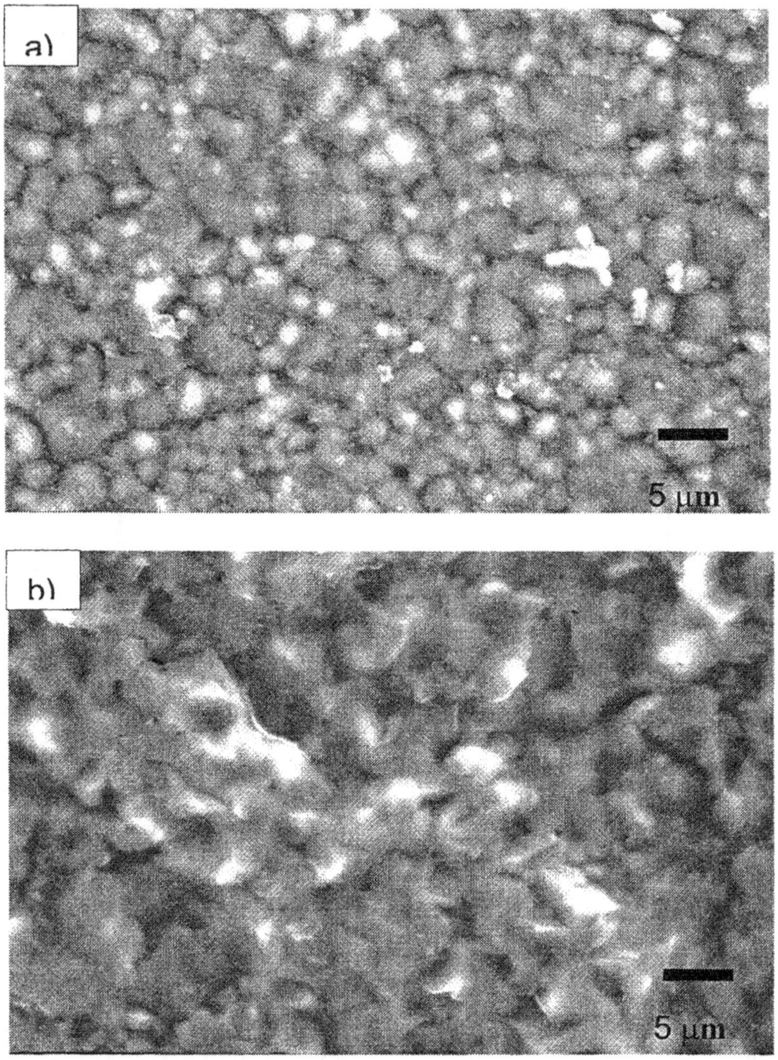

Fig. 11. SEM micrographs of (a) surface and (b) fracture surface of densified β-TCP sintered at 1200°C for 2h.

CONCLUSIONS

Hydroxy apatite (HA) and β-TCP powders of uniform particle sizes have been successfully synthesized from natural eggshells calcined at 900°C for 1h. By mixing with phosphoric acid and calcining again at various temperatures, and compositions, HA or β-TCP were formed. TEM/SAD and EDS confirmed that the powders were fine, single crystallites of the phases.

REFERENCE

[1]S.J. Lee and S.H. Oh, "Synthesis of Biocompatible Calcium Phosphate by Using an Eggshell," in *Bioceramics 15*; pp 35-38 Key Engineering Materials Series. Published by Trans Tech Publications Ltd., Uetikon a.S., Switzerland, 2003.

CALCIUM ALUMINATE/CALCIUM PHOSPHATE COMPOSITE ORTHOPEDIC BONE CEMENT

Maria L. Roemhildt
Department of Orthopedics and Rehabilitation
University of Vermont
Burlington, VA 05405-0084

Thomas D. McGee
MSE Department
Iowa State University
Ames, IA 50011

Stanley D. Wagner, D.V.M.
Department of Veterinary Clinical Sciences
College of Veterinary Medicine
Iowa State University
Ames, IA 50011

ABSTRACT

An improved cement for joint replacement surgery is needed to replace polymethylmethacrylate. A composite cement composed of calcium phosphate to control tissue response and calcium aluminate to produce set and enduring strength is described. High concentrations of $CaCl_2$ produce rapid strength and contribute to the bond by producing hydrated calcium chloroaluminates. When stored in simulated body fluids at 37°C changes in mass, dimensions, strength and composition occurs. Setting times and properties appear to warrant further investigation.

INTRODUCTION

Total joint replacements are widely used to repair defective joints. [1] Often these are cemented in place with polymethylmethacrylate (PMMA) cement. That cement has attributes needed for surgery but it has deficiencies such as excessive temperature rise in setting, lack of bonding at the cement/tissue interface, breakdown over time and inflammatory response from particulate debris. [2] PMMA cement has been identified as one of the factors that limit joint replacement life-times. There is a need for a better cement. This paper describes a composite ceramic cement that is intended to avoid the PMMA deficiencies.

Previous work on a fired ceramic composite has been based on the concept of a calcium phosphate component to control tissue response, with a second.

component to obtain enduring strength.[3] The cement described here is based on same concept, but calcium aluminate cement has been substituted for $MgAl_2O_4$ as the enduring component.

The solubility of calcium aluminates depends on the $CaO:Al_2O_3$ ratio (C/A ratio in cement notation). They are compatible with hard tissue.[4, 5, 6] Those with high C/A ratio have been studied as possible absorbable bone replacements.[8, 9] Commercial calcium aluminate cements have high early strength for concrete applications, and are resistant to dissolution in sea water.[10] Sea water is similar to salt concentrations to blood plasma. The commercial cements have C/A ratios slightly above 1:1, often with some CA_2, $C_{12}A_7$, and free Al_2O_3. The calcium aluminates may be suitable to combine with calcium phosphates to produce bioactive bone cements.

Orthopedic cements must have properties dictated by the surgical procedure and, after setting, must be strong. The requirements for PMMA cement include:[11]

Working time 5.0 min
Setting time 5-15 min
Max temperature 90°C
Min compressive strength 70 MPa at 7 days

Commercial high alumina cements set slower than required for orthopedic surgery.[12] The exothermic setting reactions do not produce excessive temperature rise. The setting reactions and hydrated products depend upon temperature.[13] Although the literature is inconsistent, accelerators such as chlorides of Li, Na, K, Ca, Mg, Sr and NH_4 either change nucleation ($LiCl_2$) or modify the setting reactions rate.[14] In general low concentrations accelerate the setting and higher concentrations retard the setting. This includes $CaCl_2$. Temperature also affects the setting behavior.[15] The effect of calcium phosphates added to calcium aluminate cements is not clear, but usually reduces strength and retards setting. Background experiments were conducted to find a suitable biologically active calcium phosphate to use with CA cement.

Initial experiments varying cement composition, finding compatible calcium phosphates, and evaluating accelerators were completed. High concentrations of calcium chloride were adopted as the accelerator.

MATERIALS AND METHODS

Calcium aluminate cement with a molar CA ratio of 0.82 containing CA, CA_2 and small amounts of $C_{12}A_7$ and A was selected. Tricalcium phosphate (β-TCP) [Fluka Chemicals] was used as the calcium phosphate component because of its bioactivity, particle size and purity. Reagent grade chemicals were used as accelerators.

The CA cement and TCP were mixed dry. The accelerator was dissolved in CO_2-free deionized water. The accelerator solution was added with stirring to the dry ingredients, using concentrations that minimized the water to cement ratio

The working time was estimated by measuring the time at which wet cement did not adhere to a small spatula when inserted and withdrawn. Setting time was estimated by determining the time when the spatula would not dent the hardened cement paste under moderate force. The cement pastes were cast in acrylic molds, vibrated and struck off. After setting they were transferred to a sealed container containing lactated Ringers solution and stored at 37°C.

Compressive strength of 2mm x 16mm height cylinders was determined with an Instron model 4202 testing instrument at 1mm/min. Diametral tension cylinders were 12mm x 4.8mm in length. Saturated masses and diameters were measured periodically. The temperature rise was measured in general accordance with ASTM F451-95 using a Styrofoam cup as an adiabatic calorimeter and a type J thermocouple. Mineralogical analyses were based on x-ray diffraction using a Siemens D-500 instrument at 50KV and 40ma.

The composition of the cement powders was 66 2/3 CA and 33 1/2 TCP weight percent. Adding $CaCl_2$ in high concentrations changed the over-all composition as reported below.

RESULTS AND DISCUSSION

Calcium chloride concentrations were varied to modify setting time. Compressive strength at 24 hours and one week were determined because accelerators affect strength (Table 1,)

Table I Effect of $CaCl_2$ on Setting Time and One Week Strength

Mols, $CaCl_2$	Set Time (min)	Strength, (MPa)
0	120	30
0.01	360	18
0.10	100	45
1.00	21	84
2.00	15	102
3.00	20	88
4.00	22	55

The maximum setting time and high strength were in accordance with surgical requirements using 2M $CaCl_2$. Including the $CaCl_2$ the composition before setting was, 64.5% CA, 37.3% TCP, and 3.2% $CaCl_2$. The temperature rise of the setting reaction for this cement was 15.5°C when cast at room temperature of 22°C. This is much lower than PMMA cements have.

The strength with time is given in Fig. 1. Note the non-linear time scale:

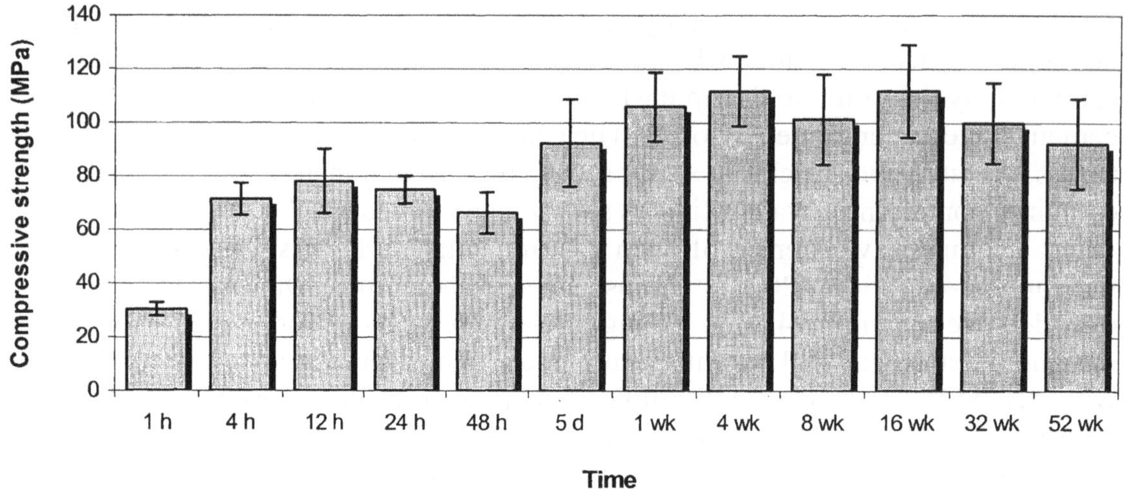

Fig. 1. Compressive Strength of O.C. Cement as a Function of Time.

The mass and dimensions of the cast cylinders stored in lactated Ringers solution increased with time (Fig. 2,3). PMMA shrinks. The small, continued expansion may prevent loosening.

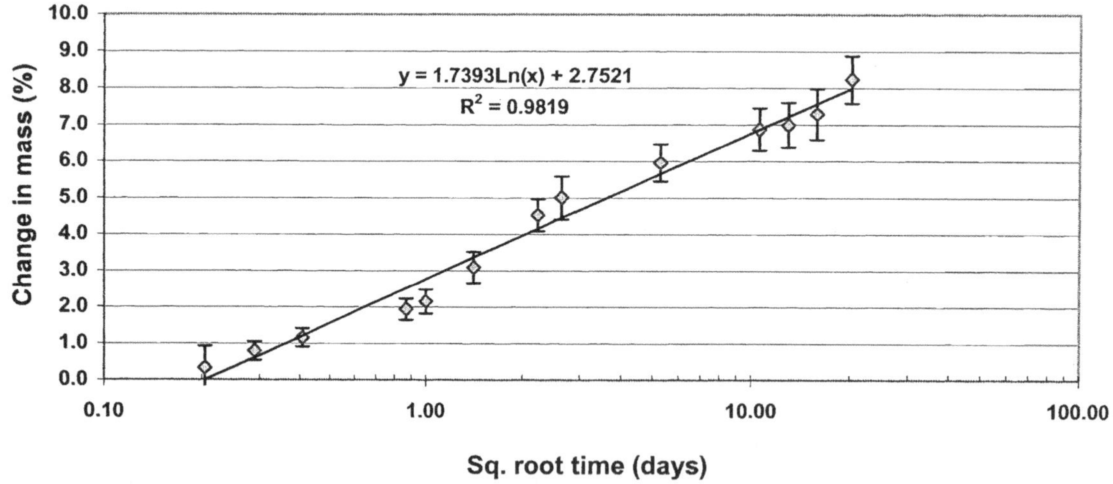

Fig. 2. Increase in Mass as a Function of Time

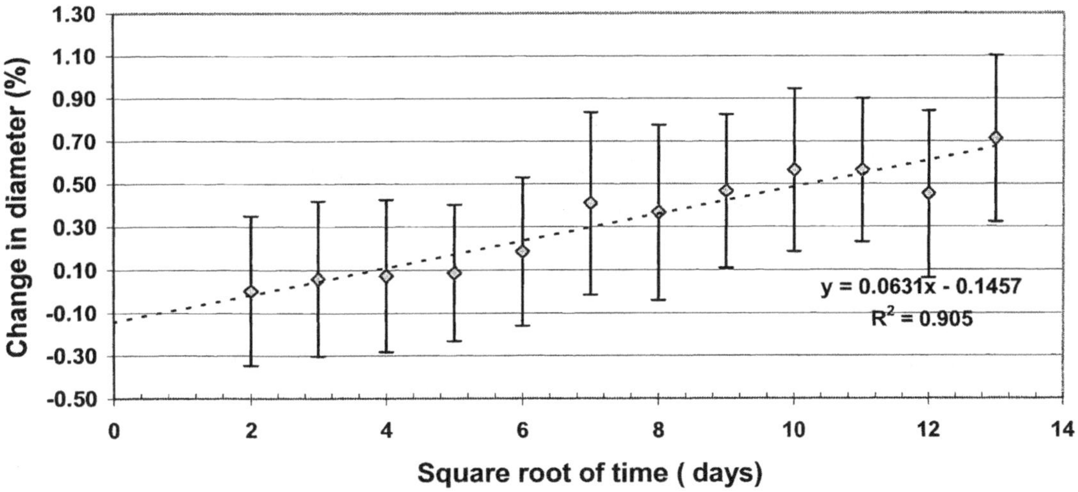

Fig. 3. Increase in Specimen Diameter as a Function of Time

The increase in both the mass and the diameter is parabolic in time, typical of a diffusion controlled reaction. This is consistent with hydration of other hydraulic cements where unreacted cement continues to hydrate. X-Ray diffraction results show a continuous increase in the concentration of AH_3, C_3AH_6 and calcium aluminate chlorohydrate and a concomitant decrease in CA and CA_2. No C_2AH_8 or CAH_{10} was found. Slow, continued hydration is normal for hydraulic cements.

CONCLUSION

A biologically-active orthopedic cement based on calcium phosphates to enhance tissue response and calcium aluminate to give enduring strength has been investigated. The resulting cement appears to satisfy the ASTM requirements for PMMA orthopedic cements. These are only the initial requirements. Tissue compatibility, long term strength and brittle fracture behavior have not been evaluated here. A patent application has been submitted.

REFERENCES

1. J.B. Park and R.S. Lakes Biomaterials – An Introduction 2nd ed. Plenum Press New York 1992
2. J.A. Planell, MM. Vila, F.J. Gil and F.M.C. Driessens, "Acrylic Bone Cements" pp. 879-922 in D. Wise, D. Trantolo, D. Altobelli, M. Yaszemski, J. Gesser & E. Schwartz, eds. Encyclopedic Handbook of

Biomaterials and Bioengineering Part B, Vol. 2. Marcel Dekker, New York, 1995.

3. T.D. McGee, "Artificial Bone and Tooth Material" US Pat. # 3,787,900, 1974
4. J.J. Klawitter & S.F. Hulbert, "Application of Porous Ceramics for the Attachment of Load Bearing Internal Orthopedic Prostheses" J. Biomed. Mat. Res. Symp. No. 2 (161-229) 1971.
5. J. Autian & J.E. Hammer, "A Toxicity Profile for Calcium Aluminate" J. Dent. Res. 51 (880) 1972.
6. G.D. Schnittgrund, G.H. Kenner & S.D. Brown, "*In Vivo* and *In Vitro* Changes in Strength of Orthopedic Calcium Aluminates" J. Biomed. Mat. Res. Symp. No. 4 (435-452) 1973.
7. A. Uchida, S. Nade, W. McCartney & W. Ching, "Bone Ingrowth into Three Different Porous Ceramics Implanted into the Tibia of Rats and Rabbits", J. Orth. Res. 3 (65-67) 1985.
8. G.A. Graves, R.L. Hentrick, H.D. Stein and P.K. Bajpai, "Resorbable Ceramic Implants", J. Biomed. Mater. Res. Symp. No. 2 (Part 1) (91-111) 1971.
9. B. Carvalho, G.A. Graves and P.K. Bajpai, "Calcium and Inorganic Phosphate Contents of Implanted Resorbable Porous Calcium Aluminate Ceramics", IRCS Medical Science: Biomedical Technology; Connective Tissue, Skin and Bone; Surgery and Transplantation 3 (185) 1975.
10. N.C. Baker and P.F. Banfill, "Properties of Fresh Mortars made with High Alumina Cements for Marine Environments" in Calcium Aluminates (R.J. Mangabhai, ed.) E. & F.N. Spon, Cambridge, Great Britain, 1990.
11. ASTM, F451-95, "Standard Specification for Acrylic Bone Cement" American Society for Testing and Materials, Conshohocken PA, 1995
12. W.H. Gitzen, L.D. Hart and G.W. MacZura, "Properties of Some Calcium Aluminate Cement Compositions" J. Am. Cer. Soc. 40 (158-167) 1957.
13. C.M. George, Manufacture and Performance of Aluminous Cement: a New Perspective, pp. 181-207 in Calcium Aluminate Cements (R.J. Mangabhai, ed.) E. & F.N. Spon, Cambridge, Great Britain 1990.
14. B.R. Currell, R. Grzeskowlak, H.G. Midgley and J.R. Parsonage, The Acceleration and Retardation of Set of High Alumina Cement by Additives" Cem. Com. Res. 17 (420-432) 1987.
15. M.R. Nilforoushan and J.H. Sharp, "The Effect of Additions of Alkaline Earth Metal Chlorides of the Setting Behavior of Refractory Calcium Aluminate Cement", Cem. Com. Res. 25 (1523-1534) 1995.

FABRICATION OF COMPOSITE FOR BONE REPAIRING FROM α-TRICALCIUM PHOSPHATE AND HYDROXYPROPYLCELLULOSE

Toshiki Miyazaki
Graduate School of Life Science and Systems Engineering, Kyushu Institute of Technology, 2-4 Hibikino, Wakamatsu-ku, Kitakyushu-shi, Fukuoka 808-0196, Japan

Chikara Ohtsuki, Haruna Iwasaki, Shin-ichi Ogata and Masao Tanihara
Graduate School of Materials Science, Nara Institute of Science and Technology, 8916-5 Takayama-cho, Ikoma-shi, Nara 630-0192, Japan

ABSTRACT

Tricalcium phosphate (TCP) ceramics is known as bioresorbable bone substitute in orthopedic field. Porous body of TCP has also high potential for application of drug delivery system in bony defect. Porous body of α-TCP can be easily fabricated through sintering β-TCP by conventional process, since α-TCP is thermodynamically stable phase at higher temperature than 1100°C. The problem is, however, that solubility of α-TCP is much higher than that of β-TCP. Therefore dissolution of the porous α-TCP ceramic is liable to progress much faster than bone repair. In the present study, we attempted to reduce dissolution rate of the porous α-TCP ceramic by coating with an organic polymer. We fabricated α-TCP porous body with continuous pores of 10-50 μm in diameter through conventional sintering process. The obtained porous body was coated with hydroxypropylcellulose (HPC). Several heat treatments were then applied for the HPC-coated porous α-TCP to increase mechanical strength and chemical durability. Chemical durability was examined in some buffer solutions with various pH by measurement of Ca^{2+} ion. Changes in crystalline phases are also analyzed with powder X-ray diffraction. The results on dissolution of α-TCP in buffer solutions showed that chemical durability increased by coating with HPC, followed by drying at 60°C and heat treatment at 100°C. Compressive strength of the porous α-TCP was also improved by coating with HPC. Thus prepared porous α-TCP is expected to be useful as a novel bone substitute by incorporating with drugs or osteoinductive factors.

INTRODUCTION

Tricalcium phosphate (TCP, $Ca_3(PO_4)_2$) is popularly known as one of bioresorbable ceramics [1-5]. TCP ceramics with continuous pores is gradually dissolved according to bone repair when implanted in bony defects, leading to complete substitution by the regenerated bone. It has been already subjected to clinical use as bone fillers. In addition, novel functions can be provided with the porous TCP, if drugs or osteoinductive factors are incorporated with it [6-8]. α-TCP is thermodynamically stable phase at higher temperature than 1100°C. Therefore porous body of α-TCP can be easily fabricated through sintering β-TCP by conventional process. Solubility of α-TCP is, however, much higher than that of β-TCP [9]. It is liable to be completely resorbed in the body before the bony defect is sufficiently repaired by the regenerated bone [10]. Therefore control of dissolution behavior of α-TCP ceramic has been desired.

In the present study, we attempted to prepare composite from porous α-TCP ceramic and organic polymer in order to improve chemical durability of the α-TCP ceramic. Hydroxypropylcellulose (HPC) with structure shown in Fig. 1 was selected as a polymer, since it has attractive features such as high ability of film formation, biodegradation, and low toxicity [11-12]. We fabricated the composites by coating with HPC on porous α-TCP ceramic, and investigated their chemical durability and mechanical property.

METHODS

β-TCP powder with particle size less than 45 μm and equivalent mass of potato starch were dispersed into distilled water to form a slurry. A polyurethane sponge 15 x 15 x 15 mm^3 in size was dipped in the slurry and dried at 60°C for 1 h. The specimen was then heated up to 1000°C at a rate of 5°C/min and kept at 1000°C for 3 h to remove the sponge. After cooling to room temperature, it was heated up to 1400°C at a rate of 5°C/min and kept at 1400°C for 12 h, followed by cooling in the furnace. Thus obtained porous body was soaked in 5 mass% of HPC aqueous solution and then dried at 60°C for 24 h. The prepared specimen is hereafter denoted as HPC60. Some specimens were further heat-treated at 100 and 140°C for 2 h. The specimens heat-treated at 100 and 140°C are hereafter denoted as HPC100 and HPC140, respectively.

Structure of the specimens was characterized by powder X-ray diffraction and scanning electron microscope (SEM) observation. In order to evaluate chemical durability of the specimens, they were soaked in 30 mL of buffer solutions at pH 4, 6 or 7.25 at 36.5°C for 7 d. Potassium hydrogen phthalate, 2-(*N*-morpholino) ethanesulfonic acid (MES) and tris(hydroxyethyl)aminomethane was used as buffer of pH 4, 6 and 7.25, respectively. Ca^{2+} concentration of the buffer solutions after soaking of the specimens was measured by a Ca^{2+} electrode. Compressive strength was quantitatively evaluated by an Instron-type material testing machine at cross-head speed of 20 mm/min.

Some specimens were then subjected to animal experiments. A hole of 4 mm in diameter was made at the medial aspect of the proximal metaphysis of the tibiae of Japanese white rabbits. The specimens 4 mm in diameter and 5 mm in length was then inserted into the hole. After 4 w implantation, the rabbits were sacrificed and the implanted specimens along with the bony tissues were extracted. The implants as well as surrounding bony tissues were observed by X-ray computed tomography (X-CT).

RESULTS

Figure 2 shows powder X-ray diffraction pattern of the porous ceramics. Peaks assigned to α-TCP were detected. This indicates that the prepared porous body was composed of only crystalline α-TCP. Figure 3 shows SEM photographs of the inside of the porous specimens. The porous body of α-TCP ceramic before coating with HPC contained continuous pores with diameter ranging from 10 to 50 μm. The morphology was almost the same even after coating with HPC and subsequent heat treatment. Figure 4 shows Ca^{2+} concentration of the buffer solutions at various pH after soaking of the porous specimens for 7 d. Release of Ca^{2+} into the buffer solutions corresponds to dissolution of porous α-TCP ceramic. HPC100 showed the lowest Ca^{2+} concentration in buffer solutions with any pH. Figure 5 shows compressive strength of the porous specimens. Compressive strength increased after coating with HPC and subsequent heat treatments. Figure 6 shows CT scanning of the porous specimens implanted in rabbit tibia for 4 w. Blank means that nothing was implanted into the bony defect as reference. Some voids were observed inside the tibia for Blank and α-TCP without coating. This indicates that the defect is not completely repaired by the regenerated bone. On the other hand, the bone defect was almost repaired by the regenerated bone for HPC60. In addition, osteocondcution was observed inside the tibia. These indicate that HPC60 was gradually dissolved and substituted by the new bone according to bone repair.

DISCUSSION

The present method easily produces porous α-TCP ceramic with continuous pores ranging 10 to 50 μm in diameter by conventional sintering. Chemical durability of porous α-TCP ceramic can be improved by simple coating with HPC and subsequent heat treatment at appropriate temperature, although further heat treatment at 140°C adversely affects (see Fig. 4). Optimum behavior of bioresorption in bony defect for HPC60 supports the results concerning the improved chemical durability (see Fig. 6). This reduced dissolution of porous α-TCP ceramic is attributed for the protective effect of the HPC coating on the porous α-TCP against surrounding buffer solutions. Therefore the skeleton of α-TCP porous body was able to sufficiently play a role in scaffold for bone regeneration.

It should be noted that increased compressive strength by the coating with HPC shows that modification with HPC has another role in improving workability during clinical use as well as chemical durability of the porous α-TCP ceramic (see Fig. 5). This is attributed to cross-linking of hydroxyl groups in HPC after the heat treatment.

CONCLUSIONS

It was found that composite fabricated from porous α-TCP ceramic and HPC showed higher chemical durability and workability than as-prepared porous α-TCP. This type of simple organic modification is expected to be applicable to another bioresorbable ceramics. Furthermore novel bone-repairing materials with ability to enhance bone regeneration can be designed by combination of drugs or osteoinductive factors.

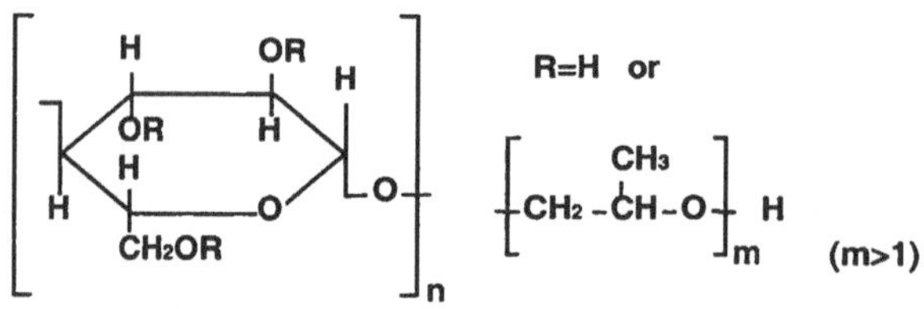

Figure 1. Structural formula of hydroxypropylcellulose (HPC).

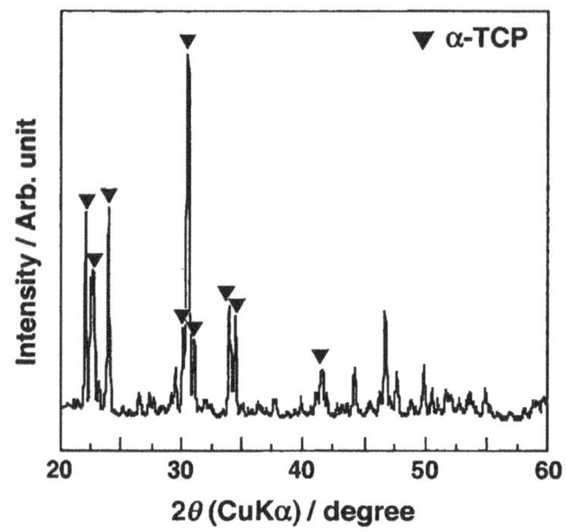

Figure 2. Powder X-ray diffraction pattern of the porous ceramics.

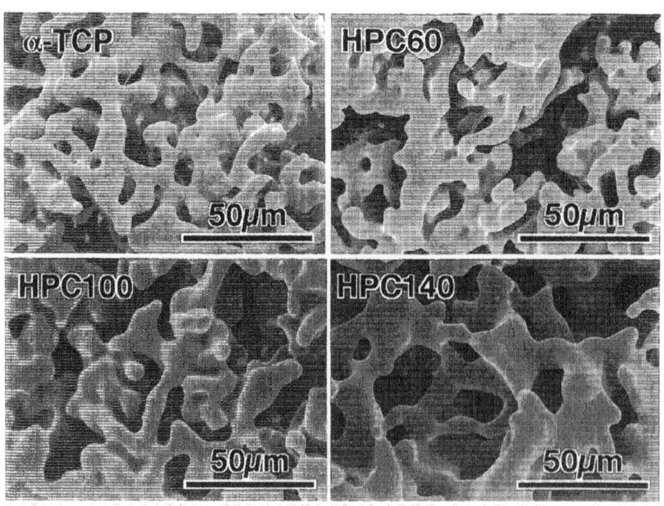

Figure 3. SEM photographs of the inside of the porous specimens. As-prepared porous ceramic is denoted as α-TCP.

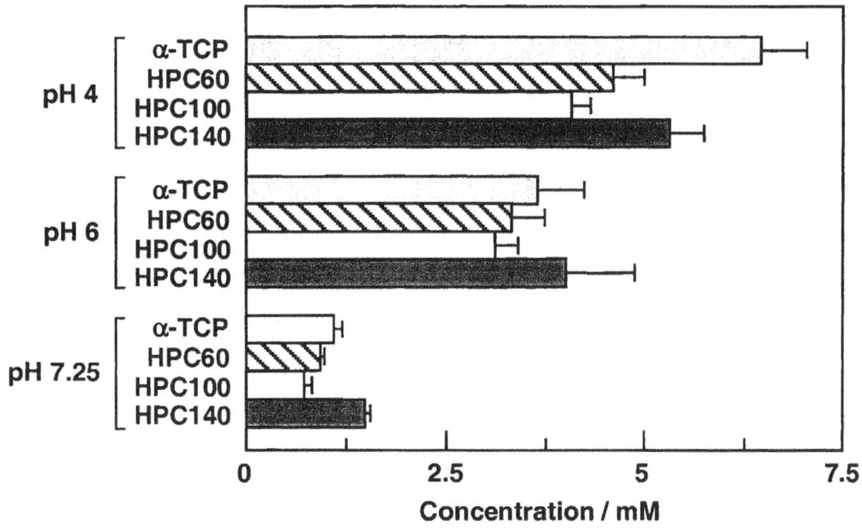

Figure 4. Ca^{2+} concentration of the buffer solutions at various pH after soaking of the porous specimens for 7 d (n=5).

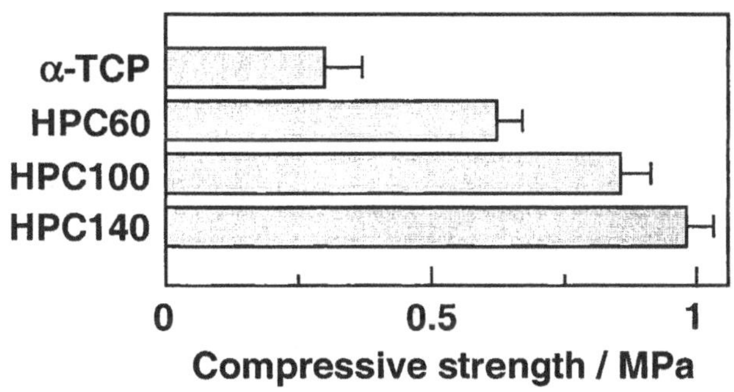

Figure 5. Compressive strength of the porous specimens (n=5).

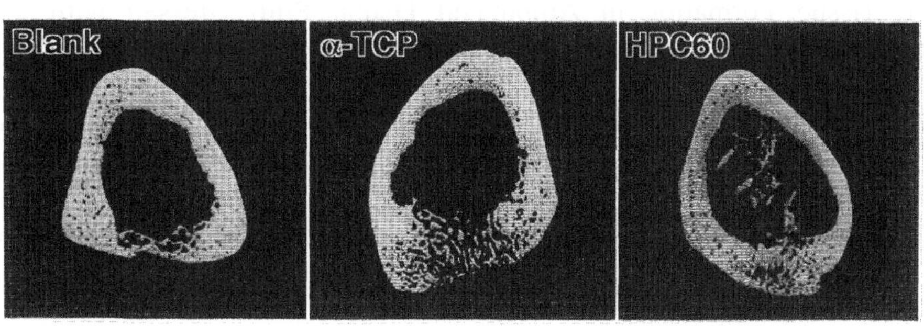

Figure 6. CT scanning of the porous specimens implanted in rabbit tibia for 4 w. Arrow indicates the implanted site.

ACKNOWLEDGMENTS

This work was supported by Industrial Technology Research Grant Program in 2001 from New Energy and Industrial Technology Development Organization (NEDO) of Japan.

REFERENCES

[1]B.V. Rejda, J.G.J. Peelen and K. deGroot, "Tricalcium Phosphate as a Bone Substitute", *Journal of Bioengineering,* **1** [2] 93-97 (1977).

[2]D.S. Metsger, T.D. Driskell and J.R. Paulsrud, "Tricalcium Phosphate Ceramic Resorbable Bone Implant Review and Current Status," *Journal of the American Dental Association,* **105** [6] 1035-1038 (1982).

[3]P. Ducheyne, S. Radin and L. King, "The effect of Calcium Phosphate Ceramic Composition and Structure on *in vitro* Behavior. I. Dissolution," *Journal of Biomedical Materials Research,* **27** [1] 25-34 (1993).

[4]H. Oonishi and H. Oomamiuda, "Degradation/resorption in Bioactive Ceramics in Orthopaedics," pp. 406-419 in *Handbook of Biomaterial Properties.* Edited by J. Black and G. Hastings. Chapman & Hall, London, 1998.

[5]H. Yuan, J.D. deBruijn, Y. Li, J. Feng, Z. Yang, K. deGroot and X. Zhang, "Bone Formation Induced by Calcium Phosphate Ceramics in Soft Tissue of Dogs: A Comparative Study Between Porous α-TCP and β-TCP," *Journal of Materials Science: Materials in Medicine,* **12** [1] 7-13 (2001).

[6]T. Gao, T.S. Lindholm, A. Marttinen and M.R. Urist. "Composites of Bone Morphogenetic Protein (BMP) and Type IV Collagen, Coral-derived Coral Hydroxyapatite, and Tricalcium Phosphate Ceramics," *International Orthopaedics,* **20** [5] 321-325 (1996).

[7]M. Itokazu, T. Sugiyama, T. Ohno, E. Wada and Y. Katagiri. "Development of Porous Apatite Ceramic for Local Delivery of Chemotherapeutic Agents," *Journal of Biomedical Materials Research,* **39** [4] 536-538 (1998).

[8]A. Scott, K. Higdon, M. Tucci, H. Benghuzzi, A. Puckett, A. Tsao, Z. Cason and J. Hughes. "The Prevention of Osteoporotic Progression by Means of Steroid Loaded TCPL Drug Delivery Systems," *Biomedical Sciences Instrumentation,* **37** 13-18 (2001).

[9]L.C. Chow, "Development of Self-setting Calcium Phosphate Cement," *Journal of the Ceramic Society of Japan,* **99** [10] 945-964 (1991).

[10]K. Ikami, M. Iwaku and H. Ozawa, "An Ultrastructure Study of the Process of Hard Tissue Formation in Amputated Dental Pulp Dressed with Alpha-tricalcium Phosphate," *Archives of Histology and Cytology,* **53** [2] 227-243 (1990).

[11]L.A. Grabowski, J.V. Bondi and R.J. Harwood, "Dissolution Rate Studies of Compression-molded Units Made from Hydroxypropyl Cellulose Films," *Journal of Pharmaceutical Sciences,* **74** [5] 540-544 (1985).

[12]E. Izeboud, "Biocompatibility of Cellulose and Cellulose Derivatives," *Papier,* **46** [12] 722-725 (1992).

PREPARATION OF BIOACTIVE INORGANIC-ORGANIC HYBRIDS BY HOT WATER TREATMENT

M. Kawashita, M. Kamitakahara, N. Miyata and T. Kokubo
Department of Material Chemistry
Graduate School of Engineering
Kyoto University
Sakyo-ku, Kyoto 606-8501
Japan

T. Nakamura
Department of Orthopaedic Surgery
Graduate School of Medicine
Kyoto University
Sakyo-ku, Kyoto 606-8507
Japan

ABSTRACT

Bioactive inorganic-organic hybrids with high flexibility are useful for a new kind of bone-repairing materials. In the present study, preparation of bioactive poly(dimethylsiloxane) (PDMS) or poly(tetramethylene oxide) (PTMO)-TiO_2 hybrids was attempted by sol-gel method and subsequent hot water treatment. Both of the hybrids showed an apatite-forming ability in a simulated body fluid with ion concentrations nearly equal to those of human blood plasma. It is considered that apatite formation is induced by anatase precipitated by the hot water treatment. The resultant hybrids showed high deformability. It can be concluded that bioactive inorganic-organic hybrids with high flexibility can be obtained by the present method.

INTRODUCTION

Some ceramics, such as Bioglass®, sintered hydroxyapatite, and glass-ceramic A-W, form bone-like apatite on their surfaces in the living body, and bond to living bone through the apatite layer. Although these bioactive ceramics are used clinically as important bone-repairing materials, they are brittle and hence, limited in their applications. It is desirable to develop new types of deformable bioactive materials.

It has been revealed that some poly(dimethylsiloxane) (PDMS)-CaO-SiO_2 and its related hybrids prepared by a sol-gel method show high apatite-forming ability in a simulated body fluid (SBF), as well as deformability [1]. This indicates a possibility that these deformable hybrids can form apatite on their surfaces even in the living body, and bond to living bone through the apatite layer. However, these CaO-containing PDMS-CaO-SiO_2 and its related hybrids show a decrease in mechanical strength by aging in SBF. The hybrids containing no CaO do not form apatite on their surfaces in SBF within 14 d.

Recently, it has been shown that apatite formation on titania gel significantly depends on its structure. Anatase type Ti-OH groups can most effectively induce apatite nucleation, whereas Ti-OH groups in the amorphous and rutile structure are not so effective [2]. It is expected that even a CaO-free hybrid can show high apatite-forming ability, if the structure of a TiO_2-based hybrid is controlled. In the present study, PDMS or poly(tetramethylene oxide) (PTMO)-TiO_2 hybrids were prepared by a sol-gel method and subsequently subjected to hot-water treatments. Their apatite-forming ability on their surfaces in SBF and mechanical properties were investigated.

EXPERIMENTAL

Preparation of hybrids

PDMS-TiO_2 hybrids: Tetraethylorthotitanate (TEOT), ethylacetoacetate (EAcAc) and ethanol (EtOH) were mixed at a molar ratio of [TEOT/EAcAc/EtOH] = [1/2/4] and stirred for 30 min under ambient conditions. Polydimethylsiloxane (PDMS, HO-[-Si$(CH_3)_2$-O-]$_n$-H, 550 in molecular weight) was then added to the mixture. After 30 min, a mixture of ultra-pure water and the rest of the EtOH was added to the solution, resulting in a solution whose composition is given in Table 1. After stirring for 30 min, the solution was poured into a cylindrical Teflon® container, 75 mm in diameter and 20 mm in depth covered with an aluminum foil having a single pinhole, and kept at 70°C for 2 d, at 100°C for 2 d, and finally at 150 °C for 3 d.

Table 1 Starting compositions of PDMS-TiO_2 hybrids

Notation	Composition in molar ratio			
	PDMS/TEOT (Si/Ti)	EAcAc/TEOT	H_2O/TEOT	EtOH/TEOT
PD2	0.27 (2)	2	2	8
PD5	0.68 (5)	2	2	8
PD10	1.35 (10)	2	2	8

PTMO-TiO_2 hybrids: Poly(tetramethylene oxide) (PTMO, HO-(-$CH_2CH_2CH_2CH_2O$-)$_n$-H, 1000 in molecular weight) and 3-isocyanatopropyltriethoxysilane (IPTS, $(C_2H_5O)_3SiCH_2CH_2CH_2NCO$) were stirred at [PTMO/IPTS] = [1/2] in molar ratio under nitrogen atmosphere at 70°C for 5 d, to obtain triethoxysilane-functionalized PTMO (Si-PTMO). Solutions with compositions given in Table 2 were prepared in glass beakers under ambient conditions. The mixture of hydrochloric acid (HCl, 35 wt%), a half amount of ultra-pure water (H_2O) and 11 ml of isopropyl alcohol (IPA), was slowly added to tetraisopropyltitanate (TiPT, Ti$(OCH(CH_3)_2)_4$). The total amount of [TiPT+Si-PTMO] was fixed at 10 g. A given mass of Si-PTMO dissolved in 7.5 ml of IPA was then added to the obtained solution. After stirring for 10 min, a mixture of the other half of the H_2O and 5 ml of IPA was slowly added to the solution, and it was stirred for another 10 min. The obtained solution was poured into a cylindrical Teflon® container 75 mm in diameter and 20 mm in depth covered with a paraffin film having several pinholes, and it was kept under ambient conditions for 4–5 w for gelation and drying.

Table 2 Starting compositions of PTMO-TiO_2 hybrids

Notation	Composition			
	Si-PTMO/TiPT (weight ratio)	H_2O/TiPT (molar ratio)	HCl/TiPT (molar ratio)	IPA/(Si-PTMO+TiPT) (weight ratio)
PT30	30/70	2	0.05	1.85
PT40	40/60	2	0.05	1.85
PT50	50/50	2	0.05	1.85

Hot water treatment

Specimens 10 × 10 × (1–2) mm^3 in size were cut from the as-prepared hybrids and polished with a #400 silicon carbide abrasive paper. They were soaked in 10 ml ultra-pure water at 80°C for 7 d or 95°C for 2 d. After various periods, they were removed from the hot water, washed with ultra-pure water and dried at room temperature.

Soaking in SBF

Specimens 10 × 10 × (1–2) mm^3 in size of as-prepared, and subjected to the hot-water treatments materials were soaked in 30 ml SBF at 36.5°C with pH 7.40 and ion concentrations (Na^+ 142.0, K^+ 5.0, Ca^{2+} 2.5, Mg^{2+} 1.5, Cl^- 148.8, HCO_3^- 4.2, HPO_4^{2-} 1.0, SO_4^{2-} 0.5 mM) nearly equal to those of human blood plasma.

Analysis of structures of hybrids

The structures of the hybrids before and after the hot-water treatment and subsequent soaking in SBF were analyzed by thin-film X-ray diffraction (TF-XRD), a transmission electron microscope (TEM) equipped with an electron diffractometer, and a field emission scanning electron microscope (FE-SEM).

Evaluation of mechanical properties of hybrids

As-prepared hybrid PD10 was abraded with a #2000 SiC abrasive paper, and then dumbbell-type specimens were stamped out using a cutting die. Rectangular specimens 3×4×30 mm^3 in size were cut from as-prepared hybrid PT40 and polished with the same abrasive paper. Hybrids PD10 and PT40 were subjected to hot-water treatment at 80°C for 7 d and 95°C for 2 d, respectively. These specimens treated with hot water were subsequently soaked in SBF at 36.5°C for 28 d. Mechanical properties were measured for the specimens before and after the hot-water treatment, and those after both the hot-water and SBF treatments, using an Instron-type testing machine. The specimens after soaking in SBF were tested within 5 min after removal from SBF.

RESULTS AND DISCUSSION

Structures of hybrids

PDMS-TiO_2 hybrids: The hybrid of composition PD2 formed many cracks. Bubble- and crack-free transparent brown hybrids were obtained for compositions PD5 and PD10. Hybrid PD5 formed many cracks after the hot-water treatment, whereas hybrid PD10 was crack-free even after the hot-water treatment at 80°C for 7 d. TF-XRD patterns of the surfaces of hybrids PD10 before and after the hot-water treatment revealed that the as-prepared PD10 hybrid is amorphous, and precipitated anatase by the hot-water treatment.

Figure 1 shows TEM photographs and electron diffraction patterns of hybrid PD10 before and after the hot-water treatment. Neither precipitates nor resolvable electron diffraction rings were observed before the hot-water treatment, whereas particles 10–20 nm in size and electron diffraction rings ascribed to anatase were observed after the hot-water treatment. This indicates that hybrid PD10 before the hot-water treatment was homogeneous and amorphous, whereas that subjected to the hot-water treatment precipitated nano-sized anatase particles homogeneously.

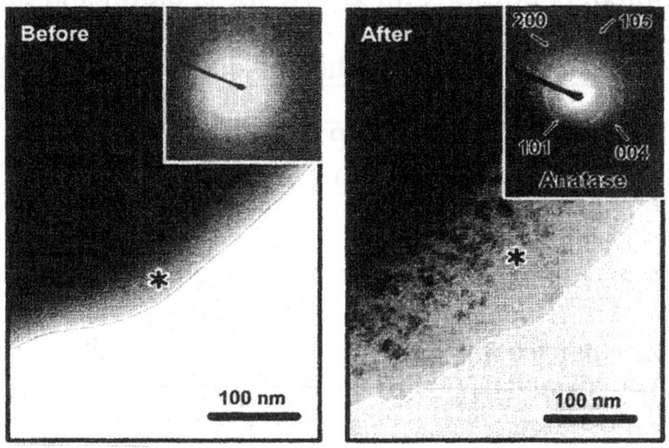

Fig. 1 TEM photographs and electron diffraction patterns of hybrid PD10 before and after hot-water treatment. (* : center of electron diffraction)

PTMO-TiO_2 hybrids: Crack-free transparent discs were obtained for all of the examined compositions. TF-XRD patterns of the surfaces of the hybrids PT30, PT40 and PT50 before and after the hot-water treatment revealed that all of the hybrids were amorphous before the hot-water treatment, but precipitated anatase after the hot-water treatment.

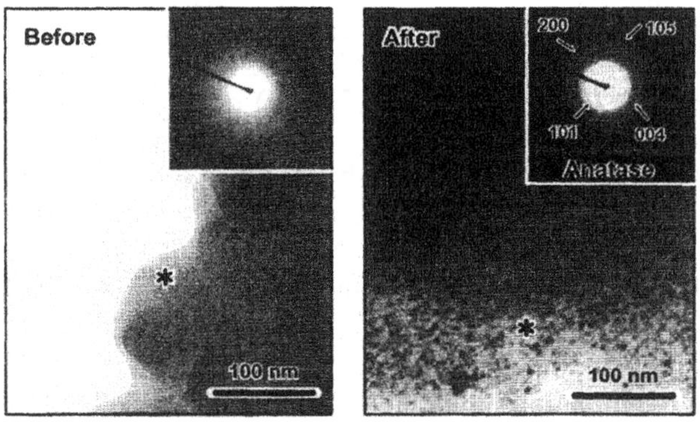

Fig. 2 TEM photographs and electron diffraction patterns of hybrid PT40 before and after hot-water treatment. (* : center of electron diffraction)

Figure 2 shows TEM photographs and electron diffraction patterns of hybrid PT40 before and after the hot-water treatment. Although no resolvable ring was observed in the electron diffraction, homogeneously dispersed particles about a few nanometres in size were observed in the TEM photograph before the hot-water treatment. These particles are speculated to be a titania-rich phase. Homogeneously dispersed particles about 10 nm in size ascribed to anatase were observed in the hybrid after the hot-water treatment. These indicate that anatase particles about 10 nm in size were precipitated in the hybrid by the hot-water treatment. The process of anatase precipitation in the PTMO-TiO_2 hybrids by hot-water treatment is considered to be similar to that in the PDMS-TiO_2 hybrid.

Apatite formation on hybrids

PDMS-TiO_2 hybrids: No apatite peaks were observed in TF-XRD pattern of as-prepared hybrid PD10 after soaking in SBF for 7 d, whereas apatite peaks were remarkably observed in that of hybrid PD10 treated with hot water and soaked in

SBF for 7 d. This indicates that the anatase precipitated in the hybrids induces apatite formation on the surfaces of the hybrids. Figure 3 shows FE-SEM photographs of surfaces of hybrid PD10 treated with hot water and soaked in SBF for 7 d. We can confirm an apatite layer on the hybrid.

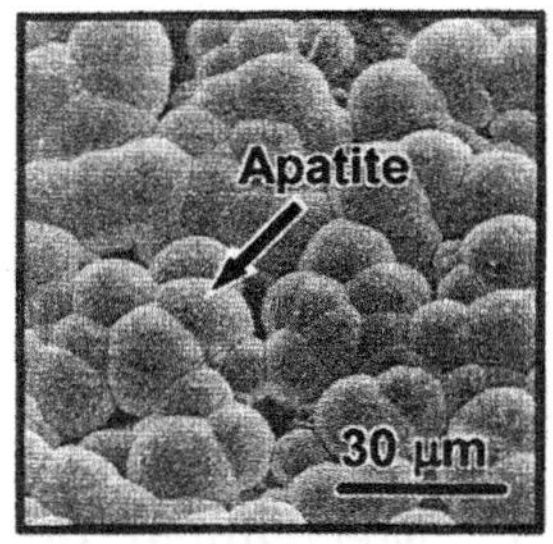

Fig. 3 FE-SEM photographs of surfaces of hybrid PD10 treated with hot water at 80°C for 7 d and soaked in SBF for

PTMO-TiO_2 hybrids: TF-XRD patterns of the surfaces of as-prepared hybrids PT30, PT40 and PT50 gave no apatite peak even after soaking in SBF for 14 d. When they are treated with hot water and soaked in SBF for various periods, apatite was formed on the surface of hybrid PT30 within 3 d and hybrids PT40 and PT50 within 7 d. Figure 4 shows FE-SEM photographs of the surfaces of hybrids PT30, PT40 and PT50 treated with hot water after soaking in SBF for 14 d. Precipitation of apatite was observed on the surfaces of the hybrids after soaking in SBF and the amount of apatite formed on them increased with decreasing PTMO content.

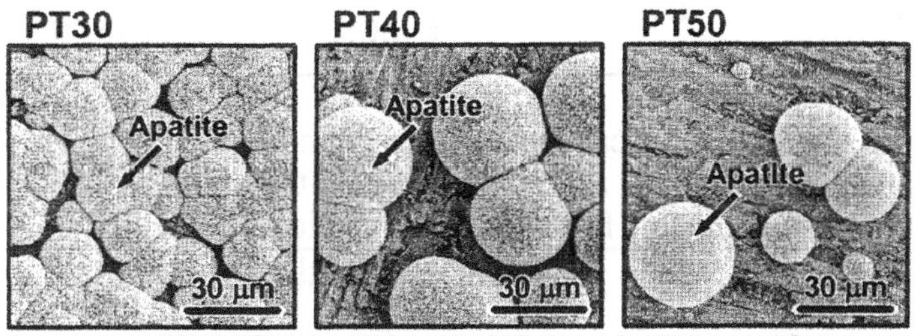

Fig. 4 FE-SEM photographs of the surfaces of hybrids PT30, PT40 and PT50 treated with hot water after soaking in SBF for 14 d.

Mechanical properties of hybrids

PDMS-TiO_2 hybrids: Table 3 shows the values of tensile strength, strain to failure and Young's modulus of the hybrid PD10 before and after the hot-water treatment, and that after both the hot-water and SBF treatments. Both of the tensile strength and Young's modulus decreased, and strain to failure increased upon the hot-water treatment. It is considered that the matrix of the hybrid was enriched with PDMS due to the segregation of TiO_2 by the hot-water treatment and hence the mechanical properties of the hybrid subjected to the hot-water treatment became close to the matrix rich in PDMS, since the continuous phase predominantly affects the overall mechanical behavior of composite materials. In contrast, the strain energies stored until failure were not significantly changed. This means that rearrangement of the hybrid by the hot-water treatment does not cause deterioration of the hybrid. A highly deformable material that can deform as large as approximately 200% until failure was obtained by the present method. After soaking in SBF, the strain to failure of the hot-water-treated specimen decreased, but its tensile strength did not change and its Young's modulus increased a little. It is considered that a increase in its Young's modulus after soaking in SBF is due to apatite formation on its surface, because apatite shows a much higher Young's modulus than the hybrid.

PTMO-TiO_2 hybrids: Table 4 shows the values of bending strength, strain to failure and Young's modulus of hybrid PT40 before and after the hot-water treatment, and that after both the hot-water and SBF treatments, in comparison with those reported for human cancellous bones. Although all of the values were decreased after the hot-water treatment, the treated hybrid still showed mechanical properties analogous to those of human cancellous bone in bending strength and Young's modulus, as well as high deformability. After soaking in SBF, both of its bending strength and strain to failure decreased, but its Young's modulus increased.

Table 3 Mechanical properties of hybrid PD10 before and after hot-water treatment, and that after both the hot-water and SBF treatments.

Specimen	Bending strength (MPa)	Strain to failure (%)	Young's modulus (MPa)
Before hot-water	0.91 ± 0.17	77 ± 19	3.4 ± 0.7
After hot-water	0.36 ± 0.05	258 ± 66	0.24 ± 0.03
After hot-water and SBF	0.36 ± 0.09	158 ± 42	0.43 ± 0.09

Table 4 Mechanical properties of hybrid PT40 before and after the hot-water treatment, and that after both the hot-water and SBF treatments, in comparison with those reported for human cancellous bone [12].

Specimen	Bending strength (MPa)	Strain to failure (%)	Young's modulus (MPa)
Before hot-water	49.6 ± 3.0	27.7 ± 7.9	468 ± 9
After hot-water	12.8 ± 1.1	24.1 ± 3.0	62 ± 2
After hot-water and SBF	7.8 ± 2.2	15.0 ± 4.5	124 ± 20
Cancellous bone	10 - 20	5 - 7	50 - 500

CONCLUSION

A highly deformable material with apatite-forming ability and durability in SBF was obtained by hydrolysis and polycondensation of PDMS and TEOT followed by the hot-water treatment to precipitate nano-sized anatase particles, although the obtained material itself shows too low a mechanical strength for application as a bone-repairing material.

A material with apatite-forming ability and mechanical properties analogous to those of human cancellous bones was obtained by hydrolysis and polycondensation of Si-PTMO and TiPT followed by the hot-water treatment to precipitate nano-sized anatase particles. The mechanical strength of the hybrid was improved by changing the organic component from PDMS to PTMO. It is expected that this hybrid will be useful as a new type of bioactive bone-repairing material.

REFERENCES

[1] Q. Chen, F. Miyaji, T. Kokubo and T. Nakamura, "Apatite formation on PDMS-modified CaO-SiO_2-TiO_2 hybrids prepared by sol-gel method," *Biomaterials*, **20** 1127-1132 (1999).

[2] M. Uchida, H.-M. Kim, T. Kokubo, S. Fujibayashi and T. Nakamura, "Structural dependence of apatite formation on titania gels in a simulated body fluid," *J. Biomed. Mater. Res.*, **64A** 164-170 (2003).

APATITE FORMATION ON THE PMMA BONE CEMENT MODIFIED WITH ALKOXYSILANE AND CALCIUM SALT IN A SIMULATED BODY FLUID

Chikara Ohtsuki and Masao Tanihara
Graduate School of Materials Science, Nara Institute of Science and Technology, 8916-5 Takayama-cho, Ikoma-shi, Nara 630-0192, Japan

Toshiki Miyazaki
Graduate School of Life Science and Systems Engineering, Kyushu Institute of Technology, 2-4 Hibikino, Wakamatsu-ku, Kitakyushu-shi, Fukuoka 808-0196, Japan

Atsushi Sugino, Akiko Mori and Koichi Kuramoto
Nakashima Propeller Co., Ltd., 688-1 Jodo-Kitagata, Okayama 700-8691, Japan

ABSTRACT

Bone cement consisting of polymethylmethacrylate (PMMA) powder and methylmethacrylate (MMA) liquid is clinically used for fixation of orthopedic implants. However it does not show bone-bonding ability. So-called bioactive ceramics show direct bone-bonding to make tight fixation. Development of bioactive PMMA cement has therefore been long desired. The essential prerequisite for an artificial material to bond to bone is the formation of apatite layer on its surface when implanted in bony defect. This type of apatite layer can be formed on bioactive materials even in a simulated body fluid (Kokubo solution) with similar ion concentrations to those of human extracellular fluid. It has been revealed that silanol (Si-OH) group and calcium ion (Ca^{2+}) act as effective constituents for apatite formation in body environment. On the basis of these findings, we modified the cement with alkoxysilane, which provides Si-OH group, as well as with calcium salts, which releases Ca^{2+}. Ability of apatite formation on the cements was examined in Kokubo solution. The cement modified with alkoxysilane and calcium salts formed apatite within 7 d in Kokubo solution. The cements modified with $Ca(CH_3COO)_2$ and $Ca(OH)_2$ kept compressive strength near the lower limit required by ISO5833, although the compressive strength decreased after exposure to Kokubo solution. Bioactive PMMA cement was successfully obtained via chemical modification with alkoxysilane and calcium salt.

INTRODUCTION

Bone cement based on poly(methyl methacrylate)(PMMA) is clinically used for fixation of implants such as artificial hip joint in orthopedic fields [1]. In this type of cement, PMMA powder and methyl methacrylate (MMA) liquid are mixed. The obtained paste is injected into the gap between the bone and the implant to be polymerized and hardened. Significant problems of the PMMA bone cement, however, include loosening at the interface between bone and the cement, since the cement does not possess ability of bone-bonding, i.e. bioactivity. Several studies have been conducted to provide PMMA bone cement with bioactivity through methods by mixing powder of bioactive ceramics with conventional PMMA cement [2,3]. In such methods, large amounts of ceramic powder are necessary to be incorporated into the cement to show bioactivity, since most of the bioactive ceramic powder particles are covered with polymerized MMA and hardly exposed to body fluid. Novel strategies for obtaining bioactive PMMA bone cements should be therefore developed.

The essential prerequisite for an artificial material to exhibit bioactivity is formation of apatite layer on its surface in the body [4]. This apatite formation can be well reproduced even in a simulated body fluid (Kokubo solution) with similar ion concentrations to those of human extracellular fluid [5]. Namely, materials which form apatite on their surfaces in Kokubo solution have a potential to be bioactive. Fundamental studies concerning apatite formation on various glasses and glass-ceramics revealed that silanol (Si-OH) group and calcium ion (Ca^{2+}) act as effective constituents for apatite nucleation in body environment [6]. These findings bring us an idea that modification of PMMA cement with Si-OH group and Ca^{2+} would make the cement bioactive.

We have been developing bioactive PMMA bone cement by modification with alkoxysilane, which provides Si-OH group, and calcium salts, which release Ca^{2+} in body environment. In this study, apatite formation and compressive strength of the some types of the modified cements were investigated by examining its ability of apatite deposition in Kokubo solution.

METHODS

Chemical reagents were used as starting materials. Calcium salts were dried in an oven for more than 12 h at appropriate temperature ranging from 120 to 220 °C to remove excessive water. The other reagents were used without further purification. Compositions of the powder and the liquid are given on Table 1. PMMA powder with molecular weight about 100,000 (Sekisui Plastics Co., Ltd., Tokyo, Japan) and average particle size about 14 μm was used. The PMMA powder was mixed with a calcium salt selected from calcium chloride ($CaCl_2$), calcium acetate ($Ca(CH_3COO)_2$) and calcium hydroxide ($Ca(OH)_2$) at 20 mass% of the powder. BPO was then added to the powder as a polymerization initiator. MMA liquid was mixed with 3-methacryloxypropyltrimethoxysilane (MPS) at 20 mass% of the liquid. N,N-dimethyl-*p*-toluidine (NDT) was then added to the liquid as a polymerization accelerator. The cement denoted as "Reference" has compositions similar to those of the commercially available bone cement (CMW®-1, Depuy, USA), containing neither MPS nor calcium salt.

The powder was mixed with the liquid at a powder to liquid ratio of 1 g / 0.5 g at 23±2°C. The paste was shaped to a rectangular specimen 10 mm x 15 mm x 1 mm in size. At a half of the setting time of the specimens, they were soaked in 35 mL of Kokubo solution (Na^+ 142.0, K^+ 5.0, Mg^{2+} 1.5, Ca^{2+} 2.5, Cl^- 147.8, HCO_3^- 4.2, HPO_4^{2-} 1.0 and SO_4^{2-} 0.5 mol/m^3) at pH 7.25 at 36.5°C for 7 d. The specimens were characterized by thin-film X-ray diffraction (TF-XRD) and scanning electron microscope (SEM) observation. Compressive strengths of the cements without and with exposure to Kokubo solution were measured with a material testing machine by applying compressive load at a cross-head speed of 20 mm / min normally to the cylindrical specimens of 6 mm in diameter and 12 mm in length until fracture occurred. In order to examine dissolution of the specimens, they were soaked in physiological saline at 36.5°C. Ca^{2+} concentration of the saline after soaking of the cements were measured by a Ca^{2+} electrode.

Some specimens were then subjected to animal experiments. A hole of 2 x 10 mm in area was made at the medial aspect of the proximal metaphysis of the tibiae of Japanese white rabbits. The mixed paste of the cement modified with MPS and $Ca(CH_3COO)_2$ before setting was then inserted into the hole to be hardened *in situ*. After 4 w, the rabbits were sacrificed and the implanted cements along with the surrounding bony tissues were extracted. The interface between the cement and the bone was observed by X-ray computed tomography (X-CT).

RESULTS

Figure 1 shows SEM photographs of the surfaces of the cements modified with MPS and various kinds of calcium salts after soaking in Kokubo solution for 7 d. Assembles of fine particles were observed on the modified cements after the soaking, but not for Reference. Figure 2 shows TF-XRD patterns of the surface of the cement with the same modification after soaking in Kokubo solution for 1 and 7 d. Broad peaks assigned to hydroxyapatite with low crystallinity were detected at about 26° and 32° for the cements modified with $CaCl_2$ and $Ca(CH_3COO)_2$ after the soaking for 1 d, while they could be detected for the cement modified with $Ca(OH)_2$ after soaking for 7 d. This means that the modified cements with $CaCl_2$ and $Ca(CH_3COO)_2$ have higher ability for apatite formation than the modified cement with $Ca(OH)_2$. Figure 3 shows Ca^{2+} concentration of normal salines after soaking of the cements modified with MPS and various calcium salts for 7 d. The Ca^{2+} concentrations relate dissolution of the calcium salts from the modified cements. Magnitude of the release of Ca^{2+} ions into the saline increased in the order: $Ca(OH)_2 < Ca(CH_3COO)_2 < CaCl_2$. Figure 4 shows compressive strength of the cements modified with MPS and various calcium salts without and with exposure to Kokubo solution for 7 d. The compressive strength of the modified cements decreased after exposure to Kokubo solution, except for the cement modified with $Ca(OH)_2$. Among the cements modified with MPS and calcium salts, those modified with $Ca(CH_3COO)_2$ or $Ca(OH)_2$ showed the compressive strength near the lower limit required by ISO5833 [7]. Figure 5 shows X-CT images of the interface between rabbit tibia and the cement modified with MPS and $Ca(CH_3COO)_2$ 4 w after implantation, in comparison with Reference. Growth of new bone was observed for the former along the surface of the cement, but not for the latter.

Table I. Compositions of the cements examined in this study

Sample	Powder in mass ratio			Liquid in mass ratio		
	PMMA	Calcium salt	BPO	MMA	MPS	NDT
Reference	0.971	0.000	0.029	0.992	0.000	0.008
Modified cement	0.776	0.194	0.029	0.794	0.198	0.008

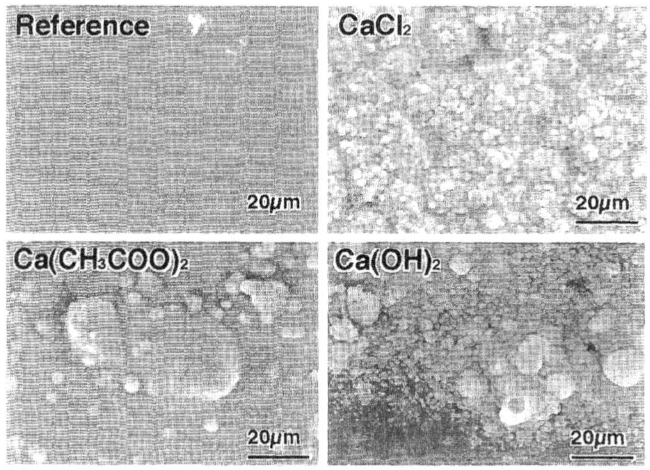

Figure 1. SEM photographs of the surfaces of the cements modified with MPS and various kinds of calcium salts after soaking in Kokubo solution for 7 d.

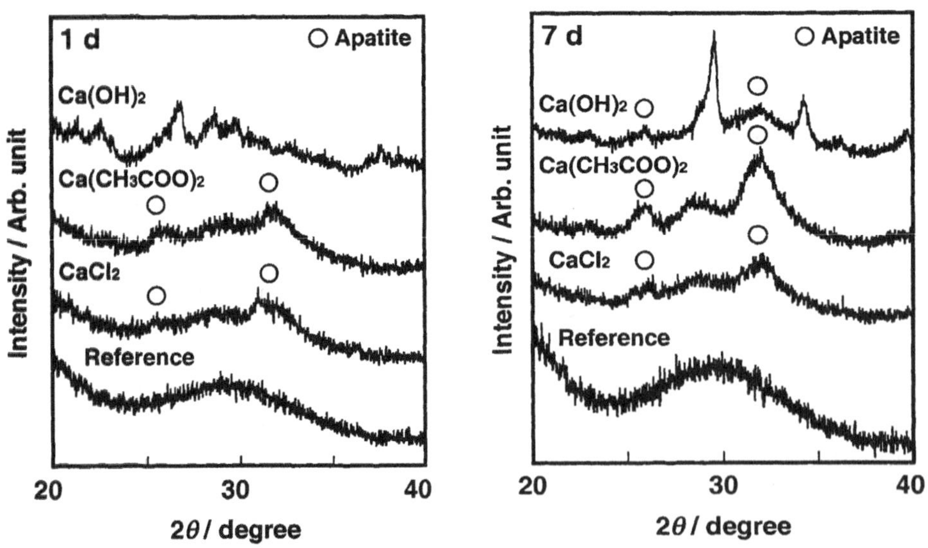

Figure 2. TF-XRD patterns of the surfaces of the cements modified with MPS and various kinds of calcium salts after soaking in Kokubo solution for 1 and 7 d.

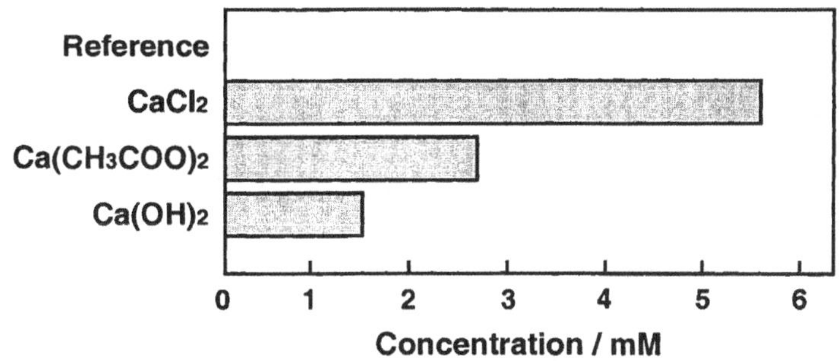

Figure 3. Ca^{2+} concentration of normal saline after soaking of the cements modified with MPS and various kinds of calcium salts for 7 d.

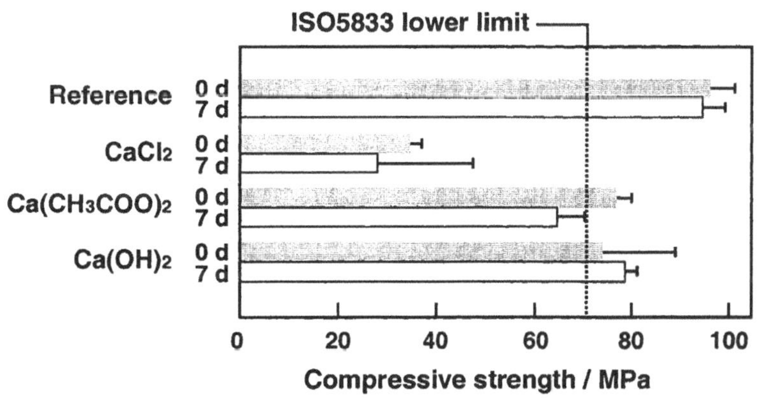

Figure 4. Compressive strength of the cements modified with MPS and various kinds of calcium salts before (0 d) and after (7 d) soaking in Kokubo solution.

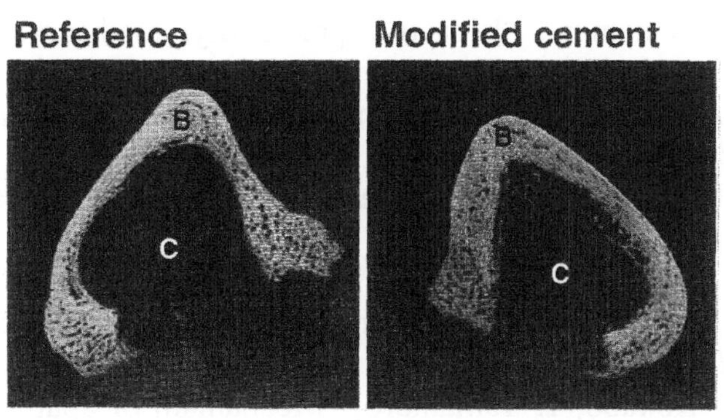

Figure 5. X-CT images of the interface between the rabbit tibia and the cement modified with MPS and $Ca(CH_3COO)_2$ 4 w after implantation, in comparison with Reference. B; bone, C; cement.

DISCUSSION

It is apparent from the results described above that modification of PMMA cement by incorporation of MPS and calcium salts makes the cement capable of apatite formation in the body environment. Improved biological affinity to the bone tissue is also confirmed by the results from Fig. 5 exhibiting higher osteoconduction of the modified cement than the Reference. The ability of apatite formation on the modified cements well supports the potential of osteoconduction on implant materials, such as Bioglass®, glass-ceramic A-W. Higher rate of apatite formation is preferred to lead higher osteoconduction.

The cements modified with $CaCl_2$ or $Ca(CH_3COO)_2$ showed decrease in their compressive strength after soaking in Kokubo solution. This is attributed to release of Ca^{2+} ions from the cement into the solution. When Ca^{2+} are rapidly released, pores would be formed inside the cement, thereby leading to decrease in compressive strength. This shows that appropriate selection of the calcium salts also important to keep a high mechanical strength in body environment. Consequently, this type of modification has a high potential for providing PMMA bone cement with bioactivity, that is useful in orthopedic fields.

CONCLUSIONS

Simple chemical modification with alkoxysilane and calcium salts was proved to be quite effective for providing PMMA cements with bioactivity. This type of cement is expected to be useful as a novel bone-repairing material in orthopedic fields.

ACKNOWLEDGMENTS

This study was supported by Grant-in-Aid for Scientific Research ((B)13450272), Japan Society for the Promotion of Science.

REFERENCES

[1]K.D. Kühn, pp. 1-5 in *Bone cements*, Springer, Berlin, 2000.

[2]E.J. Harper, "Bioactive bone cements," *Proceedings of the Institution of Mechanical Engineers, Part H*, **212** [2] 113-20 (1998).

[3]S. Shinzato, M. Kobayashi, W.F. Mousa, M. Kamimura, M. Neo, Y. Kitamura, T. Kokubo and T. Nakamura, "Bioactive polymethyl methacrylate-based bone cement: comparison of glass beads, apatite- and wollastonite-containing glass-ceramic, and hydroxyapatite fillers on mechanical and biological properties," *Journal of Biomedical Materials Research*, **51** [2] 258-272 (2000).

[4]H.-M. Kim, "Bioactive ceramics: challenges and perspectives," *Journal of Ceramic Society of Japan*, **109** [4] S49-S57 (2001).

[5]T. Kokubo, H. Kushitani, S. Sakka, T. Kitsugi, T. Yamamuro, "Solutions able to reproduce *in vivo* surface-structure changes in bioactive glass-ceramic A-W," *Journal of Biomedical Materials Research*, **24** [6] 721-734 (1990).

[6]C. Ohtsuki, T. Kokubo, T. Yamamuro, "Mechanism of apatite formation on $CaO-SiO_2-P_2O_5$ glasses in a simulated body fluid," *Journal of Non-crystalline Solids*, **14** [1] 84-92 (1992).

[7]ISO. International standard 5833/2: Implants for surgery-acrylic resin cements. orthopaedic application; 1992.

FORMATION OF HYDROXYAPATITE COATINGS ON ALUMINA UNDER HYDROTHERMAL CONDITIONS

Jung-Soo Ha
Andong National University
388 Songchun-dong
Andong, Kyungbuk 760-749
South Korea

Mohamed N. Rahaman
University of Missouri-Rolla
Department of Ceramic Engineering
Rolla, MO 65409-0330
USA

ABSTRACT

Hydroxyapatite [$Ca_{10}(PO_4)_6(OH)_2$] coatings were deposited on alumina substrates under hydrothermal conditions at 90°C from aqueous solutions of calcium nitrate and ammonium hydrogen phosphate containing EDTA disodium salt as a chelating agent and hydrogen peroxide. The influence of the solution pH and time on the deposition of the coatings was investigated. The nucleation and growth, structure and composition of the coatings as well as the bonding of the coating to the substrate were investigated using electron microscopy, X-ray diffraction, and surface chemistry techniques. The deposition mechanism of the coatings is discussed.

INTRODUCTION

Because of its high strength, low friction and wear, corrosion resistance, and biocompatibility, Al_2O_3 has been used widely as orthopedic and dental implants [1]. Commonly, bioinert Al_2O_3 and Ti implants are encapsulated by a dense fibrous tissue that prevents direct bonding to soft and hard tissues in the body, leading to loosening of the implants [1, 2]. An effective way to overcome this problem is to impart bioactivity to the implant surface through a hydroxyapatite coating. Hydroxyapatite (HA), $Ca_{10}(PO_4)_6(OH)_2$, the main mineral constituent of bone and teeth, can enhance growth of tissues around the implant, thereby promoting bonding with the implant [2]. When compared with coating methods such as plasma spraying and sputtering, the hydrothermal process has a significant advantage in that it can produce crystalline, compositionally homogeneous HA coatings without the need for high temperature calcination [3].

Hydrothermal coating of HA on Al_2O_3 has been investigated by Toriyama *et al.* [4] and Fujishiro, *et al.* [5] who used EDTA (ethylenediaminetetraacetic acid) for chelating of Ca^{2+} ions in a solution containing Ca^{2+} and phosphate ions. In the precipitation of hydroxyapatite coatings, the EDTA-Ca^{2+} chelates were decomposed by oxidation with H_2O_2 at pH = 3.9–13.9 and 90°C [4] or were dissociated thermally at pH = 6 and 160–200°C [5]. HA coatings on Al_2O_3 were obtained only with the oxidative decomposition method by Toriyama, *et al.* who found that the coating morphology and Ca/P ratio changed significantly with pH. The coatings prepared at pH = 9 or higher were granular, consisting of hexagonal, columnar HA crystals with a Ca/P ratio close to the stoichiometric value.

In the present work, the method of Toriyama, *et al.* [4] was used to deposit HA coatings on Al_2O_3 substrates and the formation mechanism of the coatings was studied as a function of the solution pH and the deposition time. The nucleation and growth, structure and composition of the coatings as well as the bonding of the coating to the substrate were investigated.

EXPERIMENTAL PROCEDURE

Solutions for the hydrothermal reaction were prepared using reagent-grade chemicals (Aldrich; Milwaukee, USA). Calcium nitrate (0.01 mol) was dissolved in deionized water and then EDTA disodium salt dihydrate (0.012 mol) was added to chelate the Ca^{2+} ions. After stirring the solution for 10 min, ammonium hydrogen phosphate (0.006 mol) was added to make a stock solution of 140 ml with the a Ca/P atomic ratio = 1.67, the value for stoichiometric HA. The pH value of the solution was adjusted to 7.2, 9.8, and 11.4 with NH_4OH. Al_2O_3 substrates were prepared by slip casting an Al_2O_3 powder (A-1000; mean particle size ≈ 0.4 μm; Alcoa, USA), followed by sintering for 2 h at 1550°C to give disc-shaped substrates (10 mm in diameter by 2.5 mm) with a relative density of 98%. The substrate surfaces were ground with SiC paper down to 600 grit.

The hydrothermal treatments were performed in a Teflon-lined autoclave (45 ml; Parr Instrument Co., USA). In the experiments, 23 ml of the stock solution was loaded into the reaction vessel after which 3 wt% H_2O_2 was added. The substrates were suspended in the solution and the vessel was heated at 2°C/min to 90°C and held for various times (0.5, 1, 3, and 12 h). After the hydrothermal treatment, the substrates were washed with deionized water for 2 min in an ultrasonic bath and dried at room temperature.

The microstructures of the top surfaces and fracture surfaces of the coatings were observed by scanning electron microscopy (SEM; JEOL T330A & Hitachi S4700). The crystalline phase was identified by thin-film X-ray diffraction (TF-XRD; Scintag 2000) with a grazing incidence angle of 1°. Surface chemical analysis of the coated samples was performed with X-ray photoelectron spectroscopy (XPS; AXIS 165, KRATOS).

RESULTS AND DISCUSSION

Figure 1 shows the surface morphology of the untreated substrate and of the substrates treated for 3 h at pH = 7.2, 9.8, and 11.4. Uniform deposition of the coating was obtained at pH = 9.8 whereas the coating deposition was very limited at pH = 7.2 and 11.4. Since the isoelectric point of Al_2O_3 occurs at 8–9 [6], the surface charge of the substrate is positive at pH = 7.2 but negative at pH = 9.8 and 11.4. It has been suggested that the nucleation of HA starts with the adhesion of Ca^{2+} ions on to negatively-charged surfaces [7], i.e., a negative surface charge of the substrate is favorable for coating formation. The uniform coating at pH 9.8 is consistent with this suggestion but the sparse coating at pH = 11.4 indicates that other parameters can also control the process. We found that homogeneous precipitation of HA in solution was considerably higher at pH = 11.4 than at pH = 9.8, presumably because of the higher OH concentration, so heterogeneous precipitation on the substrate was limited, leading to a sparse coating.

The fracture surfaces of the samples prepared for 3 and 12 h at pH = 9.8 (Fig. 2) show coatings with a thickness of ~0.7 and 0.9 μm, respectively. XRD revealed the phase composition of the coatings to be HA (Fig. 3). The coating deposited for 12 h has the strongest peak intensity for the (002) reflection at 2θ = 25.9° whereas the standard pattern (JCPDS 72-1243) has the strongest peak (211) at 31.8°. The peak intensity for the (112) reflection at 32.2° is also higher for the coating. Similar trends were observed for the coating deposited for 3 h. The X-ray data indicate a preferred orientation of the HA crystals (hexagonal structure) with their *c* axis nearly perpendicular to the substrate surface. The preferred orientation is also evident from the microstructures in Fig. 4. For the coating deposited for 12 h, HA crystals are oriented nearly perpendicular to the substrate, with hexagonal rod shapes (~300 nm wide by ~550 nm long). The orientation was not as pronounced for the coating deposited for 3 h which has finer crystals (60-80 nm wide).

The fracture surfaces [Figs. 4(b) and (d)] show the presence of a thin layer (140-200 nm thick) of fine particles adjacent to the substrates which are believed to represent the initial formation of HA crystals on the substrate. The surface morphology (Fig. 5) of coatings prepared for short times (0.5 and 1 h) indicates that the fine particles are actually rod-shaped crystals with their *c* axis oriented *parallel* to the substrate surface. For the coating deposited for 0.5 h, the fine crystals are 30-40 nm wide and 150-300 nm long. In the case of the coating deposited for 1 h, some new crystals were observed to form on the crystals oriented parallel to the substrate surface. The formation of these new crystals may represent the initial stage of the process that would eventually produce the rod-shaped crystals with a preferred alignment *perpendicular* to the substrate surface (Fig. 4).

The coatings deposited for 0.5 and 1 h were too thin for X-ray analysis of the phases (see Fig. 3) but XPS showed that the Ca and P spectra for these coatings were almost identical to those for the coatings deposited for 3 and 12 h (Fig. 6), indicating that they consist of the HA phase. Crystals oriented parallel to the substrate surface were not found for the sparse coatings deposited at pH = 7.2 and 11.4 even when these coatings were observed at high magnification in the SEM. The initial formation of the fine crystals with a preferred orientation parallel to the substrate may therefore be necessary for the deposition of uniform HA coatings.

CONCLUSION

The deposition of HA coatings on Al_2O_3 substrates under hydrothermal conditions at 90°C from aqueous solutions of calcium nitrate and ammonium hydrogen phosphate containing EDTA and hydrogen peroxide is strongly dependent on the solution pH and the deposition time. Uniform deposition of coatings is obtained at pH = 9.8, presumably due to the negative surface charge of the substrate and not too high rate of homogeneous precipitation. The coatings show preferred orientation of the HA crystals with their *c* axis perpendicular to the substrate surface. The extent of orientation increases with deposition time, giving nearly perpendicular orientation after ~12 h. The initial formation of fine HA crystals aligned parallel to the substrate surface appears to be necessary for the deposition of uniform HA coatings on Al_2O_3.

ACKNOWLEDGEMENT

One of the authors (JSH) was supported by Andong National University, South Korea, through a research visit program for 2002.

REFERENCES

[1] L.L. Hench, “Bioceramics,” *J. Am. Ceram. Soc.*, **81** [7] 1705-28 (1998).

[2] W. Suchanek and M. Yoshimura, "Processing and Properties of Hydroxyapatite-Based Biomaterials for Use as a Hard Tissue Replacement Implants," *J. Mater. Res.*, **13** [1] 94-17 (1998).

[3] M. Yoshimura and H. Suda, “Hydrothermal Processing of Hydroxyapatite: Past, Present, and Future”; pp. 45-72 in *Hydroxyapatite and Related Materials*. Edited by P.W. Brown and B. Constantz. CRC Press, Boca Raton, 1994.

[4] M. Toriyama, Y. Kawamoto, T. Suzuki, Y. Yokogawa, K. Nishizawa, F. Nagata, and M.R. Mucalo, “Hydroxyapatite Coating on Alumina Ceramics by an Oxidative Decomposition Method of EDTA-Calcium Chelate,” *J. Mater. Sci. Lett.*, **15**, 179-81 (1996).

[5] Y. Fujishiro, M. Nishino, A. Sugimori, A. Okuwaki, and T. Sato, “Coating of Hydroxyapatite on Various Substrates via Hydrothermal Reactions of $Ca(edta)^{2-}$ and Phosphate,” *J. Mater. Sci.: Materials in Medicine*, **12**, 333-37 (2001).

[6] M. N. Rahaman, *Ceramic Processing and Sintering*, Marcel Dekker, New York, 1995; p. 156.

[7] H. Takadama, H-M. Kim, T. Kokubo, and T. Nakamura, “Mechanism of Biomineralization of Apatite on a Sodium Silicate Glass: TEM-EDX Study In Vitro,” *Chem. Mater.*, **13**, 1108-13 (2001).

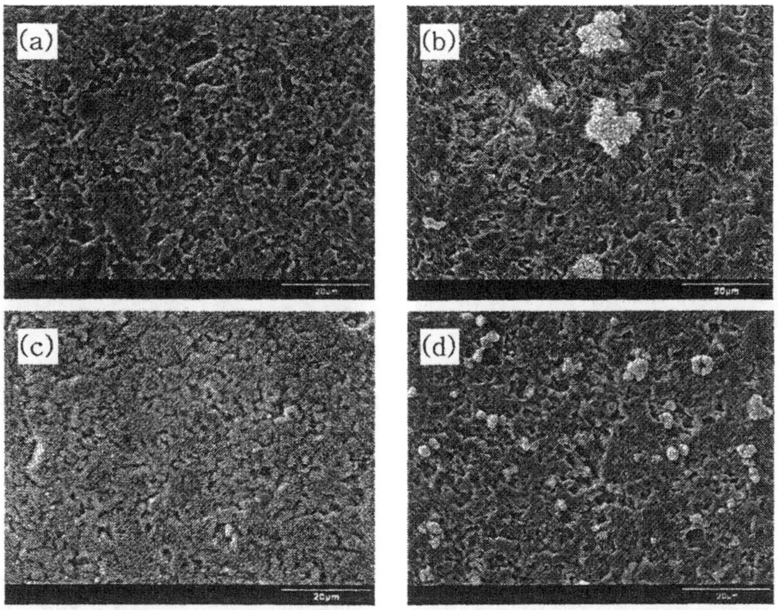

Fig. 1. Surface morphology of substrates before and after hydrothermal treatment for 3 h at different pH: (a) untreated, (b) pH = 7.2, (c) pH = 9.8, and (d) pH = 11.4.

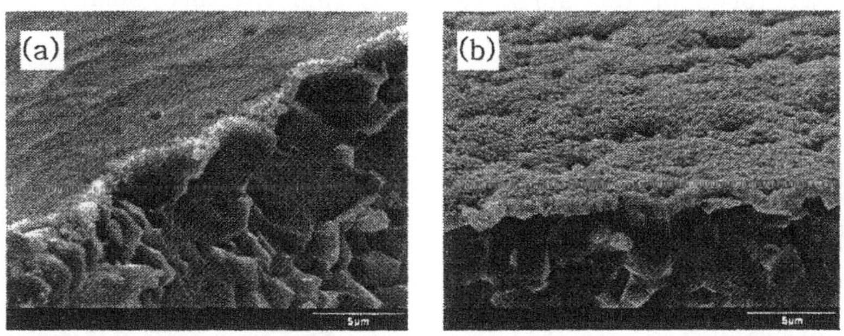

Fig. 2. Fracture surfaces of the samples treated at pH = 9.8 for deposition times of (a) 3 h and (b) 12 h, showing the HA coating.

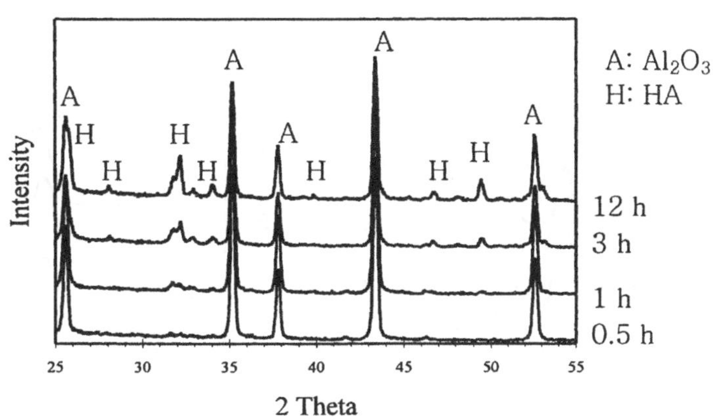

Fig. 3. XRD data for the samples treated at pH = 9.8 for various deposition times.

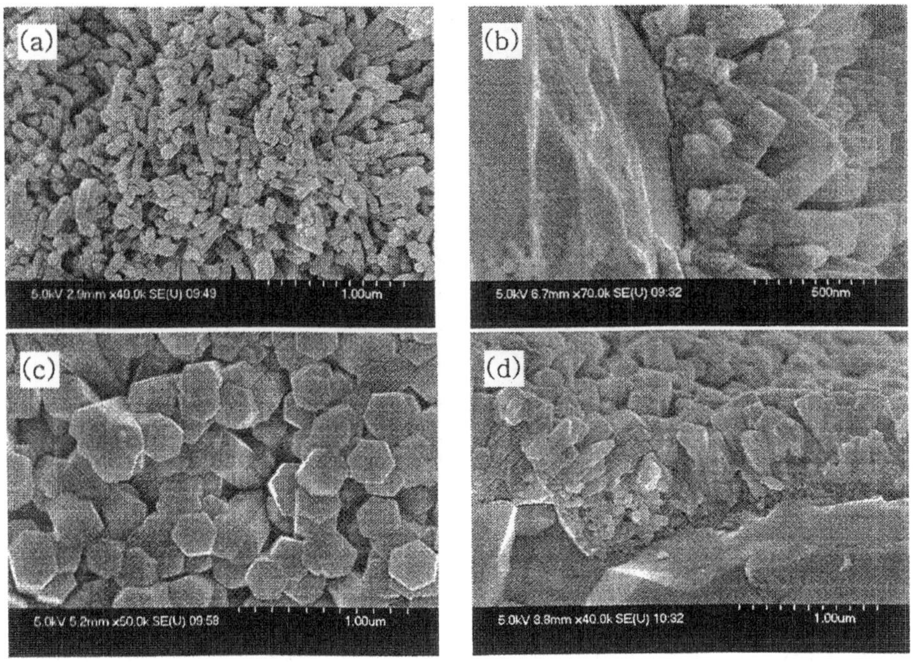

Fig. 4. Microstructures of the surfaces (a, c) and fracture surfaces (b, d) of coatings prepared at pH = 9.8 for (a, b) 3 h and (c, d) 12 h.

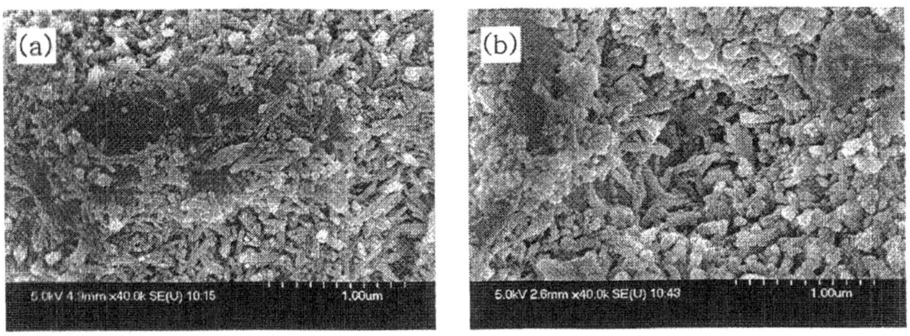

Fig. 5. Surface morphology of the samples prepared at pH = 9.8 for (a) 0.5 h and (b) 1 h.

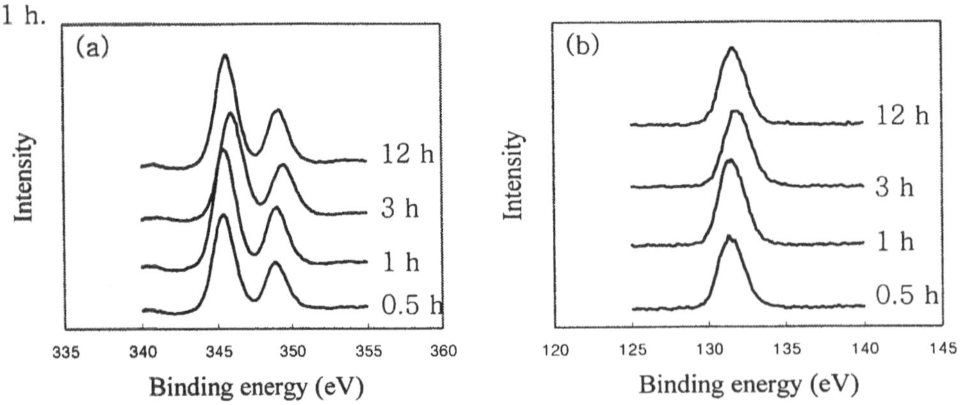

Fig. 6. XPS spectra of the surfaces of samples prepared at pH = 9.8 for various deposition times: (a) Ca *2p* and (b) P *2p*.

A MULTI-STATION HIP JOINT SIMULATOR STUDY AND WEAR CHARACTERIZATION OF COMMERCIAL HIP ENDOPROSTHESES

K. Jono, Y. Takigawa, H. Takadama and M. Mizuno
Material Research and Development Laboratory
Japan Fine Ceramics Center
2-4-1 Mutsuno, Atsuta-ku, Nagoya 456-8587, Japan

T. Nakamura
Dept. Orthopedic Surgery, Facul. Medicine, Kyoto University
54 Kawahara-cho, Shogoin, Sakyo-ku, Kyoto 606-8507, Japan

ABSTRACT

The objectives of this study are to compare ultra-high molecular weight polyethylene (UHMWPE) and closs-linked UHMWPE (cUHMWPE) wear of commercial total hip joint prostheses under identical conditions simulating a living body, and to characterize generated wear-debris using identical technique. Several prostheses with different material combinations of a head and a cup were subjected with a diluted bovine serum lubricant using a multi-station hip joint simulator. Wear rate of cUHMWPE cups against ZrO_2 ceramic head was extremely low, compared with UHMWPE cups. In this case, most of wear-debris particles of UHMWPE and cUHMWPE were less than 1 μm in size. However, slight difference was found in size distributions and in morphology between the particles from these materials. Wear rate and wear debris of CoCr-on-UHMWPE, ZrO_2-on-cUHMWPE and Al_2O_3-on- cUHMWPE were also investigated in this study.

INTRODUCTION

Wear of ultra-high molecular weight polyethylene (UHMWPE) of total hip joint prostheses is a serious problem, because the wear-debris particles induce severe osteolysis, resulting in loosening. [1] While several prostheses with different material combinations of a head and a cup have been used clinically, there is not sufficient data to compare their wear behavior and wear-debris properties directly. Because optimum methods and conditions have not been established on *in vitro* wear test, evaluation of wear has been performed using different types of simulators under different test conditions. [2]

The objectives of this study are to compare UHMWPE and cross-linked UHMWPE (cUHMWPE) wear of commercial total hip joint prostheses under identical conditions simulating a living body, and to characterize wear and generated wear-debris using identical technique.

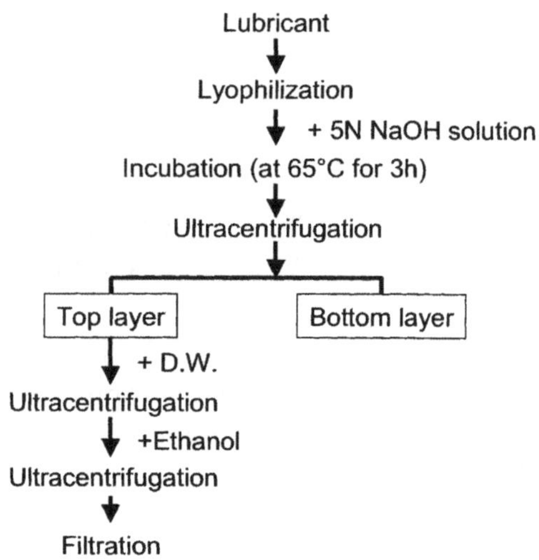

Fig. 1 Process of UHMWPE wear-debris isolation

MATERIALS AND METHODS

Materials

Fore types of commercial total hip joint prostheses, ZrO_2-on-UHMWPE, CoCr-on-UHMWPE, ZrO_2-on-cUHMWPE, Al_2O_3-on-cUHMWPE, with 26 mm femoral heads were used for simulator studies. For each type of the prostheses, three sets were studied. Sodium hydroxide (NaOH) solution and ethanol were used for wear-debris isolation. These reagent solutions and distilled water (D.W.) used in the isolation were filtered through a 0.2 μm pore size membrane prior to use in order to avoid contamination of samples by extraneous particles.

Simulator study

A 12-station hip wear simulator (MTS SYSTEM Co., USA) was used for wear studies with a frequency of 1 Hz and a peak magnitude of 2.8 kN. Heads and cups of the hip prostheses were mounted in an anatomical position. Lubricant was 7 and 25 vol% of bovine serum (SIGMA Chemical co., USA) containing 0.1% of sodiumazide, which was added to retard bacterial growth, and 20 mM of EDTA. Each chamber volume was 1000 ml, and the lubricant was completely replaced with 750 ml of fresh lubricant approximately every 500,000 cycles. After testing, the lubricant was decanted and frozen for subsequent wear particle analysis.

Isolation of UHMWPE wear-debris from lubricant

The process of UHMWPE wear-debris isolation is shown in Fig. 1. The lubricant (750 ml) after the simulator test was lyophilized in order to reduce solution volume. Approximately 20 ml of 5N NaOH was added to the lyophilized sample and the sample was incubated at 65 °C for 3 h in a shaking water bath in order to digest proteins from bovine serum. The digest was ultracentrifuged and then the top layer, containing UHMWPE particles, was collected into a new tube. The particles in the tube were washed with D.W. followed by ultracentrifugation. Contaminating lipids were removed by dissolving in ethanol followed by ultracentrifugation. Finally, the particles were recovered by filtration on a 0.1 μm pore size membrane.

Analysis of wear-debris

Characterization of UHMWPE and cUHMWPE wear-debris particles was performed by scanning electron microscopy (SEM; JSM-6330F, JEOL). Since particle size of obtained wear-debris was in a wide range from several 100 to 0.1 μm, number of the particles larger than 10 μm, 1-10 μm and 0.1-1 μm in a certain area was counted with SEM photographs taken at ×300, ×2,000 and ×10,000 magnifications, respectively. Particle size was defined as a maximum dimension of the wear-debris particle. A minimum number of 1000 particles were measured in a sample.

RESULTS AND DISCUSSION

Influence of test conditions on wear and wear-debris

ZrO_2-on-UHMWPE total hip joint prostheses tested in 7 and 25 vol% serum concentration of lubricants were used in order to study influence of the serum concentration on wear and generated wear-debris. Weight losses of UHMWPE cups at 1.0×10^6 cycles were 68.3 mg for 25 vol% and 55.6 mg for 7 vol%, although particle size distributions of recovered UHMWPE wear-debris were similar (data is not shown). This result indicated that serum concentration of lubricant affected wear rate without a change in particle size of the wear-debris. Moreover, influence of test cycles on wear and wear-debris was also investigated with a 25 vol% of serum lubricant. Weight of a UHMWPE cup constantly decreased as shown in Fig. 2 and percentage of smaller size wear-debris (0.1-1μm) increased with test cycles (Fig. 3). Therefore, wear-debris in same cycle duration should be used in comparison. These results also suggested that optimum test conditions should be selected to simulate both wear and wear-debris in a body.

Comparison of wear and wear-debris between UHMWPE and cUHMWPE

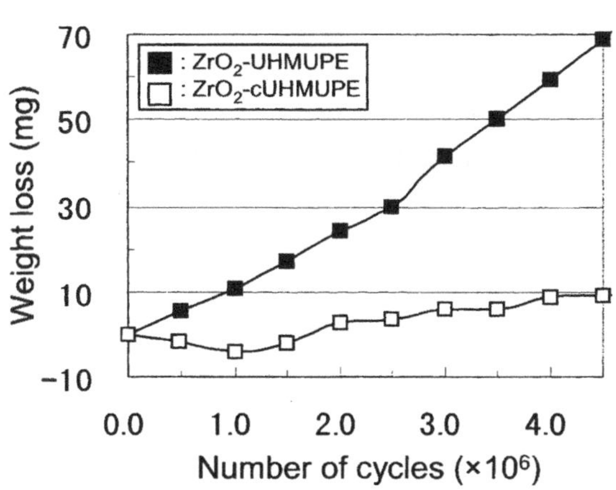

Fig.2. Weight loss of UHMWPE and cUHMWPE cups for ZrO_2 heads as a function of test cycles

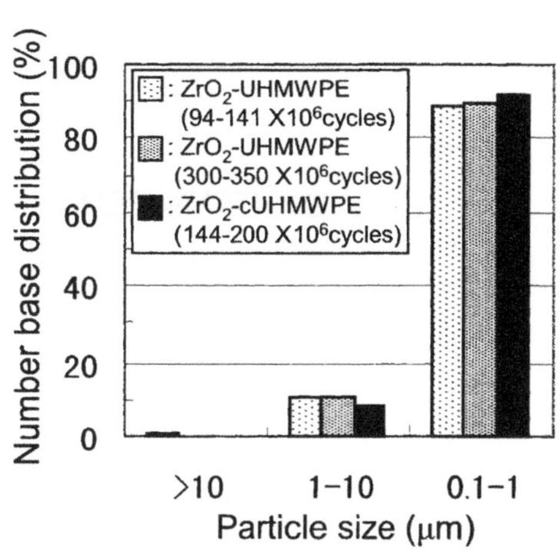

Fig.3 Particle size distributions of wear-debris generated from UHMWPE and cUHMWPE cups for ZrO_2 heads

were tested in a 25 vol% of serum lubricant. In Figs. 2 and 3, weight changes of a cup and size distributions of generated wear-debris are shown as a function of test cycles, respectively. Weight change of a UHMWPE cup was significantly large and the weight loss at 4.5 $\times 10^6$ cycles was 69 mg, while that of a cUHMWPE cup was only 9 mg (Fig. 2). Slight increase of the weight in initial stage for the cUHMWPE cup would come from its high water absorptivity. As to wear-debris, the particles ranged from sub-micron up to several 100μm in size and the large portion of particles was 0.1-1 μm in both cases, even though comparison at different test cycles (Fig. 3). There was, however, a little difference in particle size distribution; number based percentage of smaller wear-debris (0.1-1 μm) from the cUHMWPE cup seemed to be larger than that from the UHMWPE cup. Difference was found also in morphology of wear-debris between UHMWPE and cUHMWPE (Fig. 4). Shapes of UHMWPE particles were granules and twisted fibrils (Fig. 4 A and B). In contrast, the majority of cUHMWPE particles were granules and the finer particles made agglomerate (Fig. 4 C and D).

Debris in submicron size is believed to have greater osteolytic potential. [1] The wear-debris generated from cUHMWPE will have a possibility to induce osteolysis with lower concentration than those from UHMWPE in long use.

Influence of femoral head materials on wear and wear-debris

Influence of femoral head materials on wear behavior and wear-debris properties was studied with a 25 vol% of serum lubricant. ZrO_2 and CoCr heads for UHMWPE and ZrO_2 and Al_2O_3 heads for cUHMWPE were used. Weight changes of cups and size distributions of generated wear-debris are shown

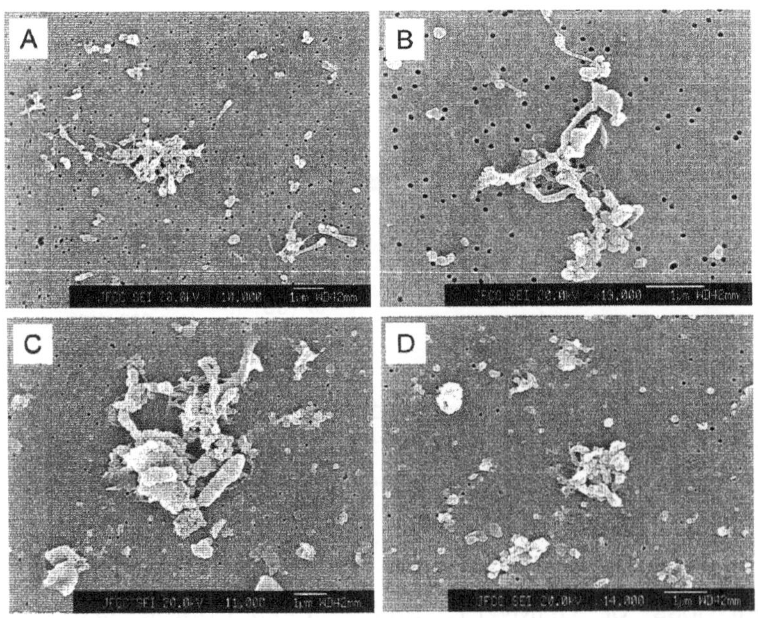

Fig.4 Morphology of wear-debris particles generated from UHMWPE and cUHMWPE cups for ZrO_2 heads
A and B, UHMWPE; C and D, cUHMWPE

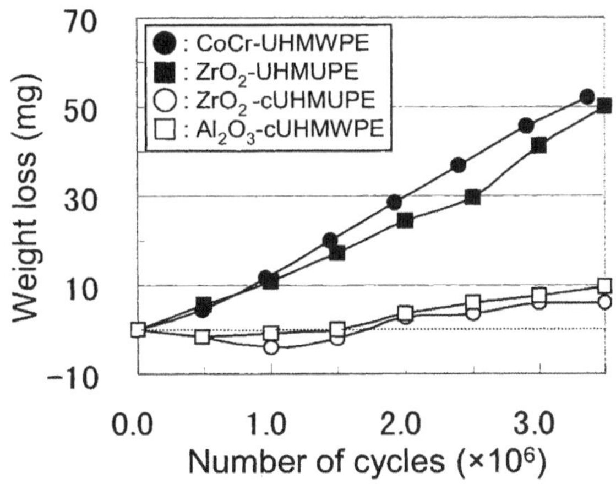

Fig.5 Weight loss of UHMWPE and cUHMWPE cups for several material heads as a function of test cycles

Weight changes of cups and size distributions of generated wear-debris are shown in Figs. 5 and 6, respectively. Weight loss of the UHMWPE cup against ZrO_2 heads was somewhat low, compared with CoCr heads (Fig. 5). In these cases, percentage of smaller wear-debris (0.1-1 μm) generated from ZrO_2-on-UHMWPE prostheses was slightly higher than that from CoCr-on-UHMWPE one (Fig. 6a). Significant difference in morphology of wear-debris was not observed between these materials. On the other hand, it was found that wear rate, size distribution and morphology of generated wear-debris particles did not depend on femoral head materials in the case of cUHMWPE (Figs. 5 and 6b).

Some authors reported that UHMWPE had relatively high wear resistance for ceramics heads, compared with a metal head in simulator and *in vivo* studies. [3, 4] The difference of UHMWPE wear rate between the CoCr and ZrO_2 heads in our study was well consistent with that. The similar wear rate and wear-debris of cUHMUPE cups for ZrO_2 and Al_2O_3 heads should be attributable to that both these heads were ceramics. As for wear-debris, it should be mentioned that the

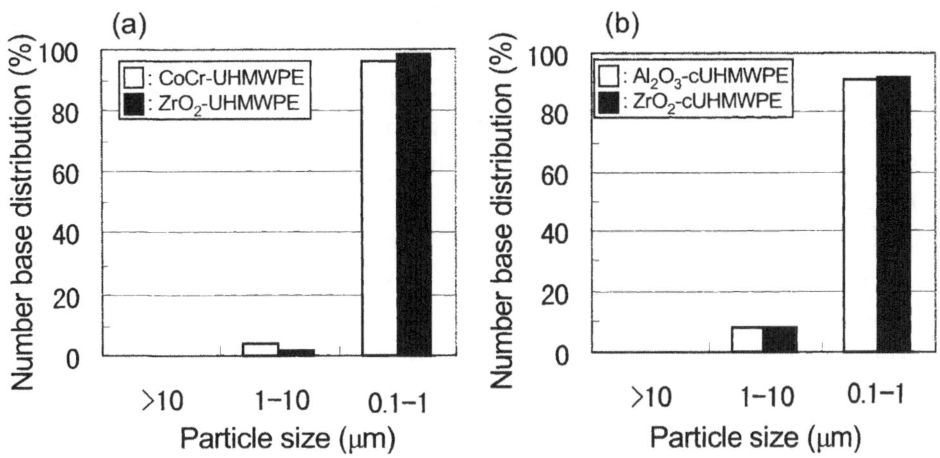

Fig.6 Particle size distributions of wear-debris generated from (a) UHMWPE and (b) cUHMWPE cups for several material heads
Number of cycles: (a), 0-0.47$\times 10^6$; (b) 1.5-2.0$\times 10^6$.

majority of the wear-debris particles generated from both UHMWPE and cUHMWPE were in the biologically active size rang, 0.1-1 μm, even if different materials were coupled.

There have been a number of *in vitro* studies of polyethylene wear and wear-debris using several types of simulator and under different test conditions. These difference means that reported results are often difficult to compare each other directly. This study, therefore, performed under an identical condition, which was basically studied [5], using a hip joint simulator. The wear and the wear-debris properties clarified in this study will be useful for comparing and understanding the properties of each commercial prostheses.

CONCLUSION

Several kinds of commercial total hip joint prosthesis with different material combinations of a head and a cup were studied using a multi-station hip joint simulator under identical condition and the wear and generated wear-debris were characterized by identical technique. It was demonstrated that wear resistance of commercial cUHMWPE is considerably high, compared with UHMWPE. The obtained properties, which could be compared directly, will be useful as information for choosing materials and as reference data for a new total hip joint prosthesis under development.

ACKNOWLEDGMENTS

This work is in part supported by the R&D Projects in "Development of artificial hip joint and its evaluation method." entrusted from the New Energy and Industrial Technology Development Organization (NEDO) to Japan Fine Ceramics Center.

REFERENCES

[1] E. Ingham and J. Fisher, "Biological reactions to wear debris in total joint replacement," *Proc. Instn. Mech. Engrs.*, **214H**, 21-37 (2000).

[2] J. A. Savio III, L. M. Overcamp and J. Black, "Size and shape of biomaterial wear debris," *Clin. Mater.*, **15**, 101-147 (1994).

[3] M. Semlitsch and H. G. Willert, "Clinical wear behavior of ultra-high molecular weight polyethylene cups paired with metal and ceramic ball heads in comparison to metal-on-metal pairings of hip joint replacements," *Proc. Instn. Mech. Engrs.*, **211H**, 73-88 (1997).

[4] I. C. Clarke and A. Gustafson, "Clinical and hip simulator comparisons of ceramic-on-polyethylene and metal-on-polyethylene wear," *Clin. Orthop.*, **379**, 34-40 (2000).

[5] Y. Takigawa, K. Jono, H. Takadama, M. Mizuno and T. Nakamura, "Wear characterization of clinically used hip joint prostheses by a hip simulator," *Ceram. Eng.&Sci. Proceedings*, **24** submitted.

PROCESSING OF BIOACTIVE CERAMICS WITH DEFINED POROSITY

Charles M. Lofton
University of Florida
225 Rhines Hall
Gainesville, Florida 32611-6400

Huiyan Huang
University of Florida
225 Rhines Hall
Gainesville, Florida 32611-6400

Wolfgang Sigmund
University of Florida
225 Rhines Hass
Gainesville, Florida 32611-6400

ABSTRACT

The current medical procedure for the fixation and stabilization of damaged bones requires the insertion and later removal of metallic pens and plates. Such a procedure damages healthy tissue and is time consuming and expensive. While there are materials that chemically bond to tissue and resorb after their usefulness, their use for fixation has been impossible because of their low mechanical strength. A new processing method shows the ability to create bone scaffolds with a mixture of chemical reactivity, functional microstructure, and good mechanical properties. This processing method uses the phase separation between polymers of two compositions to create large pores. This scaffold is a composite of sol-gel produced bioglass and a reinforcing polymer for bioactivity, resorbablity, and strength. The scaffold has a microstructure of interconnected porosity for high surface area and the possibility of integrating bone growth factors or bone cells to accelerate the repair of damaged tissue.

INTRODUCTION

The repair of skeletal system damage falls into two types of medical procedures. In one, the bone and the tissue around it are removed and replaced with synthetic materials designed to mimic the function, through not necessarily, the structure of the original tissue. Total hip replacement is an example of such a procedure. The materials in this replacement are chosen to be inert with respect to the chemistry of the body and to resist fatigue fracture due to long periods of cyclic stress. A second type of procedure seeks to stabilize the damaged bone and encourage its repair, breaking down over time to allow the tissue to return to the natural, healthy state. Such a procedure would use a bone scaffold, analogous to the porous polymer scaffolds used to repair burnt or abraded skin. The materials in this type of device require both appropriate mechanical characteristics and an appropriate chemical interaction with the chemistry of bone growth and maintenance. It seems self-evident that helping the body repair itself is a superior philosophy to the removal and replacement of tissue. Obtaining the mixture of mechanical properties and favorable chemical interactions, however, has remained elusive in tissue repair.

Of the materials compatible with human tissue, the range of glass compositions termed bioglass has demonstrated the ability of bond to bone, activate bone regrowth, and resorb into the body as harmless, soluble materials[1]. These glasses are composed of SiO_2, CaO, Na_2O, and P_2O_5, and are produced through either melting or sol-gel techniques. When placed in the body, these glasses under go a surface reaction with the surrounding fluid, leading to ion exchange and the precipitation of hydroxyapatite on the glass surface[2]. This apatite layer acts as an interface to allow the bonding of glass to the tissue, and offers the substrate for the deposition of bone cells and their construction of new bone. In this research a number of bioglass compositions, fabricated through sol-gel processing, were chosen to compose the bone scaffold.

Fundamental in the healing of bone damage with a scaffold is the rapid interlocking of the damaged tissue with the scaffold and the presence of space for the continued growth and maintenance of new tissue. This requires the scaffold possess a high volume of interconnected pores large enough (10-100 microns) for the ingrowth of bone cells and matrix.

The method of forming the interconnected porosity in the bioglass scaffold is through the spinodal decomposition of a mixture of two polymers dissolved in a liquid. As in the spinodal decomposition of a glass, a change to a multi-component system thermodynamically favors the segregation of the mixture into two phases. Unlike nucleation and growth, this process starts with the small variations in composition caused by kinetic fluctuations which grow with the lowering of the systems free energy, leading to diffusion of components against concentration gradient to form separate phases with in the bulk. The free energy of a mixture of two polymer compositions is defined as:

$$\Delta G \sim RT[(\phi_1/P_1)\ln\phi_1 + (\phi_2/P_2)\ln\phi_2 + \chi_{12}\phi_1\phi_2] \qquad (1)$$

Where ϕ is the volume fraction of each component, P is the degree of polymerization, and χ is the interaction parameter[3]. The first two term are entropic in origin, while the third is enthalpic. At low degrees of polymerization, there is a large negative contribution from the entropic terms, off setting the positive enthalpic term originating from each polymer preferring to form intermolecular bonds with its own kind. As the degree of polymerization increases, the entropic terms are reduced due to the mutual disruption in the conformational entropy of the polymer chains. When the free energy of the solution becomes positive, phase separation of the two polymers is favored. If one were to view the condensation of a metal alkoxide as polymerization, then the growth of oxide clusters in the presence of another polymer would lead to destabilization and phase separation in the sol. As the oxide clusters grow, the viscosity of the sol increases, with a rapid increase at the sol-gel transition. An increase in the viscosity reduces the mass transport in the system, making phase separation increasingly difficult. If the phase separation is controlled so that it occurs near the sol-gel transition and each phase has nearly the same volume, then a gel containing a network of interconnecting porosity will be formed.

EXPERIMENTAL DESCRIPTION

The bioglass specimens are made by sol-gel processing. First polyacrylic acid (PAA) is dissolved in the corresponding mixture of water and ethanol for 1 hour, then Tetraethyl Orthosilicate (TEOS) , Nitric Acid are added into the solvent to stir for another 1 hour. Triethyl Phosphate (TEP) is added next into the mixture and stirred for 1 hour. Finally calcium nitrate is added into the mixture and stirred for half an hour. The sol is cast into a container and gelled at a constant temperature for two days. After that the bioglass gel is washed with deionized water and put into a Teflon container covered with deionized water for near-equilibrium drying. The drying temperature is 374K. After 2 days of drying, the specimens are taken out of the oven and sintered at 1373K for 4 hours.

RESULTS AND DISCUSSION

The composition of the starting gel is the key to obtain the interconnected porous structure. The composition is expressed in a C value. C is the ratio of the number of repeat units of TEOS monomer, e.g.

$$C=\frac{\text{Concentration of PAA repeat units}}{\text{Concentration of TEOS monomer}}$$

The range of C values that led to an interconnected microstructure changes for different compostions of bioglass. (See Fig. 1)

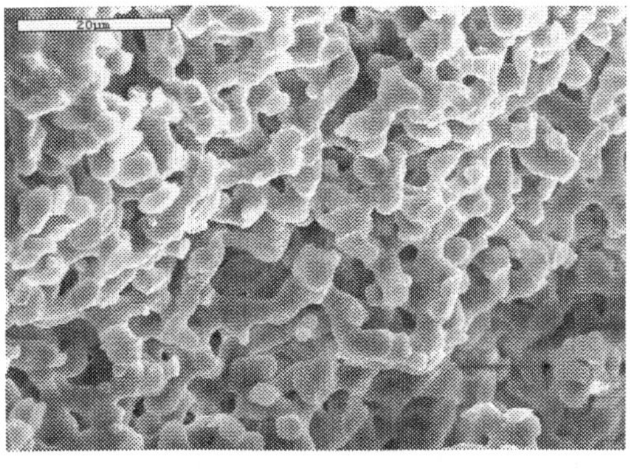

58S C=0.14

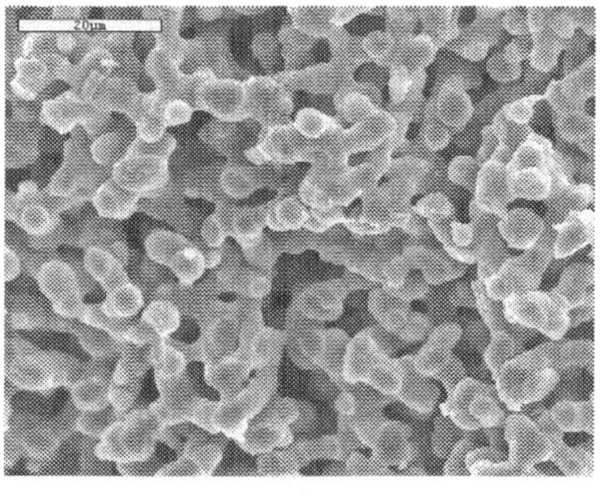

63S C=0.13

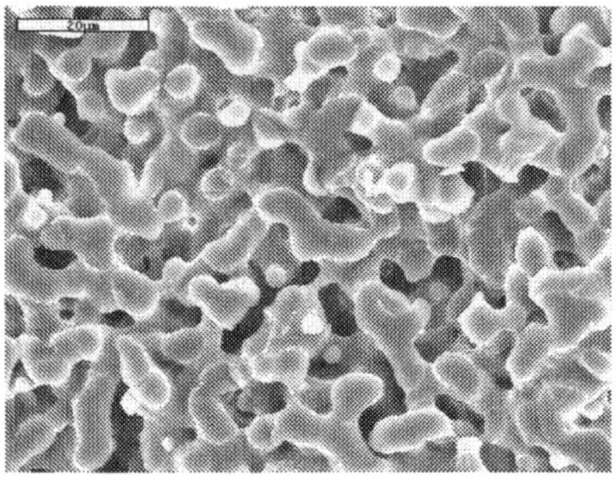

72S C=0.12

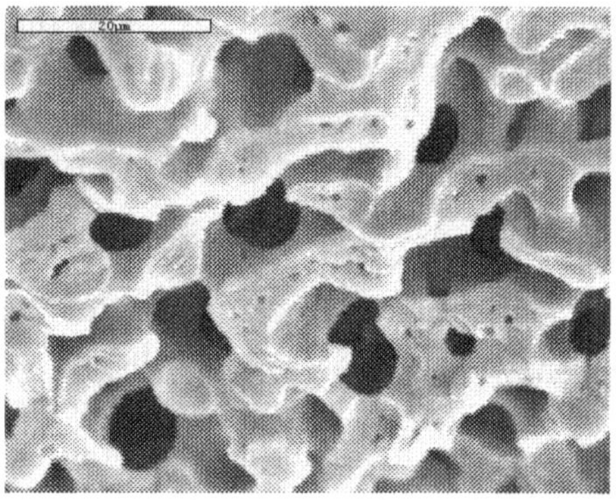

77S C=0.09

Fig. 1: SEM pictures for 58S, 63S, 72S and 77S bioglass at optimum C value, respectively. A): 58S C=0.14, B): 63S C=0.13, C): 72S C=0.12, D): C=0.09. Scale bar indicates 20 micrometers.

Sol compositions have been chosen which balance the increase in viscosity due to silica condensationand gelation and the onset of spinodal decomposition due to the phase separation of PAA and the growing silica clusters. Through controlling the kinetics of silica condensation and the mutual solubility of the silica and polymer, porous bioglass structures were formed. To achieve this, C the ratio of polymer to TEOS, and the total concentration of reactants in the solvent were controlled. In order to have the desired interconnected microstructure, the volumes of the silica and polymer rich phase must be of equal volumes. This was achieved by controlling the relative concentrations of water and ethanol, as well as the C value. Water was found to favor the silica phase, due to the highly charged silica species below pH2. Ethanol segregated more to the PAA phase, presumably due to the conversion of the polymer carboxylic acid group into the less polar ester group formed through esterification reaction of the polymer with ethanol in the presence of acid.

Several bioglass compositions were made with varying amounts of calcium oxide. Compositions with greater amounts of calcium have been found to be more bioactive than the high silica compositions[4]. High calcia glasses require larger amounts of calcium nitrate to be dissolved in the sol. This had the effect of changing the C value necessary to produce interconnect porosity. The increase in C value with calcium nitrate contend indicates the larger amounts of polymer is needed to maintain equal volume in the silica and polymer rich phases. The segregation to and the swelling of the silica-rich phase with calcium nitrate is the expected cause of this shift, requiring that more polymer be added to swell the polymer-rich phase, and maintain the equal volume situation. The segregation of calcium nitrate to the silica-rich phase expected due to the anticipation that this phase is water rich, and thus a better solvent for the salt.

The relation between gelation temperature and pore size and the relation between amount of catalyst and the pore size were also studied for the pure silica system. As the gelation temperature increased the pore size decreased. The pore size halved when the gelation temperature was increased from 333K to 343K, decreasing from an average of sixteen micrometers to eight. However, the gelation temperature must be within the range of 323K and 353K so that the sol completely gels, but the ethanol does not evaporate. The amount of nitric acid added into the sol has similar effect on the pore size. As it increases, the pore size decreases. (Table1 and Fig.2). The amount of nitric acid also must remain in a narrow range due to insure the proper mechanism of condensation and a high positive charge on the silica. Excessive acid, for example, lead to the formation of small spherical particles in the porous gel, which is undesirable.

Table 1

Pore Size (um)	PAA (g)	Ethanol (g)	H_2O (g)	HNO_3 (ml)	TEOS (g)
24.9	0.4	10	13	0.4	12.2
16	0.4	10	13	0.73	12.2
11	0.4	10	13	1.0	12.2
9	0.4	10	13	1.3	12.2

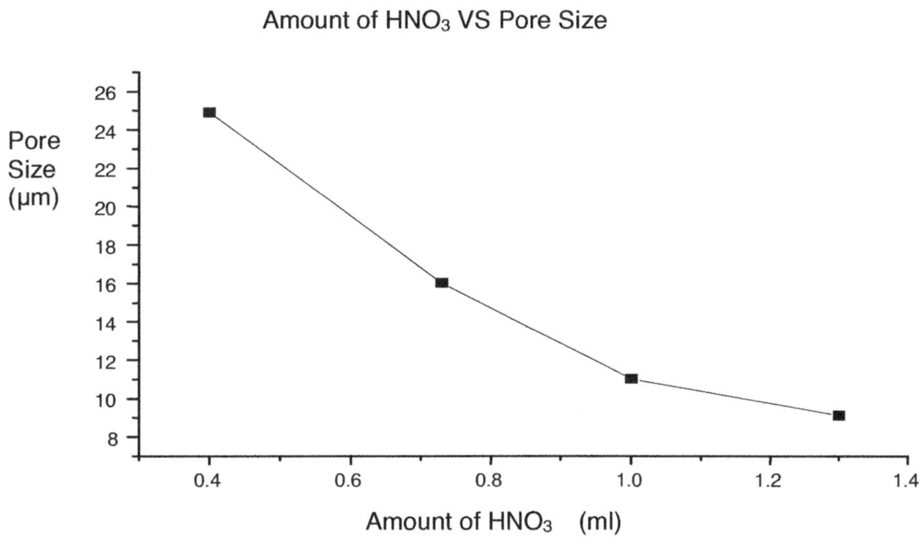

Fig. 2

The increased concentration of acid and the increase in the gelation temperature both have the effect of decreasing the pore size of the specimens. Both these factors increase the rate of silica condensation, the temperature due to kinetic factors, and the acid concentration due to the increased number of positively charged reactive silanol groups below pH 2. After gelation, phase separation leads to the formation of polymer-rich and silica-rich phase domains that grow in size through the diffusion of material in the viscous medium. The increase in condensation rate shortens the time available for the gel to phase separate due to the increase in viscosity as the silica clusters increase in size and connectivity. Both these factors control when the gel structure is frozen in place and spinodal decomposition ceases.

CONCLUSIONS

Porous, bioactive bone scaffolds have been fabricated through the spinodal decomposition of a gelling sol using an inorganic and an organic polymer to induce phase separation. Controls of the gelation temperature and catalyst concentration allow for the requiring the adjustment of the silica to polymer ratio to form the interconnected microstructure.

REFERENCE:

[1]Larry L. Hench, J. American Ceramic Society, 81 1705 (1998).

[2]June Wilson, Antti Yli-Urpo, and Risto-Pekka Happonen, "Bioactive Glass: Clinical Application"; from An Introduction to Bioceramics. Edited by Larry L. Hench and June Wilson. World Scientific, 1993.

[3]Kazuki Nakanishi, "Pore Structure Control of Gels Based on Phase Separation," J. Porous Materials, 4 67 (1997).

[4]Rounan Li, Doctoral Dissertation, University of Florida, 1991.

BIOACTIVE SURFACE FUNCTIONALIZATION: CONCEPT AND APPLICATIONS

Hyun-Min Kim

Department of Material Chemistry, Graduate School of Engineering, Kyoto University
Yoshida, Sakyo-ku, Kyoto 606-8501, Japan

ABSTRACT

Bioactive ceramics are the single material source that smartly induces biomineralization of bone mineral-like calcium phosphate, through which they integrate with bone tissue. Mechanism of the biomineralization inspires synthetic methodologies of new bioactive materials for clinical tissue repairs and replacements with enhanced physical and biological functions. This paper reviews the bioactive surface functionalization, which aims upon the surface chemistry of bioactive ceramics at surface modification for formation of bioactive structures on tough materials, sol-gel derivation of bioactive nano-hybrids, biomimetic hybridization of calcium phosphate on polymers macrotextured in 3D-structure, and bioactive matrix for tissue engineering.

INTRODUCTION

Bone diseases and defects are one of the most frequent medical conditions, which often owing to a large dimension need an extensive use of synthetic materials. Synthetic materials for bone repairs and replacements have to structurally and/or biologically function in close contact with living bone, but they are generally non-vital and poor in bonding with host bone tissue. Bioactive ceramics, represented by Bioglass®, sintered hydroxyapatite (HA), sintered β-tricalcium phosphate (TCP) and glass-ceramic A-W, are the unique material source that reveal spontaneous bone-integrating ability in bone defect.[1-3] In forms of dense and porous bulks, particulates, cements and coatings, they have provided new material strategy in clinical bone repairs and replacements, and have been documented in numerous cases of medical success in bone repairs or replacements (Fig. 1).[1,2] In fact, it appears that clinical applications of the bioactive ceramics have been largely progressed to find complaints in their performances, which mostly imply poor structural functions; the bioactive ceramics and related composites are being considered poor in fracture resistance and too stiff for load-bearing applications in compact bone defects (Fig. 2).

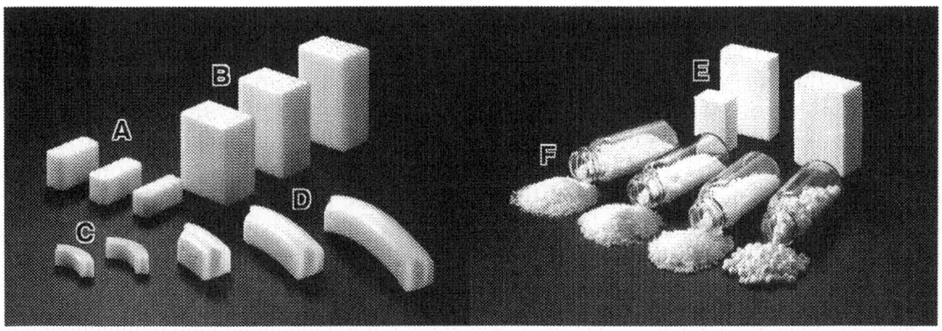

Fig. 1. Artificial bone graft sources of glass-ceramic A-W: intervertebral discs (A), artificial vertebrae (B), spinal spacer (C), iliac crests (D), porous spacer (E) and bone filler (F), (courtesy of Nippon Electric Glass Co., Otsu, Japan).

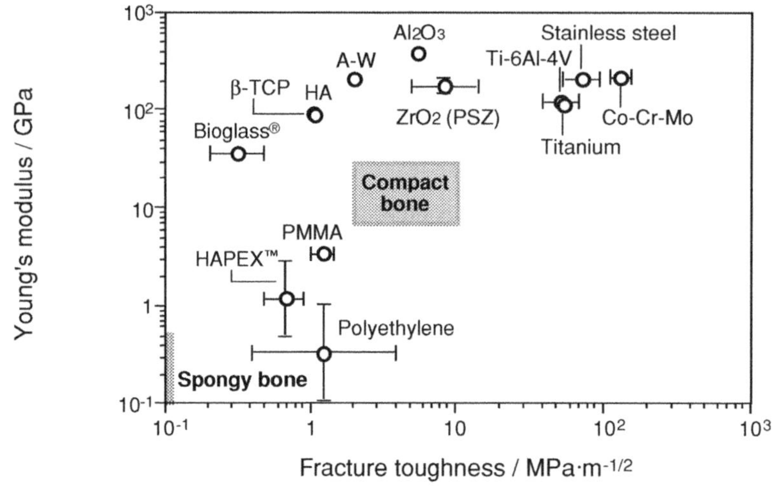

Fig. 2. Fracture toughnesses and Young's moduli of candidate materials for bone repairs and replacements, compared to those of human spongy and compact bones; note the scale.

In terms of surface chemistry of bone-integration, the bioactive ceramics are providing new challenging methodologies for bioactive materials alleviating their own problems. Among the most promising strategies for new bioactive materials with enhanced functions is the bioactive surface functionalization, which learns and mimics the induction mechanism of biomineralization of calcium phosphate on bioactive ceramics in the living body. This paper aims to introduce the concept of bioactive surface functionalization, presenting exemplified applications in designing new bioactive materials with different functions.

FUNDAMENTALS FOR BIOACTIVE FUNCTIONALIZATIONS

Mechanism of Bone-Integration of Bioactive Ceramics

General response of bone tissue to a hosted synthetic material is encapsulation by forming non-adherent fibrous connective tissue, which ensues isolation of the material. Integration of the bioactive ceramics with bone tissue is owing to a very smart surface biomineralization, of which the specification is considered essential for establishing the strategy of bioactive surface functionalization.

The interface between a bioactive ceramic and bone tissue after integration, almost independent of the type and phase of bioactive ceramics, reveals the presence of a thin layer of calcium phosphate (see Fig. 3).[1-4] Assessments in animal models are testifying that this calcium phosphate layer is formed on the ceramic surfaces at an early implantation period, and mediate thereafter the integration of ceramics with bone matrix.[5]

Characterizations has been specified that the interfacial calcium phosphate consists of nanocrystallites of apatite that subtly differs from synthetic HA in composition and structure: the apatite does contain carbonate and is structurally defective, i.e., the apatite exhibits striking resemblance to the mineral phase in bone tissue.[1, 2, 5] This type of apatite layer is not observed around non-bioactive materials in bone defects, implying that the surface biomineralization of the bone mineral-like apatite is the condition that dominates the bone-integration ability of synthetic materials. Owing to the bone mineral-like features, the apatite recruits bone-producing cells, i.e., the osteoblasts, which proliferate in preference to fibroblast to differentiate and produce an extracellular matrix (ECM) composed of biological apatite and collagen.[1-3] Bioactive ceramics are considered to have thus a surface phase equivalent to bone mineral or bone tissue, spontaneously establishing a tight chemical integration with bone to decrease the interfacial energy.

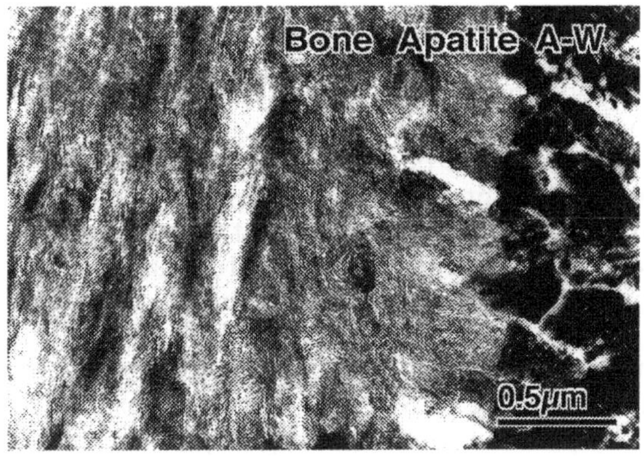

Fig. 3. Interface between glass-ceramic A-W and bone; cross-sectional TEM photograph after implantation in artificial defect of rat tibia for 8 w; see collagen fibers running transversely in the bone area.

Chemistry of Surface-Induced Biomineralization of Apatite on Ceramics

The blood plasma is the very first media that a bioactive ceramic interfaces after being hosted in bone defect. Therefore, a bioactive surface is speculated being directed toward mineralization of apatite via interaction with the blood plasma. The body fluid contains various proteins that may significantly involve in the biomineralization,[3,6] of which the cascade is too complex to mimic ex-vivo for designing new bioactive materials. But, in terms of inorganic ion species, the body fluid is solution highly supersaturated with respect to calcium phosphates, accordingly having great potential to precipitate apatite.[7] It is skillfully controlled in a metastable condition to deposit the apatite solely by means of a surface-induced heterogeneous nucleation and growth. Kokubo et al.[8] early proposed a protein-free acellular simulated body fluid (SBF) with ionic concentrations (Na^+ 142.0, K^+ 5.0, Ca^{2+} 2.5, Mg^{2+} 1.5, Cl^- 147.8, HCO^{3-} 4.2, HPO_4^{2-} 1.0, SO_4^{2-} 0.5 mM, pH 7.25 or 7.40) nearly equal to those in human blood plasma. The SBF has been extensively confirmed to produce apatite on different bioactive ceramics, as was found on them in vivo after implantation.[9]

The in vitro models using SBF are providing significant information on the compositional and

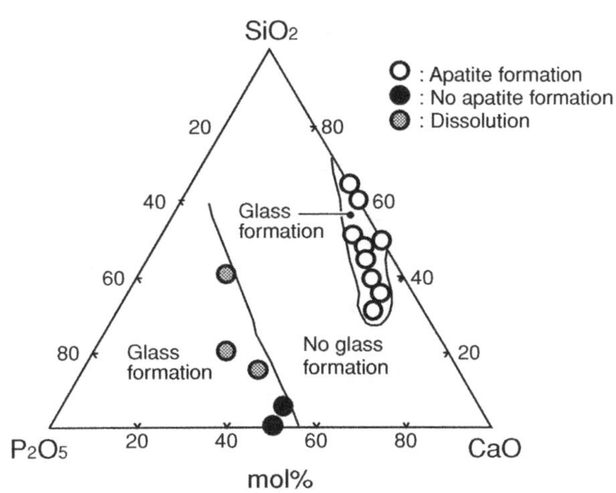

Fig. 4. Compositional dependence of apatite formation on CaO-SiO_2-P_2O_5 glasses after immersion in SBF for 28 d.

structural dependences of apatite formation on ceramic surfaces. Glasses with different compositions in the systems $CaO-P_2O_5-SiO_2$, $Na_2O-CaO-SiO_2$, $M_2O-SiO_2-TiO_2$ (M = Na or/and K) and $Na_2O-CaO-Al_2O_3$, among which the former two systems provide the basal compositions of glass-ceramic A-W and Bioglass®, have been subjected to immersion in SBF.[10-12] Basal compositions with apatite-forming ability are based upon binary systems $CaO-SiO_2$, M_2O-SiO_2 (M = Na or K) and M_2O-TiO_2 (Fig. 4), but interestingly not upon the system $CaO-P_2O_5$ nor $M_2O-Al_2O_3$. Surface characterizations of the glasses as a function of immersion time in SBF indicate that the formation of apatite is preceded not exceptionally by formation of hydrated silica or hydrated titania abun-dant in Si-OH or Ti-OH groups on their surfaces. SBF characterizations indicate that the glasses form the surface silica or titania by releasing Na^+, K^+ and/or Ca^{2+} ions via ion exchange with H_3O^+ ions in SBF. In view of the solution chemistry, the ion exchanges give an increase in the ionic activity product (IP) of apatite in SBF.[10] This implies that a bioactive ceramic induces the mineralization of apatite by providing functional groups, e.g., Si-OH and Ti-OH, effective for inducing apatite nucleation on their surfaces, being by an IP increase in the surrounding fluid.

Oxide hydrogels are immersed in SBF to provide in vitro models to determine effective compositions and structures of functional groups for apatite nucleation.[13-16] The apatite formations were known to be induced on hydrogels of silica, titania, zirconia, tantalate and niobate, but not on alumina, implying the efficiencies of functional sites composed of such as Si-OH, Ti-OH Zr-OH, Ta-OH and Nb-OH groups in apatite nucleation. Self-assembled monolayers (SAM) in SBF indicated that COOH and PO_4H_2 groups also serve as the functional groups for apatite nucleation, but not the NH_2, $CONH_2$, OH and CH_3 groups.[17] ESCA and TEM studies are indicating that the nucleation of apatite by the known functional sites progresses in process sequences: 1) formation of the functional sites on the surface, 2) early combination of calcium ions with the functional sites to form a intermediate phase of calcium compound, 3) late combination of phosphate ions with the calcium compound to form an amorphous calcium phosphate (ACP), and 4) crystallization of the ACP into apatite (Fig. 5).[18] Electrophoresis is implying that the surface potential by the functional sites is initially negative, which indicates that there involved an electrostatic interaction between the functional sites and calcium ions in initialization of apatite nucleation.[19] Therefore, functional groups able to develop negative charge at the blood plasma pH (≈7.4) are assumed approximately effective for inducing apatite nucleation in body environment. However, there is also a strong implication that the structural arrangement of the groups is also the definitive factor that determines their induction efficiencies of apatite nucleation.[20] For

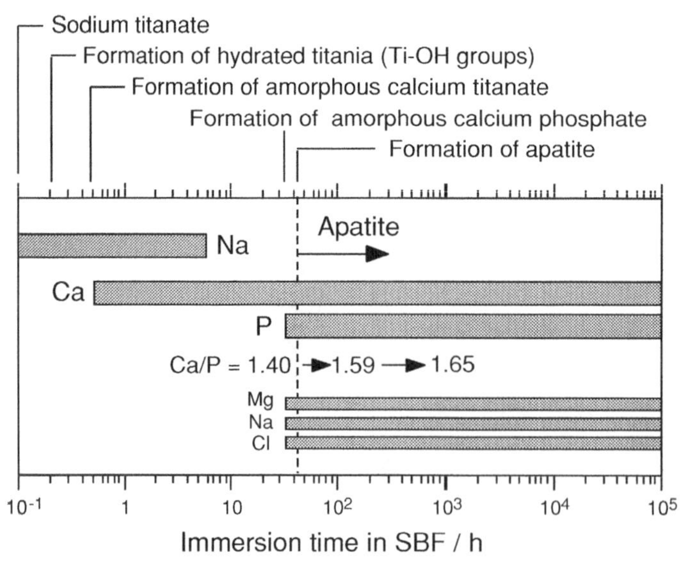

Fig. 5. Surface composition and structure of the Na_2O-TiO_2 bioactive phase as a function of immersion time in SBF; based upon XPS and TEM-EDX assessments.

example, titania gels may be precursored from tetraisopropyl titanate (TiPT) to have form an amorphous, anatase or rutile structures by thermal treatment at different temperatures. On immersion in SBF, apatite formation is much more pronounced on the anatase gels than on the amorphous and rutile gels. The nucleation of apatite appears to be processed by a certain types of nano-textures of the functional groups that provide an epitaxy site arrangement for apatite crystal.[21] In fact, this subject is one of the central challenges in bioactive ceramic research at the time being.

The bioactive surface functionalization is based upon the current knowledge of mechanism of bioactivity revelation on ceramics, and surmises functionalization of a surface of material of bio-medical interest to provide induction capability of calcium phosphate mineralization in vivo, or the production of the calcium phosphate in vitro, using one of the above the functional sites and the SBF.

APPLICATIONS OF BIOACTIVE SURFACE FUNCTIONALIZATION

Bioactivity Induction by Surface Modifications

Implants in replacement of bones such as femur and tibia are required to perform structural function under stringent load-bearing conditions, for which they need to reveal fracture strength and toughness over those of cortical bone. Metals are non-bioactive, but proper material source for this purpose (see Fig 2). Compositional review of the functional groups effective for apatite nucleation indicates, however, that many of the non-bioactive tough materials have the potential to be bioactive. Bioactive surface functionalization (BSF) schemes on the surfaces of such mater-ials to produce bioactive ceramic phase using the surface as the in situ precursor.

Chemical surface modification of titanium metal[22-24] is one of most prime BSF examples. Titanium metal is simply immersed in aqueous NaOH and subsequently subjected to thermal annealing to form a bioactive sodium titanate on its surface, which is functionally graded as a function of depth toward the substrate without phase discontinuity. Bewitchingly, this BSF pro-vokes no mechanical degradation of the titanium neither in strength nor in fatigue resistance, and can be applied to macroporous titanium to form bioactive surface along the surface and cross-sectional macrotextures. The BSF titanium metal reveals apatite-forming ability in vivo and in vitro comparable to glass-ceramic A-W. Surface and SBF characterizations indicate that the apatite formation on the BSF metal mimics the processes of those on bioactive ceramics, i.e., formation of surface functional groups of Ti-OH by ion exchange of Na^+ ion on the surface with H_3O^+ ion in the fluid, induction of apatite nucleation by the Ti-OH groups and simultaneously an acceleration of the apatite nucleation by IP increase, and spontaneous growth of the apatite nuclei consuming calcium and phosphate ions in the fluid.

The BSF titanium metal was investigated into a number of animal models, presenting pro-mising results toward clinical applications.[25-27] For example, the BSF titanium implant is im-planted into intramedullar canal of rabbit femur, eliciting much more pronounced bony formation around it than untreated implant (Fig. 6). The pronounced bony formation is clearly owing to

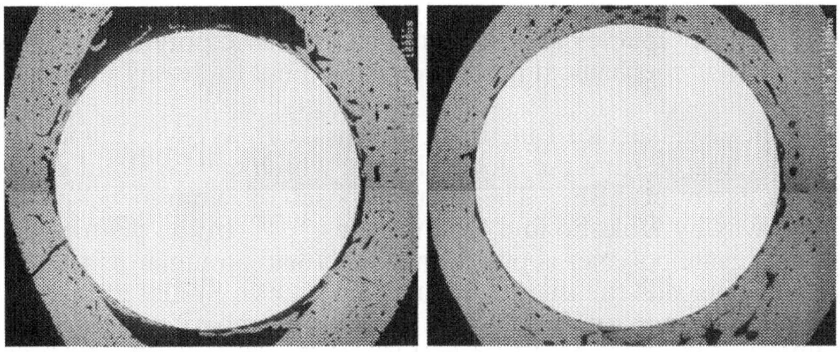

Fig. 6. Untreated (left) and BSF (right) titanium implants in artificial bone defects; cross-sectional SEM photographs after implantation in intramedullar canal of rabbit femur for 12 w.

apatite induced on its surface, where bone tissue integrates to provide a high bonding strength at the interface. The bone-bonding strength of the BSF titanium at an early implantation period of 12 w appeared over 15 times higher in tension and 8 times higher in shear than untreated titanium. Macroporous titanium is subjected to the BSF to greatly encourage bony ingrowth into the porous texture to provide chemical integration secured in biological fixation.

The chemical scheme of BSF was applied to titanium alloys such as Ti-6Al-4V, Ti-6Al-2Nb-Ta and Ti-15Mo-5Zr-3Al, and tantalum and zirconium metals, showing effectiveness in formation of bioactive surface phase of sodium titanate, sodium tantalate, or hydrated zirconia.[28-30] A Ce-TZP/Al_2O_3 nano-composite was documented to form a bioactive zirconia gel layer on its surface by BSF in aqueous HPO_4, H_2SO_4, HCl or NaOH solution. These approaches are all aim to mimic apatite nucleation on hydrogel phases of titania, zirconia, tantalite and niobate.

Synthesis of Bioactive Inorganic/Organic Nano-hybrids

In terms of Young's moduli, ceramics and metals are much stiffer than human bone (see Fig. 2). While bone has to remodel in response to mechanical stimulation to become better adapted to load, a stiff implant may give rise to stress shielding around the host bone, ensuing loss of bone tissue. Organically modified silicate (ORMOSIL) is monolithic inorganic-organic composite synthesized through sol-gel processes co-polymerizing organic components into silicate network at the molecular level. The ORMOSIL may show even a rubber-like elasticity, which is the property of much interest as biomaterial. Generally, the inorganic component of ORMOSIL is precursored from the tetraethoxysilane (TEOS) as in the bioactive silica gel, upon which it is sufficient to derive a concept of bioactive inorganic-organic nano-hybrids with high bioactivity as well as high flexibility.

The bioactive feature of the ORMOSIL was early conceived by Osaka and his co-workers.[31] Preparations of bioactive hybrids are being attempted in system polydimethylsiloxane (PDMS)-CaO-SiO_2-TiO_2.[32-34] Bioactive and physical properties of the hybrids in this system vary largely with factors such as sol-gel precursor, process and composition. Hydrolysis and polycondensation of PDMS, TEOS, TiPT and calcium nitrate give pore- and crack-free transparent monolithic hybrids with high flexibility, whose bioactivity in terms of apatite-forming ability in vitro is comparable to those bioactive glasses. The hybrids can be simply composed in the binary system PDMS-TiO_2 to reveal rubber elasticity as well as high bioactivity with an aid of the titania. Bioactive hybrids are considered as matrix materials beneficial for bioactive composites, as they can be widely controlled in flexibility to accommodate ductile or brittle materials as counter components. This approach may lead to bioactive composites with different mechanical properties.

Biomimetic Calcium Phosphate Coating on 3D-Matrices Polymer

In typical compact bone, over 99 vol% of the bone is ECM composed of 41.0 vol% (22 wt%) organic matrix of which 96 vol% is collagen, 41.8 vol% (69 wt%) apatite mineral and 17.2 vol% (9 wt%) water. Mechanical property of the bone is unique, i.e., tough as well as flexible, owing to the 3D-composite structure of the ECM: the apatite crystallites are submicroscopic and deposited on collagen fibers, which are assembled into in the form of lamellar sheets and further woven up into 3D-structure. It is therefore largely expected that even an acellular composite, in which bone mineral-like nano-apatites are deposited on synthetic polymers textured as collagen fibers in the bone, may reveal mechanical properties equivalent to those of bone, or be useful for tissue engineering.

The bioactive ceramics use surface functional groups such as Si-OH and Ti-OH to induce nucleation and growth of apatite from the blood plasma, which can be simulated biomimetically even in an acellular solution of SBF. The first proposal of biomimetic process using such polymer knit and SBF was by Kokubo and his disciples.[35-37] In the primitive version of this biomimetic process, an organic polymer is placed in contact with granular particles of a CaO-SiO_2-based glass in SBF. During this treatment, silicate ions rich in Si-OH groups release from the glass to adsorb onto the polymer surface, where they induce apatite nucleation in situ. The polymer is subsequently immersed in a solution highly supersaturated with respect to the apatite to make the apatite nuclei grow into homogeneous layer on the polymer surface. This process was shown to produce a dense and uniform bonelike apatite layer composed of nano-apatite crystallites with a desired thickness on any kind of organic polymer. Subjecting the polymer surface to pre-treatments such as glow discharge before the apatite nucleation improves adhesive strength of the apatite layer to the polymer substrate up to 10 MPa. This type of biomimetic method using nucleating agent of glass have found successes in 2D-texture of polymer knits (Fig. 7), and the in vitro apatite was proven to mediate successfully the bone-integration in bone tissue.

Biomimetic processes are now attempted to functionalize 3D-texture by specifying polymer targets and employing techniques that facilitates uniform incorporation of the Si-OH or other functional groups onto polymer surfaces. These techniques include: immersion in sodium silicate solution,[38] sol-gel incorporation of silica into silicone,[39] vapor phase photografting and hydrolysis of vinyltrimethoxysilane on polyethylene,[40] coupling and hydrolysis of iso-cyanatopropyltri-ethoxysilane on ethylene-vinylalcohol co-polymer,[41] phospholylate coupling onto polyethylene or cotton fiber,[42] attachment of SAMs or Langmuir-Blodgett films terminated with COOH groups,[43] and carboxylmethylation of chitin.[44,45]

Another interest in the biomimetic process is the control of the composition and structure of the apatite crystallites. The SBF parameters, e.g., pH, ionic concentration and temperature, sensitively affect the growth and the composition of the biomimetic apatite on the polymer surfaces.[36,46,47] The rate of apatite growth significantly increases with an increase either in ionic concentration or in temperature of SBF. Apatite with the most bone mineral-like composition is, however, produced in SBF whose ion concentrations including HCO_3^- and Cl^- are conditioned to be equal to those in blood plasma. Implication at the time being is that the composition and structure of apatite can be widely controlled by changing the SBF parameters.

Perspective in Conjunction with Tissue Engineering

Bone tissue engineering recently contemplates a synthetic bone-repairing material associated with the highly regenerative capability of bone cells. Three factors are considered vital for successful bone tissue engineering: osteoblasts to produce bone tissue, growth factors to mani-pulate cell functions, and matrix materials which have to accommodate the cells and growth factors and to provide sites for bone tissue generation. As is in most cases of tissue engineering, the bone cells and/or growth factors have to be once in vitro, whose maintenances have been very difficult. Recent biotechnology made possible the in vitro use of mesenchymal stem cell (MSC) in bone marrow, which has high capability to differentiate into osteogenic phenotypes, which can be culture-expanded in number. Significant growth factors such as bone morphogenetic protein (BMP) are commercially available by molecular cloning. Prototypically, matrix materials are required to release the growth factors in a controlled way and provide sites for bone cell attachment and bone formation, and often desired to timely degrade being replaced by regenerated bone tissue in vivo. Natural and synthetic polymers such as collagen, poly(glycolic acid), (PGA),

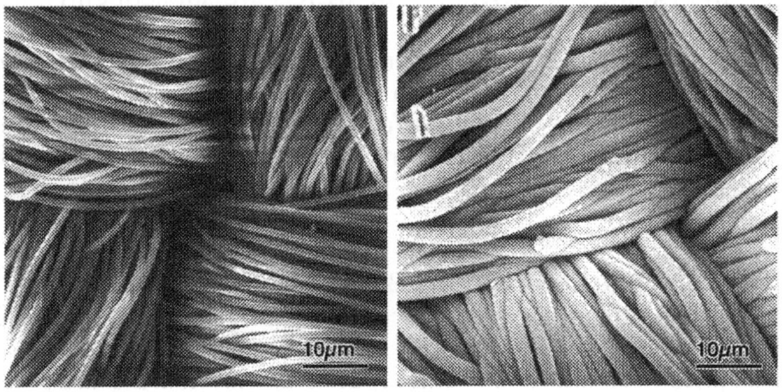

Fig. 7. SEM photographs of the polyethyleneterephthalate (PET) knit before (left) and after (right) bonelike apatite coating by biomimetic process using nucleating agent of $CaO-SiO_2$-based glass in SBF.

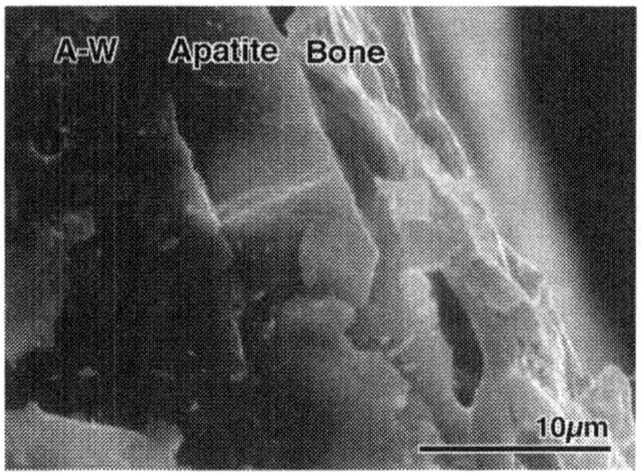

Fig. 9. In vitro bone formation on the apatite pre-formed on glass-ceramic A-W in SBF; SEM photograph after rat osteoblast cell culture for 23 d (courtesy of Dr. J.-M. Sautier, University Paris 7).

poly(L-lactic acid) (PLLA) and poly(DL-lactic-co-glycolic acid) (PLGA) are the major matrix materials for this purpose,[48] whose functions are limited in controlled release and degradation.

Recent studies are documenting experimental evidences that bioactive ceramics provide stimulation that significantly activates bone cells to generate bone tissue, implying that they are much more promising candidate matrix for bone tissue engineering. For example, Ohgushi et al.[49] showed that cultured MSCs seeded onto HA, β-TCP or glass-ceramic A-W successfully differentiate into osteoblasts to construct bone tissue tightly integrated with the ceramic surfaces. The ceramics hybridized with in vitro bone in this way are implanted in vivo to continue bony formation, implying that their biological functions are almost comparable to those of natural bone. Sautier et al.[50] reported that the surface of glass-ceramic A-W forms bone matrix on rat osteoblast cell culture, suggesting that a bioactive ceramic surface significantly facilitates the differentiation of osteogenic cells and subsequent apposition of bone matrix. This effect was, however, shown much more pronounced on bonelike apatite layer pre-formed on the glass-ceramic (Fig. 8). Using Bioglass®-type glass substrates, Ducheyene et al.[6] suggested that the bonelike apatite layer preformed in a calcium phosphate electrolyte concentrates osteoinductive growth factors on its surface in biologically active forms, thereby providing a synergistic effect on osteoblastic differentiation and subsequent bone formation. These imply that in vitro formation of bonelike apatite layer may be more advantageous than merely utilizing the bioactive ceramics.

Clinical application of the osteogenic matrix coating as termed by Ohgushi and his co-workers,[49] is considered imminent. This technique plans to collect fresh bone marrow cells from the patient's own body and isolate the MSCs. The MSCs are subsequently subjected to culture-expansion, and cultured on a bioactive implant for formation of bone matrix. The implant with in vitro bone matrix coating introduced into the surgery site is claimed as regenerative as in vivo bone. It appears, however, that the relationship among bioactive ceramics, growth factors and bone cell functions should be further identified for future advancement. Specifically, the bone tissue engineering may be greatly advanced in conjunction with 3D-matrices via the BSF techniques, which we discussed above.

SUMMARY

We reviewed above the fundamentals for BSF strategy, which learns mechanism of the biomineralization of calcium phosphate on bioactive ceramics. Proper surface functional sites that initiate nucleation of apatite by electrostatic interaction and metastable calcium phosphate solutions that has high potential to nucleate the apatite were shown to be vital in BSF. Using those is exemplified: bioactivity induction on tough substrate materials via surface modifications producing functionally graded bioactive ceramic phases, sol-gel derivation of bioactive nano-hybrids with flexibility, biomimetic processes to produce calcium phosphate coating on 3D-textured polymers, and perspective in conjunction with tissue engineering technology. These methods of BSF are believed to have great potential of producing new bioactive materials with enhanced functions for bone repairs and replacements.

ACKNOWLEDGMENTS

The author thanks Professors Tadashi Kokubo and Takashi Nakamura at Kyoto University for their long-term instructions.

REFERENCES

[1]L.L. Hench, "Bioceramics: from concept to clinic," *J. Am. Ceram. Soc.*, **74**, 1487-510 (1991).

[2]T. Kokubo, "Recent progress in glass-based materials for biomedical applications," *J. Ceram. Soc. Japan (Seramikkusu Ronbunshi)*, **99**, 965-973 (1991).

[3]L.L. Hench, "Bioactive materials: the potential for tissue regeneration," *J. Biomed. Mater. Res.*, **15**, 511-518 (1998).

[4]N. Neo, S. Kotani, T. Nakamura, T. Yamamuro, C. Ohtsuki, T. Kokubo, and Y. Bando, "A comparative study of ultrastructure of the interface between four kinds of surface-active ceramic and bone," *J. Biomed. Mater. Res.*, **26**, 1419-32 (1992).

[5]For example: T. Kitsugi, T. Yamamuro and T. Kokubo, "Analysis of A-W glass-ceramic surface by micro-beam X-ray diffraction," *J. Biomed. Mater. Res.*, **24**, 259-273 (1990).

[6]P. Ducheyene and Q. Qui, "Bioactive ceramics: the effect of surface reactivity on bone formation and bone cell functions," *Biomaterials*, **20**, 2287-2303 (1999).

[7]J. Gamble, *Chemical Anatomy, Physiological and Pathology of Extracellular Fluid*, Harvard Univ. Press, MA (1967).

[8]T. Kokubo, H. Kushitani, S. Sakka, T. Kitsugi and T. Yamamuro, "Solution able to reproduce in vivo surface-structure changes in bioactive glass-ceramic A-W," *J. Biomed. Mater. Res.*, **24**, 721-734 (1990).

[9]For example: M.R. Filguerias, G.R. Torre and L.L. Hench, "Solution effects on the surface reaction of a bioactive glass," *J. Biomed. Mater. Res.*, **27**, 445-53 (1993).

[10] C. Ohtsuki, T. Kokubo and T. Yamamuro, "Mechanism of apatite formation on $CaO-SiO_2-P_2O_5$ glasses in a simulated body fluid," *J. Non-Cryst. Solids*, **143**, 84-92, (1992).

[11] H.-M. Kim, F. Miyaji, T. Kokubo, C. Ohtsuki and T. Nakamura, "Bioactivity of $Na_2O-CaO-SiO2$ glasses," *J. Am. Ceram. Soc.*, **78**, 2405-2411 (1995).

[12] H.-M. Kim, F. Miyaji, T. Kokubo, M. Kobayashi and T. Nakamura, "Bioactivity of $M_2O-TiO_2-SiO_2$ (M=Na, K) glasses: an *in vitro* evaluation," *Bull. Chem. Soc. Japan*, **69**, 2387-2394 (1996).

[13] P. Li, C. Ohtsuki, T. Kokubo, K. Nakanishi, N. Soga, T. Nakamura, T. Yamamuro and K. de Groot, "A role of hydrated silica, titania and alumina in forming biologically active bone-like apatite on implant," *J. Biomed. Mater. Res.*, **28**, 7-15 (1994).

[14] T. Miyazaki, H.-M. Kim, T. Kokubo, H. Kato and T. Nakamura, "Induction and acceleration of bonelike apatite formation on tantalum oxide gel in simulated body fluid," *J. Sol-Gel Sci. & Tech.*, **21**, 83-88 (2001).

[15] M. Uchida, H.-M. Kim, T. Kokubo and T. Nakamura, "Bonelike apatite formation induced on zirconia gel in simulated body fluid and its modified solutions," *J. Am. Ceram. Soc.*, **84**, 2041-2044 (2001).

[16] T. Miyazaki, H.-M. Kim, T. Kokubo, C. Ohtsuki, H. Kato and T. Nakamura, "Apatite-forming ability of niobium oxide gels in a simulated body fluid, "*J. Ceram. Soc. Japan,* **109**, 929-933 (2001).

[17] M. Tanahashi and T. Matsuda, "Surface functional groups dependence on apatite formation on self-assembled monolayers in a simulated body fluid," *J. Biomed. Mater. Res.*, **34**, 305-315 (1997).

[18] For example: H. Takadama, H.-M. Kim, T. Kokubo and T. Nakamura, "Mechanism of biomineralization of apatite on a sodium silicate glass: TEM-EDX study *in vitro*," *Chem. Mater.*, **13**, 1108-1113 (2001).

[19] T. Himeno, M. Kawashita, H.-M. Kim, T. Kokubo and T. Nakamura, "Zeta-potential variation of bioactive titanium metal during apatite formation on its surface in simulated body

fluid," pp.641-644 in *Bioceramics, Vol.14*, ed. by S. Brown, I.R. Clarke and P. Williams, Trans Tech Pub., Switzerland, 2001.

[20] M. Uchida, H.-M. Kim, T. Kokubo and T. Nakamura, "Apatite-forming ability of sodium-containing titania gels in a simulated body fluid," *J. Am. Ceram. Soc.*, **84**, 2969-2974 (2001).

[21] For example: G. Daculsi, R.Z. LeGeros, M. Heughbaert and I. Barbieux, "Formation of carbonate-apatite crystals after implantation of calcium phosphate ceramics," *Calcif. Tissue Int.*, **46**, 20-27 (1990).

[22] H.-M. Kim, F. Miyaji, T. Kokubo and T. Nakamura, "Preparation of bioactive Ti and its alloys via simple chemical surface treatment," *J. Biomed. Mater. Res.*, **32**, 409-417 (1996).

[23] H.-M. Kim, F. Miyaji, T. Kokubo, S. Nishiguchi and T. Nakamura, "Graded surface structure of bioactive titanium metal prepared by chemical treatment," *J. Biomed. Mater. Res.*, **45**, 100-107 (1999).

[24] H.-M. Kim, T. Kokubo, S. Fujibayashi, S. Nishiguchi and T. Nakamura, "Bioactive macroporous titanium surface layer on titanium substrate," *J. Biomed. Mater. Res.*, **52**, 553-557 (2000).

[25] W.-Q. Yan, T. Nakamura, M. Kobayashi, H.-M. Kim, F. Miyaji and T. Kokubo, "Bonding of chemically treated titanium implant to bone," *J. Biomed. Mater. Res.*, **37**, 265-275 (1997).

[26] S. Nishiguchi, T. Nakamura, M. Kobayashi, H.-M. Kim, F. Miyaji and T. Kokubo, "The effect of heat treatment on bone-bonding ability of alkali-treated titanium," *Biomaterials*, **20**, 491-500 (1999).

[27] S. Nishiguchi, T. Nakamura, H. Kato, H. Fujita, H.-M. Kim, F. Miyaji and T. Kokubo, "Enhancement of bone-bonding strength of titanium alloy implants by alkali and heat treatments," *J. Biomed. Mater. Res. (Appl. Biomater.)*, **48**, 689-696 (1999).

[28] H.-M. Kim, H. Takadama, F. Miyaji, T. Kokubo, S. Nishiguchi and T. Nakamura, "Formation of a graded bioactive surface structure on Ti-15Mo-5Zr-3Al alloy by chemical treatment," *Biomaterials*, **21**, 353-358 (2000).

[29] T. Miyazaki, H.-M. Kim, F. Miyaji, T. Kokubo and T. Nakamura, "Bioactive tantalum metal prepared by NaOH treatment," *J. Biomed. Mater. Res.*, **50**, 35-42 (2000).

[30] M. Uchida, H.-M. Kim, F. Miyaji, T. Kokubo and T. Nakamura, "Apatite formation on zirconium metal treated with NaOH aqueous solution," *Biomaterials*, **23**, 313-317 (2002).

[31] A. Osaka, C. Ohtsuki and K. Tsuru, "Preparation of bioactive polymers modified with silanol groups," pp.441-445 in *Bioceramics Vol.8*, ed. by J. Wilson, L.L. Hench and D. Greenspan, Elsevier Sci., Oxford, 1995.

[32] Q. Chen, F. Miyaji, T. Kokubo and T. Nakamura, "Apatite formation on PDMS-modified CaO-SiO_2-TiO_2 hybrids prepared by sol-gel process," *Biomaterials*, **20**, 1127-1132 (1999).

[33] N. Miyata, Q. Chen, T. Kokubo and T. Nakamura, "Mechanical behavior of bioactive PDMS-modified CaO-SiO_2-TiO_2 hybrid materials: effects of heat treatments and TiO_2 content," pp. 441-444 in *Bioceramics, Vol. 12,* ed.by H. Ohgushi, G.W. Hastings and T. Yoshikawa, World Sci., Singapore, 1999.

[34] Q. Chen, M. Miyata, T. Kokubo and T. Nakamura, "Bioactivity and mechanical properties of PDMS-modified CaO-SiO_2-TiO_2 hybrids prepared by sol-gel process," *J. Biomed. Mater. Res.*, **51**, 605-611 (2000).

[35] Y. Abe, T. Kokubo and T. Yamamuro, "Apatite coating on ceramics, metals and polymers utilizing a biological process," *J. Mater. Sci.: Mater. Med.*, **1**, 233-238 (1990).

[36] K. Hata and T. Kokubo, "Growth of a bonelike apatite layer on a substrate by a biomimetic process," *J. Am. Ceram. Soc.*, **78**, 1049-1053 (1995).

[37] M. Tanahashi, T. Kokubo, M. Minoda, T. Miyamoto, T. Nakamura and T. Yamamuro, "Apatite coating on organic polymers by a biomimetic process," *J. Am. Ceram. Soc.*, **77**, 2805-2808 (1994).

[38] F. Miyaji, H.-M. Kim, S. Handa, T. Kokubo and T. Nakamura, "Bonelike apatite coating on organic polymers: novel nucleation process using sodium silicate solution," *Biomaterials*, **20**, 913-919 (1999).

[39] A. Oyane, K. Nakanishi, H.-M. Kim, F. Miyaji, T. Kokubo, N. Soga and T. Nakamura, "Sol-gel modification on silicone substrate to induce apatite-forming ability," *Biomaterials*, **20**, 79-84 (1999).

[40] H.-M. Kim, M. Uenoyama, T. Kokubo, M. Minoda, T. Miyamoto and T. Nakamura, "Biomimetic apatite formation on polyethylene substrate photografted with vinyltrimethoxysilane and

hydrolyzed," *Biomaterials.*, **22**, 2489-2494 (2001)

[41] A. Oyane, M. Minoda, T. Miyamoto, R. Takahashi, K. Nakanishi, H.-M. Kim, T. Kokubo and T. Nakamura, "Apatite formation on ethylene-vinylalcohol copolymer modified with silanol groups," *J. Biomed. Mater. Res.*, **47**, 367-373 (1999).

[42] O.N. Tretinnikov, K. Kato and Y. Ikada, "In vitro hydroxyapatite deposition onto a film surface-grafted with organophosphate polymer," *J. Biomed. Mater. Res.*, **28**, 1365-1373 (1994).

[43] H. Lin, W.-S. Seo, K. Kuwabara and K. Koumoto, "Crystallization of hydroxyapatite under Langmuir monolayer," *J.Ceram. Soc. Japan*, **104**, 291-295 (1996).

[44] K. Sato, Y. Kumagai and J. Tanaka, "Apatite formation on organic monolayers in simulated body fluid," *J. Biomed. Mater. Res.*, **50**, 16-20 (2000).

[45] H.-M. Kim, M. Nakao, T. Kokubo, M. Minoda, T. Miyamoto and T. Nakamura, "Spontaneous formation of bonelike apatite on carboxymethyl-chitin gel in simulated body fluid," p. 1313 in *Trans. 6th World Biomater. Cong. Vol. III*, Kamuela, HA, 2000.

[46] H.-M. Kim, K. Kishimoto, F. Miyaji, T. Kokubo, T. Yao, T. Nakamura, Y. Suetsugu and J. Tanaka, "Composition and structure of the apatite formed on PET substrate in modified SBF with various ionic activity products," *J. Biomed. Mater. Res.*, **46**, 228-235 (1999).

[47] H.-M. Kim, K. Kishimoto, F. Miyaji, T. Kokubo, T. Yao, T. Nakamura, Y. Suetsugu and J. Tanaka, "Composition and structure of apatite formed on organic polymer in simulated body fluid with a high content of carbonate ion," *J. Mater. Sci.: Mater. Med.*, **11**, 421-426 (2000).

[48] For example: R.P. Lanza, W.L. Chick and R. Langer, *Principle of Tissue Engineering*, Springer, NY (1996).

[49] H. Ohgushi and A.I. Caplan, "Stem cell technology and bioceramics: from cell to gene engineering," *J. Biomed. Mater. Res. (Appl. Biomater.)*, **48**, 913-917 (1999).

[50] C. Loty, J.-M. Sautier, H. Boulekbache, T. Kokubo, H.-M. Kim and N. Forest, "In vitro bone formation on a bonelike apatite layer prepared by a biomimetic process on a bioactive glass-ceramic," *J. Biomed. Mater. Res.*, **49**, 423-434 (2000).

AFFECTS OF ALUMINA AND TITANIA NANOPARTICULATES ON BONE CELL FUNCTION

Luke G. Gutwein and Thomas J. Webster
Department of Biomedical Engineering
Purdue University
West Lafayette, IN 47907

ABSTRACT

Proliferation of osteoblasts (bone-forming cells) and chondrocytes (cartilage-synthesizing cells) exposed to different sizes of alumina as well as titania wear debris particles were investigated in the present *in vitro* study. Such wear debris may result from friction between articulating components of orthopedic implants. Results provided the first evidence of increased osteoblast and chondrocyte proliferation in the presence of nanometer compared to conventional-dimension (*i.e.*, micron) ceramic particles. Studies revealed that the only difference between respective ceramic particles was dimension; specifically, phase, charge, and chemical properties were similar between different size alumina and titania particles, respectively. Evidence of a less detrimental affect of nanometer compared to conventional-dimension wear debris on cell function offers additional evidence that nanophase ceramics may become the next generation of bone prosthetic materials with improved osseointegrative (that is, ability to bond to juxtaposed bone *in situ*) properties.

INTRODUCTION

Investigators of the present study have previously designed, synthesized, and evaluated nanophase ceramic bone prosthetic materials with grain sizes less than 100 nm in diameter[1-10]. Nanophase ceramics can be designed to possess chemical compositions, surface properties (specifically, topography), mechanical properties (namely, ductility), and grain size distributions similar to those of hydroxapatite found in physiological bone[11]. In contrast, conventional orthopedic/dental implant materials (such as titanium and titanium alloys) do not simulate the chemical, surface, mechanical, or grain size distribution found in physiological bone[11]. It is speculated that conventional materials do not sufficiently serve as bone prostheses due to non-biologically inspired micron grain-size dimensions.

In vitro cellular models have been utilized to determine the efficacy of biologically-inspired nanophase alumina, titania, and hydroxyapatite to serve as bone prostheses[1-10]. Compared to respective conventional (or greater than 100 nm grain size) ceramic formulations, these studies provided the first evidence of enhanced adhesion of osteoblasts (bone-forming cells), decreased adhesion of fibroblasts (cells that contribute to fibrous encapsulation and callus formation events that may lead to implant loosening and failure), and decreased adhesion of endothelial cells (cells that line the vasculature of the body) on alumina, titania, and hydroxyapatite with grain sizes less than 100 nm[3]. In fact, osteoblast adhesion increased by 50% as alumina grain size decreased from 167 to 24 nm[3]. In contrast, during the same four-hour time period, fibroblast adhesion decreased by 235%[3]. Such results also indicated a 3:1 osteoblast:fibroblast adhesion ratio only when ceramic grain sizes were reduced into the nanometer regime[3]. Selective, enhanced osteoblast adhesion implies optimal new bone synthesis critical for increased implant efficacy.

Studies also provided the first evidence of enhanced osteoblast proliferation, alkaline phosphatase activity, and deposition of calcium in the extracellular matrix on nanophase compared to respective conventional alumina, titania, and hydroxyapatite formulations[5]. Specifically, three times more calcium was deposited on nano- compared to conventional alumina after 28 days of culture[5]. Lastly, compared to respective conventional ceramic formulations, these studies also provided the first evidence of enhanced functions (specifically, synthesis of tartrate-resistance acid phosphatase (TRAP) and formation of bone-resorption pits) of osteoclasts (bone-resorbing cells) on nanophase ceramics[9]. To date, these *in vitro* investigations have demonstrated enhanced functions of osteoblasts and osteoclasts that may result in the active formation and maintenance of healthy juxtaposed bone *in vivo* to improve orthopedic/dental implant efficacy.

However, when subjected to physiological loading forces (such as friction), wear debris may form from articulating components of orthopedic implants composed of ceramics. Studies have shown that wear particles induce bone loss, lead to implant loosening, and sometimes result in clinical failure of bone prostheses (such as hip, elbow, knee, ankle, *etc.*)[12-14]. To date, several *in vitro* studies have examined the response of cells (such as osteoblasts) to micron-size wear particles[15-17]. However, no studies have been conducted on osteoblast response to nano-size ceramic wear particles. The objective of the present *in vitro* study was to investigate for the first time osteoblast and chondrocyte (cartilage synthesizing cells) proliferation in the presence of alumina and titania nanometer wear particles.

MATERIALS AND METHODS

Substrates

Borosilicate glass coverslips (Fisher Scientific) were cleaned according to standard protocols[1]. Briefly, coverslips were degreased and sonicated in acetone and 70% ethanol, etched in 1N NaOH solution for 1 hour, and autoclaved at 135°C for 35 minutes before experiments with cells.

Particles and Particle Characterization

Nanophase alumina (23 nm particle size) and titania (32 nm particles size) were obtained from Nanophase Technologies, Corp. Nanophase ceramic particles were used as supplied by the manufacturer. To obtain larger conventional size ceramic particles, alumina and titania nanophase powders were separately heated (in air at 10°C/min.) to 1100°C and sintered at this temperature for 2 hours. Resulting nanophase and conventional ceramic particles were sterilized by UV light exposure for 5 minutes prior to addition to cell culture media and subsequent experiments with cells.

Nanophase and conventional ceramic phase (crystalline *vs.* amorphous) was determined using X-ray diffraction (Phillips type PW2273/20). Nickel filtered copper Kα radiation (λ = 1.5406 nm) produced at 40 kV and 35 mA was used to scan the diffraction angles (2θ) between 30° and 35° at every 0.02° for 20 seconds/angle. Diffraction signal intensity throughout the scan was monitored and processed using Scintag (Sunnyvale, CA) DMS software.

Particle size was determined through multiple point BET measurements using an SA 3100 gas adsorption analyzer (Beckman Coulter, Inc.) according to manufacturer's instructions. Agglomeration of nanophase and conventional particles in Dulbecco's Modified Eagle Medium (DMEM; Hyclone) supplemented with 10% fetal bovine serum (FBS; Gibco), 1% penicillin/streptomycin (Gibco), and 0.6% geneticin (Sigma) as well as in chondrocyte growth media (Cell Applications, Inc.) was determined using a Beckman Coulter N4 Plus according to manufacturer's instructions. The zeta potential of the particles of interest to the present study was determined using a Doppler Electrophoretic Laser Scattering Analyzer (Beckman Coulter, Inc.).

Cell Culture

Human osteoblasts (bone-forming cells; American Type Culture Collection: CRL-11372) and human articular chrondrocytes (cartilage synthesizing cells; Cell Applications, Inc.) were cultured in DMEM (supplemented with 10% FBS, 1% penicillin/streptomycin, and 0.6% geneticin) and chondrocyte growth medium, respectively. The cells were cultured under standard cultured conditions (37°C and 5% CO_2/95% air humidification). Cells were used as purchased from the vendor without further characterization at population numbers 5 – 12.

Cell Proliferation

Osteoblasts and chondrocytes were separately seeded at 2,500 cells/cm^2 on borosilicate glass substrates and were allowed to proliferate in DMEM (supplemented with 10% FBS, 1% penicillin/streptomycin, and 0.6% geneticin) and chondrocyte growth media, respectively, without ceramic particles for 42 hours under standard cell culture conditions. At that time, old medium was replaced with fresh culture media supplemented with either conventional or nanophase particles at concentrations of 10,000, 1000, and 100 μg/ml as well as 10,000, 5500, and 1000 μg/ml for alumina and titania, respectively. For controls, old medium was replaced with fresh medium without particles after 42 hours.

Cells were then allowed to proliferate for 2 and 6 hours under standard cell culture conditions. After the allotted time, substrates were rinsed with phosphate buffered saline to remove particles. Cells were then fixed with formaldehyde and stained with Coomassie Brilliant Blue. Five random fields were counted *in situ* per substrate under a light microscope. All experiments were run in triplicate and repeated at least three times.

Statistical Analysis

Cell density (cells per square centimeter of substrate surface area) was analyzed statistically using standard analysis of variance (ANOVA) techniques; statistical significance was considered at $p < 0.1$.

RESULTS

Particle Characterization

Particle diameters as quoted by the supplier (Nanophase Technologies, Corp.) were confirmed at 32 and 23 nm for titania and alumina nano-particles, respectively. Conventional particle diameters were 4,120 and 179 nm for titania and alumina, respectively. In addition, results provided evidence that nanophase titania and alumina formed spherical agglomerations 430 and 620 nm in diameter, respectively, in the presence of each cell culture media. Conventional titania and alumina particles formed much larger spherical agglomerations 6,506 and 5,831 nm in diameter, respectively, in each cell culture media. Results also provided evidence of similar crystalline phases between nanophase and conventional alumina (γ-phase) and titania (40% rutile/60% anatase). Lastly, zeta potentials were similar between respective ceramic particles of different size.

Cell Morphology in the Presence of Ceramic Particles

Compared to conventional-size particles, results of the present study provided the first evidence of a more well-spread morphology when osteoblasts and chondrocytes were cultured with nanometer-size ceramic particles. In addition, compared to 2 hours, osteoblasts and chondrocytes were less well-spread when cultured in the presence of conventional as well as nanophase ceramic particles after 6 hours. This effect was much more drastic when cells were exposed to conventional compared to nanophase particles.

Proliferation of Cells in the Presence of Alumina Particles

2 hrs.: Compared to conventional particles, there was no statistical difference in the number of osteoblasts exposed to nano-alumina particles (from 10,000 to 100 μg/ml) at 2 hours. In contrast, there were significantly ($p < 0.05$) more chondrocytes in the presence of nano- compared to conventional-alumina particles after 2 hours for all concentrations tested in the present study. There was no statistical difference in the number of osteoblasts and chondrocytes with respect to alumina particle concentration. However, there was a slight increasing trend in the number of cells with decreasing particle concentrations after 2 hours.

6 hrs.: More importantly, after 6 hours, compared to conventional alumina particles, there were significantly ($p < 0.1$) more osteoblasts and chondrocytes when incubated with any concentration of nano-alumina particles tested in the present study, respectively. There was no statistical difference in the number of cells with respect to particle concentration after 6 hours. Lastly, there was a decreasing trend in osteoblast and chondrocyte cell numbers at all particle concentrations from 2 to 6 hours.

Proliferation of Cells in the Presence of Titania Particles

2 hrs.: Compared to conventional particles, there was no statistical difference in the number of either osteoblasts or chondrocytes in the presence of nano-titania particles (from 10,000 to 1000 μg/ml) at 2 hours. In addition, there was no statistical difference in the number of osteoblasts and chondrocytes with respect to titania particle concentration after 2 hours.

6 hrs.: In contrast, after 6 hours, compared to conventional titania particles, there were significantly ($p < 0.1$) more osteoblasts and chondrocytes when incubated with any concentration of nano-titania particles tested in the present study, respectively. There was no statistical difference in the number of cells with respect to particle concentration after 6 hours. Lastly, there was a decreasing trend in osteoblast and chondrocyte cell numbers at all particle concentrations from 2 to 6 hours.

It is interesting to note that compared to titania, exposure to similar particle size (that is, nanophase and conventional) and concentration (10,000 μg/ml) of alumina resulted in no significant difference in the number of osteoblasts after 2 and 6 hours. After 2 hours, there was also no difference in the number of chondrocytes cultured in the presence of alumina and titania particles of the same size and concentration. However, compared to conventional size titania, the number of chondrocytes was significantly ($p < 0.01$) less when exposed to conventional size alumina at 10,000 μg/ml concentrations after 6 hours; this is in contrast to nanophase particles where the number of chondrocytes was similar at the same concentrations after 6 hours of alumina and titania exposure.

DISCUSSION

Aseptic loosening is the most frequent complication of orthopedic implants (such as hip, knee, *etc.*)[11, 12, 14]. Unsuitable fixation of an implant to juxtaposed bone that results in aseptic loosening could be caused by poor cementing technique during surgical implantation or insufficient osseointegration post-implantation[11]. Moreover, stress and strain imbalances around the biomaterial-bone interface during physiological loading conditions could lead to bone resorption, implant loosening, and eventual clinical failure[18]. These events may contribute to malpositioning of the implant components and subsequent generation of debris through friction of articulating surfaces; such wear debris has been associated with osteolysis and, frequent, implant failure[14].

Since conventional implants possess grain sizes in micron regime, wear particles in the range of 1 to 100 microns in diameter have frequently resulted from unstable implant formulations. Several studies have shown the influence of particle size, chemistry (*i.e.*, polymer compared to ceramic), and shape on bone cell functions[15-21]. For example, reports in the literature demonstrated a slight decrease in osteoblastic cell growth in the presence of 80 μm diameter α-alumina particles compared to 80 μm diameter polyethylene particles[21]. More importantly, studies have consistently correlated decreased osteoblast cell proliferation with smaller diameters of conventional (from 1 to 100 micron diameter) wear particles regardless of chemistry (for example, in alumina, polyethylene, titania, tantulum, *etc.*)[15, 20]. Reports indicate that wear debris between 1 and 5 microns in diameter initiate the most aggressive biological response[21].

The present study confirmed literature reports[21] of the detrimental effects of micron size particles on osteoblast and chondrocyte proliferation. However, the present study demonstrated, for the first time, that by decreasing alumina and titania particle diameters into the nanometer regime, the negative effects of particle size on both osteoblast and chondrocyte proliferation is minimized. That is to say, compared to respective conventional ceramic particles, this study provided the first evidence that osteoblast proliferation was greater when cultured in the presence of nanometer size alumina and titania particles. Furthermore, since an increase in osteoblast and chondrocyte proliferation was observed when exposed to both nanophase alumina and titania particles, the present results demonstrated that greater proliferation is independent of the specific chemistry and dependent only on the size of the ceramic particles.

CONCLUSION

In summary, compared to conventional larger-grain size ceramic compacts, reports in the literature show that nanophase (that is, those with grain sizes less than 100 nm in diameter) ceramic compacts possess a topography that selectively enhances osteoblast function leading to increased deposition of calcium-containing mineral[5]. The present study is the first of its kind to investigate osteoblast and chondrocyte function in the presence of alumina as well as titania nano-dimensional wear debris particulates. Results of a more well-spread morphology and increased cell proliferation in the presence of nanophase particles, demonstrated that wear debris resulting from bone prostheses composed of nanophase ceramics less adversely affects bone and cartilage cell function compared to larger conventional ceramic wear particles. In this manner, the present study provided additional evidence that orthopedic implants composed of nanophase ceramics have the potential to become the next generation of bone prostheses with improved osseointegrative properties.

ACKNOWLEDGEMENTS

The authors of the present study would like to thank Mr. David Detwiler for technical assistance and the Whitaker Foundation for financial support.

REFERENCES

[1]T.J. Webster, R.W. Siegel, R. Bizios, "An *in vitro* evaluation of nanophase alumina for orthopaedic/dental applications"; pp. 273-276 in *Bioceramics 11: Proceedings of the 11th International Symposium on Ceramics in Medicine* Edited by R. Z. LeGeros and J. P. LeGeros. World Scientific, New York, 1998.

[2]T.J. Webster, R.W. Siegel, R. Bizios, "Design and evaluation of nanophase alumina for orthopaedic/dental applications," *Nanostructured Materials,* **12** 983-986 (1999).

[3]T.J. Webster, R.W. Siegel, R. Bizios, "Osteoblast adhesion on nanophase ceramics," *Biomaterials,* **20** 1221-1227 (1999).

[4]T.J. Webster, C. Ergun, R.H. Doremus, R.W. Siegel, R. Bizios, "Specific proteins mediate enhanced osteoblast adhesion on nanophase ceramics," *Journal of Biomedical Materials Research,* **51** 475-483 (2000).

[5]T.J. Webster, R.W. Siegel, R. Bizios, "Enhanced functions of osteoblasts on nanophase ceramics," *Biomaterials,* **21** 1803-1810 (2000).

[6]T.J. Webster, R.W. Siegel, R. Bizios, "Enhanced surface and mechanical properties of nanophase ceramics to achieve orthopaedic/dental implant efficacy"; pp. 321-324 in *Bioceramics 13: Proceedings of the 13th International Symposium on Ceramics in Medicine* Edited by S. Giannini and A. Moroni. Trans Tech Publications, Switzerland, 2000.

[7]T.J. Webster, R.W. Siegel, R. Bizios, "Enhanced surface and mechanical properties of nanophase ceramics to achieve orthopaedic/dental implant efficacy," *Key Engineering Materials,* **192-195** 321-324 (2001).

[8]T.J. Webster, L.S. Schadler, R.W. Siegel, R. Bizios, "Mechanisms of enhanced osteoblast adhesion on nanophase alumina involve vitronectin," *Tissue Engineering,* **7** 291-301 (2001).

[9]T.J. Webster, C. Ergun, R.H. Doremus, R.W. Siegel, R. Bizios, "Enhanced functions of osteoclast-like cells on nanophase ceramics," *Biomaterials,* **22** 1327-1333 (2001).

[10]T.J. Webster, R.W. Siegel, R. Bizios, "Nanoceramic surface roughness enhances osteoblast and osteoclast functions for improved orthopaedic/dental implant efficacy," *Scripta Materialia*, **44** 1639-1642 (2001).

[11]F.S. Kaplan, W.C. Hayes, T.M. Keaveny, A. Boskey, T.A. Einhorn, J.P. Iannotti, *Orthopedic Basic Science*, Am. Acad. Orth. Surg., Columbus OH, 1994.

[12]P.C. Oparaugo, I.C. Clarke, H. Malchau, P. Herberts, "Correlation of wear debris-induced osteolysis and revision with volumetric wear-rated of polyethylene: a survey of 8 reports in the literature," *Acta Orthopaedica Scandavica*, **72** 22-28 (2001).

[13]R.M. Urban, J.J. Jacobs, M.J. Tomlinson, J. Gavrilovic, J. Black, M. Peoc'h, "Dissemination of wear particles to the liver, spleen, and abdominal lymph nodes of patients with hip or knee replacement," *Journal of Bone & Joint Surgery – American Volume*, **82** 457-476 (2000).

[14]T. Hashiguchi, T. Hirano, H. Shindo, K. Baba, "Wear of alumina prosthesis," *Archives of Orthopedic & Trauma Surgery*, **119** 30-34 (1999).

[15]C.H. Lohmann, Z. Schwartz, G. Koster, U. Jahn, G.H. Buchhorn, M.J. MacDougall, D. Casasola, Y. Liu, V.L. Sylvia, D.D. Dean, D.B. Boyan, "Phagocytosis of wear debris by osteoblasts affects differentiation and local factor production in a manner dependent on particle composition," *Biomaterials*, **21** 551-561 (2000).

[16]S.Y. Kwon, H. Takei, D.P. Pioletti, T. Lin, Q.J. Ma, W.H. Akeson, D.J. Wood, K.L. Sung, "Titanium particles inhibit osteoblast adhesion to fibronectin-coated substrates," *Journal of Orthopedic Research*, **18** 203-211 (2000).

[17]D.H. DeHeer, J.A. Engles, A.S. DeVries, R.H. Knapp, J.D. Beebe, "In situ complement activation by polyethylene wear debris," *Journal of Biomedical Materials Research*, **54** 12-19 (2001).

[18]J.B. Brunski, "Influence of biomechanical factors at the bone-biomaterial interface"; pp. 391-404 in *The Bone-Biomaterial Interface* Edited by J.E. Davies. University of Toronto Press, Toronto, 1991.

[19]A. Kobayashi, W. Bonfield, Y. Kadoya, T. Yamac, M.A. Freeman, G. Scott, P.A. Revell, "The size and shape of particulate polyethylene wear debris in total joint replacements," *Proceedings of the Institution of Mechanical Engineering. Part H – Journal of Engineering in Medicine*, **211** 11-15 (1997).

[20]D.P. Pioletti, H. Takei, D. Kwon Sym Wood, K.L. Sung, "The cytotoxic effect of titanium particles phagocytosed by osteoblasts," *Journal of Biomedical Materials Research*, **46** 399-407 (1999).

[21]M.E. Martinez, S. Medina, M.T. del Campo, J.A. Garcia, A. Rodrigo, L. Munuera, "Effect of polyethylene particles on human osteoblastic cell growth," *Biomaterials*, **19** 183-187 (1998).

A COMPOSITES APPROACH TO TISSUE ENGINEERING

Aldo R. Boccaccini, Judith A. Roether, Larry L. Hench
Department of Materials and Tissue Engineering Centre,
Imperial College, Prince Consort Rd., London SW7 2BP, UK

Veronique Maquet, Robert Jérôme
Centre for Education and Research on Macromolecules (CERM), Interfacultary Centre for Biomaterials, University of Liège, B-4000 Liège, Belgium

ABSTRACT

Composite materials based on biodegradable polymers and bioactive ceramics, including tricalcium phosphate, hydroxylapatite and bioactive glasses, are being considered increasingly as scaffolds for tissue engineering applications, especially for bone and cartilage tissue. The reason for adding bioactive phases to biodegradable polymers forming composite scaffolds is threefold: i) to enhance bioactivity, ii) to provide adequate control of the scaffold degradation rate, and iii) to enhance the mechanical properties and structural integrity of scaffolds. In the first part of this report a summary of recent composite approaches developed for bone tissue regeneration and repair is presented. In the second part a porous composite scaffold being developed and tested currently is described in terms of processing and behaviour in contact with simulated body fluid. The composite is made of a bioresorbable poly(D,L-lactide) foam impregnated and filled with bioactive glass (Bioglass®) particles.

INTRODUCTION

Tissue engineering presents an alternative approach to the repair of damaged human tissue, avoiding the need for a permanent implant. The underlying principle involved is the regeneration of living tissue where a loss or damage has occurred as a result of injury or disease [1]. A suitable temporary scaffold material exhibiting adequate mechanical and biological properties is required to enable tissue regeneration by exploiting the body's inherent repair mechanisms [2]. In general, a tissue engineering scaffold for bone tissue engineering needs to satisfy a variety of criteria which are summarised in Table I [2,3].

Table I. Criteria for an ideal scaffold for bone tissue engineering [2,3]

An ideal tissue engineering scaffold ...

1. is made from a material that is biocompatible, i.e. not cytotoxic;
2. acts as template for tissue growth in three dimensions;
3. has an interconnected macro-porous network for vascularisation, tissue ingrowth and nutrient delivery;
4. bonds to the host tissue without the formation of scar tissue;
5. influences the genes in the bone generating cells to enable efficient cell differentiation and proliferation;
6. resorbs at the same rate as the tissue is repaired, with degradation products that are non-toxic and that can be easily excreted by the body, for example via the respiratory or urinary systems;
7. is made from a processing technique that can produce irregular shapes to match that of the defect in the bone of the patient; and
8. exhibits mechanical properties sufficient to be able to regenerate bone in load bearing sites.

Numerous bioresorbable materials are being investigated as scaffolds for tissue regeneration and repair, including naturally occurring [4] and synthetic polymers [5-9]. For bone tissue engineering also bioactive porous ceramics are being considered [10].

Synthetic bioresorbable polymers have attracted increasing attention for their use as tissue engineering scaffolds in the last few years mainly because these materials have already demonstrated successful results in clinical use, for example as resorbable surgical sutures and meshes or in drug delivery systems [9]. In particular polylactic acid (PLA), polyglycolic acid (PGA), polyhydroxybutyrate (PHB) or their copolymers are being intensively investigated for developing tissue engineering scaffolds [2,5-9]. Chemical hydrolysis rather than enzymatic reactions are responsible for the degradation of polymeric chains, therefore the degradation of the material does not vary from patient to patient [11]. Some problems have been encountered however regarding the use of these polymers in tissue engineering applications due to the release of acidic degradation products leading to inflammatory responses [7, 9-11]. Other limitation of most biodegradable polymers is that they lack a bioactive function, i.e., in particular for bone tissue applications, they do not allow for bone apposition or bonding on the polymer surface [12].

Bioactive ceramics, such as hydroxyapatite (HA), tricalcium phosphate (TCP) and selected compositions of silicate and phosphate glasses and glass-ceramics, for example the commercially available Bioglass®, react with physiological fluids and form tenacious bonds to hard and soft tissues through cellular activity. These materials are therefore known as "bioactive" [13].

If biodegradability and bioactivity need be combined in an optimised tissue engineering scaffold, then the design of composite materials offers an exceptional opportunity: combinations of biodegradable polymers and bioactive phases allow for the creation of bioresorbable and bioactive composite scaffolds with tailored physical and mechanical properties. The addition of a ceramic phase to a biodegradable polymer may also be used to favourable alter the polymer degradation behaviour. It has been shown that using bioactive phases as inclusions or coatings in biodegradable polymers allows the rapid exchange of protons in water for alkali in the glass or ceramic, which in turn provides a pH buffering effect at the polymer surface, therefore acceleration of acidic degradation of the polymer will not occur [14]. Moreover composite materials can be engineered in such a way that their resorption rate in the body can be designed to match the formation rate of new tissue [15].

Numerous approaches to bioresorbable and bioactive composite scaffolds for tissue engineering applications are being investigated. Some of the most recent developments are reviewed in the next Section. As an example of the current collaborative developments between the Tissue Engineering Centre, Imperial College, London (UK) and the Centre for Education and Research on Macromolecules (CERM), University of Liège, Belgium, novel bioactive and bioresorbable composite materials based on macroporous poly(DL-lactide) (PDLLA) foams coated with and filled by bioactive glass (Bioglass®) particles are described in a subsequent section. The in-vitro response of the composites in contact with simulated body fluid (SBF) is also presented.

COMPOSITE MATERIALS FOR TISSUE ENGINEERING

A review of the different approaches intended for applications of composite materials in tissue engineering suggests a primary classification of the systems under development. This concerns the distinction between those composite materials comprising pure non-living materials and those made by the combination of a living and a non-living material, also called vital-avital composites.

In vital-avital composites a synthetic scaffold and in-growing living tissue are combined [16]. It has been proposed that in this type of composite the cellular component will generate new tissue through production of extracellular matrix while the scaffold material will provide structural integrity and mechanical stability in the short term. A recent review paper has addressed the concept, fabrication and applications of vital-avital composites [16]. In this paper only bioresorbable and bioactive composites made from totally non-living materials will be considered.

In general, one can broadly classify the developments in the area of bioactive and bioresorbable composites according to the nature of bioactive phase used, i.e. systems containing either hydroxyapatite and related calcium phosphate ceramics or bioactive silicate glasses. A further classification should consider the structure of the scaffold, i.e. if it is a dense or a porous structure. In a further distinction, the way of incorporating the bioactive phase in the composite must be also taken into account, i.e. being as filler (particle or fibre) or as a coating or external layer. Table II summarises the types of biodegradable and bioactive composite materials developed for tissue engineering applications and relevant references of recent papers dealing with the different composite approaches are given.

Table II. Types of composite scaffolds for tissue engineering applications based on resorbable polymers and bioactive ceramics or glasses

Dense (non-porous scaffold)				Porous scaffolds (foam-like structure)			
Bioactive phase: HA, TCP and related ceramics		Bioactive phase: silicate glasses (e. g. Bioglass®)		Bioactive phase: HA, TCP and related ceramics		Bioactive phase: silicate glasses (e. g. Bioglass®)	
Bioactive phase added as filler	Bioactive phase added as coating	Bioactive phase added as filler	Bioactive phase added as coating	Bioactive phase added as filler	Bioactive phase added as coating	Bioactive phase added as filler	Bioactive phase added as coating
Refs. [17-25]	Refs. [18,20]	Refs. [14, 26-30]	Refs. [31-34]	Refs. [15, 35-41]	Refs. [18]	Refs. [27,42]	Refs. [43,44]

The review of the available literature reveals that the application of bioactive silicate glasses in bioresorbable composites for tissue engineering scaffolds is not as widespread as that involving HA or related calcium phosphate ceramics. However, it is well known that bioactive glasses possess a higher index of bioactivity than hydroxyapatite [13]. It has been shown that one of the most used bioactive glasses, 45S5 Bioglass®, exhibits "Class A" bioactivity, i.e. properties of osteoconduction and osteoproduction, while HA exhibits "Class B" bioactivity, i.e. only osteoconductive behaviour [13]. Recently, Wheeler et al. [45] have confirmed that 45S5 Bioglass® has improved bone bonding and restoring effect compared with hydroxyapatite. In their study specimens of comparable structure of HA and 45S5 Bioglass® were implanted into goats to study the effect of using different bioactive surfaces. Histological and biomechanical tests were carried out on both implant materials. It was found that after several weeks of healing more bone and thicker trabeculae were measured histomorphometrically within the implant pores for the Bioglass® coated implants compared with HA-coated materials. Moreover mechanical integrity was maintained over time only for Bioglass® implants. Since Bioglass® is able to form a bond to soft tissues [3,13], the incorporation of Bioglass® and other Class A bioactive materials into resorbable polymer scaffolds is seen as a convenient way towards tissue engineering scaffolds for both hard and soft tissue engineering applications.

Preliminary results on the fabrication of composite polymer surgical sutures and meshes coated by 45S5 Bioglass® particles have been reported recently [32-34,43]. Commercially available bioresorbable polymer sutures (Vicryl®) and meshes were coated with particles of Bioglass® of diameter < 5μm. These composites were used to demonstrate that the rate of degradation of the polymer in simulated body fluid (SBF) could be adjusted by means of a protective bioactive coating. It was found that the time-dependant biomechanical properties of the composite after immersion in SBF are affected by the presence of the Bioglass® coating.

The principle of incorporation of Bioglass® particles as fillers in biodegradable polymers has been patented by Boyan et al. [27] for the use as a porous or non-porous therapeutic implant material. The implants are intended as cell scaffolds for healing of tissue defects or fixation devices and provide increased mechanical properties and pH control, exhibit desirable degradation times, elasticity and biocompatibility. However, very limited further work has been published on the use of bioactive glass phases as filler in bioresorbable polymer scaffolds [14,26,28-30]. In recent developments, bioactive glass fibres were studied by Paatola et al. [46] in terms of their potential as reinforcing elements for biodegradable polymers. The study evaluated that both mechanical properties and bioactivity could be improved significantly by addition of glass fibres into the polymer matrix. Thus, the development of bioactive glass fibres to be used as reinforcements may open new areas of applications for resorbable composites in load-bearing applications.

For completeness it must be mentioned that few other resorbable composite systems have been developed for tissue engineering, usually comprising a natural material as one of the constituents. These include, for example, hybrid sponges composed of collagen fibres in a PLLA matrix [47] and polycaprolatone (PLC) matrices incorporating chopped chitin fibres [48].

MODEL COMPOSITES BASED ON RESORBABLE POLYMER FOAMS AND BIOGLASS®

As an example of our own current developments in the area of composite scaffolds for tissue engineering a novel bioactive and bioresorbable composite material based on macroporous poly(DL-lactide) (PDLLA) foam coated with and filled by (Bioglass®) particles is described here. The in-vitro response of the composites in contact with simulated body fluid (SBF) is also presented.

Composites processing

Purasorb® (Purac biochem, Goerinchen, The Netherlands) poly(D,L-lactide) (PDLLA) with inherent viscosity of 1.52 dl/g and dimethylcarbonate (DMC) of 99% purity (Sigma Aldrich) were used. Polymers and solvents were used without further purification.The bioactive material used was a melt-derived bioactive glass powder (Bioglass® grade 45S5, US Biomaterials Co., Alachua, FL, USA). The powder had a mean particle size < 5 μm. The composition of the bioactive glass used was (in weight percentage): 45% SiO_2, 24.5% Na_2O, 24.5% CaO and 6% P_2O_5, which is the original composition of the first bioactive glass developed by Hench and co-workers [13].

The preparation of Bioglass®-filled poly(DL-lactide) (PDLLA) foams, referred here as composite foams, followed a thermally induced phase separation process, also termed freeze-drying, which has been described in detail elsewhere [8]. The process was conveniently modified for the incorporation of Bioglass® particles. The polymer was dissolved in DMC to produce a polymer weight to solvent volume ratio of 5%. The mixture was stirred overnight to obtain a homogeneous polymer solution. Determined amounts of Bioglass® powder, calculated to result in final proportions of 10 to 40wt% of Bioglass® in the composite, were added into the polymer solution, resulting in homogeneous PDLLA/Bioglass® mixtures. Each mixture was then transferred into a 150 ml lyophilisation flask and sonicated for 15 min in order to improve the dispersion of the Bioglass® into the polymer solution. The flask was then rapidly immersed into liquid nitrogen and was maintained at –196 °C for 2h. The frozen mixture was then transferred into an ethylenglycol bath at –10°C and connected to a vacuum pump (10-2 Torr). The solvent was sublimated at –10°C for 48h, and then at 0°C for additional 48h. The sample was completely dried at room temperature in a vacuum oven until reaching a constant weight.

Bioglass® particle coatings were made using a slurry-dipping technique, similar to that proposed recently to coat surgical sutures and polymeric meshes with Bioglass® particles [33,43]. The coating technique for foams similar to those used here has been optimised in previous studies [44]. Briefly, the technique involves preparation of a stable slurry with 42 wt.% of Bioglass® particles in distilled and deionised water, which is continuously stirred magnetically. Pre-treatment of the PDLLA foams with ethanol was carried out. It was shown in previous studies that better results in terms of degree of infiltration and coating homogeneity are achieved by the ethanol pre-treatment procedure because the high hydrophobicity of the PDLLA foam can be decreased [44]. Following immersion in the Bioglass® slurry for 5 min, the foam samples were carefully withdrawn to avoid damage at a withdrawal velocity of ~ 5 cm s^{-1}. The samples were subsequently dried on glass plates at room temperature in a humid-controlled atmosphere.

Characterisation and in-vitro studies

PDLLA foams and PDLLA/Bioglass® composite samples were characterised by using scanning electron microscopy (SEM) in order to assess the porosity structure of the foam and the quality of the Bioglass® coating and degree of infiltration. The morphology of a Bioglass®-filled PDLLA foam is shown in Figure 1. The foam exhibits a high porosity (> 90%), comprising two distinct pores sizes: i) macropores of ~100μm average diameter, and ii) micropores with an average diameter of 20-30μm, which form an interconnected network. The tubular macropores are seen to be highly oriented as a result of the unidirectional cooling process. It is interesting to point out that addition of Bioglass® particles of mean size < 5μm (up to 40 wt.%) had no effects on the development of a well-defined tubular and interconnected porous structure in the foam.

Figures 2a,b show SEM micrographs of Bioglass®-coated composite foams produced by slurry-dipping at different magnifications. After drying, the particles were strongly adhered to the polymer substrate as neither peeling-off of Bioglass® particles nor macro-delamination of the Bioglass® coating were observed. At low magnifications (Fig. 2a), it can be observed that Bioglass® particles homogeneously cover the outer surfaces of the foam. Using an immersion time of 5 min, the Bioglass® particles have also deeply infiltrated the pores of the foam and glass particles are deposited along the internal surfaces of the porous structure, as Figure 2b shows.

In-vitro studies in simulated body fluid (SBF) were carried out using the composition described by researchers at the University of Kyoto (Japan) [49]. The procedure followed for the in-vitro tests has been described elsewhere [44]. The PDLLA foam/Bioglass® composites and uncoated foams were left in immersion in SBF for varying time periods of 7, 14, 21 and 28 days. After immersion in SBF the samples were characterised using SEM and X-ray diffraction (XRD).

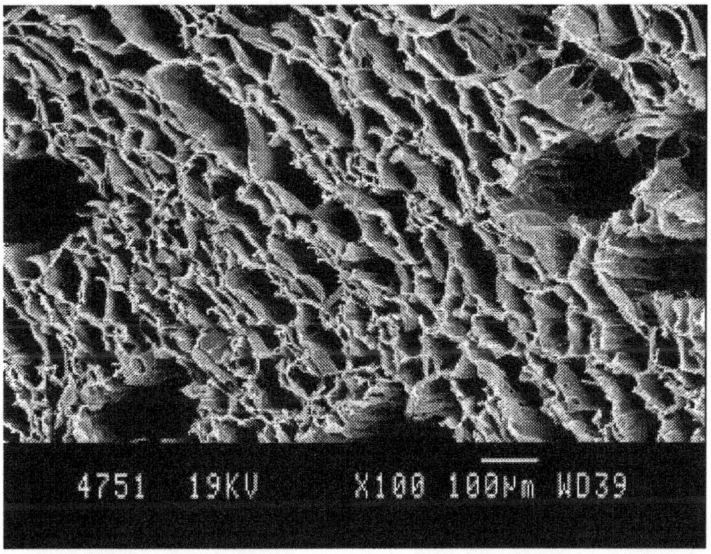

Fig. 1. SEM micrograph showing a typical cross-section of a Bioglass®-filled PDLLA foam.

The SEM micrographs in Figures 3a,b show the surface of PDLLA composite foams coated and uncoated with Bioglass® particles after 21 days in SBF. The coated sample exhibits a significant development of a HA layer, which became thicker with increasing time in SBF as shown elsewhere [42]. The SEM micrograph of the uncoated PDLLA composite foam containing the lowest addition of Bioglass® particles (10 wt%), as shown in Figure 3b, reveals also the formation of HA crystals as a result of contact of Bioglass® particles with SBF. However the HA phase remains discretely distributed on the surface of the foam and localised in the areas where Bioglass® particles have been in direct contact with SBF. No continuous layer formation, as in the case of the coated samples (see Figure 3a), is observed. However, a polymer surface exhibiting "point exposure" of HA may provide a novel and favourable substrate for primary cell attachment, as reported in the literature [20].

The crystallinity of the structure formed on the surface of the foams was investigated using XRD. For the Bioglass®-coated composite samples XRD analyses confirmed that crystalline HA formed on the composite surface after immersion in SBF for different time durations, as Figure 4 shows. Since the analysed samples varied in size and morphology, a quantitative analysis revealing the amount of HA formed in dependence of immersion time in SBF could not be carried out. Nevertheless, the in-vitro studies were successful in confirming the high ability for hydroxyapatite (HA) formation on the surfaces of Bioglass®-coated samples, which is a measure of the significant biaoctivity of the material. Raman spectroscopy investigations have also confirmed the formation of HA on the surface of the samples exposed to SBF after only 3 days of immersion in SBF [42].

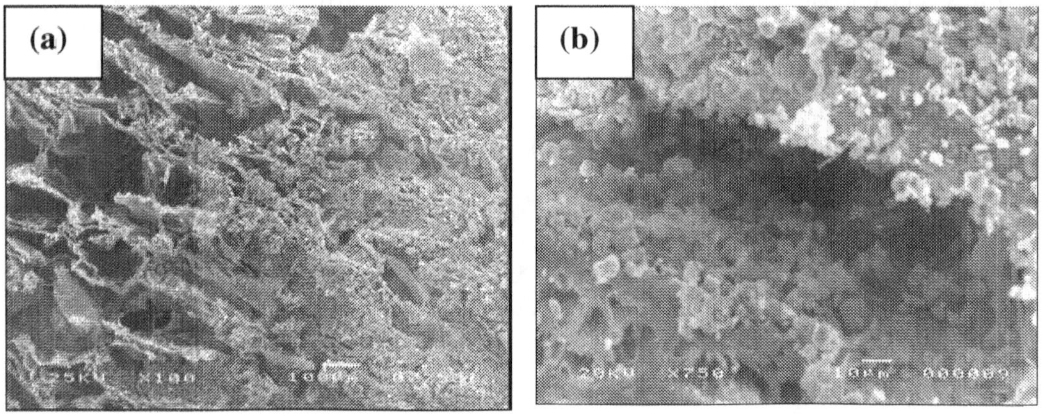

Fig. 2. SEM micrographs showing the typical microstructure of PDLLA foams coated by Bioglass® particles produced by slurry-dipping. The homogeneous coating and efficient infiltration of Bioglass® particles can be observed at (a) low and (b) high magnifications.

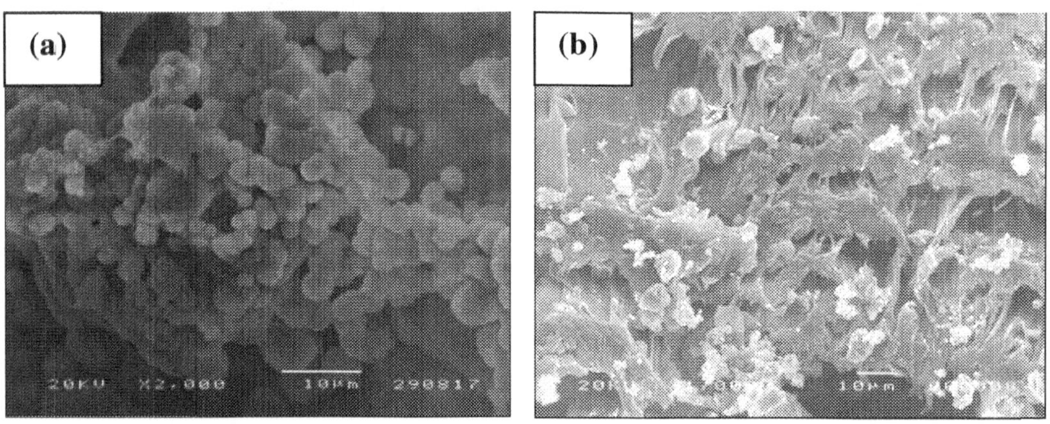

Fig 3. SEM micrographs showing the surface of (a) a Bioglass®-coated PDLLA foam and (b) an un-coated foam after degradation in SBF for 21 days. The micrographs reveal formation of a HA layer in (a) and discrete HA crystals in (b).

The HA layer formed on the Bioglass®-coated composite surfaces was relatively thick, compared to other studies on bioactive and resorbable composites reported in the literature, where HA was used as the bioactive phase (see for example ref. [35]). In the present composites, the thickness of the HA layer formed on Bioglass®-coated surfaces was increased manifold (of the order of 10 μm after 21 immersion in SBF), an indication of the enhanced bioactivity of these materials. As mentioned above, Bioglass® has a higher index of bioactivity than HA, which makes it a more suitable material for applications in bone reconstruction [3,13]. Moreover stiff Bioglass® particles used as filler can be conveniently used to enhance the mechanical properties and structural integrity of the porous constructs. Another motivation for fabricating composites both filled and coated by bioactive glass particles concerns the positive effect that the Bioglass® dissolution may have on the degradation of the polymer. This has not been yet quantitatively studied for the present composites. However, it can be speculated that the bioactive glass coating acts as a protective hydrolysis barrier affecting both the extent and rate of degradation of the polymer substrate [33]. Recent results on in-vivo and in-vitro degradation of bulk composites based on PDLLA containing bioactive glass particles seem to confirm this approach [14].

It is therefore envisaged that using Bioglass® both as filler and coating of porous resorbable polymer scaffolds will add to the possibilities of tailoring the mechanical properties and the rate of resorption of the composite scaffolds to that of the required application. Further logical steps to the optimisation of scaffolds for tissue engineering should focus on tailoring the microstructure of the composite foams for determined applications, including the development of graded porosity and graded bioactive Bioglass® coatings, this being the focus of current developments.

CONCLUDING REMARKS

As pointed out in the literature [2], the present challenge for the progress of tissue engineering, in particular for bone and cartilage tissue, is to design and fabricate reproducible biorerorbable 3-dimensional scaffolds, which are able to function for a certain period of time even under load-bearing conditions. Composite materials concepts are being explored to tackle this problem. Numerous bioresorbable and bioactive composites are being currently developed based on synthetic bioresorbable polymers and bioactive glass or ceramic phases, as reviewed in this article. Most current research and development activities focus on choosing the adequate components of the composites and on optimising the processing routes to produce the required composite architecture, including porosity, for the envisaged application. The review of the literature reveals that the ideal scaffold and matrix material has not yet been developed.

The composites presented in this paper represent a very attractive combination of bioresorption and bioactivity properties in a highly porous scaffold for hard and soft tissue engineering. In particular, the use Bioglass® instead of HA or other calcium phosphates yields composites of class A bioactivity exhibiting osteoproduction properties and the possibility to be used also in soft tissue engineering applications. Future research should focus on tailoring novel microstructures for the envisaged applications, including the development of composite foams with graded porosity and graded Bioglass® coating microstructure. The extension of the research to include soft tissue engineering, e.g. for intestinal constructs is being assessed by cell culturing work.

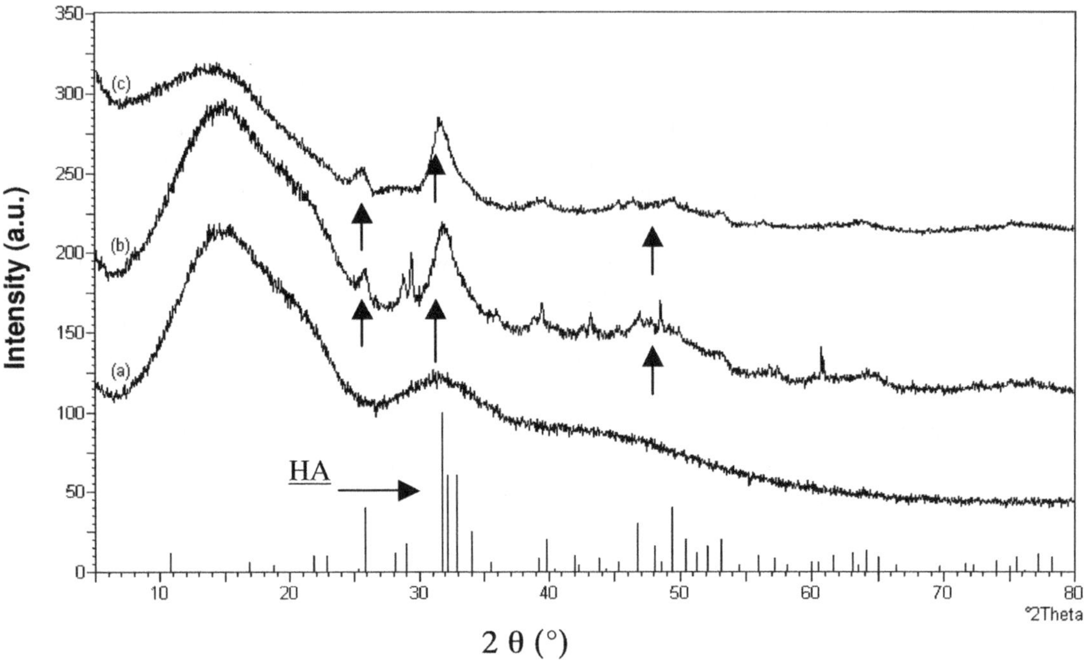

Fig. 4. XRD patterns of Bioglass®-coated PDLLA foams: in (a) as-fabricated state, and after immersion in SBF for (b) 28 and (c) 7 days. The XRD patterns demonstrate the development of crystalline HA with increasing time of immersion in SBF. Note that the intensity is given in arbitrary units, i.e. the relative height of the peaks does not correlate with the relative amount of HA present in the different samples.

REFERENCES

[1]R. Langer, J. P. Vacanti, "Tissue Engineering", *Science* 260, 920-926 (1995).

[2]D. W. Hutmacher, "Scaffolds in Tissue Engineering Bone and Cartilage, *Biomaterials* 21, 2529-2543 (2001).

[3]J. R. Jones, L. L. Hench, "Biomedical Materials for New Millenium: Perspective on the Future", *Mater. Sci. Tech.* 17, 891-900 (2001).

[4]E. Pişkin, "Biomaterials in Different Forms for Tissue Engineering: an Overview", *Materials Science Forum* 250, 1-14 (1997).

[5]V. Maquet, R. Jerome, "Design of Macroporous Biodegradable Polymer Scaffolds for Cell Transplantation", *Mat. Sci. Forum* 250, 15-42 (1997).

[6]C. M. Agrawal, K. A. Athanasiou, J. D. Heckman, "Biodegradable PLA-PGA Polymers for Tissue Engineering in Orthopadics", *Mat. Sci. Forum* 250, 115-129 (1997).

[7]S. K. Ashiku, M. A. Randolph, C. A. Vacanti, "Tissue Engineered Cartilage", *Mat. Sci. Forum* 250, 129-150 (1997).

[8]C. Schugens, V. Maquet, C. Grandfils, R. Jerome, P. Teyssie, "Biodegradable and Macroporous Polylactide Implants for Cell Transplantation: II. Preparation of Polylactide Foams by Liquid-Liquid Phase Separation", *Journal of Biomedical Materials Research* 30, 449-461 (1996).

[9]L. G. Griffith, "Polymeric Biomaterials", *Acta Mater.* 48, 263-277 (2000).

[10]P. Sepulveda, J. R. Jones, L. L. Hench, "Bioactive Sol-gel Foams for Tissue Repair", *J. Biomed. Mat. Res.* 59, 340-348 (2002).
[11]C. M. Agrawal, R. B. Ray, "Biodegradable Polymeric Scaffolds for Musculoskeletal Tissue Engineering", *J. Biomed. Mater. Res.* 55, 141-150 (2001).
[12]H. Schliephake, F. W. Neukam, et al. "Enhancement of Bone In-Growth into a Porous HA-Matrix Using a Resorbable Polylactice Membrane", *J. Oral Max. Surg.* 52, 57-63 (1994).
[13]L. L. Hench, "Bioceramics", *J. Am. Ceram. Soc.* 81, 1705-1728 (1998).
[14]H. Niiranen, T. Pyhalto, P. Rokkanen, T. Paatola, P. Tormala, "Bioactive Glass 13-93/P(L/DL)LA Composites In vitro and In Vivo", *Key Eng. Mat.* 192-195, 721-724 (2001).
[15]W. Linhart, F. Peters, W. Lehmann, C. Schwarz, A. Schilling, M. Amling, J. M. Rueger, M. Epple, "Biologically and Chemically Optimised Composites of Carbonated Apatite and Polyglycolide as Bone Substitution Materials", *J. Biomed. Mat. Res.* 54, 162-171 (2001).
[16]S. Ramakrishna, J. Mayer, E. Wintermantel, K. W. Leong, Biomedical Applications of Polymer-Composite Materials: A Review, *Composites Sci. Technology* 61, 1189-1224 (2001).
[17]K. P. Adriano, A. U. Daniels, W. P. Smutz, R. W. B. Wyatt, "Preliminary Biocompatibility Screening of Several Biodegradable Phosphate Fiber Reinforced Polymers", *J. Appl. Biomaterials* 4, 1-12 (1993).
[18]C. C. P. M. Verheyen, J. R. de Wijn, C. A. van Blitterswijk, K. de Groot, P. M. Rozing, Hydroxyapatite/poly(L-lactide) Composites: An Animal Study on Push-out Strengths and Interface Histology, *J. Biomed. Mat. Res.* 27, 433-444 (1993)
[19]J. L. Charvet, J. A. Cordes, H. Alexander, "Mechanical and Fracture Behavior of a Fiber-Reinforced Bioabsorbable Material of Orthopaedic Applications", *J. Mat. Sc.: Mater. in Medicine* 11, 101-109 (2000).
[20]S. C. Rizzi, D. J. Heath, A. G. A. Coombes, N. Bock, M. Textor, S. Downes, "Biodegradable Polymer/Hydroxyapatite Composites: Surface Analysis and Inital Attachment of Human Ssteoblasts", *J. Biomed. Mater. Res.*, Vol. 55, 475-486 (2001).
21F. L. S. Carvalho, C. S. Borges, J. R. T. Branco, M. M. Pereira, Structural Analysis of Hydroxyapatite/Bioactive Glass Composite Coatings Obtained by Plasma Spraying, *J. Non-Crystalline Solids* 247, 64-68 (1999).
[22]N. Ignjatović, K. Delijić, et al., "The Designing of Properties of Hydroxyapatite/poly-L-lactide Composite Materials by Hot Pressing, *Z. Metallkd.* 92, 145-149 (2001).
[23]X. Deng, J. Hao, M. Yuan, "Influence of Poly(d, l lactide–b–ethylene glycol) copolymer on Morphology and Tensile Moduli of Poly (d, l-lactide) Composites Containing Hydroxyapatite", *J. Mater. Sc. Letters* 20, 281-282 (2001).
[24]S. N. Nazhat, M. Kellomäki, P. Törmälä, K. E: Tanner, W. Bonfield, "Dynamic Mechanical Characterization of Biodegradable Composites of Hydroxyapatite and Polylactides", *J. Biomed. Mater. Res. (Appl. Biomater.)* 58, 335-343 (2001).
[25]X. Deng, J. Hao, "Preparation and Mechanical Properties of Nanocomposites of Poly(D,L-lactide) with Ca-Deficient Hydroxyapatite Nanocrystals", *Biomaterials* 22, 2867-73 (2001).
[26]F. Sharifi, "Bioresorbable Particulate Filled Composite for Bone Regeneration", PhD thesis Imperial College London, University of London, Mechanical Engineering Department (2001).
[27]B. D. Boyan, G. Niederauer, K. Kieswetter, N. C. Leatherbury, D. C. Greenspan, "Biodegradable Implant Material Comprising Bioactive Ceramic", US Patent nr. 5,977,204. November 2, 1999.
[28]I. B. Leonor, R. A. Sousa, A. M. Cunha, Z. P. Zhong, D. Greenspan, R. L. Reis, "Development of Highly Bioactive and Mechanically Strong Starch Thermoplastic/Bioglass® Composite Biomaterials", *Key Eng. Mat.* 192-195, 705-708 (2001).
[29]A. J. Aho, T. Tirri, J. Seppala, J. Rich, N. Strandberg, et al., "Bioactive Glass-Polymer Composite for Experimental Bone Reconstruction", *Key Eng. Mat.* 192-195, 685-688 (2001).

[30]E. Pirhonen, G. Grandi, P. Tormala, "Bioactive Glass Fibre/Polylactide Composite", *Key Eng. Mat.* 192-195, 725-728 (2001).

[31]H. Niiranen, P. Törmälä, "Bioabsorbable Polymer Plates Coated with Bioactive Glass Spheres", *J. Mater. Sc.: Mater. in Med.* 10, 707-710 (1999).

[32]A. Stamboulis, L. L. Hench, "Bioresorbable Polymers: their Potential as Scaffolds for Bioglass® Composites", *Key Eng. Mater.* 192-195, 729-732 (2001).

[33] A. G. Stamboulis, L. L. Hench, A. R. Boccaccini, "Mechanical Properties of Biodegradable Polymer Sutures Coated with Bioactive Glass", *J. Mat. Sci.: Mat. Med.* (2001) in press.

[34]A. R. Boccaccini, A. G. Stamboulis, J. A. Roether, L. L. Hench, "Herstellung neuartiger Polymer-Bioglass(R)-Komposite für Anwendungen in der Geweberekonstruktion (Tissue Engineering)". In: *Verbundwerkstoffe und Werkstoffverbunde*, ed. by B. Wielage und G. Leonhardt, Wiley-VCH, Weinheim (2001) pp. 420-423.

[35]P. X. Ma, R. Zhang, G. Xiao, R. Franceschi, Engineering New Bone Tissue in Vitro on Highly Porous Poly (a-hydroxyl acids)/hydroxyapatite Composite Scaffolds, J. Biomed. Mater. Res. 54, 284-293 (2001).

[36]C. Durucan, P. W. Brown, "Biodegradable Hydroxyapatite-Polymer Composites", *Adv. Eng. Mater.* 3, 227-231 (2001).

[37]T. Kasuga, Y. Ota, M. Nogami, Y. Abe, "Preparation and Mechanical Properties of Polylactic Acid Composites", *Biomaterials* 22, 19-23 (2001).

[38]A.A.Ignatius, S. Wolf, P. Augat, L. E. Claes, "Composites Made of Rapidily Resorbable Ceramics and Poly(lactide) Show Adequate Mechanical Properties for Use as Bone Substitute Materials", *J. Biomed. Mat. Res.* 57, 126-131 (2001).

[39]R. C. Thomson, M. J. Yaszemski, J. M. Powers, et al. "Hydroxyapatite Fiber Reinforced Poly(a-hydroxyl ester) Foams for Bone Regeneration", *Biomaterials* 18, 1935-43 (1998).

[40]H. Schliephake, T. Kage, Enhancement of Bone Regeneration Using Resorbable Ceramics and a Polymer-Ceramic Composite Material, *J. Biomed. Mat. Res.* 56, 128-136 (2001).

[41]C. Schiller, M. Siedler, F. Peters, M. Epple, "Functionally Graded Materials of Biodegradable Polyesters and Bone-like Calcium Phosphates for Bone Replacement", *Ceram. Trans.* 114, 97-108, (2001).

[42]A. R. Boccaccini, I. Notingher, V. Maquet, R. Jérôme, "Bioresorbable and Bioactive Composite Materials Based on Polylactide Foams Filled with and Coated by Bioglass® Particles for Tissue Engineering Applications" *J. Mat. Sci. Mat. Med.* (2002) submitted.

[43]A. G. Stamboulis, A. R. Boccaccini, L. L. Hench, "Novel Biodegradable Polymer/Bioactive Glass Composites for Tissue Engineering Applications", *Adv. Eng. Mat.* (2002) in press.

[44]J. A. Roether, A. R. Boccaccini, L. L. Hench, V. Maquet, S. Gautier, R. Jerome, "Development and In-vitro Characterisation of Novel Bioresorbable and Bioactive Composite Materials Based on Polylactide Foams and Bioglass® for Tissue Engineering Applications", *Biomaterials* (2002) submitted.

[45]D. L. Wheeler, M. J. Montfort, S. W: McLoughlin, "Differential Healing Response of Bone Adjacent to Porous Implants Coated with Hydroxyapatite and 45S5 Bioactive Glass", *J. Biomed. Mater. Res.* 55, 603-612 (2001).

[46]Paatola, E. Pirhonen, P. Törmälä, "Coating of Bioactive Glass (13-93) Fibers with Bioabsorbable Polymer", *Key Eng. Mater.*, Vols. 192-195, 717-720 (2001).

[47] G. Chen, T. Ushida, T. Tateishi, Hybrid Biomaterials for Tissue Engineering: a Preparative Method for PLA or PLGA-collagen Hybrid Sponges", *Adv. Mater.* 12, 455-457 (2000).

[48] A. Yang, R. Wu, Mechanical Properties and Interfacial Interaction of a Novel Bioabsorbable Chitin Fiber Reinforced Poly(e-caprolactone) Composite, *J. Mater. Sc. Letters* 20, 977-979 (2001).

[49]http://sung7.kuic.kyoto-u.ac.jp/others/SBF/SBF_E.html.

INCREASED OSTEOBLAST FUNCTION ON NANOFIBERED ALUMINA

Thomas J. Webster and Luke G. Gutwein
Department of Biomedical Engineering
Purdue University
West Lafayette, IN 47907

Frederick Tepper
Argonide Corporation
291 Power Ct.
Sanford, FL 32771

ABSTRACT

A novel nanosize form of alumina fibers has been found to be bioactive. A separate study done at Argonide Corporation (not yet published) demonstrated that such fibers attracted and retained virus particles. In this study, the adhesion and proliferation of osteoblasts (or bone-forming cells) to these fibers was completed *in vitro*. Compacts of such fibers showed improved osteoblast adhesion and proliferation as compared to notable orthopedic/dental implant materials such as commercially pure titanium and hydroxyapatite. Osteoblast adhesion on fiber compacts was determined as a function of heat treatment of the fibers, demonstrating that heat treatment at 400°C was optimal. Since adhesion and proliferation are crucial prerequisites for the deposition of calcium-containing mineral, the demonstrated activity of osteoblasts on the novel alumina fibers presents an opportunity for using them in the next-generation of orthopedic/dental implant prostheses. Such fibers could act as scaffolding in new formulations to enhance bone synthesis that is critical in the clinical success of bone prostheses.

INTRODUCTION

Sufficient bonding between an orthopedic/dental implant and juxtaposed bone is necessary to minimize motion-induced damage to surrounding tissue, to support physiological loading conditions, and to ensure implant efficacy[1]. Insufficient bonding (*i.e.*, incomplete osseointegration) of juxtaposed bone to an orthopedic/dental implant could be linked to material surface properties that do not support new bone growth. The next generation of orthopedic implants must, therefore, have biocompatible surfaces that promote bonding of juxtaposed bone; this criterion is not satisfied in materials currently utilized as bone prostheses. For example, conventional orthopedic materials (such as commercially pure titanium, Ti6Al4V, and CoCrMo alloys) possess less than optimal surface properties that often result in insufficient osseointegration to surrounding bone, a cause of clinical complications that necessitate surgical removal of these failed implants[1]. Composites based on artificial hydroxyapatite, the natural bone mineral, have not lived up to expectations[1].

Sufficient osseointegration to juxtaposed bone can be supported through the design of materials that enhance osteoblast (bone-forming cells) adhesion and proliferation. Adhesion of anchorage-dependent cells (like osteoblasts) is essential for subsequent cell functions, such as the deposition of bone. Clearly, novel material formulations are therefore needed to enhance osteoblast functions leading to sufficient osseointegration to juxtaposed bone.

Motivated by the continuous need of orthopedic implant materials with improved surface properties, we designed, synthesized, and evaluated a new form of bioactive material - compacts of nanosize alumina fiber. These fibers have dimensions similar to that of hydroxyapatite crystals found in physiological bone (10 nm in diameter and more than 50 nm length[1]). This *in vitro* study was the first ever conducted to evaluate the cytocompatible-potential of alumina nanofibers pertinent to the next-generation of orthopedic/dental implants.

MATERIALS AND METHODS

Alumina Nanomaterial Synthesis and Preparation

Alumina fibers with dimensions approximately 2 nm in diameter and >50 nm in length were synthesized by Argonide Corporation (Sanford, FL; Figure 1). The method involves the following steps. The first is a proprietary sol-gel synthesis, followed by ageing, filtration, and subsequent drying and heat treatment. Most of the fibers used in this study were heat treated at 400°C. Several lots of alumina fibers were also sintered at temperatures from 120°C to 1150°C in order to optimize osteoblast adhesion.

Previous studies showed that the surface area of the alumina nanofibers are dependent upon final heat treatment with the peak surface area greater than 600 m^2/g when heat treated to about 250°C[2]. XRD and FTIR studies have also demonstrated that the nanofibers are composed of aluminum oxide and boehmite (ALOOH)[2]. However, when heated above 465°C, results from FTIR provided evidence that the hydroxide and boehmite peaks disappear and the structure resembles gamma alumina[2].

Alumina nanofibers as received from Argonide Corporation were compacted serially in a steel-tool die *via* a uniaxial pressing cycle (0.2 GPa to 1 GPa over a 10 minute period) at room temperature according to established techniques[3]. The resulting alumina nanofiber compacts (discs 10 mm in diameter and 2 mm thick) were used in experiments with osteoblasts.

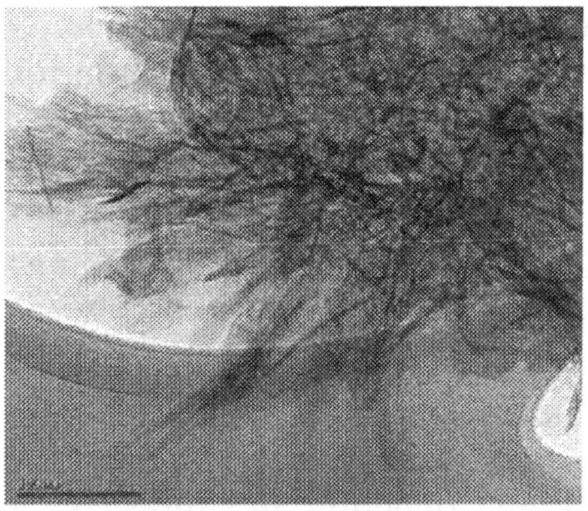

Figure 1. TEM Micrograph of Alumina Nanofibers.
The scale bar is 100 nm long.

In previous studies one of the authors showed that compacts of nanosize alumina spheres enhanced osteoblast adhesion[4], proliferation[5] and deposition of calcium-containing mineral[5]. In this study we compared compacts of the nano fibers vs. compacts of both nano and conventional spherical particle size alumina (discs 10 mm in diameter and 2 mm thick). Briefly, nanophase (23 nm spherical particle size) alumina (gamma-phase; Nanophase Technologies Corporation; Romeoville, IL) powder was compacted in a tool-steel die *via* a uniaxial pressing cycle (0.2 GPa to 1 GPa over a 10 minute period) at room temperature. Alumina grain size was controlled to less than 100 nm by heating (in air at 10°C/minute) the compacts from room temperature to a final temperature of 1000°C followed by sintering at 1000°C for two hours. Conventional substrates with grain sizes greater than 100 nm were obtained by heating (in air at 10°C/minute) alumina compacts from room temperature to a final temperature of 1200°C and by sintering at 1200°C for two hours. The average grain sizes of the resulting alumina substrates were previously determined to be 23 nm and 167 nm for the nanophase and conventional compacts, respectively[4]. In addition, previous XRD data provided evidence that both nanophase and conventional spherical grain size compacts prepared in this manner were gamma-phase alumina[4], and not a hydrated form as are the nano fibers.

Hydroxyapatite (HA; $Ca_{10}(PO_4)_6(OH)_2$) was used as a control substrate in the present study. HA was synthesized by dripping 1 M calcium nitrate and 0.6 M ammonium phosphate into a solution of distilled water and ammonium hydroxide. The solution was stirred for 24 hours at room temperature, while HA precipitated out. The solution was centrifuged and rinsed in triplicate, then dried for 24 hours in a glass-drying oven (70°C). The resulting powder was crushed, pressed into a compact (discs 10 mm in diameter and 2 mm thick) *via* a uniaxial pressing cycle from 0.2 GPa to 1 GPa over a 10 minute period, and sintered at 1100°C for 1 hour.

Commercially pure titanium (Osteonics; Allendale, NJ) currently utilized as an orthopedic implant material was used as a control in the present study. Borosilicate glass coverslips (reference material) were etched in 1 N NaOH and prepared for experiments according to standard protocols[3].

All material samples were degreased, ultrasonically cleaned, and sterilized in a steam autoclave at 120°C for 30 minutes according to standard laboratory procedures prior to experiments with osteoblasts[6].

Cytocompatibility Experiments

For adhesion experiments, human osteoblasts (bone-forming cells; CRL-11372 American Type Culture Collection) in Dulbecco's Modified Eagle Medium (DMEM; Gibco) supplemented with 10% fetal bovine serum (FBS; Hyclone) were seeded at a density of 2,500 cells/cm^2 of substrate surface area. These were allowed to adhere on the substrates of interest under standard cell culture conditions (that is, in a humidified, 5% CO_2/95% air environment) for two hours. For proliferation experiments, osteoblasts in DMEM supplemented with 10% FBS were seeded at a density of 2,500 cells/cm^2 of substrate surface area. They were allowed to proliferate on the substrates of interest under standard cell culture conditions (that is, in a humidified, 5% CO_2/95% air environment) for 1, 3, and 5 days.

After the prescribed time period, non-adherent cells were removed by rinsing in phosphate buffered saline, while adherent cells were fixed with formalin, stained with Hoeschst 33258 dye (Sigma), and counted under a fluorescence microscope. Cell counts were expressed as the average number of five random fields per square cm of substrate surface area. All experiments were run in triplicate and repeated at least three different times. Numerical data were analyzed using standard analysis of variance (ANOVA) techniques[7].

RESULTS

Enhanced Osteoblast Adhesion on Alumina Nanofibers

For the first time, we show evidence that osteoblast adhesion was significantly ($p < 0.01$) greater on alumina with either nanospherical or nanofiber particle sizes compared to the preferred bone prosthetic materials titanium and hydroxyapatite (HA) (Figure 2). More importantly, results provided the first evidence of significantly ($p < 0.05$) higher osteoblast adhesion on nanofiber than nanospherical alumina compact formulations. In fact, osteoblast adhesion was two times greater on nanofiber alumina than on titanium after just two hours. Osteoblast adhesion was similar on conventional alumina, HA, titanium, and glass.

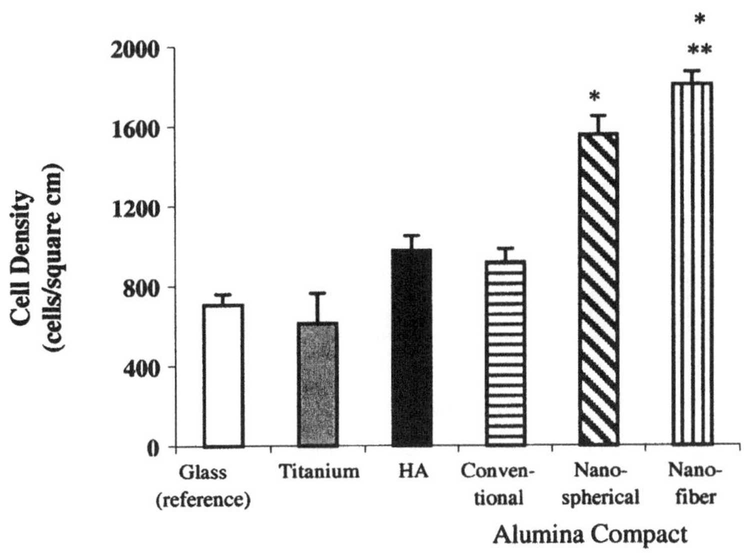

Figure 2. Enhanced Osteoblast Adhesion on Nanofiber Alumina Compacts.
Values are mean +/- SEM; n = 3; * $p < 0.01$ (compared to titanium); ** $p < 0.05$ (compared to nanospherical alumina).

These results also show that osteoblast adhesion was significantly greater on alumina nanofibers that were sintered (before compaction) at or near 400°C. There was considerable fall-off in adhesion ($p < 0.1$) for those samples heat treated above 550°C or below 400°C (Figure 3).

Enhanced Osteoblast Proliferation on Alumina Nanofibers

Although critical for subsequent functions, enhanced adhesion of osteoblasts does not always correlate to increased osteoblast proliferation[8]. However, the present study provided the first evidence that the number of osteoblasts was significantly ($p < 0.01$) greater on nanofiber alumina than on any other substrate tested in the present study after 1, 3, and 5 days of culture (Figure 4). Specifically, there were more than two, three, and four times the number of osteoblasts on nanofiber alumina than on titanium after 1, 3, and 5 days, respectively.

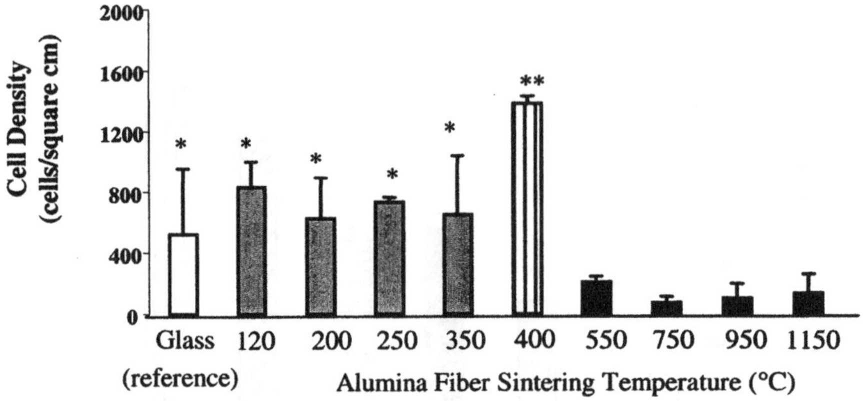

Figure 3. Enhanced Osteoblast Adhesion on Low Temperature Sintered Alumina Nanofibers. Values are mean +/- SEM; n = 3; * $p < 0.1$, ** $p < 0.01$ (compared to alumina sintered at 550°C).

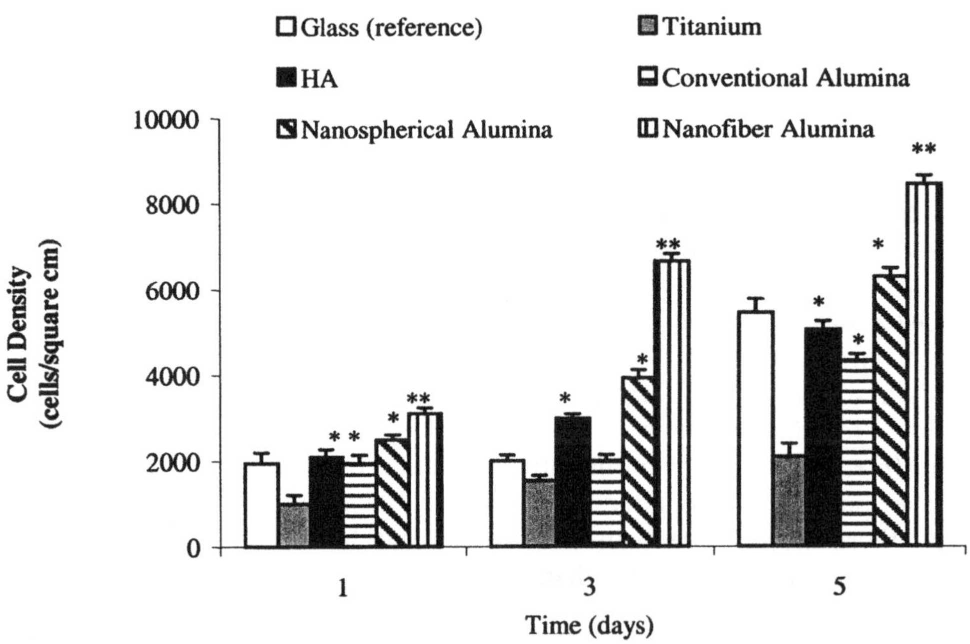

Figure 4. Enhanced Osteoblast Proliferation on Nanofiber Alumina. Values are mean +/- SEM; n = 3; * $p < 0.01$ (compared to titanium); ** $p < 0.01$ (compared to nanospherical alumina).

DISCUSSION

Promoting select osteoblast adhesion on orthopedic implant materials has been the focus of numerous recent research endeavors[3-6,8]. To date, success has been obtained by immobilizing select amino acids on material surfaces[8]. For example, glass surfaces treated with Arginine-Glycine-Aspartic Acid-Serine (RGDS)[8] have successfully demonstrated increased osteoblast adhesion. However, it remains unclear whether immobilized peptide groups will be functional *in vivo* due to either damage of delicate surface chemistry during implantation, or interaction with plasma proteins once implanted (which may compromise peptide bioactivity). The proposed compacts of nano alumina fiber materials, which do not have such delicate surface chemistry, would provide a superior approach to enhance osteoblast function.

Recently, enhanced osteoblast adhesion has also been observed on nano size (less than 100 nm in diameter) alumina compared to conventional alumina, titania, and hydroxyapatite[3-6]. For example, Webster *et al.*[3-6] showed the first evidence of enhanced adhesion of osteoblasts onto nanosize alumina, titania and hydroxyapatite. In a companion study[9], Webster *et al.* also showed decreased adhesion of fibroblasts (cells that contribute to fibrous encapsulation and callus formation) and decreased adhesion of endothelial cells (cells that line the vasculature of the body). The adhesion of fibroblasts and endothelial cells interfere with the bone growth process. That study showed that osteoblast adhesion increased by 51% as alumina spherical grain size decreased from 167 to 24 nm; in contrast, on the same substrates and during the same four-hour time period, fibroblast adhesion decreased by 235%[9]. These studies also demonstrated that an important property to selectively enhance osteoblast function is to design materials with a high degree of nanostructured surface roughness[9].

In this study, enhanced osteoblast function was also accomplished by decreasing alumina fiber dimensions. The present results of enhanced osteoblast adhesion and proliferation on alumina nanofibers provide a second example of nanostructured material surfaces that specifically increase bone-forming cell function. More importantly, functions of osteoblasts were greater on nanofibered alumina compared to nanospherical alumina. Due to changes in grain size geometry in addition to altered alumina chemistry and phase, it is unclear at this time which material properties enhance osteoblast function on nanofibered compared to nanospherical alumina.

The results also show that the surface chemistry of the fibers is important in improving osteoblast adhesion. When heat-treated above about 400°C there was deterioration in osteoblast function while at the same time the chemistry changed from AlOOH to gamma alumina. We believe that one of the contributing factors to osteoblast adhesion may be the high protonic content on the AlOOH, resulting in a high density of positive charges, thereby attracting and retaining negatively charged cells.

CONCLUSIONS

Due to grain size dimensions similar to hydroxyapatite in bone, nanostructured materials (such as alumina nanofibers) provide promise, yet widely unexplored alternatives for orthopedic implants. The present study demonstrated, for the first time, that alumina nanofibers enhance osteoblast adhesion and proliferation. These events may promote new bone synthesis leading to sufficient osseointegration between alumina nanofibers and juxtaposed bone. Deposition of bone on an orthopedic implant material is necessary to stabilize the prostheses *in situ*, support physiological loading conditions, minimize motion-induced damage to surrounding tissue, and is critical for increased implant efficacy.

ACKNOWLEDGEMENTS

The authors would like to thank the Whitaker Foundation for financial support.

REFERENCES

[1]F.S. Kaplan, W.C. Hayes, T.M. Keaveny, A. Boskey, T.A. Einhorn, and J.P. Iannotti, *Orthopaedic Basic Science,* Am. Acad. Orth. Surg., Columbus, OH, 1994.

[2]F. Tepper, "Nanosize alumina whiskers," pp. 24-27 in *Particles 2001 Conference Proceedings*, Rosen Centre Hotel, Orlando, Florida (2001).

[3]T.J. Webster, R.W. Siegel, and R. Bizios, "An *in vitro* evaluation of nanophase alumina for orthopaedic/dental applications"; pp. 273-276 in *Proceedings of the 11th International Symposium on Ceramics in Medicine,* Edited by R.Z. LeGeros and J.P. LeGeros. World Scientific Publishing Co., New York, 1998.

[4]T.J. Webster, R.W. Siegel, and R. Bizios, "Osteoblast adhesion on nanophase ceramics," *Biomaterials*, **20** 1222-1227 (1999).

[5]T.J. Webster, R.W. Siegel, and R. Bizios, "Enhanced functions of osteoblasts on nanophase ceramics," *Biomaterials* **21** 1803-1810 (2000).

[6]T. J. Webster, C. Ergun, R. H. Doremus, and R. Bizios, "Mechanisms of enhanced osteoblast adhesion on hydroxyapatite doped with yttrium," *Journal of Biomedical Materials Research* **59** 312-317 (2002).

[7]D. Montgomery, *Design and Analysis of Experiment*, John Wiley and Sons, New York, 1991.

[8]K.C. Dee, T.T. Andersen, and R. Bizios, "Design and function of novel osteoblast-adhesive peptides for chemical modification of biomaterials," *Journal of Biomedical Materials Research*, **40** 371-377 (1998).

[9]T.J. Webster, C. Ergun, R.H. Doremus, R.W. Siegel, and R. Bizios, "Specific proteins mediate enhanced osteoblast adhesion on nanophase ceramics," *Journal of Biomedical Materials Research* **51** 475-483 (2000).

BIOACTIVE GLASS-CERAMICS MATERIALS FOR BONE SUBSTITUTES

C. Vitale Brovarone, F. Smeacetto and E. Vernè
Polytechnic of Turin, Materials Science and Chemical Engineering Department, Italy
Corresponding author : vitale@athena.polito.it

ABSTRACT

Bioactive glass-ceramic powders belonging to the following system SiO_2-Na_2O-CaO-MgO were prepared via sol-gel. These powders were compacted by cold uniaxial pressing and then sintered at low temperatures in order to obtain a porous consolidated system. The biomaterials were then soaked in a simulated body fluid (SBF) to study their bioactivity. Both the as obtained samples and the soaked ones, were characterized by means of X-ray diffraction and optical and scanning electron microscopy with energy dispersive spectroscopy (EDS). In this paper , we present some preliminary results on these glass-ceramics that we believe might be successfully proposed as scaffold for bone substitutes. Future developments will involve the addition to the glass-ceramic powders of a second organic phases thermally degradable in order to obtain a macroporous structure.

INTRODUCTION

Recently, numerous scientists have proposed and developed different biomaterials to be used as bone replacements. Among them, porous hydroxylapatite and calcium phosphate ceramics [1,2] had played a major role. More recently, bioactive glasses and glass-ceramics have been proposed for repairing and reconstructing bones damaged parts [3]. An even more recent and attractive prospective is the realization of a biodegradable ceramic scaffold having a macroporous structure.

These porous implants should be characterized by an open and interconnected macroporosity that would allow the ingrowth of new bone and soft tissue within its large pores. Furthermore, these porous systems should facilitate the creation within them, of a good vascular network to allow blood supply for further bone mineralisation and remodeling [4]. Therefore, a glass-ceramic belonging to the system SiO_2-Na_2O-CaO-MgO was prepared and sintered in order to obtain a glass-ceramic block. The biomaterial was characterized from the structural, morphological and compositional point of view. An *in vitro* characterization was also performed in order to preliminarily verify its osteoinductive properties. For this purpose, the precipitation of an hydroxylapatite layer on the biomaterial surface after immersion in simulated body fluid (SBF) was investigated. In fact, the presence of this newly formed hydroxylapatite layer on the biomaterial surface is a widely accepted proof of their bioactivity.

MATERIALS AND METHOD

Glasses in the SiO_2-Na_2O-CaO-MgO system were prepared by a sol-gel method. Their preparation was carried out by hydrolysis and polycondensation of weighed amount of the following reagents: tetraethyl orthosilicate (TEOS), hydrated calcium nitrate $Ca(NO_3)_2 \bullet 4H_2O$, sodium ethoxide $2Na(OC_2H_5)$, hydrated magnesium nitrate $Mg(NO_3) \bullet 6H_2O$,1 M HNO_3 was used as a catalyst and the gel was dried in air at 220°C for 24 hours.

The obtained powders were then compacted by uniaxial cold pressing in air for 10 seconds at 4 tons obtaining a crack free and homogeneous green body.

The green bodies were then sintered in air at low temperatures ranging from 800°C to 1000°C for three hours.

The sintering process was carried out by heating the samples at 4.5°/min till the sintering temperature (800°-1000°C), allowing three hours for the sintering process to take place and then a slow cooling down till room temperature.

The samples structure was investigated by X-Ray diffraction (X'Pert Philips diffractometer) using the Bragg Brentano camera geometry and the CuKα incident radiation.

The microstructure of the samples as well as their composition were studied by scanning electron microscopy (SEM Philips 525 M) coupled with energy dispersive spectroscopy (EDS, Philips-EDAX 9100).

The bioactivity was tested by immersion in a simulated body fluid (SBF) that has an inorganic composition analogous to that of human plasma, as reported in table I. The SBF was maintained at 37°C and the samples where soaked in it for periods up to four weeks.

Table I Ionic concentration (mM) in SBF and Human Plasma

	Na^+	K^+	Ca^{2+}	Mg^{2+}	Cl^-	HCO_3^-	HPO_4^{2-}	SO_4^{2-}
SBF	142.0	5.0	2.5	1.5	147.8	4.2	1.0	0.5
Plasma	142.0	5.0	2.5	1.5	103.0	27.0	1.0	0.5

For the *in vitro* characterization, a diffractometric and microscopical characterization was carried out on the samples surfaces after the soaking in SBF, in order to verify the presence of a newly precipitated hydroxylapatite layer on them.

RESULTS AND DISCUSSION

Three different glass-ceramic belonging to the system SiO_2-Na_2O-CaO-MgO were successfully prepared and their composition is reported in table II.

Table II Composition of the three glass-ceramic prepared (molar %)

Sample	SiO_2	Na_2O	CaO	MgO
GC1	48	24.5	24.5	3
GC2	52	15	27	6
GC3	55	20	16	9

All the obtained powders showed a submicronic grain size typical of the materials obtained via sol-gel. For this purpose, in figure 1 is reported a micrograph of GC2 powder in which submicronical GC2 grains can be observed. These submicronic grains are sticked together in the micrograph to form agglomerates of some microns.

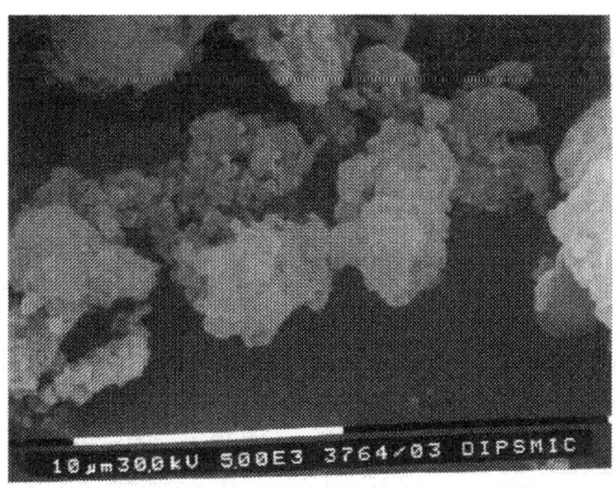

Figure 1 Micrograph of SG2 powder

The morphology and size of the powders obtained for GC1 and GC3 are analogous to those observed for GC2.

The sintering process induced a crystallization in the samples leading to the formation of two different crystalline phases, namely two silicates.

For this purpose, figure 2 depicts an X-Ray spectrum of a sintered GC2 body (900°C for 3 hours) in which all the detected peaks are identified with the two reported silicates.

Identical crystalline phases were detected for sample GC1 and GC3 and their X-Ray spectra are analogous to the one reported in figure 2.

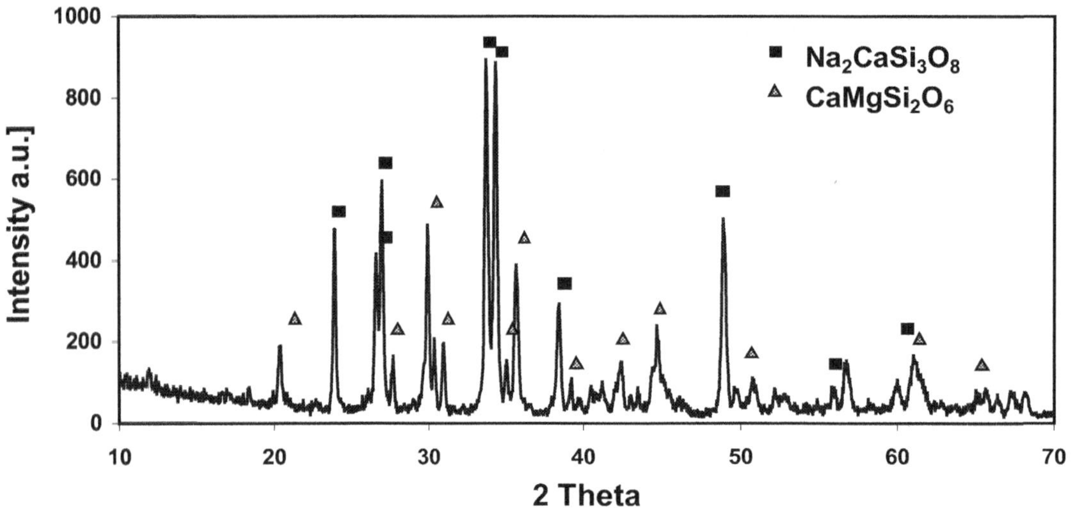

Figure 2 XRD spectrum of GC2 sintered at 900°C in air for 3 hours

The obtained XRD patterns pointed out the glass-ceramic nature of these biomaterials.
The low temperatures involved in the sintering process as well as the low pressure utilized for the preparation of the compacted green body led to a final microstructure with a certain degree of open porosity.
Figure 3 shows a general view of the sintered sample in which an interconnected macroporosity with an average dimension of 20-50μm can be observed.
The macropores dimension is compatible with the requirement of a good vascolarization of the macroporous implants, though bigger macropores (around 100μm) will be more suitable.
An increase in both the dimension and quantity of the interconnected porosity might be achieved by introducing in the sample a second phase thermally degradable (polymeric particles, starches...) and our future efforts will be focused in this direction.
Furthermore, the micrograph of figure 3 shows that the obtained compact body is cracks and thus assess the effectiveness of both the pressing and sintering processes.

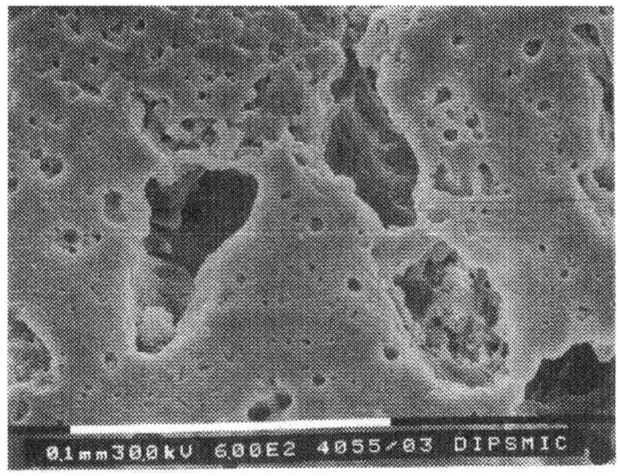

Figure 3 Micrograph of GC2 sample

The *in vitro* characterization of GC1, GC2 and GC3 showed the precipitation of an hydroxylapatite layer on their surfaces in each sample. The presence of a newly formed hydroxylapatite layer on the surface of a biomaterials is a generally accepted proof of its bioactivity.

In figure 4a and 4 b are at this purpose reported two micrographs of sample GC2 and GC3 after soaking in SBF for 4 weeks. GC1 showed an analogous behavior.

All over the surface, globular hydroxylapatite precipitates (HAp) can be observed confirming the high bioactivity of the realised samples. The globular morphology of the observed HAp is typical of the hydroxylapatite that precipitate *in vitro*.

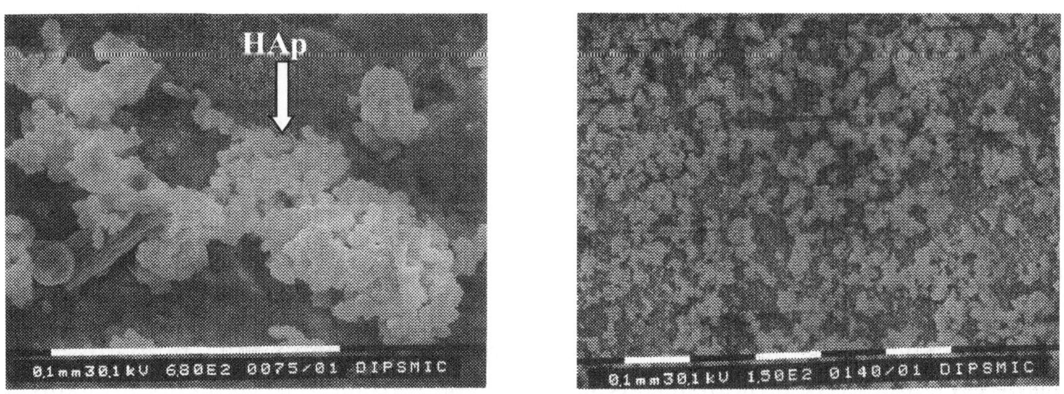

a b

Figure 4 Micrographs after 4 weeks in SBF a) GC2 b) GC3

Compositional analysis (EDS) performed on the precipitated layer showed the presence of only calcium and phosphorus in relative amount analogous as those found in hydroxylapatite.

Figure 5 depicts at this purpose the results of an EDS analysis performed on the whole area of figure 4b.

The formation of a silica rich gel layer on the surface of samples soaked in SBF is the first step involved in the complex mechanism which end with the precipitation of HAp. The presence of small amounts of Silicon is then related to the formation of this silica gel and can be still detected in the areas that are not yet completely covered by HAp.

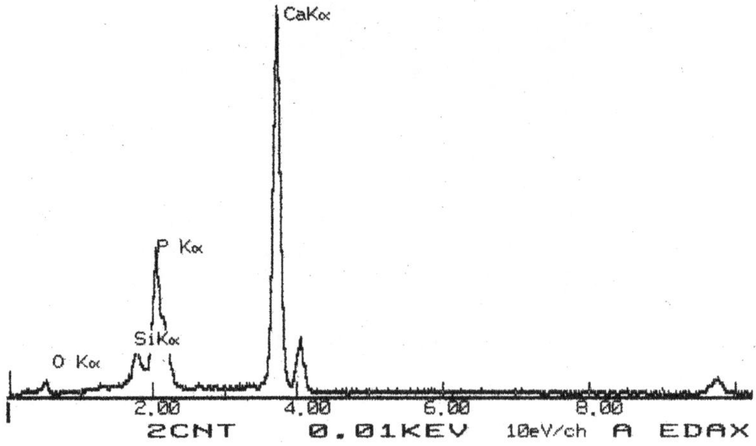

Figure 5 EDS analysis on GC3 after soaking in SBF for 4 weeks.

CONCLUSIONS

The proposed compositions and experimental route allowed to obtain crack free macroporous glass-ceramic bodies.

The obtained materials showed an interconnected macroporosity, which is suitable for the proposed aims. Though, an increase in both the dimensions and quantity of the macroporous would be desirable.

The sintering process leaded to the crystallization of two different silicates that didn't affect the final bioactivity and in fact, all the samples showed highly satisfactory *in vitro* results with the precipitation, in all samples of an HAp layer.

REFERENCES

[1] W Suchanek and M. Yoshimura "Processing and properties of hydroxylapatite- based biomaterials for use as hard tissue replacements implants", J Mater Res; **13**, 94-117 (1998)

[2] C. Klein, K De Groot, C. Weiquin, L. Yubao and Z, Xingdong, "Osseous substance formation induced in porous calcium phosphate ceramics in soft tissue", Biomat, **15**,31-34 (1994)

[3] H. Yuna, J. De Bruijn, X. Zhang, C. Van Blitterswijk and K. De Groot, "Bone induction by porous glass ceramic made from Bioglass (45S5)", J Biomed Mater Res **58**: 270-276, (2001)

[4] U. Ripamonti, "Osteoinduction in porous hydroxyapatite implanted in heterotopic sites of different animal models", Biomater; **17**:31-35 (1996)

FATIGUE PROPERTY OF ZIRCONIA FOR HIP JOINT PROSTHESES

Y. Takigawa, Y. Yasutomi and M. Mizuno
R & D Laboratory
Japan Fine Ceramics Center
2-4-1 Mutsuno, Atsuta-ku, Nagoya
456-8587, Japan

K. Shirakihara

Graduate School
Nagoya University
Furo-cho, Chikusa-ku, Nagoya
464-8603, Japan

ABSTRACT

Uniaxial bending fatigue tests are conducted on biomedical grade zirconia for hip joint prostheses at room temperature in air and in physiological saline solution. Zirconia ceramics exhibit better fatigue resistance than alumina ceramics, which have been actively used for hip joint prostheses. In the test in saline solution, the number of cycles at fracture decreases to 95% against that obtained in air at the same stress level. The slight decrease of the number of cycles must be the effect of stress corrosion. Analysis by Raman spectroscopy reveals that phase transformation from tetragonal to monoclinic phase is observed at some conditions. Since the specimen always fails when the amount of *m*-phase reaches to almost 30%, it seems to be the critical amount of phase transformation for failure.

INTRODUCTION

Zirconia ceramics have been used for 15 years now in orthopedic surgery as material for ball heads for total hip prostheses system. This material is attractive because of its high strength and fracture toughness. The most commonly use biomedical grade zirconia is doped with 3mol% of yttria, which stabilizes zirconia in its tetragonal phase. For yttria-stabilized tetragonal zirconia polycrystal (Y-TZP), required physical and chemical properties for use as material for surgical implants have been specified in an international standard ISO 13356. However, it seems to be the question that the required mechanical property is only flexural strength by biaxial or 4-point bending in ISO 13356, although the material is required a high degree of reliability for more than 20 years in living body. It should also be considered the effect of phase transformation on mechanical properties by stress or by aging in wet environment [1]. Thus, the characteristics and corresponding test method for mechanical properties over a long period such as fatigue must be provided for Y-TZP for surgical implants. In the present study, cyclic fatigue property is examined and the effect of phase transformation on the fatigue lifetime is discussed in biomedical grade 3Y-TZP as the basic step for standardization.

EXPERIMENTAL PROCEDURE

The material used in this study is a 3Y-TZP, ZR1, distributed as a standard material by Japan Fine Ceramics Center. ZR1 is not developed as bioceramics, but the properties satisfy the requirements in ISO 13356. The comparison between the properties in ZR1 and the requirements in ISO 13356 is summarized in Table I.

Uniaxial bending cyclic fatigue tests are conducted by 4 point bending with the upper span of 10mm and the lower span of 30mm. The tests are made at room temperature in air or in physiological saline solution at 36°C under a frequency of 20Hz or 1Hz and stress ratio of 0.1. The limit number of cycles is set to 1×10^7 cycles in these tests. Analysis of phase transformation from tetragonal to monoclinic phase is conducted by Raman spectroscopy. Monoclinic molar fraction is determined from the Raman intensities for the tetragonal peak at 260cm^{-1} and the monoclinic peak at 177cm^{-1} [2].

Table I. Properties in ZR1

Property	ISO	ZR1
Bulk density	≥6.00	6.07
Chemical composition:		
ZrO_2+HfO_2+Y_2O_3	>99.0	>99.65
Y_2O_3	4.5 to 5.4	5.09
HfO_2	≤5	-
Al_2O_3	<0.5	0.238
Other oxides	<0.5	0.07
Microstructure		
Mean linear intercept distance (μm)	≤0.6	0.37
Strength:		
4-point bending (MPa)	≥800	1,100

RESULTS AND DISCUSSION

Figure 1 shows the relationship between maximum stress and number of cycles at fracture in ZR1 and a biomedical grade alumina ceramics, which has been actively used for hip joint prostheses. The number of cycles to failure gradually increases as maximum stress decreases in both materials. From this figure, it is clearly shown that zirconia ceramics exhibit much better fatigue resistance than alumina ceramics. Assuming that the relationship between the maximum stress, σ_{max}, and the number of cycles, N, are represented as $\sigma_{max}{}^{n} N = Const.$, the exponent of crack propagation n is estimated to be about 200 and 35 in zirconia and alumina, respectively. Since this value of zirconia is very large in comparison with general ceramics and fracture does not occur even after 10^7 cycles at 800MPa, it is demonstrated that high degree of reliability is expected as well as high strength in Y-TZP.

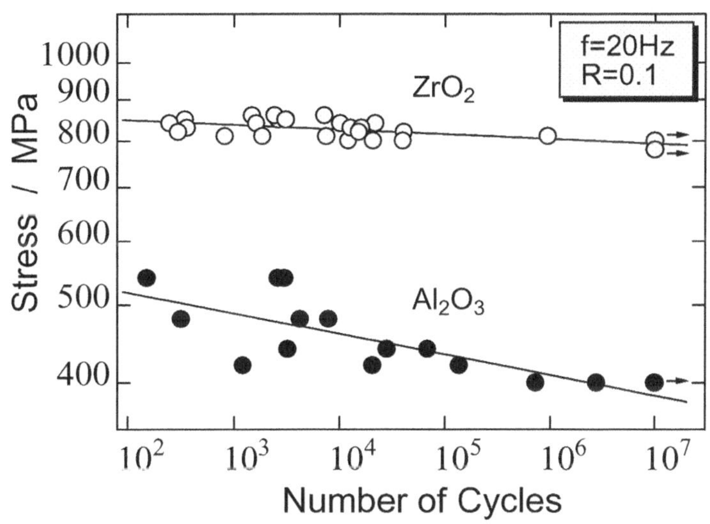

Fig. 1 Relationship between maximum stress and number of cycles in ZR1 and a biomedical grade alumina ceramics

Figure 2 shows the relationship between maximum stress and number of cycles in ZR1 at two conditions, *i.e.*, the tests at room temperature in air under a frequency of 20Hz and those in physiological saline solution at 36°C under a frequency of 1Hz. In the test in saline solution, the number of cycles decreases to 95% against that obtained in air at the same stress level. The slight decrease of the number of cycles must be the effect of stress corrosion [3].

Next, analysis of phase transformation from tetragonal (t) to monoclinic (m) phase is conducted to clarify its effect on fatigue lifetime. Figure 2 shows typical Raman spectra obtained from lower side of the tested specimen. In the specimen tested at 780MPa up to 1×10^7 cycles, the peaks of only t-phase are observed and no phase transformation occurs. In contrast, in the other two specimens, the peaks of both *t* and *m*-phase are observed. Thus, the amount of phase transformation depends on the applied stress level.

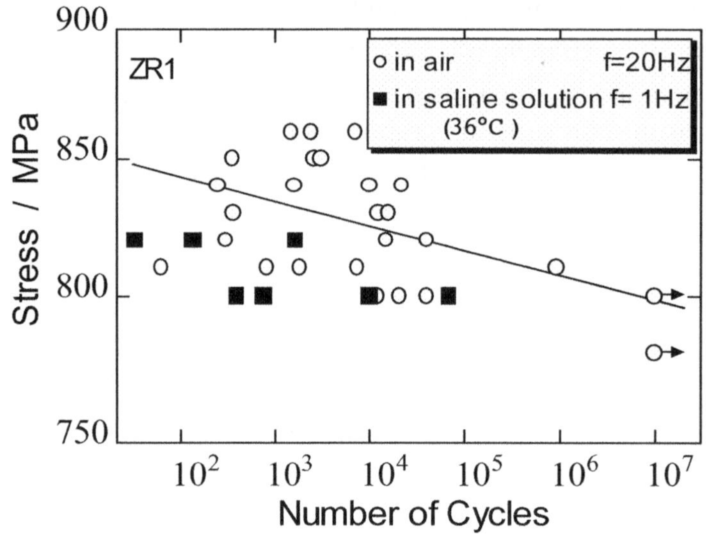

Fig. 2 Relationship between maximum stress and number of cycles in ZR1 at two conditions

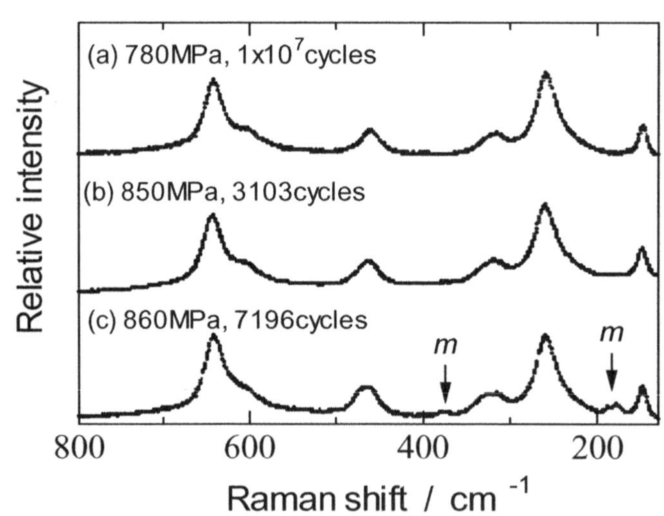

Fig. 3 Typical Raman spectra obtained from lower side of specimens tested at several conditions

As shown in Fig. 3, the amount of phase transformation depends on the testing conditions. Then, the amount of phase transformation is estimated to discuss its effect on fatigue lifetime. It has been reported that the ratio of molar fraction x of the t and m-phase are represented by the following equation [2],

$$\frac{x_t}{x_m} = \frac{1}{1.8}\frac{I^{260}}{I^{177}} \tag{1}$$

Where I^{177} and I^{260} are intensity of the peaks at 177 and 260cm^{-1}, which are originated from m and t-phase, respectively. By using this equation, the molar fraction of m-phase is estimated in the specimens tested at several conditions. For example, the molar fraction of m-phase is estimated to be 5% in the specimen shown in Fig. 3 (b) and 30% in the specimen shown in Fig. 3 (c).

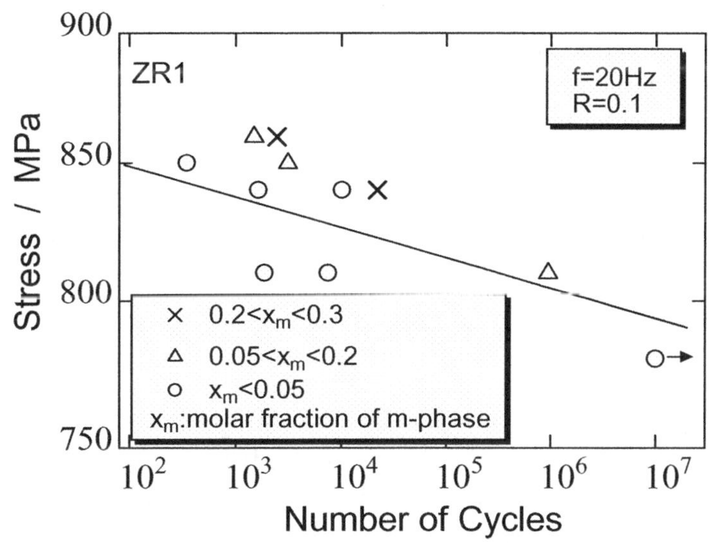

Fig. 4 Relationship between testing condition and molar fraction of m-phase

Figure 4 shows the relationship between testing condition and molar fraction of m-phase. In the figure, three symbols represent the molar fraction of m-phase of 20 to 30%, 5 to 20% and less than 5%, respectively. The molar fraction of m-phase increases as the maximum stress or number of cycles increases. Since the specimen always fails when the amount of m-phase reaches to almost 30%, it seems to be the critical amount of phase transformation for failure. Although the fracture by phase transformation seems not to be a major problem in the case tested in air because the phase transformation is not observed in the specimens tested at low stress or exhibiting short lifetime, this value must be important in the case of phase transformation by aging in wet environment. The results on the effect of phase transformation on fatigue lifetime during the tests in saline water will be clarified in future works.

CONCLUSION

Cyclic fatigue property is examined and the effect of phase transformation on the fatigue lifetime is discussed in biomedical grade 3Y-TZP. The results are summarized as follows:

(1) Zirconia ceramics exhibit better fatigue resistance than alumina ceramics, which has been actively used for hip joint prostheses. Since the exponent of crack propagation *n* of zirconia is very large in comparison with general ceramics and fracture does not occur even after 10^7 cycles at 800MPa, it is demonstrated that high degree of reliability is expected as well as high strength in Y-TZP.

(2) In the test in saline solution, the number of cycles at fracture decreases to 95% against that obtained in air at the same stress level. The slight decrease of the number of cycles must be the effect of stress corrosion.

(3) Analysis by Raman spectroscopy reveals that phase transformation from tetragonal to monoclinic phase is observed at some conditions, which depends on the testing conditions. Since the specimen always fails when the amount of *m*-phase reaches to almost 30%, it seems to be the critical amount of phase transformation for failure.

ACKNOWLEDGEMENT

This work is now being conducted in the program "Standardization of test evaluation method for fine ceramics for living body" which is consigned to Japan Fine Ceramics Center by New Energy and Industrial Technology Development Organization, under the Research and Development for International Standards for Supporting New Industries Program.

REFERENCES

[1] T. Sato and M. Shimada (1984) *J. Am. Ceram. Soc.* 67:C212-213.

[2] C. G. Kontoyannis and M. Orkoula (1994) *J. Mater. Sci.* 29:5316-5320.

[3] A. G. Evans (1972) *J. Mater. Sci.* 7:1137.

Printed and bound by CPI Group (UK) Ltd, Croydon, CR0 4YY

15/09/2026

14962415-0001